Judo Master Reference

An Anthology

Compiled by
Michael A. DeMarco, M.A.

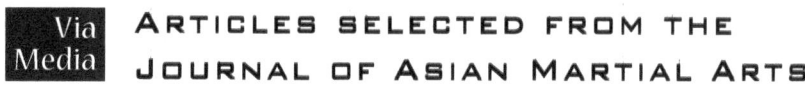
Articles selected from the
Journal of Asian Martial Arts

Disclaimer
Please note that the author and publisher of this book are not responsible in any manner whatsoever for any injury that may result from practicing the techniques and/or following the instructions given herein. Participation in martial arts activities can be dangerous and can lead to serious injury. The material presented in this book is intended for reference only, and the reader assumes all risks associated with attempting to perform any of the activities described herein. Before attempting any of the physical activities described in this book, the reader should consult a physician for advice regarding their individual suitability for performing such activity.

All Rights Reserved
No part of this publication, including illustrations, may be reproduced or utilized in any form or by any means, electronic or mechanical, including photocopying, recording, or by any information storage and retrieval system (beyond that copying permitted by sections 107 and 108 of the US Copyright Law and except by reviewers for the public press), without written permission from Via Media Publishing Company.

Warning: Any unauthorized act in relation to a copyright work may result in both a civil claim for damages and criminal prosecution.

Copyright © 2025
by Via Media Publishing Company
941 Calle Mejia #822
Santa Fe, NM 87501 USA

Book and cover design
by Via Media Publishing Company
Background texture Japanese_Pattern_33_D
courtesy of www.freepik.com

ISBN 979-8-218-68528-7

www.viamediapublishing.com

Dedication

To all those who have contributed to the
Journal of Asian Martial Arts (1992–2016)
providing articles of high academic standards
that will continue to inspire research and practice.

Table of Contents

Preface vii

- The Masters Contest of 1926: An Epiphany in Judo History 1
  Robert W. Smith, M.A.

- Jujutsu: The Gentle Art and the Strenuous Life 5
  Joe Long, B.A.

- The School of Hard Knocks: Seattle's Kurosaka / Tentoku Kan Dojo 1928–1942 17
  Joseph R. Svinth, M.A.

- Masato Tamura, Ryoichi Iwakiri, and The Fife Judo Dojo, 1923–1942 35
  Joseph Svinth, M.A.

- Origins of the British Judo Association, the European Judo Union and the International Judo Federation 49
  Richard Bowen

- Repercussions from the Douillet v.s. Shinohara's Final Judo Bout at the 2000 Olympics in Sydney 61
  David Finch

- Judo and Character: Moving from the Hard to the Gentle Way 67
  James Behrendt

- Ulla Werbrouck: Olympic and European Judo Champion Retires 71
  David Finch

- Sport, Industrialism, and the Japanese "Gentle Way": Judo in Late Victorian England 77
  Geoffrey Wingard, M.A.

- American Judo Pioneer Vince Tamura and Heike-ryu Jujutsu 87
  James Webb, M.A.

- Isao Okano's Impact on Judo Since the Lausanne World Championships 95
  David Finch

- Jujutsu's Image in Spain's Wrestling Shows: A Historic Review 99
  Carlos Gutiérrez, Ph.D., and Julián Espartero, Ph.D. Trans. from Spanish by Dave and Sonia Katz

- Haragatame: Judo's Rare Stomach Armlock 121
  David Finch

- Kataguruma: Judo's Spectacular Shoulder Wheel Throw 124
  David Finch

- Competition, Kata, and the Art of Judo 127
  Llyr C. Jones, Ph.D.

- North Korean Kye Sun Hui: An Extraordinary Olympic Judo Player 141
  David Finch

- Competition Versus Tradition in Kodokan Judo 146
  S. Biron Ebell, M.A.

- The First Kodokan Judo International Competition and Its Katas 156
  W. Lance Gatling, M.A., M.P.S.

- Building Men on the Mat: Traditional Manly Arts 165
  and the Asian Martial Arts in America
  Geoffrey Wingard, M.Ed.

- Judo Comes to California: Judo vs. Wrestling in the American West, 1900–1920 177
  Matt Hlinak, M.A., J.D.

- The Way of Kata in Kodokan Judo 190
  Llyr C. Jones, Ph.D., and Michael J. Hanon, Ph.D.

- A Taxonomy of Principles Used in Judo Throwing Techniques 210
  Linda Yiannakis, M.S.

- Rhythm, Patterns, and Timing in Martial Arts as Exemplified Through Judo 221
  Linda Yiannakis, M.S.

- Kodokan Judo's Self-Defense System: Kodokan Goshin-jutsu 234
  Llyr C. Jones, Ph.D, Martin P. Savage, B.Ed., and W. Lance Gatling, M.A., M.P.S.

- The Logic of Kodokan Judo Kata 282
  Llyr C. Jones, Ph.D.

- The Budokwai Centennial 285
  Brian N. Watson

- Budokwai Kime-no-kata: Budokwai Form of Decisive Techniques 294
  Llyr C. Jones, Ph.D., H. John Bowen and David W. V. Finch

- "Treasure Chivalry, Despise Cowardice, and Esteem Straight-Living": 342
  Culture and the Origins of The Budokwai
  Michael Callan, Ph.D.

- One Hundred Years of The Budokwai 347
  John B. Goodbody, M.A.

Sources of Original Publication 353

Index 354

Preface

Via Media Publishing was founded in 1992 in order to produce the peer reviewed quarterly *Journal of Asian Martial Arts* (1992–2012)—the first publication of its kind to focus on martial traditions in an academic format. Many of the authors were scholar–practitioners, who utilized their unique talents to present articles from various specializations, such as Asian Studies, kinesiology, history, anthropology, philosophy, and physical education.

Those who were serious about this field subscribed to the journal to read articles noted for their high academic and aesthetic standards. Most were in the United States, Canada, and Europe, but also in other areas of the world. Subscribers naturally included martial art schools and individual practitioners. There was a strong base among university and public libraries too.

As founder of Via Media, I've decided to assemble this anthology of articles relating to the martial arts associated with judo. There are millions of judo practitioners worldwide, drawn to the art mainly for sport, self-defense and a form of exercise. Researchers can benefit from this handy anthology, particularly for the information and analyses presented, including the rich bibliographic listings. Judo practitioners will also gain insights to benefit their own practice, be it for competition, health and/or self-defense.

A total of twenty-nine chapters are conveniently compiled in this volume. In addition to 1,780 illustrations, there are glossaries, charts, and bibliographies. *Judo* is the term representing the general category of study, but it can be subdivided into its branches, such as the original Kodokan and the competitive Olympic sport.

The variety of material in this anthology reflects in-depth scholarly research and the experience of master practitioners. It will be a valuable source for karate enthusiasts for future decades. By making this book available to individuals and libraries, we hope this rare material will greatly contribute to further research in this field and inspire many to learn the history and culture of judo with aspirations to mastery.

Michael DeMarco, Publisher

chapter 1

The Masters Contest of 1926: An Epiphany in Judo History
by Robert W. Smith, M.A.

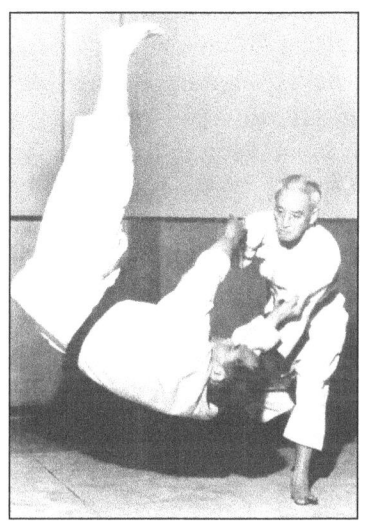

Mifune Kyuzo executing a "corner drop" (*sumiotoshi*).
All photos courtesy of R. Smith.

    The Biblical phrase "There were giants in those days" is exemplified by the judo masters of the Kodokan. Some of their past exploits indicate an extraordinary mental and physical capacity.
    In 1926, a contest (*shiai*) occurred that was the equal of any preceding and without peer in any following tournament. Thirty-seven of the finest judoka in Japan competed before the Emperor Hirohito. But the championship eliminations were eclipsed by the appearance on the mat of eight of the greatest judo masters in history:[1] Mifune Kyuzo, Tabata Shotaro, Goto Ichizo, Kurihara Tamio, Samura Kaichiro, Iizuka Kunizaburo, Isogai Hajime, and Nagaoka Shuichi.[2] All were highly-graded teachers well along in years, probably not at their contest best, but willing to demonstrate their ability in the face of age and its concomitant slowing reflexes. The four matches in which they participated are an epiphany in judo history.

Note: This chapter was first written in 1953. Readers must take this into consideration to clearly understand the chronology of events and the respective ages of the practitioners discussed.

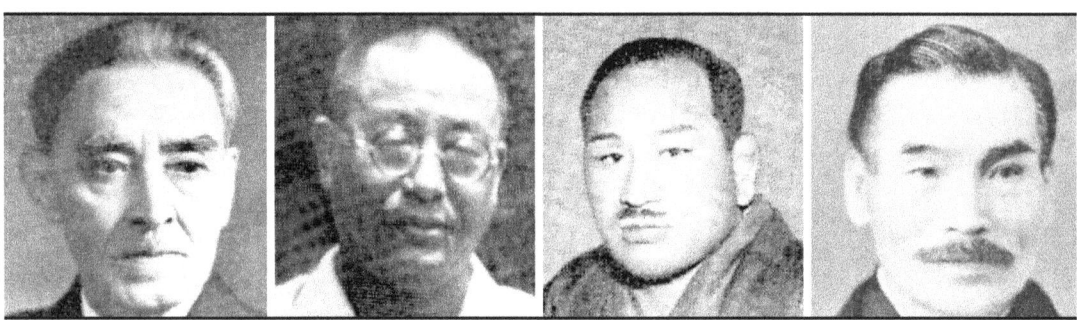

Left to right: Mifune Kyuzo, Tabata Shotaro, Kurihara Tamio, and Iizuka Kunizaburo.

Mifune vs. Tabata

Mifune (5 foot 3 inches, 135 pounds) was dwarfed by the stocky Tabata (5 foot 6 inches, 190 pounds). Mifune was a decided underdog—to everyone but Mifune, that is. No sooner had the two taken hold than Mifune, with no show of strength, lashed out with a foot sweep (*okuriashi-hari*), causing Tabata to stumble and temporarily lose his balance. Tabata recovered before Mifune could follow up his advantage. Both held lightly, stood straight, and moved gracefully. Tabata took the offensive with a well-placed blocking foot-lift pull throw (*sasae-tsurikomi-ashi*), which caused Mifune's body to rock precariously. Quickly regaining his balance, Mifune shortly after attempted a circle throw (*tomoe-nage*), but this was blocked easily by Tabata. With three minutes remaining, Tabata tried a side sacrifice throw (*yoko-sutemi*), failed, and immediately tried it again. Mifune's feet left the mat and *ippon* (full point) seemed a certainty. Midway in its arc, however, Mifune's body turned like a cat and he rolled onto his side. It was a close escape, and Yamashita Yoshitsugu, that whitehaired exemplar of pure judo, the referee, called out nothing. Shortly afterward, time ran out and Yamashita declared the match a draw.

Goto vs. Kurihara

Next, Goto and Kurihara, each 39 years of age, squared off. Immediately Kurihara, renowned in the Kyoto area for his groundwork, tried a circle throw (*tomoe-nage*) and, when this failed, attempted a body drop (*taiotoshi*). Goto shook off both attempts easily. It was obvious to the spectators that Kurihara was trying to lead Goto into *ne-waza* (groundwork).[3] But this time, Goto, seeing his antagonist supine, leaped into groundwork. Kurihara turned from underneath at Goto's approach and began a strangle. Adroitly, Goto escaped and stood up. On again taking hold, Goto speedily struck with a lift-pull hip throw (*tsuri-komi-goshi*). But Kurihara remained upright. After several feints, Kurihara tried a combination of smaller inner reap (*ko-uchi-gari*) and side sacrifice (*yoko-sutemi*) throws, against which Goto defended successfully. With time expiring, Kurihara essayed a volley of throws—circle, big outer reap, and side sacrifice—but in his concern over the time, his coordination was lacking and Goto never lost his balance. After time expired, referee Yamashita called the match a draw.

Isogai vs. Nagaoka

The last bout of the day brought together the two greatest experts of that era, Isogai and Nagaoka. The spectators leaned forward on the edge of their seats. Here was the zenith of judo!

With a fierce *kiai* (spirit shout), Isogai seized Nagaoka's jacket. There was no aimless walking about, both moved with the utmost caution. Isogai stepped in beautifully with a

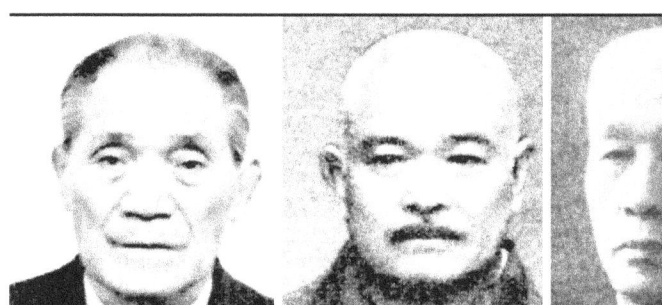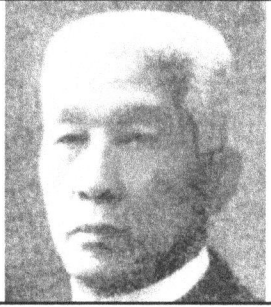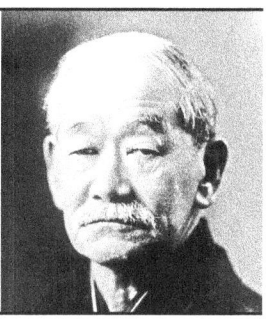

Left to right: Samura Kaichiro, Isogai Hajime, Yamashita Yoshitsugu (referee of the 1928 Masters Contest). He taught President Theodore Roosevelt at the White House (1903–1907), and Kano Jigiro, founder of judo.

side sacrifice throw (*yoko-sutemi*), but, just as beautifully, Nagaoka evaded the attempt. In escaping, he did not push, but rather skipped outside the trajectory of Isogai's pull. Isogai stood up and they again took hold. While neither tried a great deal, it was clear that the minds of both were racing apace. Suddenly, Nagaoka spun into a leg wheel (*ashi guruma*) but Isogai did not waver. A silence permeated the crowd. Time was on the move and the watchers knew that neither of the masters could be content with a draw. They were right. After some maneuvering, Nagaoka tried his terrible favorite left-side sacrifice throw (*hidari-yoko-sutemi*). This was the technique that had enabled him to reach the judo heights. It was yoko-sutemi that succeeded when other throws (*te*) failed. But it did not succeed this day against Isogai. That master did not lose his balance. Isogai's backers breathed easier. At this point, referee Yamashita declared the match over and announced it a draw. Probably neither Nagaoka nor Isogai was content but each had to be in the face of the merit of the other.

    The principals of these bouts lived to further the concepts developed by Kano Jigoro, the creator of judo. Mifune, our "grand old man," is on the wrong side of seventy, but still engages in daily free practice (*randori*) and teaching. Before his death, Tabata wrote an occasional article for the Kodokan monthly magazine *Judo*. Kurihara (ninth-dan) lives in Kyoto and in 1951 traveled to Europe with Kano Risei's Kodokan party, where he gave masterly kata demonstrations with his prize student Awazu Shozo (sixth-dan). Awazu, predictably, is also a ground specialist and currently assists Kawaishi Mikonosuke (seventh-dan), the leader of French judo since 1936.

    Samura, at an advanced age, teaches tactical theory through a regular section in the Kodokan *Judo* journal. In this, his esteemed collaborator was, until his recent death, the incomparable Nagaoka. So far as this writer knows, Iizuka is still living, and a member of the faculty of a Tokyo university where he has taught judo for many years.

    Nagaoka has passed on. Shortly before his demise, a picture of this mighty master, walking in a flower garden with a cane much in evidence, appeared in a French publication. I experienced a mild pang on seeing it, for not too long before this I had seen Nagaoka in the 1950 Kodokan judo film, in which he tossed a younger, heavier opponent with ease and grand *waza* (techniques). *Tempus fugit*, and "before one realizes it, one is in the sere and yellow leaf," as E. J. Harrison, quoting the Bard, commented in a recent missive. And it is a pity.

    Isogai is gone also. But he left a legacy in the form of two judo texts. I have been unable to ascertain the present status of Goto (eighth-dan).

    So much for the men. Now, what of their techniques? I think the reader will readily discern at least two points emerging from the above descriptions of their bouts:

1) The predominant use of tomoe-nage and yoko-sutemi, throws now seldom achieved or even tried.
2) The few throwing techniques tried during the course of a match.

In respect to the first point, the implications are easy to grasp. All of these masters had the "feel" of sacrifice and foot techniques to such an extent that a throw such as tomoe-nage or yoko-sutemi was as much a major weapon for them as the inner thigh throw (*uchi-mata*) is for Yoshimatsu Yoshihiko[4] or the big outer reap (*osoto-gari*) is for Daigo Toshiro[5] at the present. In other words, they relied more on subtle unbalancing than on strength.

Regarding the second point, the masters "thought" during a match. Only when there was a concrete likelihood of a full point was a throwing attempt made. The fact that no *kaeshi-waza* (counterattacking techniques) occurred and the ease with which they escaped their antagonists' overtures attest to good initial unbalancing and body control (*tai-sabaki*) beyond the ken of most judoka.

In closing, I venture the opinion that these eight masters came to the art with no extraordinary physical equipment. Nor did they reach their high estate in the judo hierarchy by remarkable brainwork. Without a doubt, they all held in common (though in varying degrees, certainly all high) a will to win. This will sufficed to make their ordinary bodies perfect servants of their nimble minds, minds which had been made sharp by repetitious physical practice.

We see a complementary, reciprocating process at work—the will driving the mind, which works the body, which in turn, refurbishes the mind and, in the end, rewards the will. The process is exemplified in each of the masters we have discussed, and if the reader must have a moral, it is probably this: the merit of the masters began—and continues to begin—with the will, and in the end, their merit was and is proportionate to that will.

ACKNOWLEDGMENT
Special thanks to Warren Conner, Russ Mason, and Joseph Svinth for reading and commenting on this article in its preliminary stages.

NOTES

[1] The summaries of these bouts were taken from *Showa Tenran Shiai* (Judo and Kendo Matches Before the Emperor in the Showa Period), Tokyo: Kodansha, 2 volumes, 1934, 1981 pages. The writer thanks Ben Ishii (first dan, Seattle) for the translation. The article itself was first written in 1953 and appeared in the *Budokwai Judo* quarterly (London).

[2] The personal names cited are rendered in the conventional Japanese style, with the surnames first.

[3] Ground techniques allowed in judo include holding techniques (*osae-waza*), joint-locking techniques (*kansetsu-waza*), and choking techniques (*shime-waza*).

[4] Yoshimatsu won the All Japan Championships in 1952 and 1953.

[5] In 1950, Daigo was the youngest man ever to be awarded a sixth-dan. He was 24 at the time. He was noted for various reaping throws and won the All Japan Championship in 1951.

chapter 2

Jujutsu: The Gentle Art and the Strenuous Life
by Joe Long, B.A.

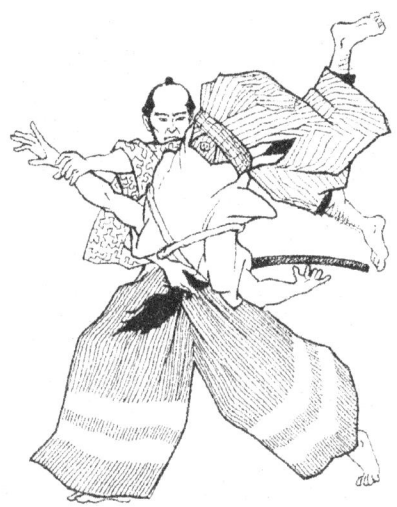

All illustrations by Tony LaMotta.

Introduction

When the Japanese art of jujutsu was introduced to the United States at the turn of the century, Americans largely misinterpreted it. Jujutsu could have been an improvement upon Western pugilism and wrestling, and more importantly provided vital insights into Japanese psychology and strategy as the Japanese-American rivalry in the Pacific began. Instead, jujutsu was transformed to fit American preconceptions and its origins were shrouded in unnecessary and often sinister myth. Western practitioners took on the difficult task of transplanting jujutsu away from its Japanese context while preserving its physical and philosophical essence. Several factors contributed to their essential failure to do so in the first decade of the twentieth century.

At the end of the nineteenth century, jujutsu was a peculiarly Japanese method of unarmed combat, partially derived from Chinese sources but developed in relative isolation throughout Japan's feudal period. Individual schools taught variations of the art, usually as a supplement to swordsmanship, and the jujutsu methods of each school were jealously guarded against rivals, and restricted from common citizens by the nobility. Sweeping social changes in Japan eased these restrictions and introduced both the Japanese citizenry and the world to the art as the century closed.

Although Rudyard Kipling made reference to "devilish art and craft and wrestling tricks" (McKenzie, 1906:225) encountered by rowdy British sailors who fell afoul of Japanese police in 1892, the first Western reaction to a formal demonstration of jujutsu was published by Lafcadio Hearn in 1895. His description is instructive:

> To the uninitiated it looks like wrestling ... A professional wrestler would observe more ... the grips, holds, and flings are both peculiar and risky. In spite of the care exercised, he would judge the whole to be dangerous play, and would be tempted, perhaps, to advise the adoption of Western 'scientific' rules.
> – Hearn, 1895:185

Hearn explained that jujutsu was, in fact, not a sport at all, and went on to describe the terrible prowess of a master of the art.

> By some terrible legerdemain he suddenly dislocates a shoulder, unhinges a joint, bursts a tendon, or snaps a bone—without any apparent effort. He is much more than an athlete; he is an anatomist ... The fact, however, to which I want to call attention is that the master of jiujutsu [sic] never relies upon his own strength ... Then what does he use? Simply the strength of his antagonist. The force of the enemy is the only means by which the enemy is overcome ... I may venture to say, loosely, that in jiujutsu there is a sort of counter for every twist, wrench, pull, push, or bend: only the jiujutsu expert does not opposes such movements at all. No: he yields to them. But he does much more than yield to them. He aids them with a wicked sleight that causes the assailant to put out his own shoulder, to fracture his own arm or, in a desperate case, even to break his own neck or back.
> – Hearn, 1895:186–187

The fundamental principle of jujutsu described here by Hearn is reflected in the translation of the term itself. *Jutsu* refers to methods or techniques (Lattimore, 1904:431); *ju* or *jiu*, to yielding, blending, or even gentleness (Ratti and Westbrook, 1973:347); in context, jujutsu becomes the art of yielding for the purpose of self-defense, or as Hearn translates, "to conquer by yielding" (Hearn, 1895:187). Individual jujutsu techniques involved blending with the momentum of an attack in order to draw the opponent off-balance and subdue him. This contrasted sharply with Western wrestling and boxing, which were both understood as contests of applied force.

The fundamental techniques of jujutsu were those directed toward unbalancing the foe, consisting primarily of throws and "trips" or "sweeps." Two significant secondary categories were the so-called "chokes" (which were very different from actual strangulation) and the *atemi*, open-handed strikes associated with some jujutsu styles (Clark, 1992:138). Mechanically jujutsu resembled wrestling much more than boxing, and had very little at all in common with contemporary foot-oriented fighting styles such as the Korean tae-kwondo or the French savate.

The introduction of jujutsu to the West coincided with the heyday of "Lancashire," or "catch-as-catch-can" wrestling in the English-speaking countries (Britannica, 1911). This rough-and-tumble sport had supplanted the more restrictive Greco-Roman style in the public imagination, and was well on its way to acceptance as a collegiate and Olympic sport. This form of wrestling had several throws which corresponded closely to jujutsu techniques, particularly the "buttock" and "cross-buttock" throws, and Hugh Leonard, recognized as the leading authority on wrestling by the *Encyclopedia Britannica*, went so far as to state after a jujutsu exhibition by Katsukama Higashi that he had "been unable to find anything in jujutsu [sic] which is not known to Western wrestling" (Leonard and Higashi, 1905:33). The perceived similarity between jujutsu and catch-as-catch-can would bring the two into competition, both in exhibition matches for the curious and in an ongoing contest for public favor.

Catch-as-catch-can developed into modern collegiate wrestling, and also into the entertaining spectacles of "professional wrestling." Jujutsu is still practiced today in ways very much resembling those imported from Japan during this period, and is also recognized as the foundation of the modern sport of judo. Judo was synthesized during the 1880's by Dr. Jigoro Kano, a Japanese reformer steeped in the lore of Western physical education (Clark, 1992:138). Kano's new sport had a terrific impact on the teaching of jujutsu in Japan, just as the first foreign students were being introduced to the art. Kano had adapted jujutsu's safest techniques to a Western-style competitive environment, allowing matches to proceed at full speed and force with minimal risk of injury. Chokes as well as many throws and trips were retained; for sport judo, however, all forms of striking and most joint-holds were discarded.

Kano also framed his sport within a larger context of education and philosophy, describing judo as a way of life. The renaming was very deliberate, as Kano explained:

> I named the subject I teach jiudo instead of jiujutsu ... *Jiu* means gentle or give way, *jutsu*, an art or practice; and *do*, way or principle, so that *jiujutsu* means an art or practice of first giving way in order to gain final victory; while *jiudo* means the way or principle of the same.
> – Hancock and Higashi, 1905:200

Since the Japanese government officially sanctioned the resulting sport, many foreign observers concluded that judo was a superior form of "scientific" jujutsu. Sometimes the terms jujutsu, jiujitsu, judo, and jiudo were used interchangeably, although judo enthusiasts were swift to assert their distinction from and superiority to older schools.[1]

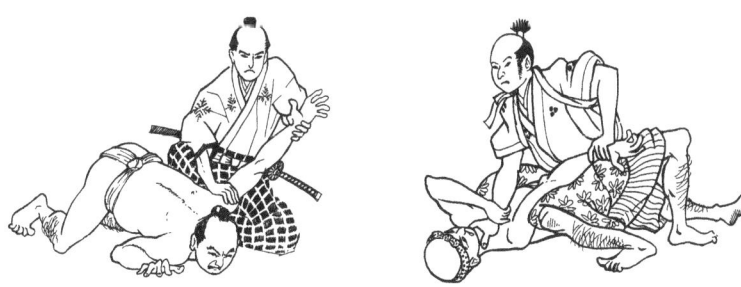

"National Jujutsu:" A Strategic Insight

Beyond jujutsu's significance in physical education or as an improvement on conventional American fisticuffs lay its implications about Japanese psychology and national strategy. Perceptions about the ethics and mechanics of conflict, as well as the notion of force and the balance of power, were bound to be vastly different between the Japanese with their jujutsu paradigm and the Westerners, whose metaphor for contest tended to be boxing. Lafcadio Hearn concluded this immediately as he observed jujutsu in its native land. He coined the phrase "national jiu-jutsu" (Hearn, 1895:193) to describe the larger strategic implications of the concept.

In Hearn's view, this aptly described the rapid yet very deliberate selective modernization that Japan underwent once her self-imposed solitude was broken by contact with the Western powers. Various benefits of modern science were diligently sought after by Japan with the intention of adapting them to Japanese culture, but the culture itself was kept intact by the conservative policies of the Imperial government. Japan had decided to "blend" with technological forces much as a jujutsu practitioner might blend with the force of an incoming physical threat.

Hearn's evaluation shows considerable insight, much more insight than is apparent in the written works of some of his contemporaries who (unlike Hearn) actually laid claim to a certain degree of mastering the art.

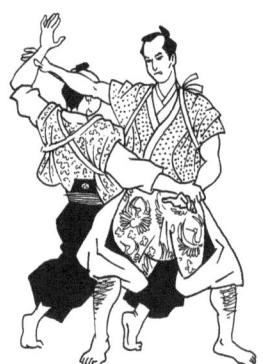 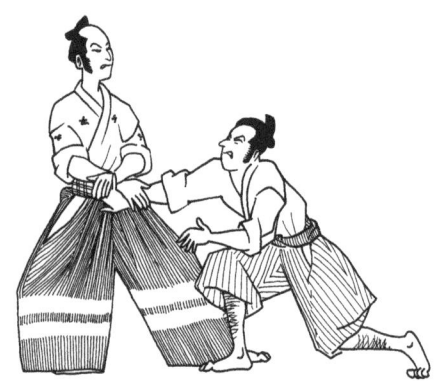

The Strenuous Life

President Theodore Roosevelt was the most prominent jujutsu student in the United States, and responsible for the surge in public interest that followed his importation of Kano-certified instructors. However, his "Strenuous Life" doctrine led him to publicly promote native martial arts (especially boxing) instead.

Roosevelt requested Yamashita Yoshiaki to be his personal instructor in the White House where the President's recreation room became the first official dojo in the United States. As part of his personal commitment to "the strenuous life," Roosevelt was already wont to box, fence, and wrestle with a wide range of sparring partners there, and apparently he had received some sort of introduction to jujutsu before Yamashita's arrival in 1904. ". . . I had Professor Yamashita teach me the 'jiudo'—as they seem now to call Jiu Jitsu" (Bishop, 1919:113), he wrote in a personal letter, and his awareness of the name change may lend credence to the claim of one John J. O'Brien, a policeman, to have actually been the first to introduce jujutsu to the United States and to have been Roosevelt's first instructor (O'Brien, 1905:3). Yet another account cites Charles Perry (Stevens, 1984:7), an American traveller in Japan, with exciting State Department interest in the art. In any case Roosevelt established a regular workout schedule with Yamashita and included Commander Takashita, the Japanese naval attache, and a Japanese youth named Kitagaki who would subsequently attend the United States Naval Academy at Annapolis (Bishop, 1919: 113).

Roosevelt's interest was probably excited purely by the prowess of his instructors rather than any philosophical implications in their art, for his vaunted "strenuous life" had an essential martial bias. He believed in seeking out physical challenges in order to grow stronger through struggle against them, and conflict sought for this purpose must oppose physical force with force in order to achieve its goal. Roosevelt took great pride in the caliber of his opponents in combative sports, the vigor of his training, and even the multitude of his injuries. He was an outspoken advocate of amateur boxing for American youth, for both the physique- and character-building qualities of the sport.

As a combative sport enthusiast, Roosevelt seems to have trained intensively in his new art. Despite his extensive experience he seems to have been manhandled by Yamashita rather convincingly, for he wrote his son Kermit:

> I am wrestling with two Japanese wrestlers three times a week. I am not the age or the build one would think likely to be whirled lightly over an opponent's head and batted down on the mattress without damage. But they are so skillful that I have not been hurt at all. My throat is a little sore, because once when one of them had a strangle hold I also got hold of his windpipe and thought I could perhaps choke him off before he could choke me. However, he got ahead.
> – Bishop, 1919:93–94

The vigor of Roosevelt's training seems to have been considerable, although his windpipe-clutching tactics may well have tried the patience of his partners! (Proper judo uses only the side of the neck.) Before his course of instruction was done he was ranked at least as a "brown belt" (Kano introduced a system of designating judo proficiency with a series of colored belts from white to black, with darker colors showing more advanced students). Yamashita, his personal instructor, was assigned to develop judo training for the midshipmen of the Naval Academy in 1905 (New York, 1905) thus founding the Navy judo team (which is still in existence) a decade before the Navy began a collegiate wrestling program.

Yet Roosevelt, for all his apparent personal enthusiasm, did little for the public promotion of judo or jujutsu in America, continuing instead his strong advocacy of Western martial arts. His autobiography dedicates page after page to the joys and benefits of boxing and wrestling, while summing up his jujutsu experience in a sentence and implying that it was an art he found suitable mostly because advancing age was gradually restricting his participation in rougher pursuits (Roosevelt, 1924:41).

Had Roosevelt not believed strongly in the efficacy of the Japanese art, it is very doubtful that Yamashita's next assignment would have been as the Navy's first judo coach. However, Roosevelt's lack of enthusiasm for judo as physical education makes sense in the light of the beliefs he articulated about the Western combatives. Yielding to aggressive force (even in an advantageous manner) may have been good strategy, but it could never be a Roosevelt principle, and Roosevelt could bring himself to be a student of the art but not its public advocate.

Jujutsu and the American Occult

While some Americans might have found jujutsu difficult to reconcile with their own philosophies, there were those who insisted upon making it difficult to reconcile with reality. The first reports and the earliest demonstrations of jujutsu arrived on American shores during a heyday of spiritualism and of interest in the occult here, and some observers immediately inferred supernatural forces at work.

As an esoteric Eastern art in which, by secret knowledge, a man could manifest apparently superhuman powers, jujutsu could certainly be classified among occult phenomena. For jujutsu, the association could only be an unfortunate one, creating on the one hand unrealistic expectations on the part of the credulous and, on the other, suspicion of charlatanry or even evil supernatural influences.

Impressed by the art's startling effectiveness and novelty, laymen often colorfully compared jujutsu to supposed mystical phenomena. Outlandish claims for the art were made, which publicity-hungry experts were loathe to contradict; thus jujutsu acquired an unnecessarily mysterious and even sinister air. In the long run, sensationalism proved counterproductive, drawing ridicule or censure on various occasions.

One enduring myth linking jujutsu with occult powers was (and is) the legendary "death touch." By this method, it was believed, a master of the art could slay an opponent instantly with a light stroke to pressure points on his victim's body.

"The science is far more potent than hypnotism," wrote one American, making an obvious comparison to another 'supernatural' phenomenon then in vogue, "for by a swift physical touch a victim's brain can be benumbed, his hips or shoulders dislocated, an ankle unhinged, or a tendon burst or twisted. By a single lightening-like stroke of the operator one can be made instantly helpless..." (Terry, 1902:18).

This ludicrous claim may well be an imported Oriental superstition. Hearn reported that a master "knows also touches that can kill––as if by lightning" (Hearn, 1895:186). Since he did not report witnessing any such performance, the idea probably was passed on to him verbally by his Japanese hosts. However, it may have been an incidence of misunderstanding on Hearn's part, for although he may have been the first he would not be the last Westerner to read the concept of a "death touch" into Japanese sources which imply no such thing.

One phenomenon consistently confusing to the Western observer was the unconsciousness and subsequent revival of those who fell prey to judo or jujutsu choking techniques. These constriction holds were distinct from strangulation, for no pressure was applied to the windpipe of a receiver (except by Theodore Roosevelt!) nor was the victim's breathing impeded at all. Instead one or both of the carotid arteries in the sides of the neck were pressured, cutting off blood to the brain and inducing swift unconsciousness. Far from being especially brutal or dangerous, jujutsu chokes were retained in judo as humane finishing holds and were certainly far less risky to the recipient's future health than any knockout boxing blow (Clark, 1992:55).

To the unschooled Westerner, however, these techniques were apparent instances of murder by strangulation, and the victim's revival by another set of jujutsu techniques was nothing short of miraculous. H. Irving Hancock, an early American jujutsu instructor, ascribed to the Japanese jujutsu man utter fearlessness in the face of death itself, and attributed this to the student's being "many times... 'killed' and... brought back to life by his teacher. Hence, it is schooled into him to be indifferent about such a petty detail as death" (Hancock, 1905:204).

As promoter of the art and of his own elaborate system of diet and "physical culture" (nominally founded on Japanese principles), Hancock had a vested interest in the art's (and his own) sensational reputation. He thus encouraged the "death touch" legend with misleading allusions such as this one from the *American Review of Reviews*:

> Included in the one hundred and sixty feats of the Kano system are the "serious tricks," by which death may be caused at the will of the adept. Included also in these one hundred and sixty feats are the processes of *kuatsu* [*katsu*], or revivification, by which an opponent who has been apparently killed is brought back to full possession of his functional powers.
> – Hancock, 1905:204

The initiate will recognize this as a reference to the chokes of judo and the first aid which restores the unconscious unfortunate afterward. However, in this article intended for the general public, Hancock neglected to put "death at will" into the limited context of knockout chokes, leaving the reader to infer a claim of more generalized lethal powers at the command of the "adept." Hancock more blatantly laid claim to personal occult powers in his first book, *Japanese Physical Training*. Here, after lecturing a bit on the moral imperative of entrusting the science of jujutsu only to the worthy, he went on to state:

> There are no fewer than six blows known to native practisers of the art that will cause death. Although the author has been taught these blows, for obvious reasons he will not explain them.
>
> – Hancock, 1903:54

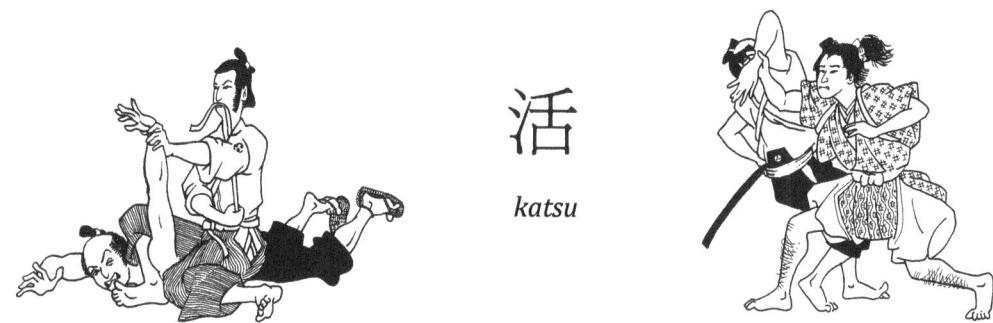

katsu

Since this work does explain the mechanics of the Japanese choke, as well as edge-of-the-hand and one-knuckle jabbing strikes, Hancock is again implying a secret, higher jujutsu more akin to magical than physical education. Again there is no blatant lie here; certainly at least six potentially lethal hand blows are possible, and in fact at least that many could be surmised by any astute reader who recognized that Hancock's recommended edge-of-hand blows could be sped toward vital areas of the anatomy rather than toward the arms and shoulders as Hancock advocated. Still it seems that Hancock's reference to these deadly blows is meant as a coy revelation of his mysterious powers.

It was left to a Japanese jujutsu emissary, Katsukama Higashi, to detail the fabled "death touch" more forthrightly in print. Higashi noted that jujutsu did indeed include blows of devastating power ("blows," not "touches," though precision was valued over raw force). However, these strikes were not delivered to a foe until other means had already made his defeat certain! Higashi explained that "the jiu-jitsu expert first trips his opponent and then strikes him as he is falling" (Higashi, 1905:320). In true jujutsu form, the foe would himself provide most of the force of a Higashi strike; indeed, the blow itself is less a technique than a flourish upon an already-successful technique of some other kind.

Significantly, Higashi and the American, Hancock, espoused the same jujutsu style and co-authored the volumes which followed Hancock's original jujutsu treatise. *The Complete Kano Jiu-Jitsu* which they eventually authored covered orthodox judo in great detail, but also included an appendix purporting to chart the vital points for "serious and fatal blows" by which "the processes of life are mechanically stopped." Resuscitation (*katsu*) alone will reverse this effect, which may be initiated by striking (among other specified points) the coccyx (point 23). None of Higashi's previous candor about downing an opponent before striking is evident here, nor are there accompanying photos of Higashi demonstrating atemi techniques as he demonstrates all of the others (and the katsu revivification). Instead the occult implications of the secrets of atemi are left intact, lending jujutsu both the attraction and the stigma of a quasi-mystical art.

Lost in Translation: Jujutsu in Print

As unfortunate for jujutsu as the occult associations were the approximate and unflattering translations of some common jujutsu terms. Already a foreign system and one which flouted the conventions and "civilized" rules of boxing and wrestling, jujutsu suffered greatly at the hands of translators.

Again the enthusiastic Hancock was an offender. It is difficult to see how an instructor laying claim to seven years resident study of jujutsu in Japan could translate the name of the art itself as "muscle-breaking" (1903:2), yet Hancock did. Techniques in Hancock's written descriptions lost all trace of the jujutsu principles of blending or yielding, as if "muscle-breaking" was indeed the essential nature of the art:

> First of all the tricks taught is the hand-grip that is used in throwing an opponent. The hand is seized ... at the same time the man who attempts to make the throw presses his own thumb severely over a muscle that may be found just below the base of the opponent's third finger ... As soon as the hand is so seized the man who has secured the grip gives his enemy's wrist a violent wrench outward and over, and endeavors to throw him.
> – Hancock, 1903:100

While this passage generally outlines the mechanics of the wrist throw known as *kotegaeshi*, it can readily be seen that this technique performed as described would be a blatant departure from jujutsu principles. No allowance is made for the strength of an opponent's attack to be redirected to make this technique work; in fact, the Hancock student is apparently himself the aggressor, beginning the sequence by seizing the foe's hand. Following this up with severe pressure and a violent wrench leaves no room at all for characteristic jujutsu grace or strategy on the part of Hancock's man!

A description of kotegaeshi in a more accurate modern manual (an aikido manual, but reflecting the jujutsu form which that art was derived) begins with a strike thrown by the opponent, and uses a parry to "lead" the striking hand into a similar hold. Once the offensive force has been "guided" into the wrist hold, the defender is advised that his right hand "will assist in extending his fingers over and down" to complete the throw (Ratti and Westbrook, 1970:202). This careful language is not euphemism but precision, for in jujutsu and its derivative arts non-resistance is not an ethic but an enabling tactic of the arts themselves.

More subtle influences in written jujutsu descriptions were exerted by individual terms. As noted earlier, "choke" described a constrictive neck-hold distinct from Western strangulation, but the word itself implied an unfair and murderous tactic. "Trip" was another unfortunate choice much in favor with both Hancock and Higashi, used to describe any technique in which the opponent's feet were taken out from under him. Unfortunately, no matter how sneaky the technique itself (judo players now prefer to call them "sweeps" or "reaps," and they are generally employed while face-to-face with the opponent) the implication is one of trickery. Even worse-sounding is "wrist-pinch," Hancock's choice for describing what is normally referred to as a "joint-lock" today (Higashi, 1905:321).

Worst, however, was the use of the word "trick" for *waza*, now generally translated "technique." Waza were the basic units of jujutsu, the elements of proficiency gained one at a time to be employed in contest or conflict. That the art should consist of a great many "tricks" emphasized the idea of unfairness once more, besides conjuring up the image of that turn-of-the-century icon, the stage magician.

In the case of jujutsu, at least, written language seemed to merely impede communication. For the Japanese expert Higashi, the attempt to communicate the art physically was to have pitfalls as well.[2]

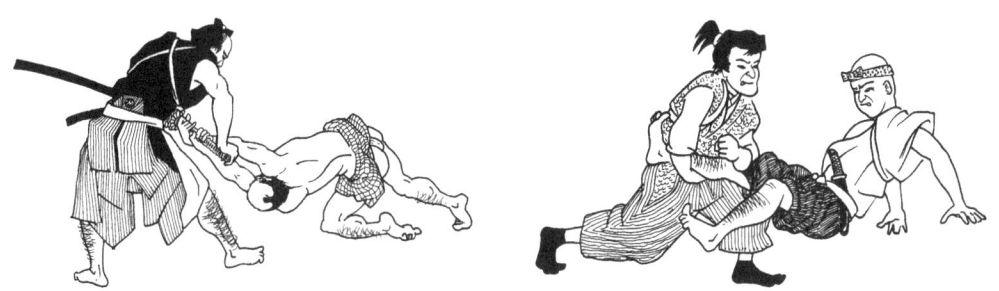

Jujutsu's Collision with Sports

Katsukama Higashi was a man of twenty-three years, 110 pounds, and terrific prowess when he embarked upon his American odyssey (Leonard and Higashi, 1905:33). His initial demonstrations, presented to the professional audience of the New York City Police Department, were completely successful in showing the practicality of jujutsu. His comrade Hancock could later claim that, when Higashi was confronted by the Department strong man who could casually manhandle pianos, "each of the three bouts was won in an instant by the Japanese" (Hancock, 1905:202). Moreover, the contests were concluded with very basic techniques, "only the simplest feats known to adepts," supposedly because Higashi did not consider the police champion a difficult enough opponent for more advanced ploys (Hancock, 1905:202) (Of course, in conflict as in other endeavors, the simplest approach may also be the best, but whether or not Higashi gave away any advantage by restricting himself to elementary technique, he made a strong impression).

Higashi thus established his reputation, a reputation that would be spread through his own writings and Hancock's as they introduced jujutsu to the American public. Although the two published the first Kano-style manual in the United States in 1905, Higashi's connection with orthodox judo before that seems to be tenuous. Certainly he preferred the term "jujutsu" for his own practice, and described with some pride aspects of his art inconsistent with Kano's sport, including the atemi strikes, dangerous wristlocks, and techniques employing sticks and ropes offensively (Higashi, 1905:320). Judo included no armed techniques, although traditional jujutsu schools always had, and while Higashi gave his allegiance to Dr. Kano's style at some point (possibly with the Japanese adoption of judo as the "official" national system) he certainly received his initial training elsewhere.

Kano's judo, however, greatly influenced Higashi's career and his approach to teaching in the United States. Kano's rules for competition allowed Higashi a framework within which to test himself competitively against Western fighters. This led to his great public misadventure on a Thursday evening in April, 1905.

Higashi had arranged to take on the United States lightweight wrestling champion, George Bothner, before a large crowd at the Grand Central Palace in New York City. Perhaps he intended to prove the superiority of jujutsu through this contest; in any case, the crowd and the *New York Times* chose to view the match as a contest between Eastern and Western grappling methods rather than between two athletes.

The rules to be followed generated much confusion. Both combatants had agreed to "Japanese rules" (New York, 1905b), including the wear of the heavy cotton jackets customary in judo. The *Times* was under the impression that Higashi's vaunted strikes and joint-locks were legal under foreign rules (New York, 1905b), but Higashi employed none during the course of the bout nor would they have been permitted in a judo match. The boisterous crowd was clearly on Bothner's side in the contest and would judge the match based on their experience of catch-as-catch-can wrestling. One of the judges was John J. O'Brien, another American jujutsu proponent and allegedly Roosevelt's first teacher. However, since O'Brien had no connection with Dr. Kano or judo, Higashi contended that techniques the American judges disallowed fall outside the familiar native rules without any regard to the Japanese rules that competitors had explicitly agreed upon.

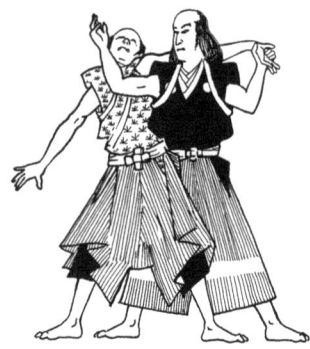

According to the *New York Times*, the first round went swiftly to Bothner, who took Higashi down cleanly after the jujutsu man had failed in an attempt to apply a standing choke. During the second round, a long and tedious one for both combatants and spectators, it became clear that Bothner had sufficient understanding of jujutsu tactics to frustrate Higashi severely. Bothner went to his knees, sank his weight back onto his heels, and would commit no energy to any offensive attempt for more than an hour. Higashi could not prevail over this inertia, for Bothner was aping his own strategy, and each man waited for committed force from the other.

Apparently, however, Bothner tired of the static situation first, for the round concluded with a shoulder-throw by Higashi. In the Japanese competitor's mind, this was a decisive fall—in fact, by judo rules, an *ippon* or match-winning throw. According to Higashi, it was this sort of fall which represented a "real" victory (New York, 1905b) (Recall that in non-sport application, Higashi advocated that a falling foe, while unbalanced, be finished with a powerful strike. Therefore, if an opponent falls during an actual fight with Higashi the outcome would be predictable).

The American judges did not count this fall at all, nor two others during the third round even though the final one Higashi followed up with a pin (legal under judo but not wrestling rules). At the end of the third round, Bothner scored his second takedown, a half-Nelson, and the match was over (New York, 1905b). Bothner had won by American rules and the judges' ruling, but Higashi had won by Kano's rules, while the spectators in the crowd and in the press were filled with nationalistic pride but also with profound disappointment that Higashi had not worked any spectacular Oriental magic during a basically boring fight.

Higashi had made a mistake in his quest for publicity, and jujutsu would pay for it in the New York press. Thereafter the *Times* took a strong editorial stance against jujutsu, opining that it was useless against superior strength and unethical in application (New York, 1905b). When an American jujutsu student was injured in practice, the Times lamented his "sacrifice . . . on the altar of an uncanny Eastern rite" (New York, 1905a). Mainstream American opinion had dismissed jujutsu, and the practice of Oriental martial arts in the United States would languish until their re-introduction by returning servicemen after the Second World War.

Conclusion

The attempted transplantation of Japanese jujutsu to the United States as the twentieth century dawned was hindered by a variety of factors. The art itself was based upon ideas about conflict antithetical to Roosevelt's "strenuous life" and contrary to combative traditions in the American culture. Translation of these new ideas was imprecise and further confused by suggestions that the art had sinister occult aspects. Finally, Katsukama Higashi's attempt to prove jujutsu's superiority in a wrestling ring was inconclusive, disappointing public expectations and turning the press against the art.

Successful communication of this uniquely Japanese art might have improved American understanding of Japanese psychology and strategy, as it had aided Lafcadio Hearn in his speculation on Japanese national strategy in the 1890's. Instead, the public impression of the art contributed to stereotypes of the Japanese as treacherous, ruthless, possibly evil but still ineffectual against Western strength. Had the initial public amazement at jujutsu been followed by deeper understanding rather than disenchantment, it would surely have been reflected in a better understanding of a great national rival in the twentieth century.

NOTES

[1] In reality the distinctions between the arts were blurry. The use of the terms judo and jujutsu was sometimes indiscriminate even among advanced practitioners in judo's early years. Kano's creation would progress further from its jujutsu roots and almost completely into the realm of athletics as the century progressed, but during Roosevelt's day the two arts were much more closely related and must be considered together. Where it is possible to distinguish between the sport of judo and the combat methods of jujutsu I have attempted to do so. One relatively reliable clue to the distinction in early English-language references is that, while "jujutsu" was often used to refer to Kano's style, no form of jujutsu devoid of Kano's influence was called "judo" by practitioners or informed observers.

[2] In the cases of Hancock, Higashi, and the other budo pioneers in the West, however, it is easy to be unduly judgemental. Hindsight's harsh light reveals flaws in descriptions of highly specialized Japanese terms, for which no English equivalents even existed. The comprehension and presentation of the technical concepts of the martial arts remains challenging even today, after almost another century of contact between the American and Japanese cultures. That Americans today have had a century of exposure to Japanese martial arts is due to men like Hancock and Higashi, and they were the first to publish extensively in English; whatever their foibles or flaws, today's American martial artists owe them a great deal. At first, however, written language seemed merely to impede communication in the case of jujutsu. For the Japanese expert Higashi, the attempt to communicate the art physically was to have pitfalls as well.

REFERENCES

Bishop, J. (Ed). (1919). *Theodore Roosevelts' letters to his children*. New York: Charles Scribner's Sons.

Clark, R. (1992). *Martial arts for the university*. Dubuque, Iowa: Kendall/Hunt Publishing Company.

Encyclopedia Britannica, (1911), Vol. 15, Ju-jutsu (sic), pp. 546–547; Vol. 28, Wrestling, pp. 844–845.

Hancock, H. (1903). *Japanese physical training*. New York: G. P. Putnam's Sons.

Hancock, H. (February 1905). The Japanese art of jiu-jitsu. *The American Monthly Review of Reviews*, 202–205.

Hancock, H., and Higashi, K. (1905). *The complete Kano jiu-jitsu (jiudo)*. New York: G. P. Putnam's Sons.

Hearn, L. (1895). *Out of the east: Reveries and studies in new Japan*. Boston: Houghton Mifflin Company.

Higashi, K. (9 February 1905). Wonderful jiu-jitsu. *The Independent*, 319–322.

Lattimore, D. (2 June 1904). Ju-jutsu. *The Nation*, 431.

Leonard, H., and Higashi, K. (May 1905). American wrestling vs. jujitsu. *Cosmopolitan*, 33–42.

McKenzie, R. T. (December 1906). The legacy of the samurai, *American Physical Education Review*, 215–230.

New York Times, (12 March 1905a).

New York Times, (8 April 1905b).

O'Brien, J. (1905). *A course in jiu-jitsu and physical culture*. Chicago: American College of Physical Culture and Jiu-Jitsu.

Ratti, O., and Westbrook, A. (1973). *Secrets of the samurai: The martial arts of feudal Japan*. Rutledge, VT: Charles E. Tuttle.

Ratti, O., and Westbrook, A. (1970). *Aikido and the dynamic sphere: An illustrated introduction*. Rutledge, VT: Charles E. Tuttle.

Roosevelt, T. (1924). *Theodore Roosevelt: An autobiography*. New York: Charles Scribner's Sons.

Stevens, J. (1984). *Aikido: The way of harmony*. Boston: Shambhala Publications.

Terry, T. (October 1902). Jiujutsu: Japanese self-defense without weapons, *Outing*, 12–18.

chapter 3

The School of Hard Knocks:
Seattle's Kurosaka / Tentoku Kan Dojo 1928-1942
by Joseph R. Svinth, M.A.

Winter seclusion
Kotatsu* reverie
Faces of childhood.
  – Richard Hayes

* Low table with heater beneath

At 8 p.m. on Sunday, 11 November 1928—the coronation date of the Japanese Emperor Hirohito—the Kurosaka Dojo opened at 900 Yesler Way in Seattle. Its name was that of its chief instructor, Kurosaka Hiroshi, 3rd-dan. Permission to open the school had been granted by Nagaoka Hidekazu, 8th-dan chief instructor at the Tokyo Normal School, and stylistic leader of the Hojin Dai Nippon Butokukai, a Kyoto martial art association whose politics were often at odds with those of the Tokyo-based Kodokan.[1]

Kurosaka believed that judo was the best kind of exercise, both physically and mentally, for young people. Americans who wished to learn the art were welcome in his club, he said, as this would give them a better understanding of Japanese people. Nevertheless, all of his approximately twenty students were *nisei*.[2]

From the mid-1920s until November 1928, Kurosaka had been chief instructor at the Seattle Dojo. His split with the Seattle Dojo came over a number of small grievances. Money probably played a role. The Seattle Dojo was trying to raise money to build a new dojo on Washington Street (it was then located in the basement of the Tacoma Hotel), and Kurosaka apparently disagreed with the way the money was being allocated. Additionally, there were the usual dojo politics. Kurosaka was a Butokukai man, and the Seattle Dojo was a Kodokan school. As noted above, the Butokukai and the Kodokan were rivals even in Japan, and apparently their rivalry carried over to Seattle. Finally, there seem to have been personality conflicts between Kurosaka and the Seattle Dojo's leadership.[3]

The split between Kurosaka and the Seattle Dojo was acrimonious. The boys in one club would call the boys from the other club *yogore* ("dirty guys"), and claimed that what they did wasn't real judo. Of course this was not true. While Butokukai schools may have placed more emphasis on ground wrestling than Kodokan schools, their technical standards were virtually identical. Meanwhile, the boys' parents muttered calumnies against the leaders of the other school, and said that their teachers did things which did not set good examples for children. Once again, this wasn't true. Nevertheless, such bitterness led to significant disharmony in Seattle judo. Matters improved over time, but it wasn't until June 1938 that the *North American Times* could say:[5]

> Tentokukwan Dojo and Seattle Dojo were at forks' end with each other for several years. Rivalry approached the fight stage, as each fought to gain more new members to increase its own prestige.
>
> Now, however, things are different. There is, of course, rivalry between the local groups, but it is of the friendly, competitive kind. The coming of the present judo instructors, Sakata and Kumagai, as well as the formation of the all-star black belt team to tour California, were no doubt factors which brought about the more peaceable era in the judo front.

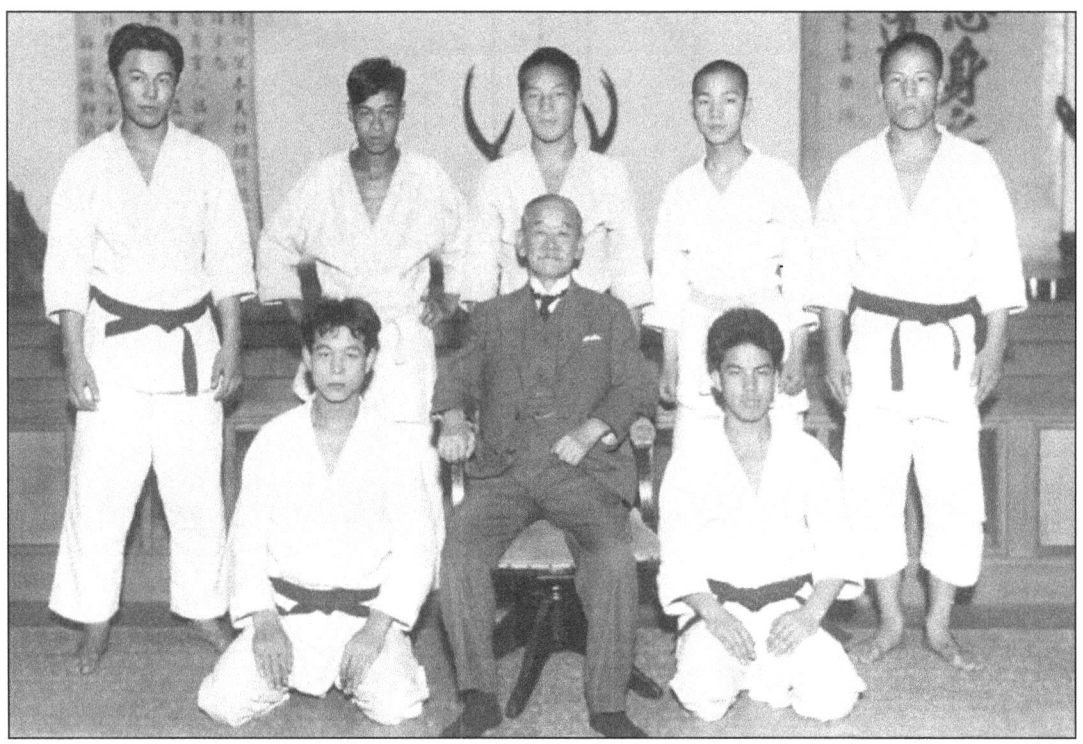

Young judoka pictured with Kano Jigoro. Professor Kano sits in the middle, while Seattle's Uzo Shiji stands at the far left. The others are unidentified. Photo courtesy of Kuqo Shinji.

Kurosaka Dojo made its first important tournament appearance in Vancouver, British Columbia, on Sunday, 9 February 1930. With only about twenty members, mostly teenaged or younger, it was hard for the Kurosaka Dojo to make much of a dent on bigger clubs with older, more experienced members. However, Kurosaka was a first-rate coach, and his young men tried.[6] Tad Kuniyuki, one of those original students, later recalled:[7]

> Mr. Kurosaka was the best judo instructor for the young students because he taught each of the students the name of the *waza* [technique] and why the waza worked when applied properly (the laws of physics) and also how to counter it. He also started the use of colored belts for the young teenagers and younger so they would have a higher belt to work for before getting a brown belt.

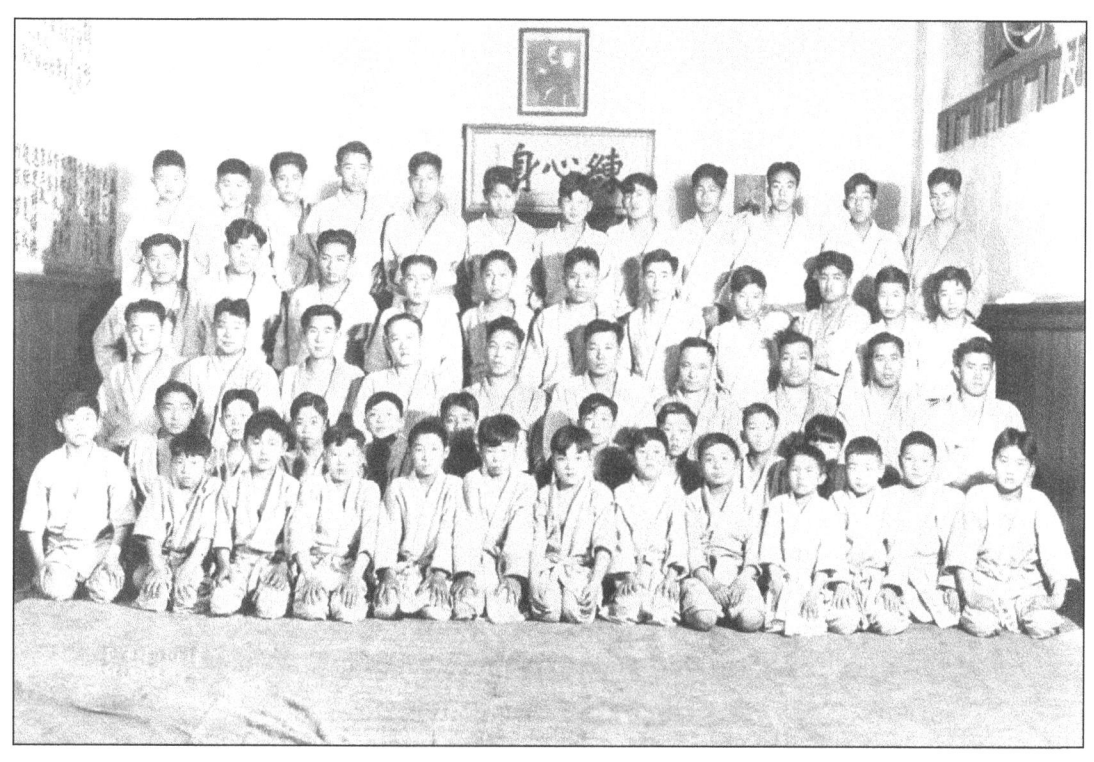

The Seattle Dojo group photo circa 1929 at its "old location" under the Tacoma Hotel shortly before Mr. Kurosaka split away from Kurosaka Dojo. Photo courtesy of Kozu Shinji.

First row, kneeling, L to R: Sam Kozu, Ben Terao, Tom Kubota, Abe Mitsuji, Kozu Shinji, Tom Mayeda, Asakura Yukio, Terumasa "Pan" Furuta, Elmer Tazuma, Taka "Tom" Okazaki, Ihashi Mamoru, Kubo Kazuo, Iseki Tsutomu, unidentified, George Ogishima, Furuta Yoshio, Henry Uyehara, unidentified, unidentified, Kimura Michio, Frank Yoshitake, George Hasegawa; **Second row,** seated, L to R: unidentified, Sakano Ichiro (1st-kyu), Kanda Yoshiharu (1st-kyu), Masachi "George" Maniwa, (1st-kyu), Suzuki Eitaro (3rd-dan), Kurosaka Hiroshi (3rd-dan), Masataro "John" Shibata (2nd-dan), Hama Hideo (2nd-dan), Mochizuki Goro (1st-kyu), Kudo Kaimon, 1st-kyu); **Third row,** standing, L to R: unidentified, Kaname "Ken" Kuniyuki, unidentified, Yoshijima Takeo (?), unidentified, Hamamoto Kiichi, unidentified, Bill Yorozu, unidentified, unidentified, Kubota Takeshi; **Fourth row,** standing, L to R: unidentified, Nitta Susuma, Sakuma Takeo, Hideo "Lindy" Uyehara, Horiuchi Takeo, Tad Kuniyuki, Iwana Shiro, Iwana Saburo, Sam Asanuma, Yorita Tatsuo, Nakagawa Nobushi, unidentified. Identification courtesy of Tad Kuniyuki.

Sometime during the spring of 1930, Kurosaka discovered he had tuberculosis. He went to Los Angeles to see doctors, which caused the newspaper to prematurely report that he died there of the disease. Yet, while his condition was fatal, and would soon cause his death,[8] Kurosaka did not quit judo until the very end. Said the *Japanese American Courier*, "Kurosaka had an easy time taking the '*yodan*' or fourth grade title by defeating eightmen in about seven minutes" during a tournament at the Nippon Kan Theater on 18 January 1931.[9] In April 1931, he also gave what seems to have been his final public demonstration to the members of the posh Washington Athletic Club in Seattle.[10]

In February 1931, the Kurosaka Dojo opened a satellite dojo at the Seinen Kai (Youth Club) Hall of the Nichiren Buddhist temple. The reason was to get better facilities. "When Tentokukan was on Yesler Way," says Koiwai Eichi, "we had a dressing room but no showers. In the back of the dojo were hard straw tatamis while in front was a softer canvas mat which of course we practiced on whenever we could."[11] In 1934, Kurosaka Dojo vacated the premises on Yesler altogether, and with the move into the Seinen Kai facilities changed its name to Tentoku Kan.[12] Although I haven't found anyone who remembers what the name means—most Seattle nisei spoke little Japanese and read less—it probably means "Heavenly Virtue Hall."[13]

In October 1931, Torigoye Kanezo became Tentoku Kan's first junior star. He accomplished this by winning the junior division of a tournament held at the Tacoma Buddhist Temple. Four months later, in February 1932, Seattle judoka celebrated twenty five years of Kodokan judo in the northwest by holding a huge tournament at the Nippon Kan Theater in Seattle.[14]

This was a single-elimination tourney, starting with the juniors. Red and White Contests (*kohaku shobu*) were included. White Team was Seattle Dojo, South Park, and White River Dojo. The Red Team was Kent, Tentoku Kan, Tacoma, and Fife. In *Fighting Spirit of Japan* (1982), E.J. Harrison described Red and White competitions as follows:[15]

> The competitors are divided into two teams (red and white), each team having its leader and being arranged according to the degree of skill possessed by the members. Thus the contest will begin with the least proficient and youngest opponents of the lower grades, and each bout is decided by the first fall or point scored instead of the best two out of three.... Ultimately the two best men on either side meet and fight it out.... At such moments, not unnaturally, intense excitement prevails.

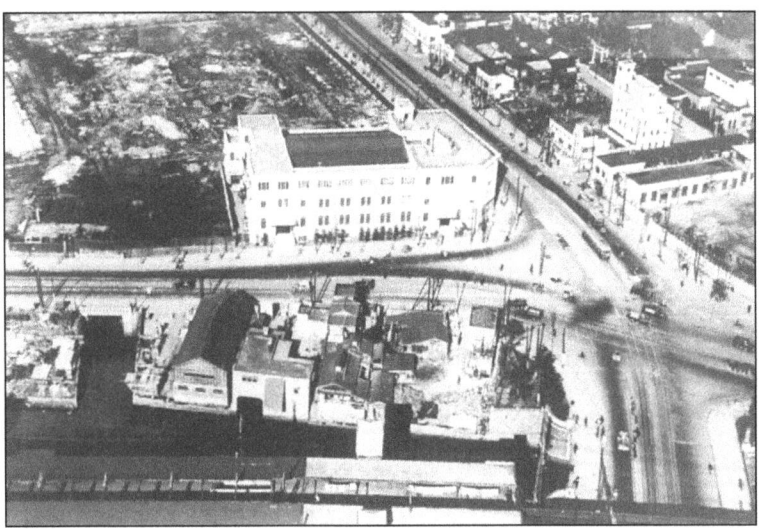

Aerial view of the Kodokan 1935.
Photo courtesy of Koqu Shinji.

In other words, everyone screamed and shouted. However, during individual competition, strict silence was maintained in the auditorium, much to the surprise of European-American observers.

It was during such a Red and White contest in Fife in February 1932 that Kuniyuki Kaname became Tentoku Kan's second nisei star. For, on the strength of the twenty-two-year-old former football star's victory, Tentoku Kan won its first ever senior division pennant.[16]

In October 1932, Yorita Tatsuo, who had just been promoted to 1st-dan, sailed to Japan.[17] In Tokyo, he trained under Professor Iizuka Kunisaburo, 8th-dan (later 10th-dan), a man E.J. Harrison once described as "a miniature Hercules in physique and possessed of astonishing skill and agility."[18] In April 1933, Yorita was promoted to 2nd-dan, making him the first Seattle nisei to receive that rank in Japan.[19] Kuniyuki Kaname followed Yorita to Japan in October 1934. There he too studied with Professor Iizuka.[20] However, while going to Japan was good for Kuniyuki and Yorita, their departure left just five black belts at the Tentoku Kan, none of whom were highly ranked. These were Sakano Ichiro, supervisor, 2nd-dan; Hama Hideo, 2nd-dan; Nitta Susumu, 1st-dan; Horiuchi Takeo, 1st-dan; and Torigoye Kanezo, 1st-dan. Reflecting the changing demographics of the times, the first two men were issei, while the latter were nisei.

Undaunted, the Tentoku Kan men persevered, and even hosted their own regional tournament at the Nippon Kan Theater on Sunday, 29 January 1933. Explained Sakano to a *Japanese American Courier* reporter: "It is understood the meet will be made into a competitive tournament in which every participant will be forced to give his utmost from the start to the finish."[21]

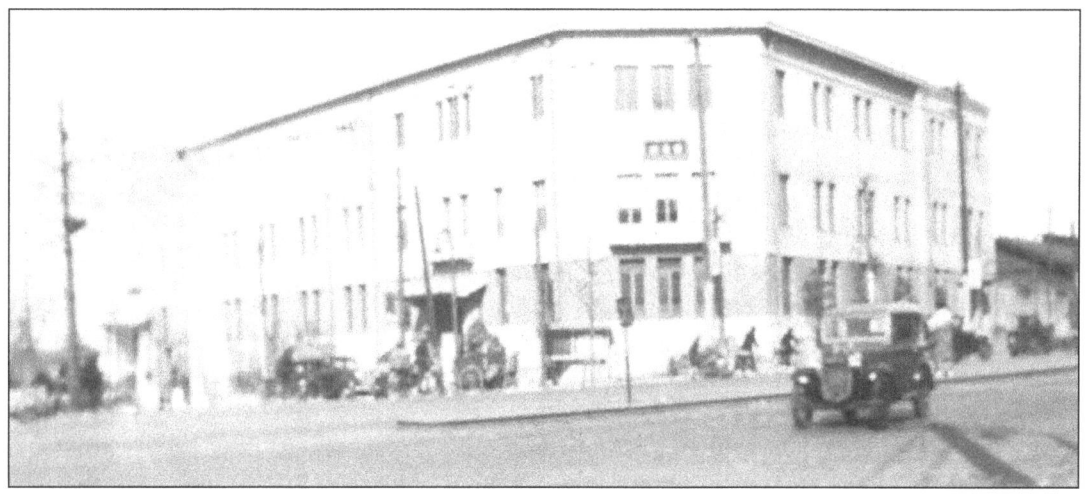

The Kodokan (1935) at street level. Notice the scarcity of automobiles and the absence of neon. Photo courtesy of Kozu Shinji.

Although White River Dojo, a Seattle Dojo affiliate, won that particular tournament, Tentoku Kan's never-say-die attitude was soon rewarded. At a judo tournament held at the Nippon Kan Theater on Saturday, 3 March 1934, Nitta Susumu, who was still three weeks away from his fifteenth birthday, took first in men's black belt competition. At a Seattle Dojo tournament held 10 February 1935, Nitta took second in the senior division while Frank Yoshitake took first in the junior division. A week later, however, the best any Tentoku Kan player did during their own tournament was a second place, taken by Frank Takeshita of Kent. Evidently beating the host school in its own tournament was the chief attraction of intraclub competition.[22]

About the same time (early 1934), Kiyoshi "Kelly" Uno went to Japan to study judo. Despite an appendectomy in May 1934, Uno earned his 1st dan in November by throwing one brown belt and three 1st-dans in a row, then tying a fourth. Six months later, he was promoted to 2nd-dan.[23] Kozu Shinji of the Seattle Dojo was in Japan about the same time. As Kozu recalled his year at the Kodokan:[24]

The dojo was open every day. Since Kodokan was the headquarters, there were many hundreds of black belts training daily. All one had to do was go up to a judoist and ask to practice. Every month there was a tournament for the first four judo ranks. Depending on the record of the individual over a space of time, he was promoted to the next rank. That was how I attained the *ni-dan* [2nd-dan] belt rank.

Technically, added Kozu:[25]

Judo training was much harder at Kodokan than in Seattle. In Seattle there usually was one or two *yo-dan* [4th-dan] and *go-dan* [5th-dan] judoists. At Kodokan on any day there were many high ranked judoists present throughout the day. There was no formalized sessions that I know of and so one got out of training only how much effort one put in.

Still, concluded Kozu, high school football training was often more physically demanding than judo training, and much more likely to cause debilitating injuries.[26]

Elmer Tazuma, a Tentoku Kan judoka who went to Japan on 9 September 1934, had similar experiences, saying: "I participated in judo at the high school and also visited a dojo in Kure, Japan, where I stayed with my uncle. Since I never planned to be an instructor, I only learned the fundamentals and was never outstanding like some of the students who I thought were really great."[27]

While many nisei made this trip to Japan, most did not find it an entirely pleasurable experience. Many did not speak Japanese well, and when they spoke English, they were ridiculed for their accents and their pretensions.[28] Further, flush toilets were rare, houses rarely had central heating, and the newsreels blared little but news of Japanese victories in China. Fortunately, the music was familiar. Said University of Washington graduate Kobayashi Shin in a letter home in 1937:[29]

When I took a bath in the public bath the other day (since we have no bath in this house), the woman attendant (yes, a woman attendant in the men's section of the bath) turned on 'Singing in the Rain' and some Bing Crosby numbers. The radios have symphonies and recorded programs in the best American fashion.

Meanwhile, back in Seattle, Tentoku Kan celebrated its seventh anniversary with a tournament at the Nippon Kan on 3 March 1935. Over two hundred judoka from nine schools attended. The Tentoku Kan team, composed of Frank Yoshitake, Kato Hiroshi, and Nitta Susumu, defeated a Kent team to win the senior team trophy. Tentoku Kan juniors took second place. A scheduled and highly anticipated rematch between Kudo Kaimon and Nitta Susumu failed to happen, however, when Nitta injured his leg earlier in the evening.[30]

During a tournament at South Park on 10 March 1935, Kato Hiroshi of Tentoku Kan threw three opponents and tied a fourth to win individual honors in the team competition. This was quite an honor, as Tamura Masato of Fife led the second place finishers.[31]

A few weeks after this tournament, Nitta Susumu, Kato Hiroshi, and Shibuya Masanori traveled to Portland, Oregon, to attend Obukan Dojo's annual tournament. About the same time, Tentoku Kan's Frank Yoshitake, a star athlete in baseball, basketball, and judo, also left for Japan. Before he left, however, a special intradojo meet was held in which Yoshitake distinguished himself by throwing five opponents.[32]

On Thursday, 9 May 1935, Nitta Susumu and Kato Hiroshi gave a judo demonstration at the posh Washington Athletic Club in Seattle. They were featured on a card including boxing, wrestling, and fencing matches that was intended to raise money for the Sea Scouts. Five days later, a thirty-one-year-old Japanese businessman named Sakata Chuji arrived in Seattle.[33] Ranked 5th-dan in judo, Sakata quickly assumed the role of chief instructor at Tentoku Kan. To honor his arrival, over one hundred judoka and their friends greeted him with a banquet at the Kin Ka Low restaurant.[34]

Sakata's first official actions included awarding some well-deserved promotions. For example, on 7 June 1935, he promoted Nitta Susumu to 2nd-dan and Kato Hiroshi and Nitta Masaru to 1st-dan. Nitta Susumu was also recognized for having thrown Kudo Kaimon during a Seattle Dojo tournament held 10 February 1935, thus giving Tentoku Kan an unexpectedly easy victory.[35] The promotion ceremony coincided with the opening of Tentoku Kan's new home, which was inside the Murakumo Hall at the Nichiren Buddhist Temple.

Sakata also proved his personal skills as a grappler during a tournament held on 22 September 1935.[36] His specialty was ground wrestling, or *ne-waza*, something many of the Seattle judoka hadn't practiced much.[37] Said the *Great Northern Daily News* afterward:[38]

Sakata, who holds a *go-dan* [fifth black] rank, proved his right to the title by downing ten men in a row in the feature event of the evening. He started out with a win over Frank Takeshita, Kent strongman; and when he had finished, the following had gone down to defeat: Susumu Nitta, Miyake, *ni-dans* [second black]; George Hiranaka, Takeo Horiuchi, Toregoe, Mas Tominaga, Hiroshi Kato, and younger Nitta *sho-dans* [first black]; and Ted Takeshita, *ikkyu* [first brown].[39]

Kuniyuki Kaname, by now ranked 3rd-dan, returned from Japan on 15 December 1935. As Sakata was often out of town on business, Kuniyuki became the usual instructor. One of his first students was fifteen-year-old Katsumi ("Jim") Yoshida. Yoshida did not want to do judo, but his father told him that if he wanted to keep playing football, he would have to learn either judo or kendo. As young Yoshida didn't like the idea of being whacked on the head with a stick, he decided on judo. He chose Tentoku Kan rather than Seattle Dojo because his father was friends with Tad Kuniyuki's father.[40]

There were about two dozen youths training at the Tentoku Kan during the winter of 1935–1936. Classes met Monday, Wednesday, and Friday from 7 p.m. to 9:30 p.m. Training involved learning to kneel Japanese style and throwing and being thrown almost without break. About once a month the Tentoku Kan held an intraclub tournament. These contests were single elimination, with the winners staying up and the losers sitting down. During an internal tournament held in May 1936, Yoshida, who stood about 5'9" and weighed about 170 pounds (approximately six inches taller and forty pounds heavier than his peers), threw seven men in a row, including two black belts. For this feat, he was promoted from white belt to black belt.[41]

After class on Friday nights, if they had money, Yoshida and his friends would go to the Paramount Cafe on Jackson Street, where Pete Fujino's sister worked as a waitress, and eat pie, drink milk, and play the pinball machines with their nickels. If they didn't have money, then they would go to the Nakamura house on Yesler Way, and play penny-ante poker and sing. "We did all the things white kids our age did for fun," Yoshida later told Bill Hosokawa, "but we never forgot we were Japanese-Americans."[42]

Tentoku Kan sponsored its eighth anniversary tournament at the Nippon Kan

Theater on 1 March 1936. According to the *Japanese American Courier*, "Three hundred agile athletes, their bulging biceps hidden in the padding of judo jackets, took part."[43] Nitta Masaru, Kato Hiroshi, and Frank Yoshitake won the team title for Tentoku Kan. Kuniyuki Kaname had a disappointing day, however, being thrown by Masato Tamura of Fife during a demonstration match.[44]

Tentoku Kan normally closed during the summer because the young men got jobs in Alaskan fish canneries. Judo men were in demand both as workers (they were usually fitter than other youths were) and as foremen (in these preunion times, foremen were expected to keep their work gangs in line, physically if necessary). Tentoku Kan men working at the Nakat Packing Corporation cannery in Waterfall, Alaska, in the summer of 1936 included Kuniyuki Kaname, Nitta Susumu, Jim Yoshida, and Koiwai Eichi. "We practiced judo on the wooden floor (no mats) in the warehouse to keep us in top condition," says Koiwai.[45] They also watched movies; played craps; and, on Sundays and Mondays, the Alaskan days of rest, danced with the nisei women employed in the warehouses. "Until we get one choice gal to each man, I know there is no alternative, but to rotate them around," explained George Takigawa in 1940.[46]

Such hijinks only took place when there were no fish, of course. When the boats were in, everyone worked until the fish were processed. Pay was low, overtime was rare, and the food was little but rice and salmon. Still, no one got tired of the diet, in part because only the choicest cuts were eaten. (Indeed, former cannery men still debate which tasted better, the lean cheeks of a sockeye or the fat-laden abdominal steaks of an Alaskan king salmon.) They also supplemented their meager wages of about $75 a month by salting their favorite cuts into wooden boxes, then smuggling their booty home in duffel bags.[47]

Regular training resumed in late August or early September, after the salmon runs ended, and everyone returned to Seattle.[48] By October, everyone was back in shape. In October 1936, twenty three northwest judoka drove to California to participate in a big interstate tournament. In part because they had received their ranks in Japan, Kuniyuki Kaname and Kelly Uno were the northwest team captains. Supervision and planning was provided by Sakata Chuji and Sakano Ichiro of the Tentoku Kan, and Kumagai Yasuyuki and Miyazawa Yasutaro of Seattle Dojo.[49]

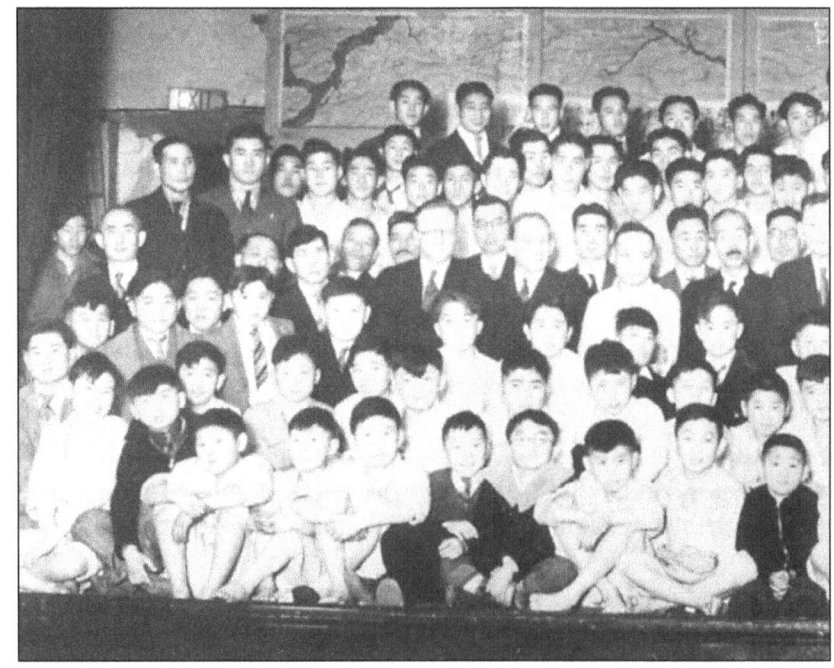

Tournament at the Nippon Kan Theater on Sunday, 1 February 1934. The lone European American judoka in the back row was probably Stanley MacDonald of the Seattle Dojo. Photo courtesy of Kozu Shinji.

As a group, the California judo clubs gave the visitors a cool reception. Said the *Japanese American Courier* upon their return to Seattle: "The traveling team found themselves practically ignored in Los Angeles until Kaz Nishimura, former Seattlite, and Kimon Kudo, Seattle wrestler, came to their rescue."[50] San Francisco judo groups were worse: they ignored the visitors altogether. At an individual level, however, the northwesterners had nothing but praise for the California judoka, and they were especially impressed by the skill of Kano Jigoro, founder of judo, who happened to be in Los Angeles at the time. The actual meet took place in San Pedro on 24–25 October 1936. The match was about even, the California judoka winning Saturday and the northwesterners winning on Sunday. Individual stars included Masato Tamura of Fife and Nitta Susumu of Tentoku Kan. In fact, these two did so well that Professor Kano personally promoted both to 3rd-dan.

"Following the tournament in 1936," says Larry Kobayashi, a longtime student and friend of Kuniyuki Kaname,[51]

> Kuniyuki Sensei was approached by Mr. Jack Wada, an astute businessman on the west side of Los Angeles, to take over the duties of head instructor of Seinan Judo Dojo. Sensei accepted and became the head instructor in 1936. He was also offered the same duties at Uemachi Dojo in the Uptown district. So, Sensei actually taught at the two dojos until the war broke out. At Uemachi, all the students were Japanese-Americans, while at Seinan Dojo the students were mostly Japanese-Americans but occasionally police officers like Jack Sergel (who later acted in a few movies as a Japanese military officer because of his judo background) and other Caucasian students used to come to practice because of our close proximity to the University of Southern California. Because of Sensei's training in Japan, we would have visitors from Japan who worked out at our dojo while in Los Angeles. When Sensei took over Seinan, it was a comparatively weak dojo. Gradually it was transformed into a powerhouse under the teachings of Kuniyuki Sensei.

奉祝皇子殿下御降誕紀念柔道大會

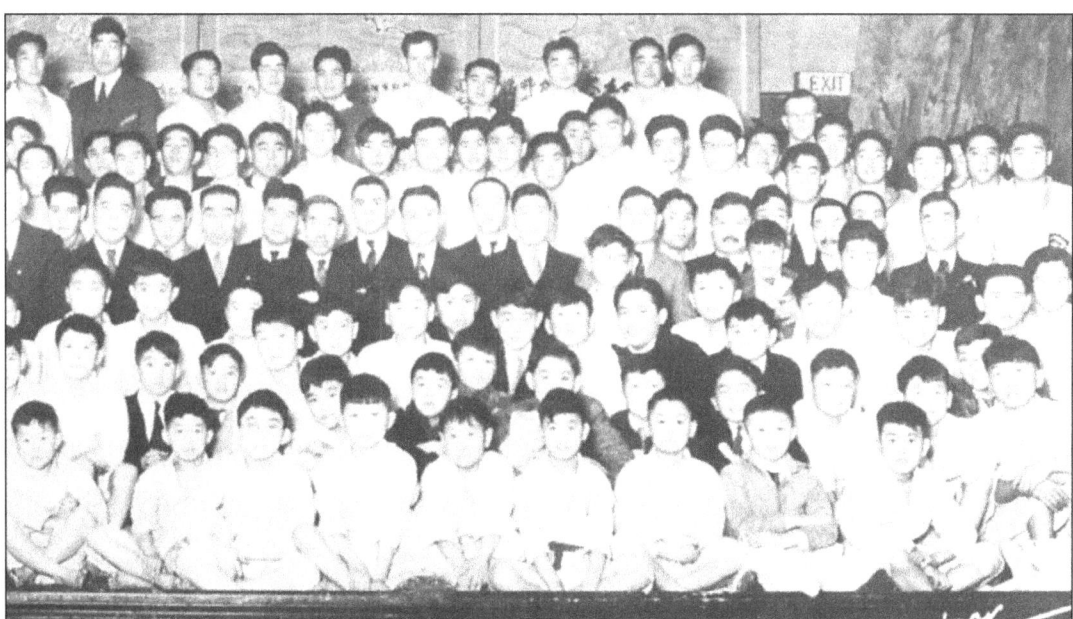

Kobayashi adds: "Kuniyuki Sensei was outstanding in standing wrestling. I've never seen anyone better."[52] This skill was based in part on sweat, and in part on research and study. Says Kobayashi, "He had a lot of books on judo, mostly in Japanese. It was the best collection I've seen."[53]

Meanwhile, back in Seattle, Tentoku Kan hosted a tournament at the Nippon Kan Theater on 13 December 1936. Junior players from Tentoku Kan included Bob and Ben Ikeda, Hayashi Meiji, Higashi Akira, Shibuya Tadao, Tanemura Toshikazu, and Shimada Masayuki. Senior players included Nitta Masaru, Kato Hiroshi, Sumioka Shigeo, Jim Yoshida, Harry Sekiya, Momoda Shigeru, and Mizuki Mitsuo.[54]

Tentoku Kan also gave exhibitions. For example, Shimada Masayuki, Mamiya Sumio, Kato Hiroshi, and Nitta Susuma gave an exhibition to the Veterans of Foreign Wars at the Green Lake Fieldhouse on Wednesday, 31 January 1937. The club even took its entire cast of black belts to the Seattle YMCA on Sunday, 17 January 1938. There members gave demonstrations and explained that judo prepared one not just for self-defense but for life as well. And on Friday, 21 May 1938, Tentoku Kan supported a judo and kendo exhibition at the American Legion Hall. Judoka taking part in this show included Sakata Chuji, T. Bun, Mamiya Satoru, and Tsuchikawa Kiyoshi.[55] As the American Legion was usually very anti-Japanese, the show was undoubtedly meant to ease tensions between the Legion and Japanese-Americans.

Tentoku Kan held its ninth anniversary tournament at the Nippon Kan Theater on Sunday, 14 February 1937. The Japanese consul and the president of the Japanese Association spoke on behalf of the community, while Sakata Chuji and K. Yoshitake spoke on behalf of the judo club. Joe Nakatsu, of Tentoku Kan's Sunnydale branch, was also honored as the first Japanese-American to earn a varsity letter at Highline High School in Des Moines, Washington (large for a nisei, he played halfback.)[56]

"Joe was about as big as Pete [Fujino], and we met through judo," Jim Yoshida recalled.[57]

> Joe didn't say much, but we got along famously. He and I were usually the top boys in judo tournaments, which meant that often we faced each other. In one match we were fooling around, each not wanting to throw the other, and the referee was about to call it a draw when Joe's dad jumped up and shouted: "Yoshida, if you're good enough to throw my son, I want you to throw him and win." Well, we both went at it, and I threw Joe. As soon as he hit the mat Joe jumped up and embraced me, and I cried because I had defeated my friend. We were that kind of buddies.

Of course, such parental behavior sometimes embarrassed the young men to whom it was directed. One Tentoku Kan father was notorious for yelling at Seattle Dojo officials during tournaments. A Seattle Dojo judoka asked the man's son if this behavior didn't bother him. The son replied that it embarrassed him tremendously, but that there was nothing he could do to stop his father from yelling that wouldn't hurt the man's feelings. And, as there weren't many places that this hard-working farmer could vent his frustrations, his son didn't feel right telling him to restrain himself at tournament.[58] To minimize such unseemly behavior, both Mr. Kumagai and Mr. I Sakata worked hard at judging matches so fairly that there would be no reason for anyone to complain. This explains much of their popularity with the parents and players of both Tentoku Kan and Seattle Dojo.

A California judo team visited Seattle in April 1937. The meet was held at the Seattle

Chamber of Commerce hall on 3–4 April 1937. The northwest judoka won 7–6 in team competition, but lost 11–9 in individual competition. Tentoku Kan judoka who won their individual matches in this tournament included Torigoye Kanezo and Nitta Masaru.[59]

On Sunday, 12 December 1937, White River Dojo held its tenth anniversary tournament at the White River Buddhist Temple in Auburn. Higashi of Tentoku Kan won first place in the senior division while Kitajima of Green Lake took first in the junior.[60]

With such a record, Tentoku Kan went to the Nippon Kan Theater on 24 January 1938 intending to keep the team pennant it had won the year before. However, its members went home disappointed. While Jim Yoshida made it to the semi-finals, no Tentoku Kan player made it any further. Meanwhile, Bainbridge Island took first in senior team competition while Green Lake took first in junior.[61]

The Tentoku Kan hosted its tenth anniversary tournament at the Nippon Kan Theater on 27 February 1938. Having started with just twenty players in 1928, ten years later, counting its affiliates in Bellevue, Kent, and Sunnydale, it now boasted more than one hundred players.[62] Although they had not done well during the Seattle Dojo's thirty-first anniversary tournament two weeks before, Tentoku Kan players outdid themselves in this tournament, winning three of the top five spots in the senior competition.

Bellevue players dominated the junior division. Tom Okazaki, 2nd dan, especially distinguished himself during the team competition by throwing two men and drawing with a third.[63]

The *Seattle Post-Intelligencer* sent a reporter to this tournament. Afterward, the reporter wrote, "Judo's purposes as explained by Coach Sakata of Seattle, is manifold: to develop the body, to develop character, and to protect oneself."[64] Photographs showing Koiwai Eichi of Tentoku Kan throwing Ted Hachiya of Portland accompanied the article.[65]

Kano Jigoro flew into Seattle on Tuesday, 19 April 1938. He was on his way back to Japan from International Olympic Committee meetings that had been held in Greece and Egypt. Meeting him at Boeing Field were Kumagai Yasuyuki of Seattle Dojo and Sakata Chuji of Tentoku Kan. The next day, Kano ate dinner at the Gyokko Ken as the guest of the Seattle Yudanshakai (Black Belt Association). Afterward, Kano watched a judo exhibition at Washington Hall, and awarded various promotions, including a 2nd-dan ranking for Koiwai Eichi. Kano died on 4 May 1938, and Sakata Chuji sent the Seattle judokas' condolences to Kano's family in Tokyo.[66]

In November 1938, Sakata Chuji left Seattle. His employer may have transferred him to Los Angeles. This left Hama Hideo (3rd-dan) as chief instructor at Tentoku Kan. Hama's assistants included Torigoe Kanezo, Kato Hiroshi, Tom Okazaki, Sumioka Shigeo, and Elmer Tazumaa[67] Despite Sakata absence, Tentoku Kan went to the third annual Yudanshakai tournament two weeks later in Seattle and took second overall. Jim Yoshida was the individual Tentoku Kan star of this tournament, making it to the quarterfinals before losing to Masato Tamura of Eatonville.[68]

Sakata was in Los Angeles for the February 1939 all-star tournament. Tentoku Kan leaders accompanying the team included Hama Hideo (3rd dan). Leading Tentoku Kan players on the all-star squad included Kato Hiroshi (3rd dan), Jim Yoshida (2nd-dan), and Joe Nakatsu (2nd-dan). The Tentoku Kan players did not enjoy any individual success in California: Joe Nakatsu got a draw, and Jim Yoshida and Kato Hiroshi lost to the Californians on Saturday, 4 March 1939. However, they were part of the team victory the following day, and so got to fondle the 36" high trophy that commemorated the win. On the way back, they also made a side trip to visit the World's Fair in San Francisco.[69]

Tentoku Kan hosted its eleventh anniversary tournament at the Nippon Kan Theater on Sunday, 19 February 1939. This was the first tournament attended by Tentoku Kan's

Spokane affiliate. And a good thing, too, as otherwise Tentoku Kan would have lost almost all their trophies to Seattle Dojo affiliates.[70]

Nitta Susumu, who had gone to Japan in 1937, returned home ranked 4th dan in September 1939, making him Tentoku Kan's highest-ranking nisei judoka (while Hama Hideo was 3rd-dan, he was also issei, which gave him cultural seniority). Nitta's welcome home banquet was held at Seattle's Nikko Low restaurant on Sunday, 24 September 1939.[71] Nitta, who was known to his friends as "Baby Beef" (his even brawnier older brother Masaru was "Beefo"), remained active in northwest judo following his return, and soon became supervisor at Tentoku Kan's Bellevue, Sunnydale, and Kent affiliate.[72]

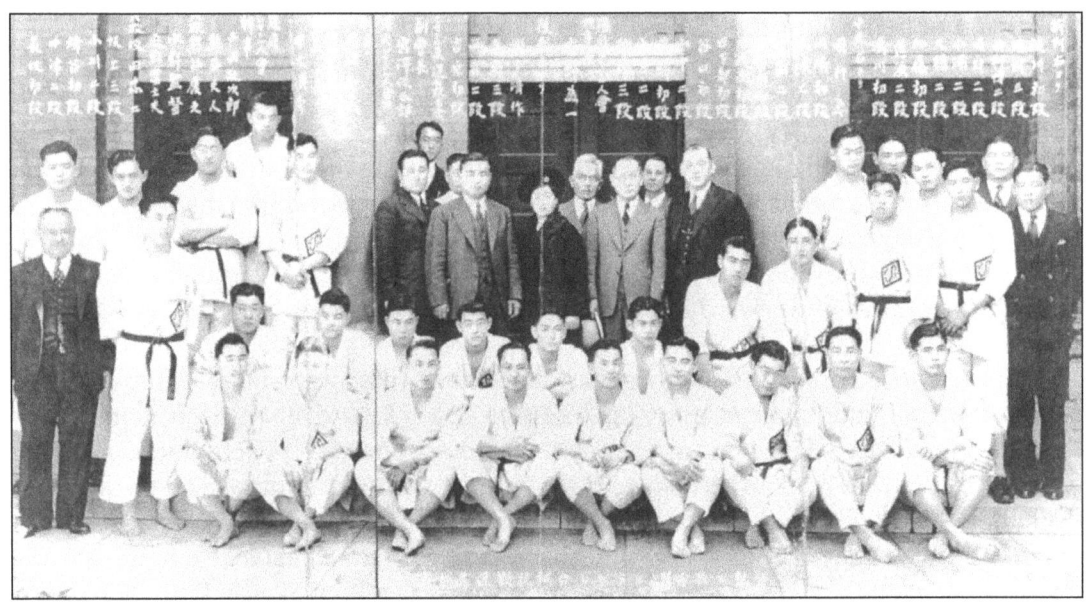

The Northwest Judo All Star Team in Los Angeles, 1939.
Photo courtesy of Masato Tamura Collection.

On 15 December 1939, Yorita Tatsuo, another Tentoku Kan 4th-dan, also returned to Seattle from Japan.[73] Like Nitta, Yorita was initially active in dojo activities, but unlike Nitta, his involvement didn't last long, as he found himself engaged to Yonemura Yoshiko of Wapato in October 1940, and married soon after.[74] Tentoku Kan's twelfth anniversary tournament was held in Seattle on Sunday, 4 February 1940.[75] The results were not listed in the Seattle newspapers. About the same time, the Nichiren Temple moved, and the club moved with it.

The Seattle Dojo's thirty-third anniversary tournament took place three weeks later. The champion in the 2nd-dan competition was Jim Yoshida, whom the *North American Times* described as "another who relied principally on his physical prowess."[76] Hank Ogawa of Bainbridge Island, who was Yoshida's friendly opponent during those days, adds, "You didn't try to sweep him. He was too big. His legs were like tree trunks."[77]

During Seattle's fifth annual yudanshakai tournament on Sunday, 10 November 1940, Jim Yoshida won another individual championship and the Consul's Cup. In junior competition, Ikeda (its unclear whether it was Bob or Ben), Komorita Shozo, Nitta Masaru, and Shibuya Tadao also placed first or second in their divisions.[78]

Tentoku Kan's thirteenth anniversary tournament was held in Seattle on 23 February 1941.[79] Soon after, Jim Yoshida accompanied his mother on a trip to Japan, where she was taking his father's ashes for burial. While there, Yoshida studied judo at the Kodokan. There was no horseplay at the Kodokan in 1941, Yoshida said, "only intense, dedicated concentration on judo."[80] Training lasted eight hours a day, six and a half days a week, with fifteen-minute breaks for lunch. On the mat:[81]

> Anyone could come up to you and request a practice bout... [and] the rule was that you couldn't refuse... Eventually, as I worked out day after day, the truth of what Kenny Kuniyuki had tried to teach dawned on me: Judo is not a test of strength alone; judo is a sport of skill and its essence is timing.

Of course, all was not hardship. Otherwise no one would have done it. Instead, said the English judoka Trevor Leggett, who left the Kodokan in 1940, when the teacher was in the room, then the formality and solemnity were palpable, and hardly a word was exchanged anywhere. But once the teacher left the room for his bath:[82]

> Immediately everyone relaxes, and their natural Japanese cheerfulness comes out. The practice is over, and you can smoke and talk freely, and joke as much as you like. In the next room is a huge bath of steaming hot water where one can soak, and afterwards return to cool off clad in nothing but a towel. Some tea and cakes are brought in, and you spend a pleasant half hour with some of the jolliest, kindest, and most unaffected friends you could meet anywhere in the world.

Shortly before he was scheduled to return to the United States in August 1941, Yoshida threw a line of Japanese Navy 3rd-dans who had come to the Kodokan seeking promotion. As a result, Yoshida was rewarded with promotion to 4th-dan. Unfortunately, the Japanese preparations for the attack on Pearl Harbor interfered with Yoshida's plans for returning to the United States, and after a year teaching judo in a Japanese high school, he found himself serving in a Japanese artillery unit in China. As a result, Yoshida did not get his American citizenship back until 1953.

Tentoku Kan's final tournament appearance took place in Seattle on Sunday, 16 November 1941. The occasion was the third annual Kumagai Cup competition, which honored the memory of Seattle Dojo's Kumagai Yasuyuki, who had returned to Japan in 1940. While Dick Yamasaki of Seattle Dojo won the cup, Tentoku Kan tied with Bainbridge Island for second place in the junior team competition. Fourteen-year old Komorita Shozo was Tentoku Kan's star player of the day.[83]

Like most Japanese-American athletic organizations, Tentoku Kan closed following Pearl Harbor. Starting in May 1942, Seattle's Japanese-Americans began to be sent to a temporary assembly center located at the Puyallup Fairgrounds.

In August 1942, the internees started relocating from Puyallup to Hunt, Idaho. As Minidoka Camp was still under construction and mates were not available, formal judo classes did not resume until 14 February, 1943. Tentoku Kan judoka, including Nitta Masaru, Nitta Susuma, and Sakano Ichiro, were at the forefront of the plan to turn Recreation Halls 5, 17, and 39 into dojos.[84] Jackets were always something of a problem, however, as the younger players outgrew their old jackets while in camp, and new jackets were not commercially available. And while new jackets could be sewn using white canvas duck, such jackets were rarely as strong as prewar commercial uniforms.[85]

Wartime judo training at Minidoka was geared mostly for building character in school-aged boys, as after mid-1943, most older judoka went into military service or found agricultural work outside the camps. The agricultural work was physically demanding and paid terribly (depending on one's skills, wages averaged $12–$14 a month), but it beat sitting inside a prison camp with nothing to do. Meanwhile, military service attracted eight hundred Minidoka nisei, which was more than any other relocation center. Tentoku Kan judoka were especially well represented among both the volunteers and the casualties.[86]

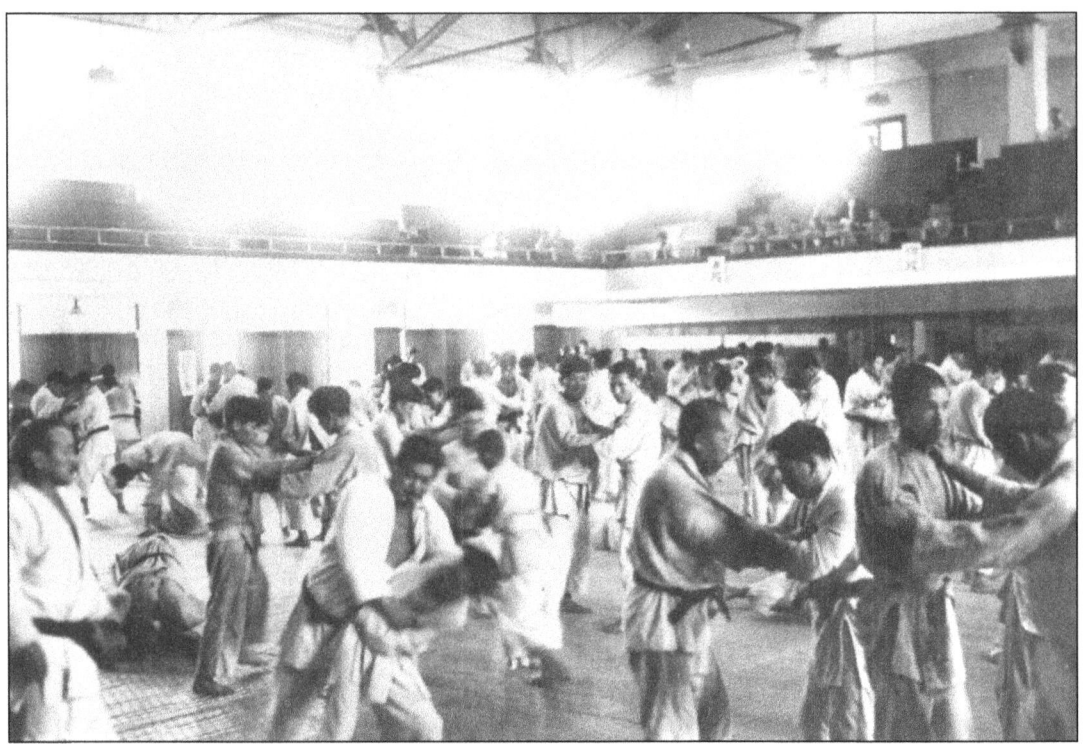

Interior of the Kodokan 1935. There were no classes at the Kodokan in 1935. Instead, you walked up to anyone you wanted (or dared) and asked him to show you a technique or to grapple. Photo courtesy of Kosu Shinji.

Although Tentoku Kan did not reopen in Seattle following the war, afterwards, its members helped spread judo throughout the United States. For example, Jim Yoshida helped introduce judo into Honolulu high schools. Ken Kuniyuki became a leader in the Nanka Kodokan Judo Yudanshakai in southern California. Koiwai Eichi was active in establishing judo in Philadelphia, and later became a leader in Shufu Yudanshakai and US Judo Inc. Locally, Nitta Susumu also played a key role in the reestablishment of the Seattle Dojo.

NOTES ON REFERENCES

Research was supported by the King County Landmarks and Heritage Commission and Hotel/Motel Tax Revenues. Research was conducted at the National Archives and Record Administration in Seattle, the Sno-Isle Public Libraries, and the Suzzallo-Allen Libraries at the University of Washington. The assistance of the following individuals is gratefully acknowledged: Fujiko Tamura Gardner, Al C. Holtmann, William K. Hosokawa, S. Chris Kato, Larry Kobayashi, Koiwai Eichi, Kojima Tats, Art Koura, Kozu Shinji, Tad Kuniyuki, Patrick Lineberger, Tom T. Matsuoka, Hank Ogawa, Robert W. Smith, Suzuki Yanagimachi Nobu, Elmer S. Tazuma, D.B. Waterhouse, Yaguchi Kenji, Yamanaka Toshio, and Richard I. Yamasaki.

ENDNOTES

[1] The Zaidan Honin Dai Nippon Butokukai ("Federation of Greater Japan Martial Virtue Society") was established in Kyoto in 1895. Its leaders were as a group more nationalistic and militaristic than the leaders of the Kodokan, and as a result, the Butokukai was closed following the war. The organization encouraged Japanese youth to practice all martial arts, not just judo, and as a stylistic rule, Butokukai judoka emphasized ground grappling (*ne-waza*) while Kodokan judoka emphasized standing grappling (*tachi-waza*). For additional details, see Jeffrey L. Dann, "Kendo in Japanese Martial Culture: Swordsmanship as Self-Cultivation," Ph.D dissertation, University of Washington, 1978, 62–63, fn. 61, 119.

[2] *Japanese American Courier*, 29 Sep 1928, 2; *Japanese American Courier* 13 Oct 1928, 2; *Japanese American Courier*, 26 Feb 1938–4.

[3] *Japanese American Courier*, 7 Jan 1928, 2; *Japanese American Courier,* 21 Jan 1928, 2; *Japanese American Courier*, 16 Jun 1928, 2; Letter from Tom T. Matsuoka, 9 Jul 1997.

[4] Politics: Interview with S. Chris Kato, 28 Mar 1997; Matsuoka letter, 9 Jul 1997; Name-calling: Interview with Art Koura, 3 May 1997.

[5] *North American Times*, 28 Jun 1938, 1.

[6] *Japanese American Courier*, 7 Jan 1928, 2.

[7] Letter from Tad Kuniyuki, 16 Jun 1997.

[8] *Japanese American Courier*, 29 Mar 1930, 2; *Japanese American Courier*, 26 Feb 1938, 4.

[9] *Japanese American Courier*, 24 Jan 1931, 2.

[10] *Japanese American Courier*, 2 May 1931, 2.

[11] Letter from Koiwai Eichi, 12 Jul 1997.

[12] *Japanese American Courier*, 21 Feb 1931, 2. While the *Courier* usually called the club "Tentokwan," and the *Great Northern Daily News* called it "Tentokukwan," Polk's City Directory for 1940 shows the club's name as "Tentoku Kan." For consistency, I have used the latter transliteration. Canadian scholar D.B. Waterhouse, of the University of Toronto's East Asian Studies Department, says *kwan* "is an old-fashioned romanisation of Japanese, reflecting the old-fashioned pronunciation of that syllable." Letter from D.B. Waterhouse, 23 Jul 1997.

[13] Waterhouse letter, 23 Jul 1997.

[14] While the establishment of the Seattle Dojo is traditionally dated 1907, there were qualified jujutsu instructors living in Seattle at least a decade earlier. Sakamoto Osamu, father of newspaper editor James Y. Sakamoto, is Seattle's first qualified jujutsu instructor of whom I am aware.

[15] E.J. Harrison, *The Fighting Spirit of Japan* (New York: Overlook Press, 1982), 51.

[16] *Japanese American Courier*, 5 Mar 1932, 2.

[17] *Japanese American Courier*, 15 Oct 1932, 2.

18 Harrison, 1982, 47.
19 *Japanese American Courier*, 15 Jul 1933, 2.
20 *Great Northern Daily News*, 17 Oct 1934, 8.
21 *Japanese American Courier*, 14 Jan 1933, 2.
22 *Great Northern Daily News*, 11 Feb 1935, 8; *North American Times*, 21 Feb 1935, 1.
23 *Japanese American Courier*, 30 Jun 1934, 4; *Japanese American Courier*, 15 Dec 1934, 3.
24 Letter from Kozu Shinji, 22 May 1997.
25 Letter from Kozu Shinji, 31 May 1997.
26 Ibid. Hank Ogawa (31 May 1997 interview) and Yaguchi Kenji (22 Jun 1997 interview) concur with this observation.
27 Letter from Elmer S. Tazuma, 21 May 1997.
28 Interview with Suzuki Yanagimachi Nobu, 31 May 1997.
29 *University of Washington Daily*, 21 Oct 1937, 4. The public baths, or *firoya*, in the basement of the NP Hotel in Seattle had male attendants in the male sections.
30 *Great Northern Daily News*, 20 Feb 1935, 8; *Great Northern Daily News*, 4 Mar 1935, 8.
31 *Great Northern Daily News*, 11 Mar 1935, 8.
32 *Great Northern Daily News*, 14 Mar 1935, 8; *Great Northern Daily News*, 15 Mar 1935, 8.
33 "List or Manifest of Alien Passengers for the U.S. Immigration Officer at Port of Arrival," Heian Maru, 14 May 1935, M1383; "Passenger and Crew Lists of Vessels Arriving at Seattle, Washington, 1891–1957," Roll 204, Apr 22, 1935, Screw Beatrice – June 1, 1935, SS Tantalus.
34 *Great Northern Daily News*, 15 May 1935, 8; *Great Northern Daily News*, 24 May 1935, 8.

   Many years later, Sakata told Kazuo Ito: "I graduated from Tokyo Fisheries Institute. I gave judo lessons to nisei and sansei youths at Seattle.... At that time Japanese were living shrunken lives under the storm of anti-Japanese feeling. The tall white men frequently insulted the Japanese with their small body and mind by saying, 'Harro Chary!' and roughing up our hair... [But I] am 5'5" tall, and I was never insulted or excluded. My ears were cauliflowered due to hard training. Noticing them, whites always said: 'Are you a wrestler?' 'No, I'm a professor of judo.' 'You strong man! Shake hands!'" In Kazuo Ito, *Issei: A History of Japanese Immigrants in North America*, translated by Shinichiro Nakamura and Jean S. Gerard (Seattle: Japanese Community Service, 1973), 133.
35 *Great Northern Daily News*, 11 Feb 1935, 2.
36 *Great Northern Daily News*, 21 Sep 1935, 8.
37 Koiwai letter, 12 Jul 1997.
38 *Great Northern Daily News*, 23 Sep 1935, 8.
39 *Japanese American Courier*, 21 Dec 1935, 3.
40 Jim Yoshida with Bill Hosokawa, *The Two Worlds of Jim Yoshida* (New York: William Morrow, 1972), 24–25.
41 Ibid., 26–27.
42 Ibid., 18–20.
43 *Japanese American Courier*, 7 Mar 1936, 3; *Japanese American Courier*, 9 Mar 1935, 3; *Japanese American Courier*, 16 Mar 1935, 3.
44 Masato Tamura collection.
45 Koiwai letter, 12 Jul 1997.
46 *Great Northern Daily News*, 14 Aug 1940's. See also *Great Northern Daily News*, 13 Aug 1940, 8.
47 During the 1930s, about seven hundred Seattle nisei spent their summers working in

Alaskan or Aleutian canneries. Base pay was about $90–$100 a month, from which living expenses were deducted. In 1940, overtime (at $.90 an hour) was paid employees who worked eight hours on Sunday, or more than sixteen consecutive hours a day; Interview with Hank Ogawa, 31 May 1997; *North American Times*, 25 May 1940, 1; Paul Yee, *Saltwater City: An Illustrated History of the Chinese in Vancouver* (Seattle: University of Washington, 1988), 59, 62–63; Yoshida, 1972, 28.

[48] *Great Northern Daily News*, 6 Sep 1941, 8.
[49] *Japanese American Courier*, 24 Oct 1936, 3.
[50] *Japanese American Courier*, 7 Nov 1936, 3.
[51] Letter from Larry Kobayashi, 19 Aug 1997.
[52] Interview with Larry Kobayashi, 8 Aug 1997.
[53] Ibid.
[54] *Japanese American Courier*, 12 Dec 1936, 3.
[55] Tsuchikawa's younger brother "Mud" (Masakatsu) was Jim Yoshida's friend, and another Tentoku Kan junior player.
[56] *Japanese American Courier*, 13 Feb 1937, 3. A photograph of Nakatsu Jintaro's family, in which Joe Nakatsu appears fifth from the right, appears in the book, Hokubei Nenkan, lower plate [32], which is located in the University of Washington's East Asia Library. The call number is N979.5N79y.
[57] Yoshida, 1972, 18–19.
[58] For obvious reasons, the individual who told me this story requested anonymity for all concerned. The interview was conducted 27 Jul 1997.
[59] *Japanese American Courier*, 3 Apr 1937, 3; *Japanese American Courier*, 10 Apr 1937, 3.
[60] *Great Northern Daily News*, 13 Dec 1937, 8; *North American Times*, 8 Dec 1937, 1.
[61] *Great Northern Daily News*, 24 Jan 1938, 8.
[62] *Japanese American Courier*, 26 Feb 1938, 4; *North American Times*, 26 Feb 1938, 1.
[63] *Great Northern Daily News*, 7 Feb 1938, 8; *Great Northern Daily News*, 22 Feb 1938, 8; *North American Times*, 7 Feb 1938, 1; *North American Times*, 28 Feb 1938, 1. Okazaki died in France during World War II.
[64] *Seattle Post-Intelligencer*, 20 Mar 1938, 5.
[65] Koiwai letter, 12 Jul 1997.
[66] *Japanese American Courier*, 23 Apr 1938, 4; *Japanese American Courier*, 7 May 1938, 3; *Japanese American Courier*, 14 Sep 1940, 4; Koiwai letter, 12 Jul 1997.
[67] *Great Northern Daily News*, 7 Nov 1938, 8.
[68] *Great Northern Daily News*, 21 Nov 1938, 8.
[69] *North American Times*, 6 Mar 1939, 1; *North American Times*, 11 Mar 1939, 1; *North American Times*s, 13 Mar 1939, 1.
[70] *North American Times*, 16 Feb 1939, 1; *North American Times*, 18 Feb 1939, 1.
[71] This was a Chinese restaurant rather than a Japanese restaurant. Letter from William K. Hosokawa, 4 Sep 1997.
[72] *Japanese American Courier*, 23 Sep 1939, 3; *North American Times*, 22 Sep 1939, 1; *North American Times, 23 Jan 1939*, 1; *North American Times*, 10 Jan 1940, 1.
[73] *North American Times*, 14 Dec 1939, 1.
[74] *Great Northern Daily News*, 19 Oct 1940, 8.
[75] *North American Times*, 31 Jan 1940, 1.
[76] *North American Times*, 26 Feb 1940, 1.
[77] Ogawa interview, 31 May 1997; Letter from Toshio Yamanaka, 17 Sep 1997.
[78] *North American Times*, 11 Nov 1940, 1.
[79] *Great Northern Daily News*, 20 Feb 1941, 8.

[80] Yoshida, 1972, 41.
[81] Ibid., 42.
[82] *Japanese American Courier,* 28 Sep 1940, 3.
[83] *Great Northern Daily News*, 17 Nov 1941, 8.
[84] *Minidoka Irrigator*, 27 Feb 1943, 7. "Many of the builders," says historian Leonard Arrington, "coming from farms rather than cities, lived in houses and shacks without running water, and they used outhouses. As they constructed the camp's communal kitchens, laundries, and bathhouses they were envious: the incoming 'Japs' were being given such 'luxuries' as public toilets at public expense. It would never have occurred to the workers what a God-forsaken place this would seem to people from Portland and Seattle forcibly exiled into the Idaho desert." Leonard J. Arrington, *History of Idaho, vol. 11* (Moscow, ID: University of Idaho Press, 1994), 88.
[85] Conversation with Fujiko Gardner, 7 Jun 1997; interview with S. Chris Kato, 28 Mar 1997; Koiwai letter, 12 Jul 1997; Ogawa interview, 31 May 1997; "JiuJitsu Institute," two letters in "Henry H. Okuda," Accession Number 2345, Box 1, University of Washington Manuscripts and University Archives Division, University of Washington, Seattle, WA.
[86] Ibid.; Arrington, 1994, 88–92.

chapter 4

Masato Tamura, Ryoichi Iwakiri, and The Fife Judo Dojo, 1923–1942
by Joseph Svinth, M.A.

The father I thought so strict
Where did he conceal
Such tender feelings
Revealed in those gentle letters?
Many days I cried.
– Teiko Tomita (Nomura, 1987:19)

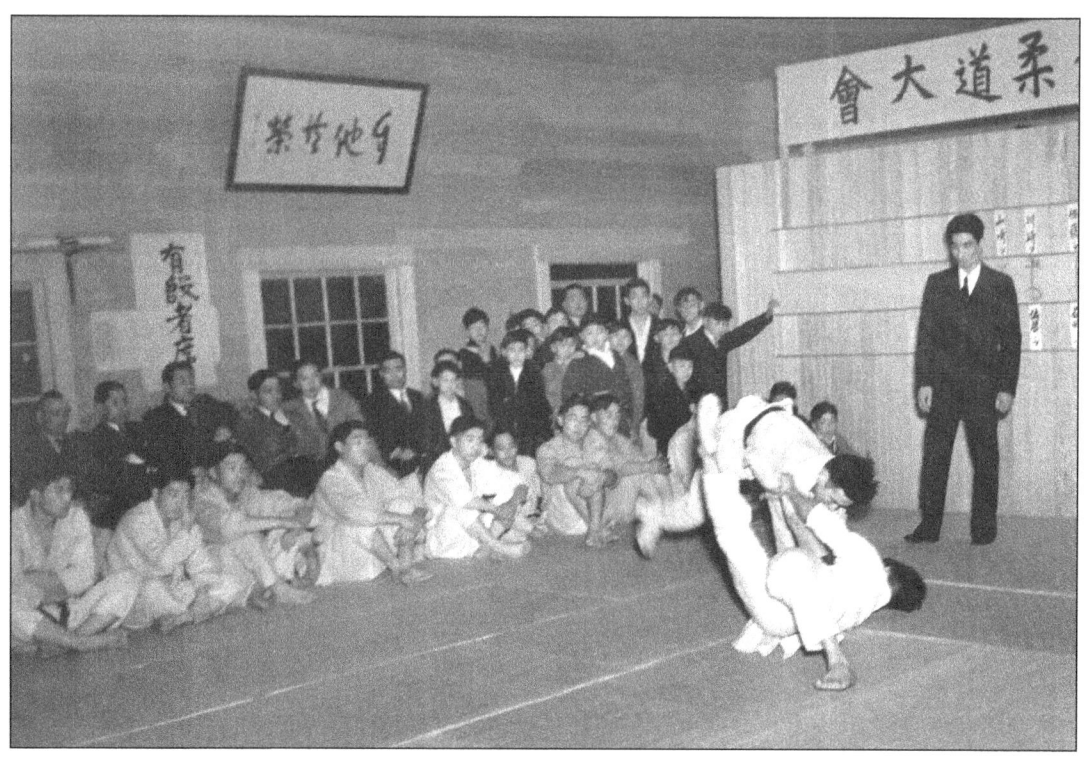

Judo Tournament at the Fife Dojo, March 1938.
Photo from the Boland Collection, courtesy of the Washington State Historical Society, Tacoma, Washington.

Fife is a farm town located about two miles northeast of Tacoma, Washington. The first Japanese immigrant (*issei*) to farm the region was probably Heishiro Mihara,[1] who leased twenty acres from the Puyallup Indians Mary Charley and William McShill in 1897. Mihara then brought over his brothers-in-law Gorimatsu, Heisuke, Toichi, and Tokichi Ohashi to help him clear and work the property. Other pioneers included Soroku Kuramoto, Shintaro Mukai, and Yokichi Nakanishi (Watanabe, 1986:86–88; Magden, 1998: 35–36).

A local landowner, John McAleer, believed that having people of different races work together would overcome racism and nationalism. By 1907, there were about thirty issei families working McAleer properties in the area. By the mid-1910's, this number had grown to about one hundred and thirty, plus more than two hundred children. From 1910 to 1930, Japanese comprised the largest group of non-European ethnic females in Washington State (Watanabe, 1986:86–88; Magden, 1998:35–36; Nomura, 1987:15).

To educate these children in Japanese culture, history, and language, sixteen issei farmers organized a Fife Language School Support Association in June 1909. The teachers were Tomehachi Nagai and his wife Yoneko (Magden, 1998:69–70).

A schoolhouse capable of holding thirty-five students was built in late 1912. A Seinen Kai (Young People's Club or Association) was added in July 1915. The club's missions included cultivating lofty ideals and character in young people, teaching an appreciation for traditional Japanese values, and improving relations between Japanese and European-Americans. Members paid about a dollar per child per month. With that money, club leaders paid rent and bought books and sports equipment. While the outdoor sport of choice was baseball, indoor sports included judo and kendo. The club met every Sunday, and had about thirty members in 1917 (Magden, 1998:69–70; Watanabe, 1986:95–96).

Parents soon found that American-born sons usually preferred playing sports to attending language school. So, in 1923, Fife farmers Hikozo ("Harry") Kawasaki and Kichigoro ("Kay") Yamamoto donated a barn and some mats to the Seinen Kai, and arranged for a local man to teach judo to community youths. From late September until mid-May, the Fife Dojo was open three nights a week. Like most rural judo clubs, the Fife Dojo closed during the summer. The reason was, of course, that the barn was needed for storing crops and the boys and men were busy with the harvest (Edith Kuramoto, personal communication, September 25, 1997).

Ryoichi Iwakiri was the local man who taught at the Fife club. Born in Ehime Prefecture, Japan, in 1899, Iwakiri started studying judo at the St. Paul and Tacoma lumber company's judo club around 1917. His early students included George Kawasaki, Jack Ohashi, and Masato Tamura (*Japanese-American Courier*, hereafter referred to as JAC, February 12, 1938:4).[2]

His first dojo was far from fancy. For instance, the original mat consisted of canvas stretched from wall to wall over sawdust. The walls had no insulation, and "on cold winter nights," said the *Japanese-American Courier* many years later, "many can hark back to those times when we used to toast our toes at spots which glowed red hot on an old cracked stove" (JAC, February 12, 1938:4). Still, it beat walking a couple miles into Tacoma two or three nights a week. "We went to school in Tacoma," recalled former Fife resident Joe Kosai in 1998, "and used to walk there and back every day. Just the other day I walked the route for the first time in years. It was a lot longer than I remembered. The hills were steeper, too" (Joe Kosai, personal communication, March 16, 1998).

Although Fife judoka surely participated in tournaments in Tacoma and Seattle from 1924 to 1927, I have seen no record of the results. Iwakiri was evidently an active tournament player. He later told his student, Jerry Dalien, that the only Seattle judoka who could beat him was Kaimon Kudo, a Seattle Dojo star who later became a well-known professional wrestler (Dalien, 1988:23). Therefore, Fife Dojo's recorded history begins with Jack Ohashi's victory over Seattle Dojo's Michio Shinoda on November 18, 1928 (JAC, September 22, 1928:2; JAC, November 24, 1928:2). During another Seattle tournament held on January 18, 1931, Masato ("Mac") Tamura was the star (JAC, January 24, 1931:2). As a result, he received promotion to first dan. His teacher, Iwakiri, simultaneously received promotion to second dan (JAC, February 20, 1931:2; JAC, March 11, 1933:2).

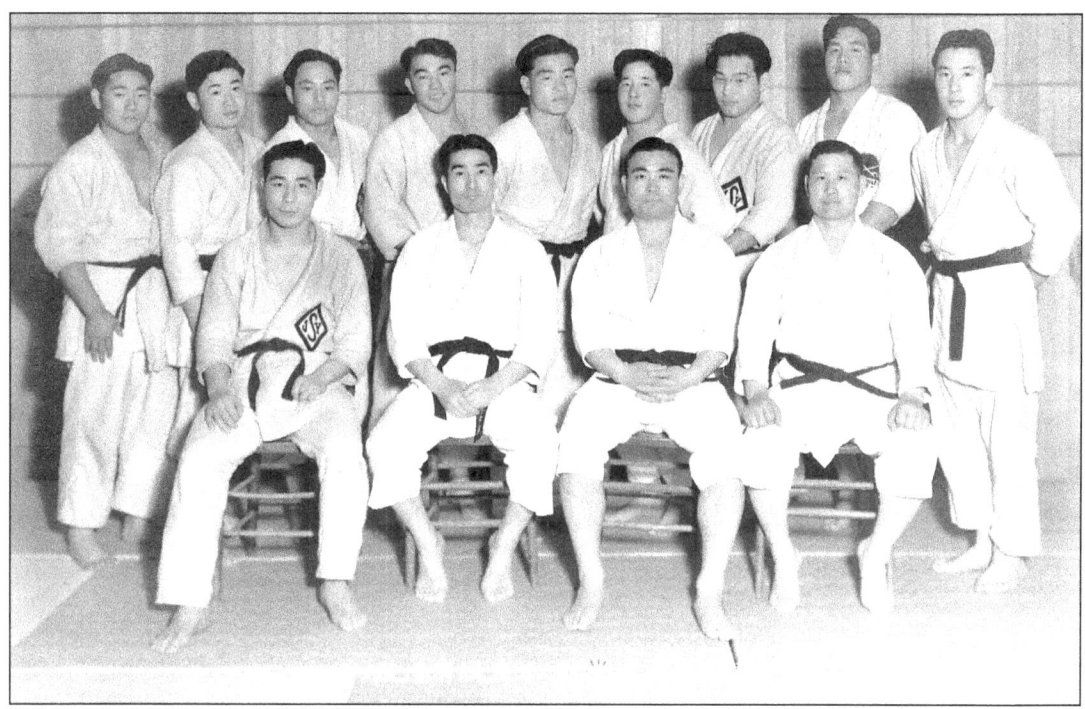

Fife Yudansha (judo black belts), 1940. Front row, left to right: Masato Tamura, Richard Hayashi, Yasuyuki Kamagai (Seattle Dojo supervisor), Ryoichi Iwakiri. Second row, left to right: George Iwakiri, Leo Kawasaki, Jack Ohashi, Seiichi Yamada, Masaru Tamura, Joe Mizumoto, Hikaru Tamura, Hiroshi Masuda, Sunji Dogen. Photo courtesy of George and Risa Kawasaki.

Note: The SJY patch stands for "Seattle Judo Yudanshakai." It was worn by men who were part of the team that went to Los Angeles in 1939. The other patch is that of the Eatonville Dojo (Eatonville is a logging town southeast of Tacoma whose club was led by Masato Tamura. An article about this club should appear in Columbia: The Magazine of the Washington State Historical Society, in late 2000).

In those days, belts were white, brown, or black, and the chief promotion criterion was tournament success. Traditional throwing forms (*kata*) and meditation were taught only to boys who asked—and boys being boys, few asked (Shinji Kozu, personal communication, September 21, 1997; Hank Ogawa, personal communication, September 22, 1997). Instead, what schoolboys wanted was outward recognition. Accordingly, in February 1931, Fife Dojo members voted to award varsity-style letters to deserving members. "The qualifications," said an article in the *Japanese-American Courier*, "were to be decided upon later. Its purpose was to create more interest in the sport, and to set a goal for the younger boys to strive toward" (JAC, February 13, 1931:2).

On September 26, 1931, nineteen-year old Masato Tamura took over day-to-day instruction at the Fife Dojo. The stated reasons for this change were that Ryoichi Iwakiri had recently started a commercial produce business, and therefore lacked the time to attend every practice (JAC, September 26, 1931:2; *Tacoma News Tribune*, hereafter referred to as TNT, May 27, 1987:B2). However, the unstated reason was that Mrs. Iwakiri did not support Mr. Iwakiri's love of judo. Like most issei men, Iwakiri worked ten to twelve hours a day, six days a week. Add judo classes three nights a week, plus a tournament most Sundays from January to April, and Mrs. Iwakiri's disapproval becomes eminently understandable. Indeed, to keep peace, says Iwakiri's daughter Chiyo Iida (Fujiko Gardner, personal communication from Chiyo Iida, May 4, 1997):

> Judo was rarely mentioned in our house. I never heard anything about the judo tournaments from my family. My friend, Kiyoko Yamada, kept me informed about who won. It was from her I learned about Masato's brilliant participation in judo and also about my brother's accomplishments.

For the boys in the Fife club—their ages ranged from eight to twenty—Iwakiri's absence was probably something of a blessing. Tamura was an older brother rather than a father figure, and he greatly preferred tussling on the mats to lecturing. On the other hand, Iwakiri was more of a father figure. He never learned to speak English well, and when he did speak English, it was usually to stress the importance of having strong character. The following summarizes his favorite speech. The version quoted here was given in Japanese during the 1950's, and later translated into English (Dalien, 1988: 25–26).

> As an integral part of our instruction, we are taught among other things patience, courtesy, humility, and self-discipline. What passes for acceptable conduct from some athletes should not be our goal, but rather our minimum. Self-discipline and courtesy dictate that we respect the rights of others. We are not loud, ill-mannered, or boorish. We lose graciously and win with humility. We act and dress like ladies and gentlemen both on and off the mat.
>
> We take great pains to inform the public that judo is different from other sports. We read about it, talk about it, write about it. We tell boys' and girls' mothers and fathers that judo will make a lady or gentleman of their son or daughter, and that judo is the missing cog in a well-rounded education. In our drive to bring judo closer to the American philosophy of competition, we must not lose sight of these basic principles which make our sport unique.
>
> Nothing is more striking and impressive as a tournament or practice where the players are neat, reserved, and dignified, and the judging is sincere, honest, and honorable. There is the lasting impression and the principle of judo at work. Actions do speak louder than words.

Still, with the combination of lectures, good examples, and sweat, the Fife youths soon dominated local judo tournaments. At a tournament held at the Tacoma Buddhist Church on October 11, 1931, for example, Masato Tamura, Jack Ohashi, Hiroshi Tamura, George Kawasaki, and Masaomi Kibe all won pennants (JAC, October 10, 1931:2; JAC, October 17, 1931:2).

While instruction was always in English at the dojo, the names of techniques were taught in Japanese. Upon entering or leaving the mat, students were expected to bow toward the instructors. Students also were expected to sit quietly when not practicing, avoid horseplay, and keep unnecessary talking to a minimum (Kenji Yaguchi, personal communication, October 3, 1997).

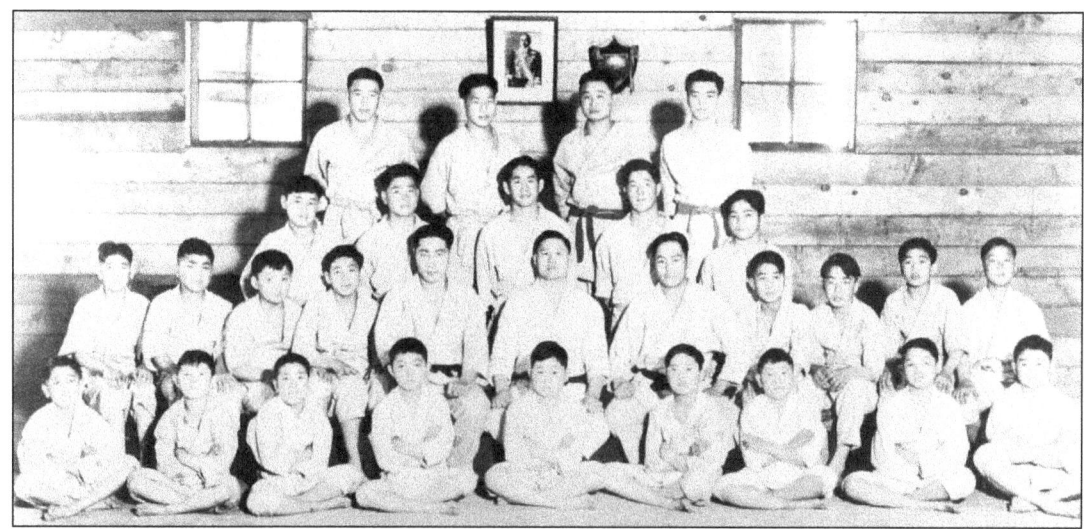

Fife Dojo March 5, 1934. Front row, seated left to right: Kiyoshi Kuramoto, Mitsuru Tamura, Bob Watanabe, Harry Morisaki, Leo Kawasaki, Hiro Yaguchi, unidentified, unidentified, Don Kawasaki. Second row, seated, left to right: Atsushi Kuramoto, unidentified, unidentified, Sam Uchida, Masato Tamura, Ryoichi Iwakiri, Jack Ohash, Sakahara, Seiichi Yamada, unidentified, S. Teranishi. Third row, kneeling left to right: Jin (?) Sagami, Masaru Tamura, Kimio Watanabe, Joe Mizumoto, unidentified. Fourth row, standing, left to right: Sunji Dogen, P. Tamura, George Kawasaki, Masachi Kibe. Photo courtesy of George and Risa Kawasaki.

Note: The photo on the back wall shows judo founder Kano Jigoro in his court uniform. The significance of the shield is not known. Note the canvas mats. The knotty lumber used in the construction of the barn suggests that it was built from scrap from the St. Paul and Tacoma lumber mill, which was then the world's largest.

As money was always tight, in October 1931, the Fife Seinen Kai decided that it would raise money by holding Japanese movie nights. Excepting the refreshments sold by the local Girls' Club (Fuyo Kai) during these movie nights, Fife youth were not exposed to club fund-raising activities. Instead, finances were handled entirely by adults. Parents whose children didn't do judo complained that judo diverted money from other youth activities. So, in January 1935 the Fife Seinen Kai and the Fife Dojo split into separate organizations (Kenji Yaguchi, personal communication, October 3, 1997; JAC, October 17, 1931:2; JAC, January 26, 1935:3).

The Fife Dojo hosted a tournament inside the Fife High School auditorium during the weekend of February 28 thru March 1, 1931.[3] Fife hosted another tournament at Fife High School on February 27–28, 1932. The highlight of this tournament involved Ito, a fifth-dan from a ship visiting Tacoma, throwing six local judoka during a handicap match. In competition, Masato Tamura also threw five men to take first place in his division. *The Japanese-American Courier* noted, "In promoting and making a success of the big tournament, the local mothers' group, Girls' Club and the men cooperated in every way" (JAC, March 5, 1932:2).

So that people could work on their farms, the dojo normally closed between May and September. However, when judo's founder Kano Jigoro announced that he was going to visit Pacific Northwest Japanese language schools in late August 1932, the Fife Dojo resumed training on August second that year (JAC, August 6, 1932:2). The extra effort paid off, too, as during the welcoming tournament held in Seattle, Jack Ohashi earned a promotion to first dan awarded by Professor Kano himself (JAC, October 15, 1932:2).

Oral tradition has it that Professor Kano visited the Fife Dojo during the 1932 Northwest US visit. Although I have seen no photos or newspaper articles to prove either the visit or the timing, I suspect that it did take place, on August 18, 1932. Kano had a documented speaking engagement at the Tacoma Japanese Language School that evening, and while en route he probably visited the dojos in Kent, Auburn, and Fife.

In 1933, the club resumed training at its normal time, late September. In early November, Ryoichi Iwakiri loaded the boys in his truck and took them to a small tournament on Bainbridge Island. George Kawasaki returned to Fife with the first place trophy (JAC, September 29, 1933:2; JAC, November 11, 1933:2).

Fife was always a popular stop on the local tournament circuit. The reason was that the school auditorium held two mats rather than one, as was typical elsewhere. Therefore meets ended somewhat earlier in the evening (JAC, February 18, 1933:2). As elsewhere, speeches, announcements, and the award of service trophies usually prefaced the bouts. For example, on March 17, 1934, Kichigoro Yamamoto and Ryoichi Iwakiri both received silver cups in appreciation of their support throughout the years. Then, to the local crowd's delight, Masato Tamura, Hikaru ("Polka") Tamura, and Joe Yamamoto went out and won medals in their respective divisions (JAC, March 17, 1934:2).

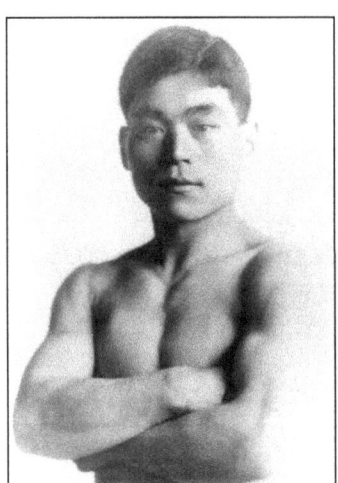 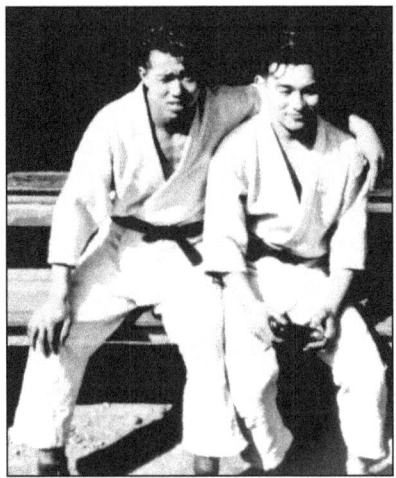

Left: Kichigoro ("Kay") Yamamoto, future patron of the Fife Dojo, after winning the Northwest AAU wrestling championship at 125 pounds in 1912. Photo courtesy of Edith Yamamoto Kuramoto. Right: Hank Ogawa and Hiroshi Tamura resting during the training preceding the 1939 all-star tournament in Los Angeles. Photo courtesy of Hank Ogawa.

The 1935 season was among Fife's best. George Kawasaki received an honorable mention at a February 10, 1935 tournament at the Seattle Dojo (JAC, February 16, 1935: 3). Daizo ("Dykes") Itami of Fife, a former Cleveland High School four-sport letterman, took his turn by winning first place during a Tentoku Kan tournament held March 3, 1935 (JAC, March 9, 1935:3). Finally, Masato Tamura won an upset victory over Seattle Dojo's Kaimon Kudo at South Park on March 10, 1935, and came home with second place (JAC, March 16, 1935:3; *Great Northern Daily News*, hereafter referred to as GND, March 11, 1935:8).

In 1936, a small child playing with matches started a fire that razed the Fife Dojo (Edith Kuramoto, personal communication, September 25, 1997). Since Japanese-American boys provided the backbone of the Fife High School football, wrestling, and track teams, the judo club had no trouble arranging temporary sanctuary at Fife Junior High School. The Tacoma Dojo also welcomed Fife judoka. However, living on charity wasn't the same as having a dojo, and the Fife community responded to the disaster by building a judo wing to the Fife Japanese Language School (Edith Kuramoto, personal communication, September 25, 1997).

Other than the loss of its dojo, 1936 was another good year for the Fife Dojo. In March 1936, Masato Tamura, 2nd-dan, threw Kuniyuki Kaname, 3rd-dan, of Tentoku Kan in a well-publicized match.[4] In October 1936, a twenty-three-man Northwest all-star judo team that included Masato Tamura, Jack Ohashi, and George Kawasaki went to Los Angeles for a tournament with a California all-star team. Said the *Great Northern Daily News* afterward (October 27, 1936:8):

> Wins were scarce [for the Northwest team] until Masato Tamura, who ranked fifth on the Seattle team, turned the tables and hurled three men to the mat. He drew with Warren Lewis, Negro judoist.[5]

As a result of this outstanding performance, Professor Kano personally promoted Tamura to third dan in California (JAC, October 31, 1936:3). Although this meant that Tamura was now technically senior to Iwakiri, the rank inversion did not affect their friendship. Says Iwakiri's daughter, Chiyo Iida, "My father was very proud to have the Tamura family participating in the Fife judo. Of course, Masato was the number one judoist in the region, as well as other regions. The other brothers did very well too" (Fujiko Gardner, personal communication from Chiyo Iida, May 4, 1997; Fujiko Gardner, personal communication, July 12, 1997). Tamura was equally proud of his teacher, and after the war, whenever visiting his family in Tacoma, he would visit Iwakiri at his house. Adds Stewart Bush, one of Iwakiri's postwar seniors, "And Mr. Iwakiri didn't let anybody inside his house!" (Stewart Bush, personal communication, August 30, 1997; Fujiko Gardner, personal communication, October 28, 1997).

Besides doing judo, Fife *nisei* (people born in America of issei parents) were also active in the Fife High School wrestling team, where they dominated the lower weights. With the exception of heavyweight Joe Yamamoto, Swiss-Americans dominated the upper weights (Leslie Sandvig, personal communication, August 14, 1997). Prewar all-Northwest wrestling champions from Fife High School included Don Kawasaki, Leo Kawasaki, and Kenji Yaguchi. George Makoto Iwakiri was also active in both wrestling and judo.[6]

Les Sandvig was the wrestling coach at Fife. Due to federal salary subsidies, Sandvig earned $150 a month while his principal earned just $90. To be sure, Sandvig earned all that extra money, the principal assigned him every extra duty he could find, including wrestling coach. (Few Northwest high schools of the 1930's had wrestling teams.) As Sandvig later recalled:

> The teachers did a lot of after school hours of work—with school programs, P.T.A. meetings, etc. There was no such thing as overtime!
>
> The wrestling coach job was enjoyable—working with the kids. Joe Yamamoto at 165 pounds, had no partner to work out with, so he and I spent a lot of time working out (my weight at that time was 170, 175). The things he taught me—together we made a great team, and he made a better coach of me.

> Often there would be judo exhibition matches to raise money for the athletic departments. The Japanese who had graduated from Fife and lived in the community were available for these events. Masato Tamura and Sunji Dogen were glad to support this effort.
> – Sandvig, personal communication, August 14, 1997

On January 31, 1937, the Fife and Tacoma clubs held a joint tournament at the Tacoma Buddhist Church. This was in preparation for a rematch with the Californians to be held in Seattle over the weekend of April 3–4, 1937. In the individual competition, Hikaru Tamura lost to California's Hikaru Nakao and Masato Tamura drew with California's Mitsuo Kimura. In the team competition, Hikaru Tamura drew with California's Oseko and Jack Ohashi drew with California's Asano (JAC, April 10, 1937:3).[7]

On February 7, 1938, Fife Dojo celebrated the opening of its new judo hall. The master of ceremonies was Tsugio Yaguchi, and speakers included the head of Kodokan judo in the Northwest, Yasuyuki Kumagai of Seattle. *The Japanese-American Courier* described the new facility, which was attached to the Japanese Language School, as "well-lighted, well-heated, and the mat consists of rubber-cushioned imported tatami—a veritable judoist's paradise" (February 12, 1938:4).

On March 20, 1938, Fife celebrated the opening with a tournament. Spectators included Tacoma photographer Marvin Boland, who hoped to get some action photos for *Life* magazine,[8] and officers from the Pierce County Sheriff's Department and the Washington State Patrol (*North American Times*, hereafter referred to as NAT, March 17, 1938:1).

Judo founder Kano Jigoro visited the Northwest for the last time in April 1938. During this visit, Kano promoted Iwakiri to third dan and his fourteen-year old son George Makoto Iwakiri to 1st dan. While Dennis Helm has claimed these as Kano's last promotions, that is probably not the case. For one thing, other Northwest judoka, including Ei'ichi Koiwai of Seattle, received promotion the same night. It seems petty to argue about who stood last in line. More importantly, Kano visited Vancouver, British Columbia, on April 21–22, 1938, and probably promoted someone there before leaving (Dalien, 1988: 13–14; Ei'ichi Koiwai, personal communication, July 12, 1997).

The certificates that Kano left behind also caused some confusion. Kano had signed them using the phrase "*kiichi sai*," which means, "return to the original way." In 1977, Dennis Helm speculated that Kano meant that the Northwest judoka, many of whom were Christian, should take up Zen Buddhism (Helm, 1977:16). Of course, Kano meant no such thing. Kiichi Sai was simply a pen name he adopted upon turning seventy. Therefore, when he visited Seattle in 1938, he unsurprisingly signed promotion certificates, "Kano Kiichi Sai" (Dalien, 1988:14; Nakayama, 1984:201).

Fife hosted another regional tournament on February 12, 1939. The purpose of this tournament was to decide who would represent the Northwest during an upcoming tournament in California. Seven of the thirty players sent to Los Angeles came from Fife. These were Masato Tamura, Hikaru Tamura, Hiroshi Tamura, Jack Ohashi, Sunji Dogen, George Kawasaki, and Joe Yamamoto. The Northwest team trained hard, and while they lost the individual matches 7–11 on March 4, 1939, its members evened things up the following day by winning the team competition (JAC, February 25, 1939, p. 3; NAT, March 6, 1939:1).

As many of these young Northwesterners had never been south of Portland, Oregon, the two days spent visiting San Francisco's Golden Gate International Exposition on the way back from Los Angeles were the true highlight of the trip. Auburn judoka Toshio

Yamanaka recalled:

> The Japanese Pavilion and Hawaii Exposition were the team's favorite places to meet and get together. That's because the many girls working at the two places were nisei students at U.C. Berkeley and were there helping and working to help pay their college expenses. They were very friendly and treated us extra good so our car drivers drove them to their homes when it came time for them to get off work. The rest of us had to wait over an hour longer than the time set to leave to get a ride back to our hotel. Most of us in those days were rather girl shy, but the girls were all pretty and very nice and friendly and treated us like we were a special group. So we weren't upset to wait for the guys to take them home. But when we got back [Yasuyuki] Kumagai Sensei had us all stand in the main hotel lobby and gave us a lecture to never do such a thing again, to make all of us wait. It was the first and only lecture that we got from our sensei. This world's fair was really the greatest.
> – Yamanaka personal communications, February 3, 19 and March 11, 1998

Being otherwise responsible young men, the travelers bought souvenirs for their stay-at-home friends. Recalled Ryoichi Iwakiri's daughter, Chiyo Iida (Fujiko Gardner, personal communication from Chiyo Iida, May 4, 1997):

> I have a good memory about our [family's] relation with them [Hiroshi and Hikaru Tamura, both of whom were years older than she]. In 1939 they went to the World's Fair in San Francisco (Treasure Island) and brought us a lot of mementos from the Fair. I was so proud I wore my bracelet to school and everyone was so envious.

In January 1941, Masato Tamura's sister, Tadako,[9] saw an advertisement announcing a full-time job teaching judo at Chicago's Jiu-Jitsu Institute (GND, January 15, 1941:8). She mentioned this to her brother, who immediately applied. He got the job and left for the "Windy City" in March 1941 (GND, February 28, 1941: 8; JAC, March 1, 1941:3). Besides being lauded in the local papers, Tamura received various honors at local tournaments plus a send-off banquet from the Fife Dojo (GND, September 24, 1940:8; NAT, November 17, 1938:1). The latter likely took place at Fife's Poodle Dog Cafè on a Friday night in late February. The main course was probably chicken, with the men drinking beer and the youths drinking apple cider. And afterwards there were likely speeches culminating in a stirring rendition of "Auld Lange Syne" (NAT, 1940, September 30:1).

During World War II, Fife's Japanese-Americans were relocated to concentration camps in California and Idaho. Because he lived in Chicago, Masato Tamura avoided being relocated. Hiroshi, who had been drafted in 1940, also avoided relocation. However, the rest of the Tamura family was sent to Minidoka Relocation Center in Hunt, Idaho.

During the summer of 1943, Masato Tamura received permission to visit his family at Minidoka. There he found his brothers active in the camp judo club, and even arranged for his mother to stitch judo jackets for his Chicago judo students (Fujiko Gardner, personal communication, June 8, 1997). Mrs. Tamura always was an enthusiastic supporter of her sons' judo practice (Fujiko Gardner, personal communication, March 16, 1998). Soon after, both Masaru and Mitsuru Tamura enlisted in the US Army and served in the 442nd Regimental Combat Team. Masaru was killed in Italy in April 1945.

After the war, most of the surviving Tamura boys stayed in the Midwest. Ryoichi

Iwakiri returned to Fife in 1947. While his first postwar judo dojo was a friend's garage, around 1952 he moved it inside the old Tacoma Japanese Language School. His dojo was in the basement. The floor area measured about 20' x 20', and the tatami were provided by friends (NT, August 16, 1952:2; Washington 1995).

Although Iwakiri retired from active training around 1957, he remained affiliated with the Tacoma-Fife Dojo until his death in May 1987. Most of what he taught during the last thirty years of his life was philosophy. Favorite sayings included, "Success is like your eyebrows. It's in front of you all the time, you just can't see it," and "Victory even before the battle is for the person who is embraced with compassion and no thought of himself" (Stewart Bush, personal communication, March 10, 1998).

A prospective student once asked Iwakiri what it took to become a judo master. Three things, he replied: the first two were practice, and the third was more practice. "That's not what I meant," said the student; "what is the key to mastering the long run?" Replied Iwakiri, "In the long run, we are all dead." Another student asked what he would be taught. To which Iwakiri replied, "I can't teach you very much, but you can learn a lot" (Stewart Bush, personal communication, November 28, 1997). And, shortly before his death, Iwakiri told his longtime student Jerry Dalien:

> [Kano Jigoro] told me once that I must be strong in mind and body always, and help others in life. I appreciate all you peoples who come and see me. I am old now and peoples have no time for them. Mr. Yamashita, Mr. Bush, Mr. Demorest, and you Mr. Dalien are fine students of Kano's judo.[10] Mr. Uchida, he is important mans in judo—you tell him good-bye for me. I am not important persons, I have done nothing great, I have no schooling. You please make any honor for me, just judo. Okay? I do not have long time left to live anymore, but want you to keep my judo, please? Okay? – Dalien, 1988:23–24

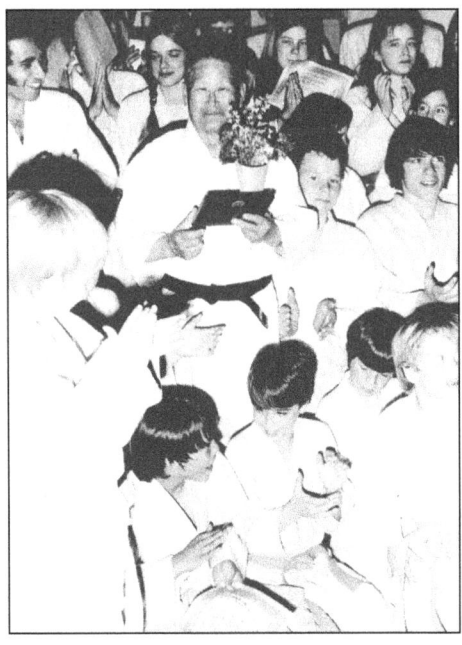 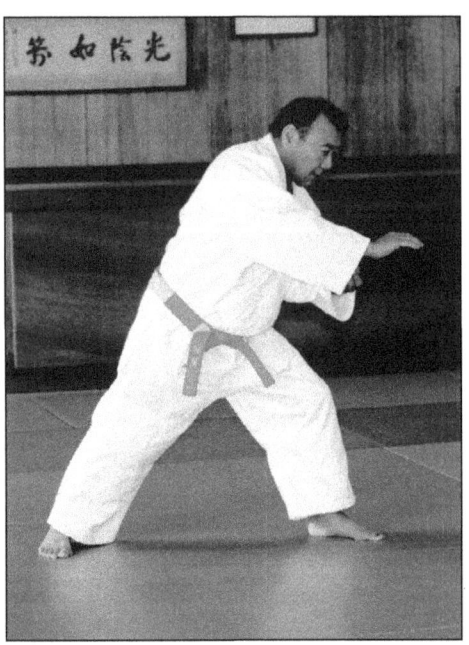

Left: Ryoichi Iwakiri, mid-1960s. Photo courtesy of Hank Ogawa.
Right: Vince Tamura, three time U.S. AAU judo champion, training at his dojo in Dallas, Texas, in 1997. Photo courtesy of Fujiko Tamura Gardner.

Following the war, Masato Tamura also remained active in judo. In 1944, he bought the Jiu-Jitsu Institute of America from Harry Auspitz. In 1949, he was elected president of the Chicago Judo Black Belt Association, and in 1958 he became president of the US Judo Federation. Yet he was not just another judo politician, for as late as 1964 he was still winning US masters championships.[11] More importantly, he remained a friend and mentor to his many students. As one of them wrote following Tamura's death on June 10, 1982, "With modesty and humility he characterized the true judo spirit" ("Masato Tamura, Hachidan," in Masato Tamura collection).

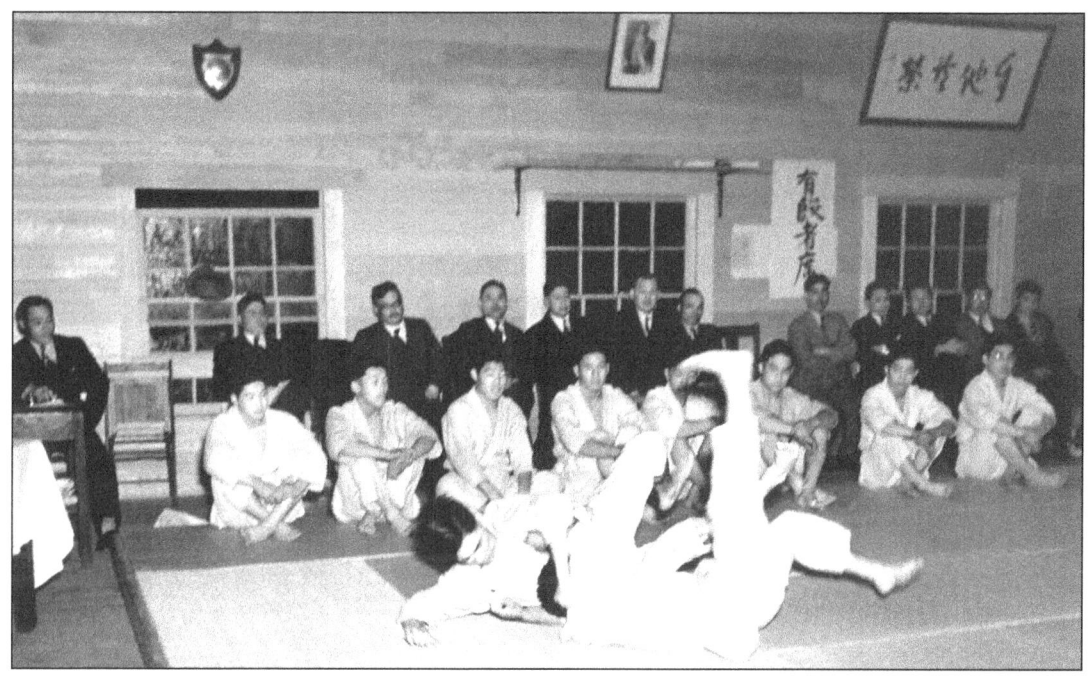

Judo tournament at the Fife Dojo, March 1938.
Photo from the Boland Collection, courtesy of the Washington State Historical Society, Tacoma, Washington.

Other former Fife judoka also remained with judo until age or infirmity forced their retirement. For example, Vince Tamura moved to Chicago in June 1945. After completing high school and military service in Korea, he went on to become a three-time AAU national judo champion. In August 1960, he relocated to Dallas, where he was still teaching judo in 1998. After separation from the service, Mitsuru Tamura also moved to Chicago, where he was an instructor at his brother's Jiu-Jitsu Institute for many years. Hikaru Tamura taught judo in Ogden, Utah. Hiroshi Tamura taught judo in Chicago and France. George Iwakiri, George Kawasaki, and Leo Kawasaki taught judo at the Tacoma-Fife Dojo. Finally, Kenji Yaguchi taught judo in Ontario, Oregon, and was chairman of the Oregon AAU Judo Committee from 1958 to 1966 (Stewart Bush, personal communication, November 28, 1997; Kenji Yaguchi, personal communication, June 22, 1997).[12]

And so the falls first learned in Mr. Yamamoto's barn in the 1920's continue to echo throughout North American judo.

ENDNOTES

1. Although Japanese put family names before personal names, most of the people named in this paper were or eventually became US citizens. Therefore, it better reflects the way they described themselves if their names are written personal name, family name rather than the other way around. To keep things simple, the occasional Japanese names are also written in the American fashion.
2. The history of the Fife Dojo—given in Helm (July 1977) and reprinted almost verbatim (albeit without any attribution to Helm's editorial team or acknowledgment of US Judo Federation copyright) by Corcoran and Farkas (1988:212-214, 217)—is wrong in almost every detail. On the other hand, the history given in Helm, Armetta, and Wickham (May 1973:14-15) is generally accurate except for spellings.
3. Photograph (cir. 1931-3) of a Fife High School tournament in the Joseph Svinth collection.
4. Published articles and photographs owned by Mr. Tamura's widow, Rose Tamura.
5. Reasonable numbers of early twentieth-century judoka were not of Japanese ancestry. In California, for example, non-Japanese judoka included San Jose State's Emilio Bruno, Los Angeles' Jack Sergel and Warren Lewis, and Stockton's Robert E. West. In British Columbia, there were a number of Royal Canadian Mounted Police judoka, and in Washington State, there was Stanley McDonald in Seattle and Vernon Anderson in Winslow. There were of course more non-Japanese jujutsu teachers and students elsewhere, especially in New York City and the upper Midwest. While most teachers and students were male, there were female students in New York City and Los Angeles, plus at least one female instructor in Wisconsin.
6. See Fife High School's Trojan, 1935-1942. Fife nisei did equally well in postwar AAU wrestling. For example, Hisashi Watanabe lettered in wrestling at Fife in 1946 and 1947, and qualified for the US AAU Nationals in Ames, Iowa, in 1948 (*Northwest Times*, hereafter referred to as NWT, May 1, 1948:3).
7. See the Keigi Horiuchi collection. The first names for the California judoka were not noted in the reporting.
8. While Boland's records at the Washington State Historical Society in Tacoma date the surviving photographs to March 30, 1938, that was probably the day he developed them, as the tournament took place a week earlier. Unfortunately, the pictures were too blurred to make *Life* magazine.
9. Tadako Tamura is an excellent writer, and examples of her essays appeared in the *North American Times* on January 4, 1938 and May 14, 1938, and the *Great Northern Daily News* on January 1, 1940. Her postwar pen name was Thea Mori. For a brilliant example of her mature style, see "Salmon Creek This Week" in the *White Center News*, May 26, 1960.
10. Stewart Bush, Robert Demorest, and Jerry Dalien were among Iwakiri's postwar seniors. Masao Yamashita was a prewar friend from Auburn who later established the Boise Valley Judo Club in Caldwell, Idaho. George Uchida was a former San Jose State University judo coach who took a job teaching judo in the Kent-Meridian High School program after one day realizing that the spirit of judo was not found in winning medals, but in working with kids.
11. Tamura became known nationwide through television. The most famous television appearances included his daughter Diane. The act was usually nothing more than Tamura doing a few throws and falls with his daughter, and then talking about judo. The first took place on Chicago television on February 10, 1952. The popularity of their act lead to national television exposure beginning in June 1952. For contemporary

accounts of Tamura's postwar career, see NT, November 3, 1948:1; NT, August 20, 1949:4; NT, August 31, 1949:3; NT, February 16, 1952:4; NT, June 18, 1952:4.

[12] "Members of the Tamura Family Involved with Tacoma-Fife Dojo," unpublished typewritten document in the Fujiko Gardner collection.

BIBLIOGRAPHY

Corcoran, J. and Farkas, E. (1988). *Martial arts: Traditions, history, people.* New York: W. H. Smith.

Dalien, J. (1988). *Judo: The life, the way, the concept.* Spanaway, WA: Self-published.

Helm, D. (Ed.). (1977, July) The history of American judo. *Judo USA, 3*(3):16–17.

Helm, D., Armetta, P. and Wickham, D. (1973, May). The Pacific North West 1907 to 1941. *Judo Illustrated, 7*(1):14–15.

Magden, R. (1998). *Furusato: Tacoma-Pierce County Japanese.* Tacoma, WA: Tacoma Japanese Community Service: 35–36.

"Masato Tamura, Hachidan," unpublished document in Masato Tamura collection.

"Members of the Tamura Family Involved with Tacoma-Fife Dojo," unpublished typewritten document in Fujiko Gardner collection.

Mori, T. (1960, May 26). Salmon Creek this week. *White Center News.*

Nakayama, G. (1984). *Issei: Stories of Japanese Canadian pioneers.* Toronto: NC Press.

Nomura, G. (1987). Tsugiki, a grafting a history of a Japanese pioneer woman in Washington State. *Women's Studies, 14*(1):19.

Trojan, 1935–1942. (n.d.). Fife, Washington: Fife High School.

Washington State Judo 1995 Hall of Fame (n.d.). No city or publisher given.

Watanabe, J. (Trans.) (1986). *History of the Japanese of Tacoma.* Seattle: Pacific Northwest Council, Japanese American Citizens League.

NEWSPAPERS

Great Northern Daily News (referred to as GND).
Japanese-American Courier (referred to as JAC).
North American Times (referred to as NAT).
Northwest Times (referred to as NWT).
Tacoma News Tribune (referred to as TNT).

ACKNOWLEDGMENTS

Research was conducted at the Japanese Canadian Museum and Archives, Sno-Isle Public Libraries, Tacoma Buddhist Temple, Tacoma Public Library, University of British Columbia, University of Washington, and Washington State Historical Society Research Center.

The assistance of the following individuals is gratefully acknowledged: W. Stewart Bush, Jerry Dalien, Shane Foster, Fujiko Tamura Gardner, Tsuneharu Gonnami, Richard Hayes, Keigi Horiuchi, Chiyo Iida, George and Risa Kawasaki, Ei'ichi Koiwai, Joseph Kosai, Shinji Kozu, Edith Yamamoto Kuramoto, Ronald Magden, Hank and Yo Ogawa, Charles Payton, Leslie A. Sandvig, Robert W. Smith, Curtis and Cynthia Stanley, Rose Tamura, Vince Tamura, Joy Werlink, Kenji Yaguchi, Mae Iseri Yamada, and Toshio Yamanaka.

Financial support included a grant from the King County Office of Cultural Resources and the Hotel/Motel Tax Revenue Program.

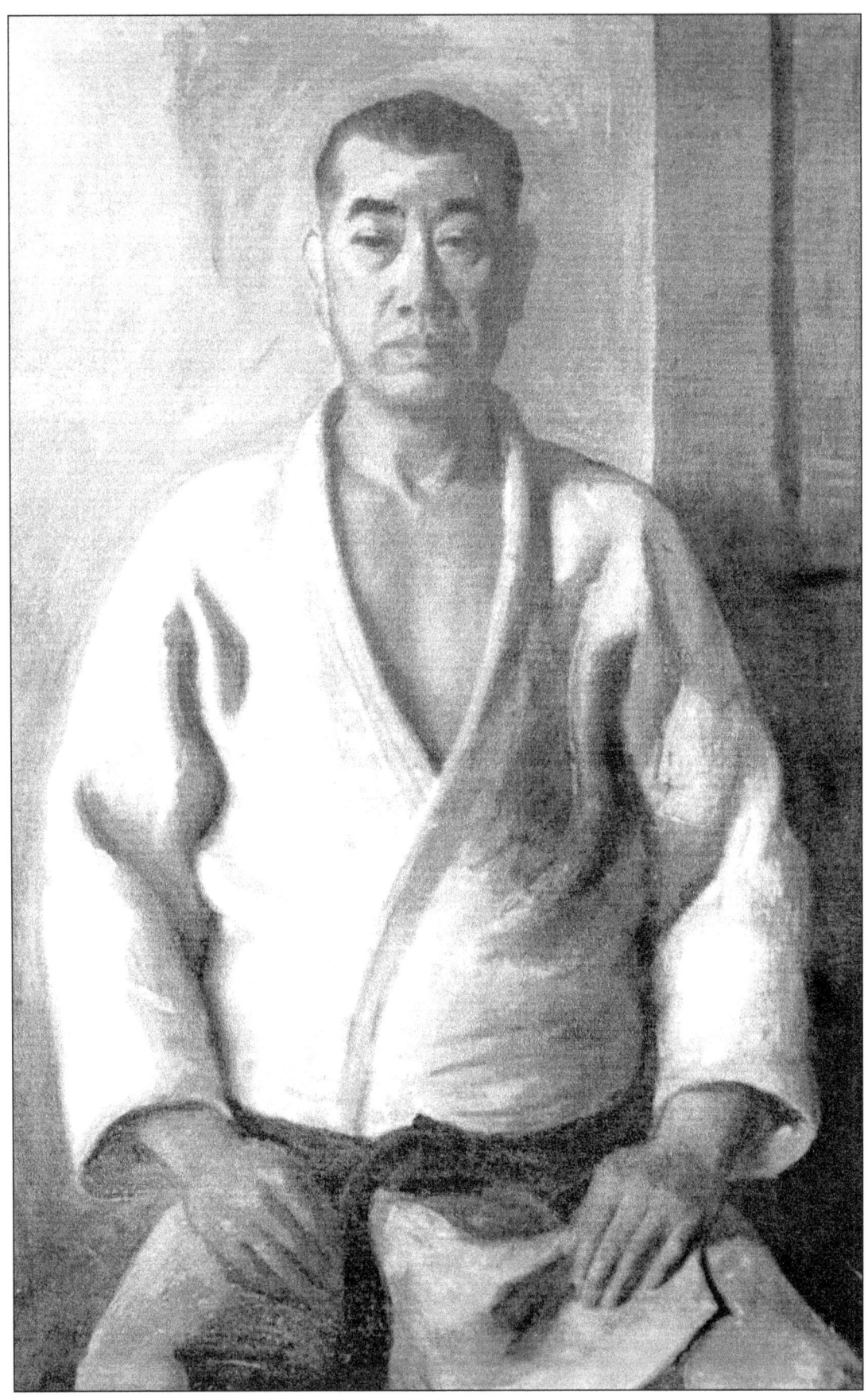

chapter 5

Origins of the British Judo Association, the European Judo Union and the International Judo Federation
by Richard Bowen

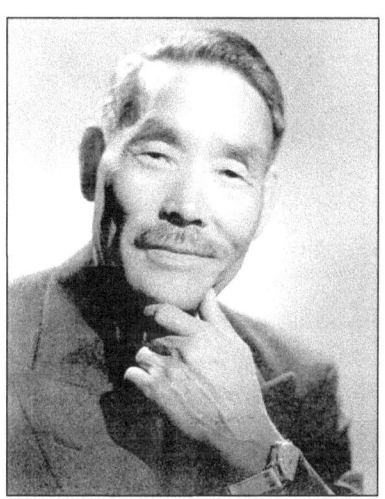

Above: G. Koizumi, 1950s. Previous page: Painting of Yukio Tani, 1930s.
All photographs courtesy of Richard Bowen.

The years slip by and much which should be remembered is forgotten. This is a brief account of the creation of three judo organizations, two founded over fifty years ago and the third a few years short of that period.

The story starts with Gunji Koizumi. In the early 1930s, he suggested to a group of judo friends on the European continent that a union should be formed to facilitate international judo matters. It is quite likely that the concept originated earlier in discussions between Koizumi and Jigoro Kano, these taking place during the five visits, from 1920 to 1933, which the founder of Kodokan Judo made to the Budokwai in London.

Much is known about Jigoro Kano, but what about Gunji Koizumi? Koizumi arrived in London in 1906 and some nine months later went to the United States of America. By 1910, he was back in London where he set up an antique business. Wishing to contribute something to his adopted country (although he never became British), he organized at his own expense a martial arts society in London, the Budokwai, which opened its doors on January 26, 1918. This was, and is, a strictly amateur and democratic body, which is run by and owned by the members.

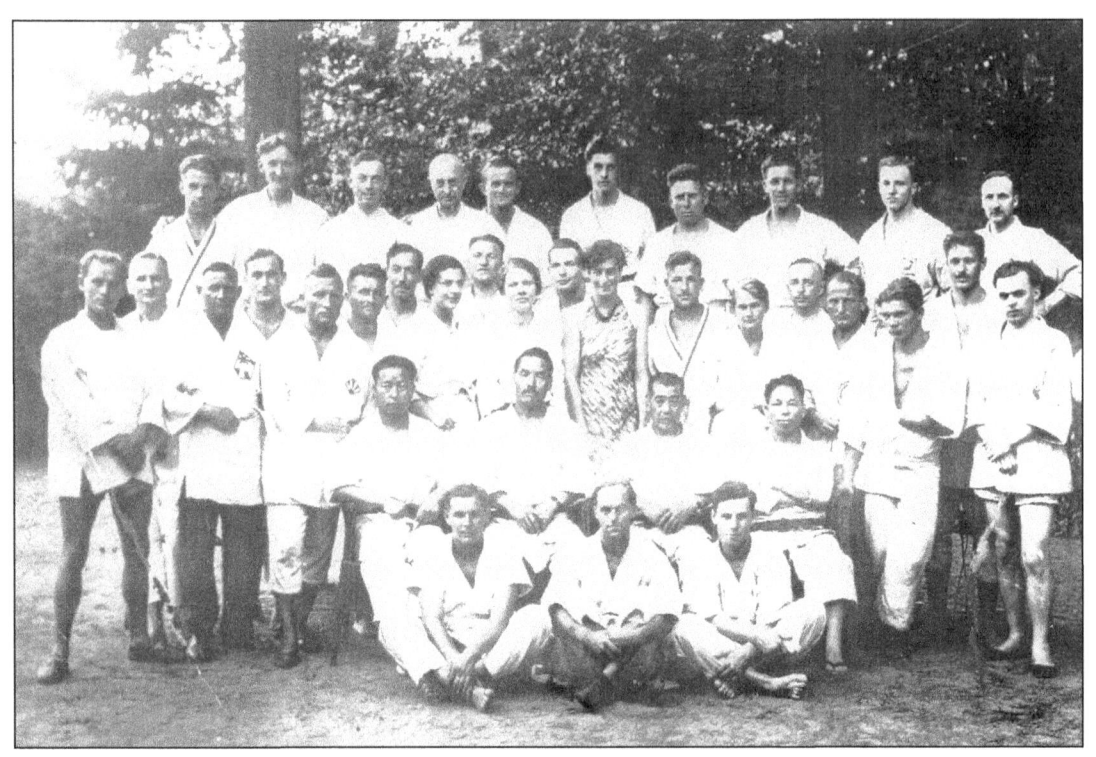

Judo Summer School in Germany, 1933.

In 1929, the first international judo contests took place in Germany between the Budokwai and the Frankfurt-am-Main and Wiesbaden clubs. It must be recorded that the initiative for this came from the Frankfurt Jujutsu Club. While these started as interclub matches, by 1931 they had assumed the character of full international contests. Within a year or two Judo Instructional Summer Schools were taking place in Frankfurt and it would have been at these that plans were made for some form of European union. A skeleton organization was indeed formed, but came to naught with the rise of the Nazis and the threat of war. In later years Koizumi was prone to say, "The European Judo Union was formed but never matured." At times he would refer to this early organization as the First European Judo Union.

In passing, the instructors at the three or four pre-Second World War summer schools were: Gunji Koizumi, Yukio Tani, and Masutaro Otani, all from the Budokwai; M. Kawaishi from Paris; Dr. Rhi from Switzerland; and Dr. Kitabatake from Berlin. All, with the possible exception of Dr. Rhi, were members of the Kodokan.

After the war, Koizumi discussed with the Budokwai Committee the possibility of forming a British national judo body and of reviving a possible European organization. Early in 1948 he decided to act, and John Barnes, then Chairman of the Budokwai, sent out invitations for a conference to all known British clubs. A invitation to a second conference was sent to all known judo/jiujutsu clubs in Europe. These two conferences were timed to coincide with a Judo Summer School run by the Budokwai in London in July 1948, a suitable time for matters international as the first post-war Olympic Games were being held in the city.

The British conference took place in Committee Room A, at London University's Imperial College Union, Prince Consort Road, on Saturday, July 24, 1948. The meeting convened at 2:30 p.m. Those present were:

Miss Barbara Ball (later Dr.) .... Liverpool University
Mr. G. Dawson-Grove .... Imperial College, London
Mr. Hylton Green .... Imperial College, London
Mr. John Barnes .... Budokwai
Mr. Michael Bell .... Budokwai
Mr. Frederick Kauert .... Budokwai
Mr. Gunji Koizumi .... Budokwai, and representing
                                           the South Shields Judo Club
Mr. Eric Dominy .... South London Judo Society,
                                           (later the London Judo Society),
                                           Budokwai, and representing
                                           Bristol Judokwai
Mr. Stan Bissell .... Budokwai
The Manchester Y.M.C.A. Judo Club sent apologies.

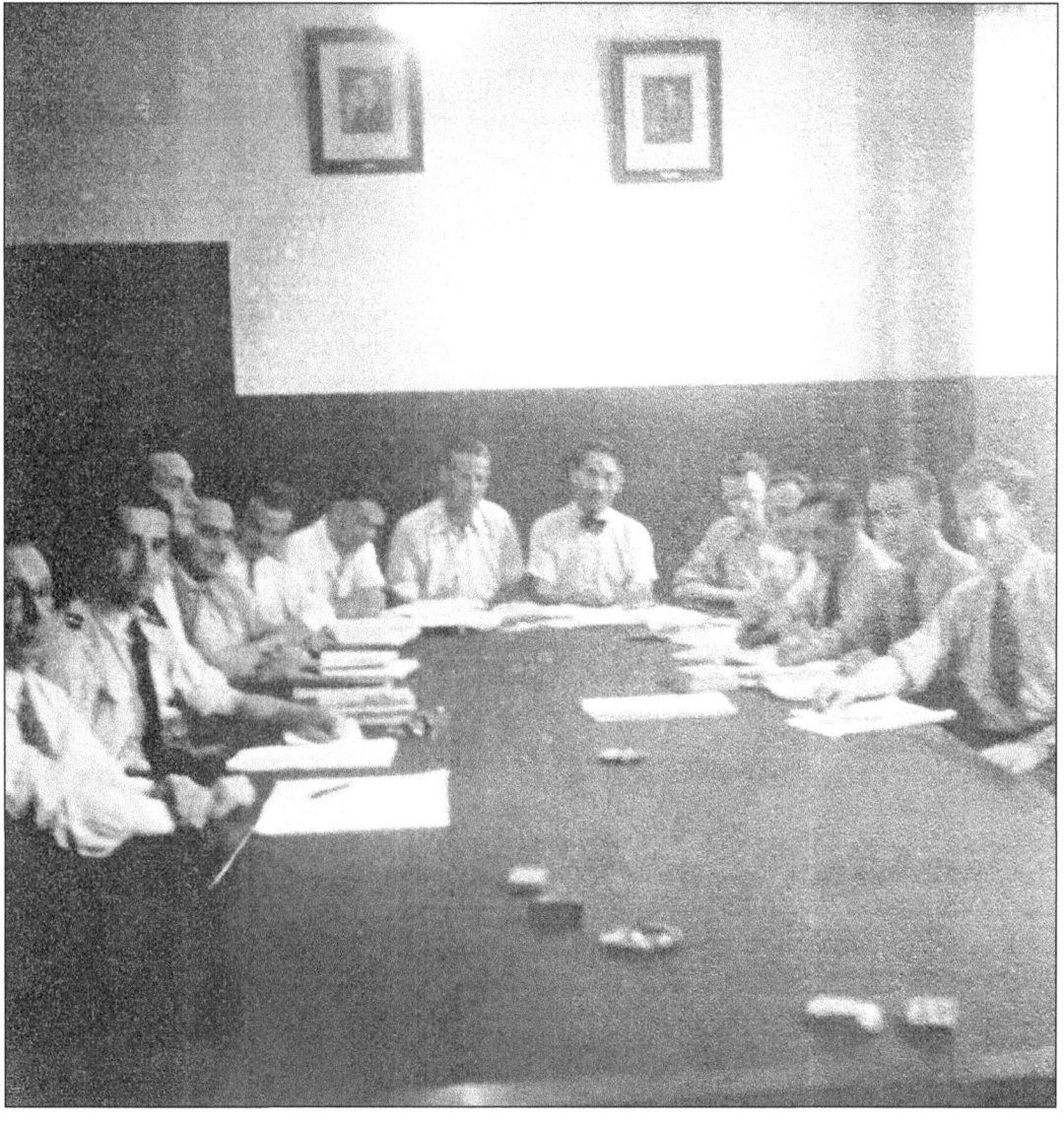

International Conference on the proposed European Judo Union, 1948.

The meeting examined a proposed constitution put forward by Koizumi which, after some amendments and additions, was unanimously adopted. This is not the place to set out the agreed constitution, but it could hardly be called lengthy, running to twenty-nine lines. How nice! With the British Judo Association (BJA) now formed, the meeting went on to elect the following: Committee members Koizumi, Barnes, Green, Dominy, and Bissell; Barnes was elected Chairman, Green Honorary Secretary, and Bissell Honorary Treasurer. But the Treasurer had nothing to treasure, so Koizumi lent a few pounds to allow the baby Association to stagger forward.

The Association then got down to discussing ideas for the forthcoming international conference on the proposed European Judo Union. A draft constitution was formulated to be presented at the international conference. And that was that, with the meeting closing at 5:30 p.m.—three hours to form the first amateur national judo association in the world.

The number of clubs attending gives an indication of the size of judo in Britain at that time. There were probably eighteen clubs affiliated to the Budokwai. Doubling that number gives the likely number of clubs in the country in 1948. A few years later there were a hundred and ten clubs affiliated to the Budokwai and about forty in the BJA. But then the number of clubs in the Association gradually overtook the Budokwai affiliates.

On Monday, July 26, 1948, the International Conference was convened in the same Committee Room A at the Imperial College Union, commencing at 2:45 p.m. Those present were:

Mr. John Barnes	Budokwai
Mr. E. Kauert	Budokwai
Mr. G. Koizumi	Budokwai
Mr. T.P. Leggett	Budokwai
Mr. H. Green	Imperial College
Mr. AT Scala	South London Judo Society (LJS)
Mr. EA. Vincent	Interpreter
Mr. P. Buchelli	Austria
Mr. E. Nimfuhr	Austria
Lt. M. Thieme	Holland
Mr. Alfonso Castelli	Italy
Mr. Stott	Interpreter for Mr. Castelli
Dr. Feldenkrais	The Minutes do not give in what capacity he attended
Mr. de Jarmy	Observer from France

Only four votes were allowed, equaling the number of countries present (Britain, Austria, Holland, and Italy, France being an observer).

Leggett was elected Chairman for the Conference, and Hylton Green was appointed scribe. The Budokwai's draft constitution, which was actually based on a proposed constitution from the thirties, was presented. Leggett then explained that the object of the proposed Union was the standardization of judo rules and procedures and the establishment of an international body for arbitration.

As it was generally agreed by those present to form a Judo Union, the members went on to examine the draft constitution. A detailed examination followed, with each section being scrutinized, hacked about, taken out, put back in, altered, and put to the vote; all no doubt with varied expletives in various languages. At one point Mr. de Jarmy tried to vote until he was reminded that he was there as an observer and not as a member of the conference. By 5:25 p.m., everyone had enough, so the meeting was adjourned until the following Wednesday, giving the delegates time to recover and to examine further details at leisure.

The adjourned meeting took place on Wednesday, July 28, at 2:30 p.m. in the same Committee Room. G. Chew of the South London Judo Society joined the conference as a new delegate, otherwise membership remained unaltered, apart from Mr. Castelli who was unable to attend. Leggett continued to chair the conference. The French delegate, who was allowed to express opinions but not to vote, continued to raise objections about certain points although the delegates had already approved them. Finally, Britain put forward the motion: "That the European Judo Union be now formed on the basis of the Constitution as approved, and that all other European countries be circulated with a copy of it and be invited to join." This was seconded by Holland and approved unanimously.

First General Meeting of the European Judo Union

The meeting then resolved itself into the First General Meeting of the European Judo Union (EJU), and proceeded to the election of officers. This resulted in Leggett being appointed Chairman and Mr. Thieme of Holland as Vice-Chairman. The next move was to form a Judo Council (a technical body as opposed to the General Committee). Those elected were:

        Mr. G. Koizumi   Dr. M. Feldenkrais
        Mr. P. Bonet-Maury   Mr. E. Mossom
        Mr. T.P. Leggett

France intervened with the suggestion that each of the important judo countries should be represented on the Council. As Chairman, Leggett pointed out that the purpose of the Council was not to represent national interests but to be composed of real judo experts. Just before the meeting closed, Holland issued a formal invitation to the EJU for the next General Meeting to be held in Holland. The meeting concluded at 4:30 p.m. with a vote of thanks to Britain for taking the initiative in organizing the Union. Shortly after the close of the meeting, Leggett relinquished the position of Chairman of the General Committee (but retained his position on the technical body) as mat judo was more important to him than political waza. As the position of Chairman was now vacant, it was suggested that Mr. John Barnes should act as pro tempore Chairman until the Holland gathering. This was agreed. The first Constitution of the EJU was naturally more comprehensive than the twenty-nine lines of the BJA's Constitution as, including titles and sub-titles, it ran to sixty-eight lines. A triumph of judo over bureaucracy.

No doubt the creators of the first continental judo union then retired to the Union bar to celebrate, in the time honored manner of judo folk everywhere, with tankards of weak lemonade.

2nd General Meeting of the European Judo Union

This was held in Bloemendaal, Holland, on October 29, 1949. Those present were:

        Mr. J. Barnes .... Britain
        Lt. H. Thieme .... Holland
        Dr. Aldo Torti .... Italy
        Mr. Jorn Aabrink .... Denmark
        Messrs. Marcelin and Lagaine were present as observers for France.

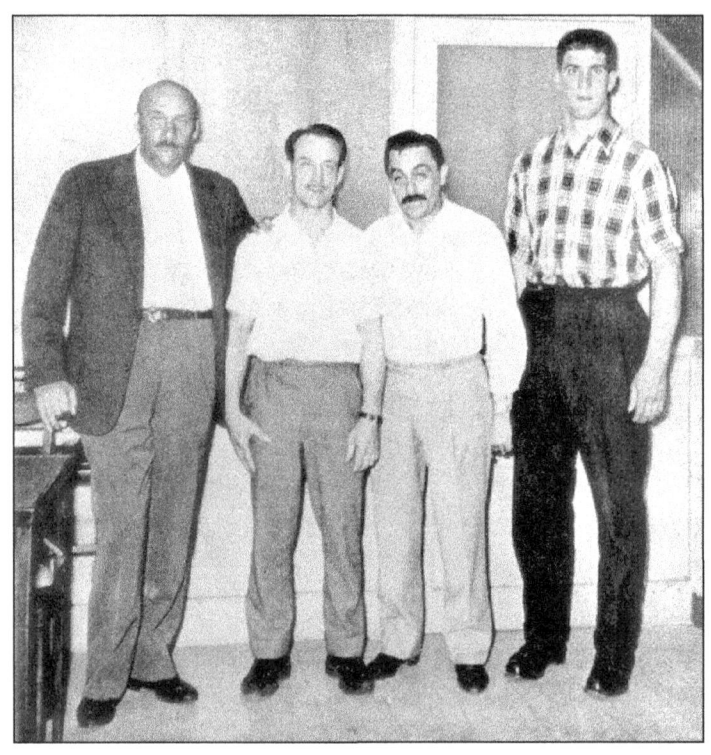

From left to right: Dr. Torti (President of the European Judo Union), Mr. Nauwelaerts de Age, Mr. Genolini and the young judoka Anton Geesink. Photo courtesy of Luni Editrice.

Denmark, who earlier had applied for membership to the Union, was unanimously elected. Most of the discussions centered around contest rules; it was decided that in international contests between Union members the Kodokan contest rules should be used. Italy was elected Chairman for the coming year with Denmark as the Vice-Chairman. Mr. Kawaishi of France and Dr. Rhi of Switzerland were elected to the Judo Council, the other members being Messrs. Koizumi, Leggett, Bonet-Maury, Mossom, and Dr. Feldenkrais.

In 1989, an account appeared in an official Union publication stating not only that this was the First Annual General Meeting, but that it was at this meeting where the Union was formed. The English version (which was accompanied by French and German versions) reads:

> On October 29, 1949, in Bloemendaal (Holland) the EJU was founded and the following countries were present Denmark, France, Great Britain, Holland and Italy, Mr. Torti (ITA) was elected President.

That the EJU was founded on that date and place is false. And an earlier paragraph says that a meeting was held in London on July 26, 1948, to prepare the basis for the foundation of the EJU. It is correct to write that a meeting took place, but the rest of the report is false. I have the minutes of the 1948 meeting. There was also a report in the October 1948 issue of the *Budokwai Bulletin* on the founding of the Union, and there is other documentary evidence. The matter was eventually taken up with the Union by John Barnes, a Vice-President, and it is hoped that these errors, which surely are the result of inadequate research, have now been remedied in the official records.

3rd General Meeting of the European Judo Union

This was held in Venice on Sunday, October 29, 1950, with delegates from Italy, Britain, Holland, Belgium, Austria, and Switzerland, under the Chairmanship of Dr. Torti. It was thought that the term of chairmanship was too short, so it was extended to four years. The General Committee was enlarged to include three Vice-Presidents and two Advisors. Britain and Austria were elected Vice-Presidents with Holland and Switzerland as Advisors. The third Vice-Presidency was left vacant pending the Chairman's invitation to France to join the Union.

I do not possess the minutes of this meeting and, while I do have a long report in three languages by Dr. Torti, this does not give the names of the delegates. It is certain that John Barnes represented Britain and Dr. Torti Italy. The identity of the others is yet to be resolved. France sent an observer in the person of Mr. Marcelin. Switzerland, Belgium, and Germany, were elected to membership of the Union, and a fourth language, German, was added to the official languages (French, Italian, and English) of the Union.

The French observer explained the failure of France to join the Union. France had four separate judo organizations: two amateur and two professional. As a consequence there were difficulties in forming a single national body to represent France. And, of course, the Union would only accept a single national body. Similar trouble arose with Holland where two organizations were competing for national supremacy. The Union solved this by rejecting the claims of one body for non-payment of the Union fees, and accepting the other body as the new representative for Holland. This General Committee meeting was relatively short, not so the meeting of the Judo Council which ended five hours after the other group's discussion had finished. The Council went through the contest rules with the diligence of an elephant searching for fleas. It ended with the adoption of the Budokwai's contest rules, which were based on those of the Kodokan, with some minor alterations of wording to avoid ambiguity.

Things change little. After offering some praise for the British attitude to judo, the report of the Chairman, Dr. Torti, continued with, "... though I deplore their lack of a federal outlook." As one of the bloody-minded islanders, who am I to contradict his judgement?

A few weeks after the Venice conference, France managed to reconcile its internal differences and applied to join the Union. And at about the same time Argentina also applied, with others outside Europe having similar thoughts. The Statutes of the Union had already been widened to allow for this. Europe was very stretchable in those days.

4th General Meeting of the European Judo Union and the
1st General Meeting of the International Judo Federation

This important meeting was held in a private room at Choy's Chinese Restaurant, Frith Street, Soho, London, on Thursday, July 12, 1951, no doubt to the comforting rattle of chopsticks. Eight countries were present: Italy, Britain, Belgium, France, Holland, Germany, Austria, and Switzerland. Here too, I lack the names of all the delegates. But again, John Barnes was the British representative, Dr. Torti (the Chairman) represented Italy, Mr. Scharfer Germany, Mr. W. Graf Switzerland, and Mr. J.J. Moes Holland.

With others outside the European ambit just as keen, the desire of Argentina to join required serious thought. A proposal, which had been circulated earlier with a suggested constitution, was presented. After discussion and agreement on the proposed constitution for a new organization, the European Judo Union was formally dissolved and replaced by an International Judo Federation. Instead of holding individual elections for officials to serve on the new Federation, it was agreed that the officials of the now extinct EJU take up similar positions on the new body. How sane, how peaceful, how logical!

The other main subject was the position of the judo colossus in the Far East-Japan. Koizumi, who had been corresponding with Risei Kano (the President of the Kodokan and son of the founder), read a letter from him in which he explained that he regretted being unable to attend the meeting or to send a delegate. The letter contained the suggestion that the headquarters of a world federation should be in Tokyo. The meeting declined this on the grounds that Japan was too distant. Furthermore, Japan was not a member of the Federation.

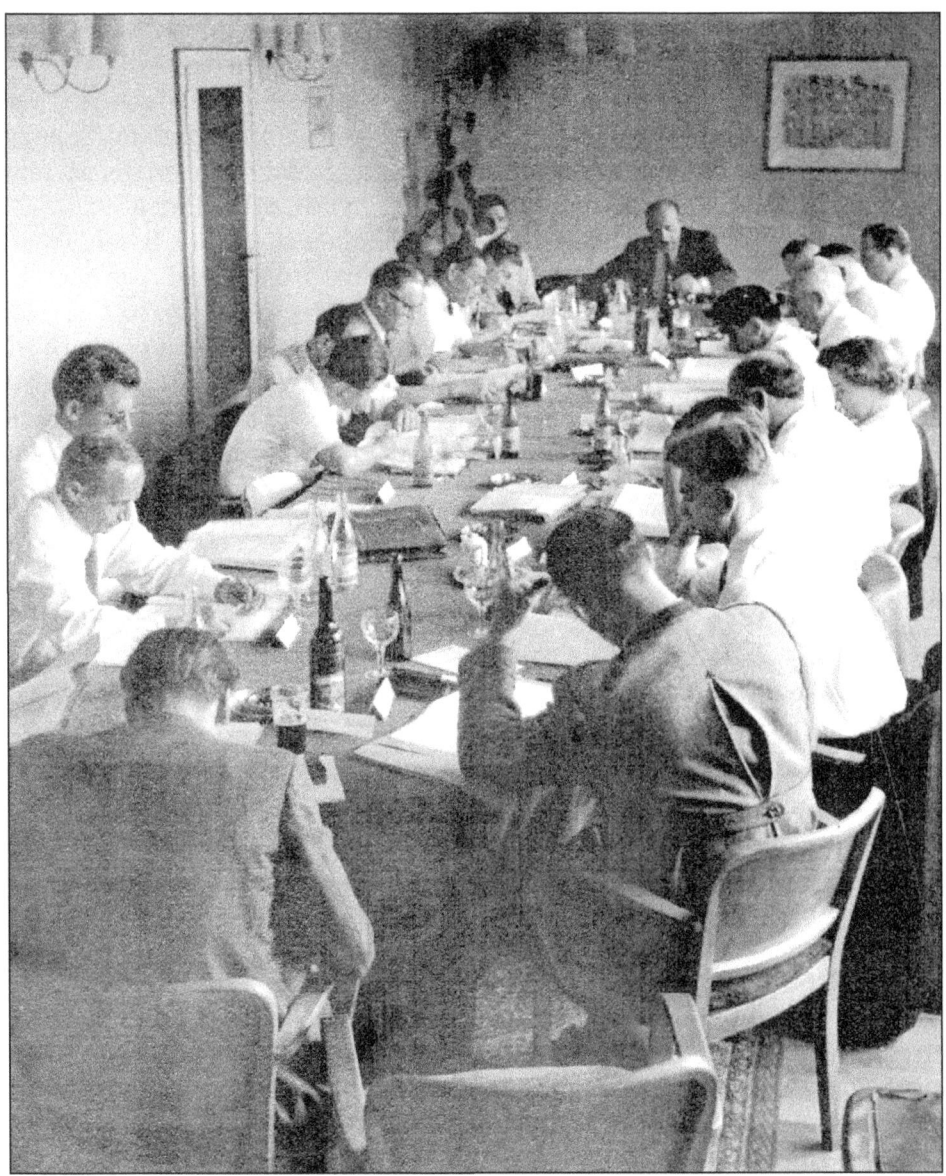

2nd general meeting of the International
Judo Federation in Zurich, 1952.

2nd General Meeting of the International Judo Federation and the Resurrection of the European Judo Union

This meeting, a real humdinger, was held in Zurich on Saturday, August 30, 1952. It started at 10:00 a.m. and continued, apart from breaks for food, to midnight. "Discussion raged!" The outstanding problem was how to find a way for Japan to enter the Federation; the problem was the same as France had earlier faced—there was no single national body. It was finally decided to offer Risei Kano the Presidency of the International Judo Federation. A diplomat acting on behalf of the Japanese Ambassador, who had been asked by Mr. Kano to represent him at the conference, thanked the meeting.

With the Presidency of the Federation now in the hands of Japan, the conference dealing with the Federation came to an end and discussion switched to Europe. But without a Union, nothing could be done, so the European Judo Union was re-established. Bonet-Maury expressed the wish that France should become the President of the European Judo Union as France's importance in Europe was on a parallel with that of Japan in the East, and that it was essential for the progress of the movement in Europe that France assume this important role and, failing this, France might not take a very active part in the Union. This subtle and canny diplomatic statement resulted in Italy being elected to the Presidency. France and Britain were elected Vice-Presidents with Belgium as Treasurer.

Among other problems was the application of East Germany to join the EJU. This was temporarily solved by admitting East Germany as an Observer for one year, without voting rights but the right to participate in competitions. Further discussions ranged about the question of weight categories, which Britain, France, Belgium, and Holland opposed. A French proposal was eventually adopted, this being that those nations who wished to have weight category competitions do so in their own countries, and in the European Championships special weight category events should be held for them which were not to interfere with the customary non-weight category competitions of Britain, France, Belgium, and Holland.

> On more than one occasion, differences of opinion in four or five quarters I occasioned a full scale battle of words, the contestants excitedly flinging their arms in the air. Suddenly, a split-second silence. Somebody smiled and the whole room dissolved into laughter!
> – meeting minutes

Those present were:

Messrs. Hartmann	Switzerland	Mr. Oletti	Italy
Mr. Plee	France	Mr. Genolini	Italy
Mr. Lasshan	E. Germany	Mr. Nauwelaerts	Holland
Mr. Johannson	Denmark	Mr. Nimfuhr	Austria
Mr. Koizumi	Britain	one unknown	Austria
Mr. Barnes	Britain	Mr. Schafer	Germany
Mr. Bonet-Maury	France	Mrs. Schafer	Germany
Mr. Marcelin	France	Dr. Torti	President, Italy
Mr. Verlinde	Belgium	Dr. Castelli	General Secretary
Mr. Callier	Belgium		

Strictly speaking some were not delegates but present as advisers or in some other capacity. Koizumi was one example of this. He was present as a Technical Adviser, as Barnes was the official British Judo Association (BJA) delegate.

The young lions of the time took little interest in the first tottering steps of the three new organizations; apart from lacking the experience and seniority necessary, they were far more interested in forwarding their personal prowess on the mat. This was certainly the case in Britain and it is unlikely that their counterparts on the European continent differed. It was during the decade starting in 1950 that Leggett encouraged and helped many on the trek to Japan, some sixteen from the Budokwai including myself. The next largest number of "Exiles" was provided by France, with other countries supplying smaller numbers. But to return to the Zurich meeting of 1952, Koizumi, who had been at a separate technical meeting, was invited by the Chairman Torti to address the delegates. This is what he said:

> When I was coming along this morning I was sorry, not only for myself but for all of you, that I was the instrument of your not being able to enjoy this lovely country and lovely weather today [A reference to his founding of the EJU in 1948]. From the way you have been struggling to solve the pressing problems at this conference, it seems that you are suffering from a sort of toothache which you do not know how to cure! That means that all these problems arose from the basis of competition championships and international contests. For a cure, I should like to advise you to extract this tooth—that is, to do away altogether with championships and international competition.
>
> To appreciate judo, its benefits and value, you must actually taste and digest it. That means you must partake of judo training. Like food, unless you eat and digest and enjoy the flavour and the quality of the food, you cannot appreciate its goodness. So it was on Friday, after two or three hours' hard struggle discussing technical problems of this conference, we were invited to go to Mr. Graf's dojo, and there on the mat we all mixed—seven nations—practising judo and partaking of training together. You ought to have seen the effect of that completely changed atmosphere, and the feeling of the people! There was no question of weight categories or other problems.
>
> We enjoyed the beer afterwards and the taste of the food, which completely changed after those two hours' training on the mat. That is judo. Without that there is no judo. You cannot express the realities of life. However wise or clever, they are always insufficient in terms of human language. Any move you may bring forward, if it is not to produce the result judo aims at, you are defeating its own end. Therefore, you must be very careful what you do today.
>
> Good positive work has been accomplished here, that is absolutely certain. Please do not make rules that are too hard and too fast. That is all I have to say.
>
> Thank you.

A few words of explanation are required here. Koizumi was not against contests per se. Like Jigoro Kano, he was against championships as they tend to deceive people into believing that contests of this nature are the ends rather than the means of training. Contests are a form of training and nothing more. Failure to see this is really a failure to fully understand judo. For those who never had the privilege of knowing Koizumi; he was teaching until the day before he died in April 1965. Altogether he spent over sixty-four years in judo and, apart from nine months in 1906 and 1907, he was a strict amateur for the rest of his life. At his death, he held the Kodokan grade of 8th dan.

Much more could be written about the early years, but this short chapter will suffice to acquaint readers of the origins of the three organizations. Before closing, here is an opinion from Mr. Somsak of Bangkok, a Kodokan 2nd dan, contained in a letter to E.J. Harrison in 1948:

> Emphatically judo should not be a mass movement. Its confinement to a select membership will curtail abuse which will result if it is an open affair to all and sundry. To cover up their inferiority complex or to feed their egoistical sense of importance, those with a rudimentary grasp of it are liable to make a detrimental use of this art, thus violating the Kano principles. It should not be taken up lightly and treated as any other game or sport. Just look what has been done to wrestling.

Was he was right? Many years later I wrote to the General Committee of one of the three bodies about its abuse of Jigoro Kano's principles, saying, "The Committee is striving to attain mediocrity—without much success." A remark which could apply to all three.

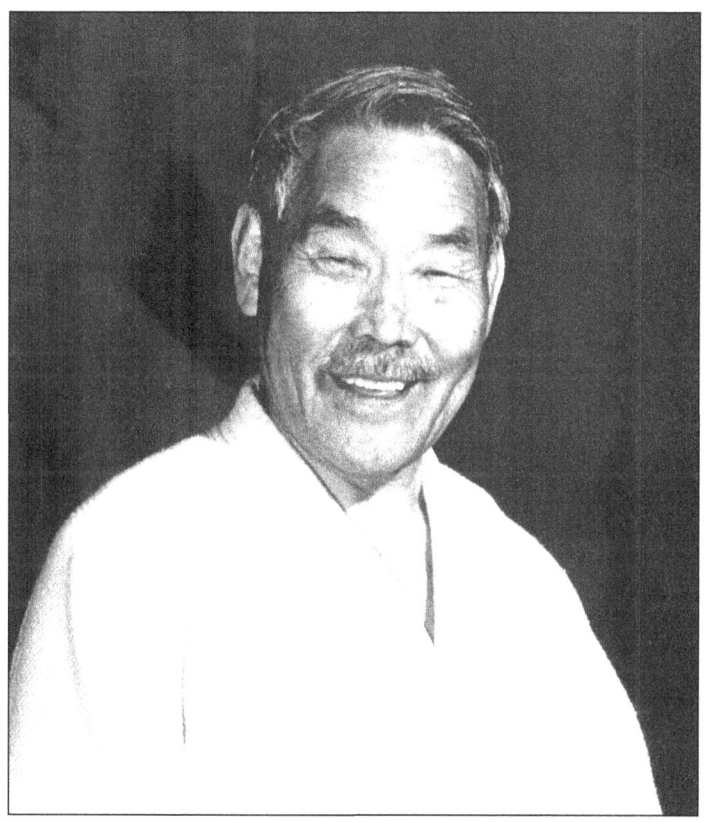

G. Koizumi, day before he died.

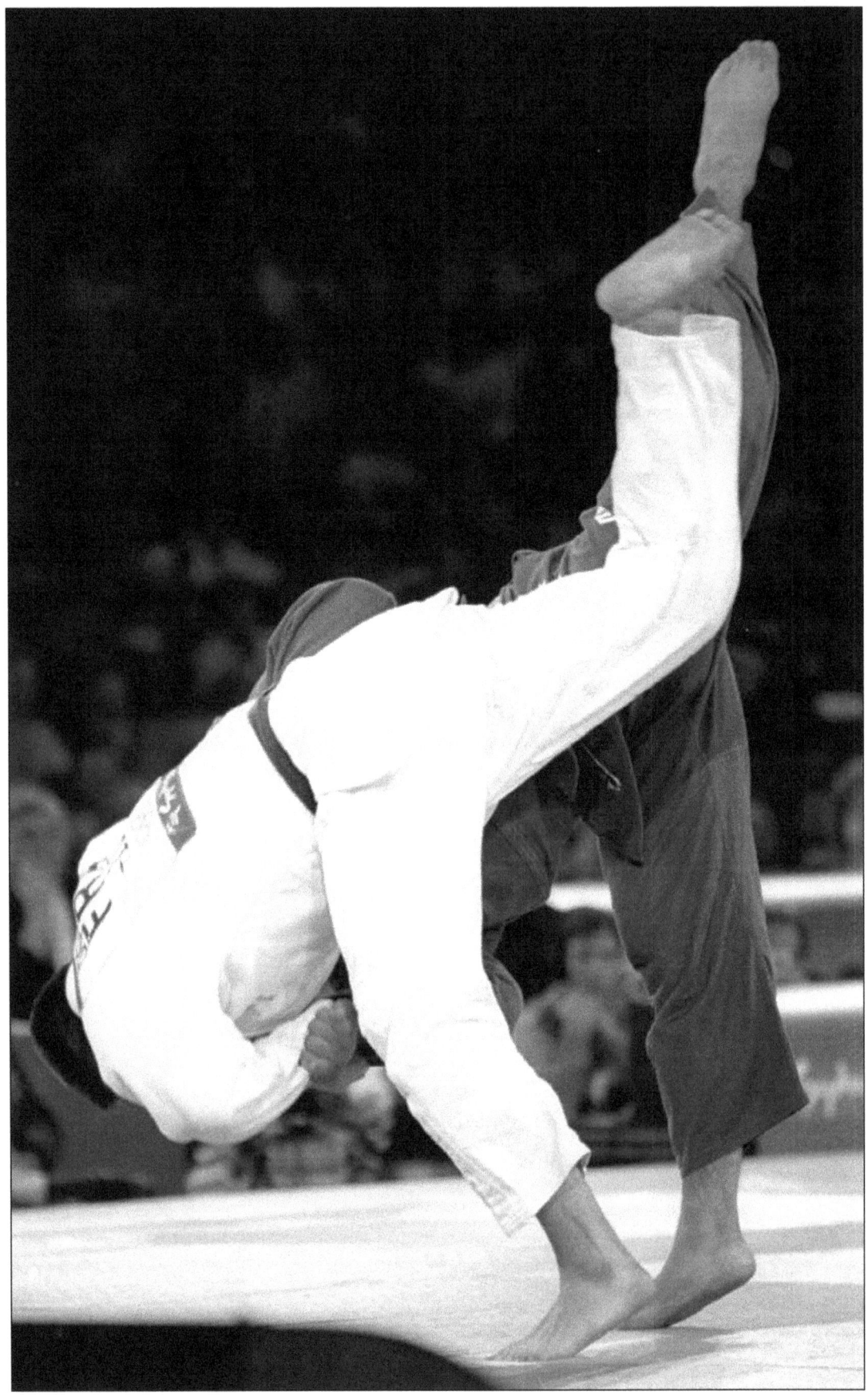

chapter 6

Repercussions from the Douillet v.s. Shinohara's Final Judo Bout at the 2000 Olympics in Sydney
by David Finch

Previous page: Douillet and Shinohara caught nicely by the camera in mid-technique. All photographs by David Finch.

Introduction
Frenchman David Douillet was not expected to retain the heavyweight Olympic title that he won at Atlanta. This was only his third competition in three years because of a recurring back injury following a motor cycle accident shortly after the 1996 Games.

Of those three competitions, the most important had been the May 1999 European Championships at Bratislava. There he had lost easily in the early rounds and succumbed to a winning score (*ippon*) in the repercharge (*the repercharge is a system used in tournament judo where the contestants beaten by the four semi-finalists in each weight category fight each other to fight the loser of the semi-final contests. This contest is then known as the "bronze medal contest" and there are two bronze medals in judo). After that, most people did not expect him to return to international competition.

Douillet had always intended retiring after the Sydney Games, and he waited until the very last minute to join the French team following a tournament in August that did not aggravate his back injury. Unlike his name, which means "wimpish" in French, Douillet is big in heart and in stature and as the reigning champion had an automatic right to defend his title. Injury or no injury, he did not miss the chance.

It was expected that Douillet's main opponent would be Shinohara of Japan who in the previous year had won the Birmingham World Championships in both the heavy and open weight categories with a unprecedented 11 winning scores from 11 contests. The last time the two had met was at the 1997 Paris World Championships. There, Shinohara was given an undeserved penalty and as a consequence Douillet won his second world title. However, this time Shinichi Shinohara was favorite.

Douillet progressed through to the final with only two fights, due to a withdrawal, and each was won easily by a winning point. Shinohara had a little more difficulty. He had three fights but could only manage a technical point win in the quarter final against the experienced Sanchez of Cuba.

The Exhibition Hall at Darling Harbour was full to capacity when both men stepped onto the mat. Their grips were opposite, Douillet right, Shinohara left, but the favorite throw of both was the inner thigh throw (*uchi-mata*), and it was to have a dramatic effect on the match.

One and a half minutes into the contest, Douillet hooked onto Shinohara's left leg for uchi-mata with his right. Being taller than the 134 kg Japanese, Douillet had his right arm over Shinohara's back and held his belt tightly. Both hopped to the left as the Frenchman tried to lift Shinohara with his right leg.

Shinohara is a predominantly left-handed player and at the Birmingham World Championships nearly half of his victories came from his left uchi-mata. Here, he could either try to block the attack by pushing his hip forward, releasing his own grip and driving his body weight across the line of attack in an attempt to collapse Douillet, but potentially risking an even heavier throw if Douillet succeeded with the thrust of his leg. Or, he could slip his left leg off of the attack and, as every judo man knows, use Douillet's attacking movement to his own advantage.

Shinohara chose the latter course and used uchi-mata-sukashi to counter the Frenchman. He cleanly slipped his left leg from the apex of Douillet's attack while, at the same time, pulling Douillet's right sleeve and pushing his chest with his left hand. It was at this stage that the Frenchman's over-shoulder grip on Shinohara's belt at the back prevented a perfect stance for the throw that ended with Douillet being flipped a full 180% to land squarely on his back.

Fractionally after Douillet hit the mat squarely and forcibly on his back, Shinohara was pulled down by the over-shoulder belt grip. As a consequence he fell on his right shoulder. Here the confusion started.

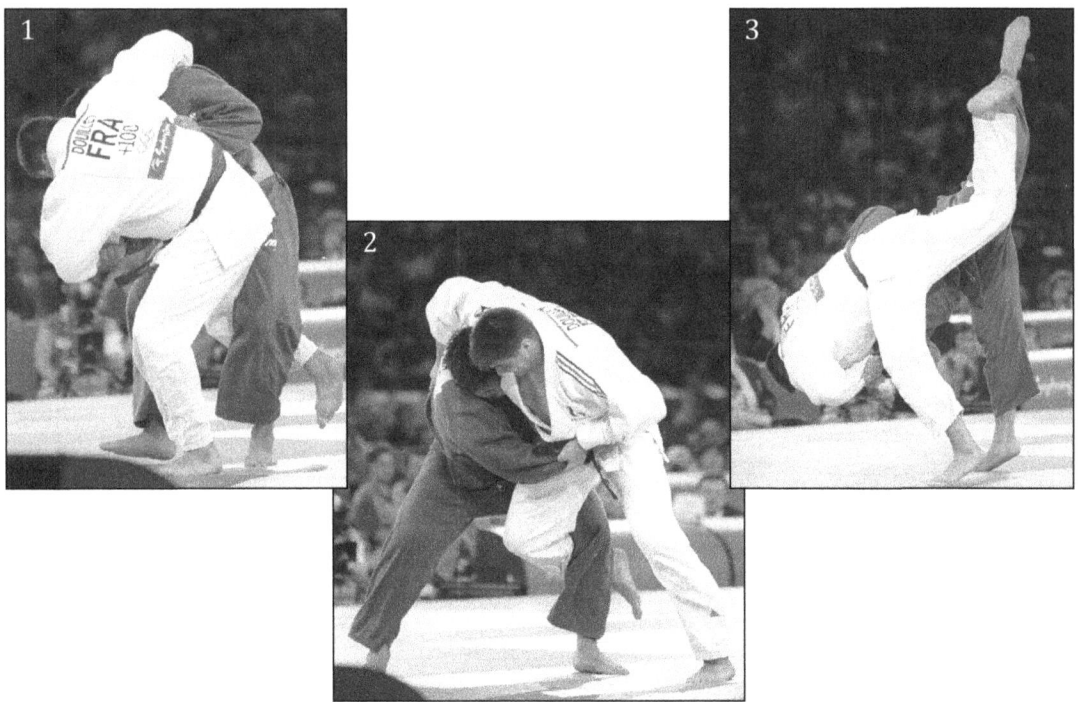

Photo #1-2: The initial attack by David Douillet shows him gripping Shinohara's belt with his right hand and inserting his right leg in readiness for the full inner reap (*uchi-mata*).
Photo #3: As Douillet lifts his right leg to throw Shinohara, Shinohara holds Douillet's left sleeve and pulls upwards while pushing with his left hand against the Frenchman's chest. At the same time Shinohara lifts his left leg higher than Douillet and performs uchi-mata-sukashi. With Shinohara still on his right foot, Douillet is flipped on his back but manages to unsettle Shinohara by still pulling on his belt.

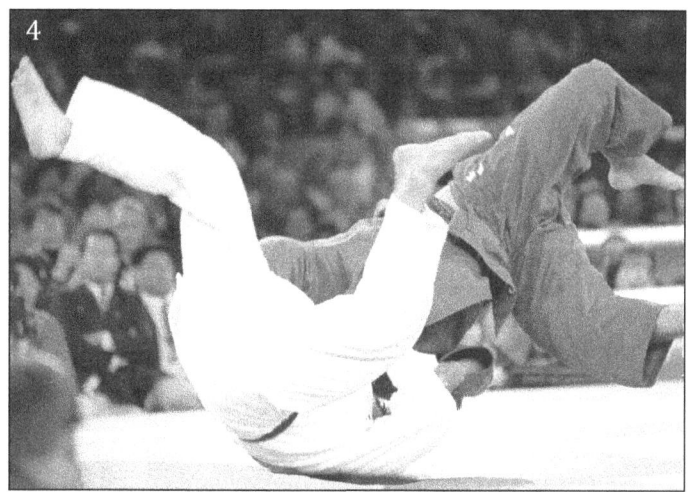
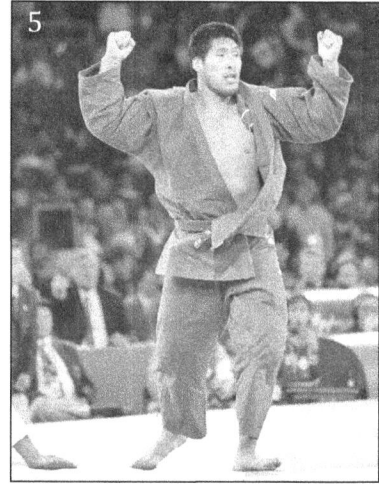

Photo #4: David Douillet is thrown cleanly onto his back but causes Shinohara to collapse by continuing to hold Shinohara's jacket at the rear.
Photo #5: Shonohara rises from the mat with his arms raised in a gesture of triumph after the corner judge with the best view of the throw signals an ippon score.

Immediately the corner judge nearest the pair stood and raised his arm to indicate a scored winning point throw by Shinohara. Shinohara also quickly leapt to his feet with both arms raised in a gesture of victory while Douillet regained his composure on his hands and knees. Seconds later the Frenchman got to his feet and looked incredibly guilty. It was not the worried look of a contestant who thought that the referee was going to award an undeserved point against him, but the look of a man who had made a bad mistake knowing that he had been thrown cleanly on his back. It was a shocked look of guilt and remorse.

The referee however, took an entirely different and, in the opinion of the writer, perverse view, signaling a technical point score to Douillet! He was not overridden by the other corner judge, who may have had his view obscured by the referee, and had not clearly seen the throw. The score stood. At the end of the contest, Douillet was pronounced the winner based on the following scores:

Douillet	Time	Shinohara
Technical Point	1:39 min.	
Minor penalty (*shido*)	1:55 min.	"Small" scored point (*koka*)
Serious penalty (*chui*)	2:40 min.	Technical Point or repeated shido
Technical Point	4:14	

TOTAL
2 Technical Points to
1 Technical Point and a koka

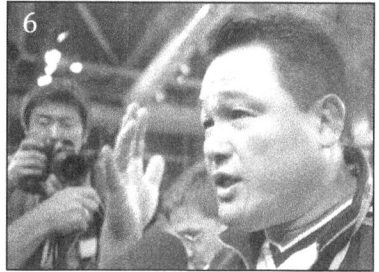

Photo #6: Legendary Olympic 1984 Champion and manager of the Japanese team, Yasuhiro Yamashita, talks to the press about the Douillet v.s. Shinohara contest. The press interviews continued late into the evening and went on for four hours!

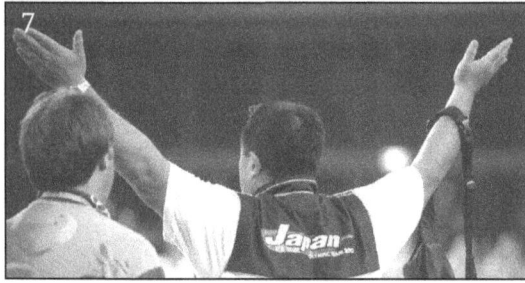

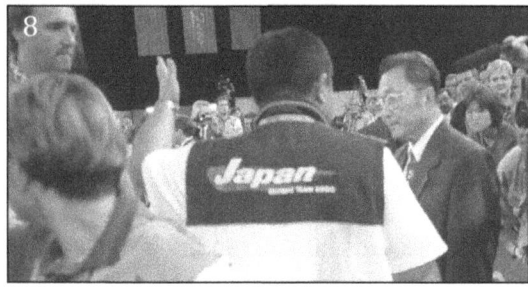

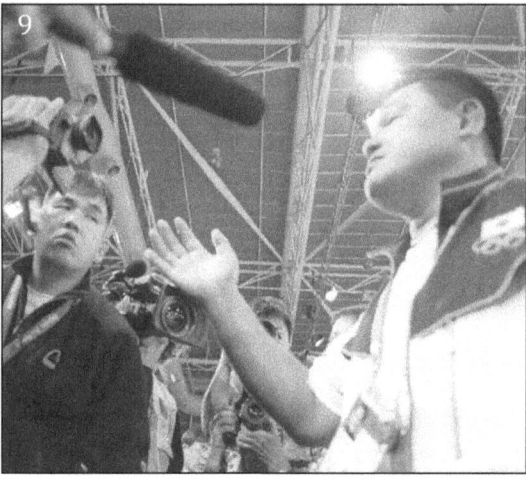

Photo #7: Throughout the contest Yamashita had sat quietly at the mat side instructing and supporting Shinohara in his fight with Douillet. When the contest finished and the referee awarded the fight to the Frenchman, Yamashita appealed beyond the referee and judges to the IJF Committee seated on the other side of the mat shouting "Ippon? Ippon? Ippon?!"

Photo #8: Yamashita appeals to the IJF refereeing director Jim Kojima of Canada. Kojima was heard to agree with Yamashita's assertion that the throw was a winning point for Shinohara, and this was even reported by the BBC in its Daily Olympic Round Up.

Photo #9: Yasuhiro Yamashita talking to reporters.

As Douillet was awarded the result at the end of the contest, he looked towards Shinohara and shrugged his shoulders. It was the look of a man that could not believe his luck!

The Repercussions

Both contestants bowed to each other. Douillet tried to console Shinohara with a hug, but Shinohara was totally dejected as he walked away. Had he been other than Japanese he would not have left the mat. In fact he would have remained to complain to the referee, the judges and all those in the stands that could not believe the result.

Legendary 1984 Olympic Champion and successful current Japanese team manager, Yasuhiro Yamashita, jumped to his feet, climbed the barrier and shouted across the mat to the International Judo Federation (IJF) Commission opposite. "Ippon?" he shouted with arms outstretched. "Ippon?" he shouted again, and the Japanese spectators joined in chorus with him, waved their flags and stamped their feet. In answer, Frenchmen with tricolor painted faces increased their shouting and cheers for Douillet's unbelievable victory.

Unlike Douillet, Yamashita does not have two Olympic gold medals. He only has one because of the Japanese boycott of the 1980 Moscow Olympics. But he does have an unbeaten international record in that makes him one of the most successful and respected athletes in the world with more than 200 international wins to his credit, tying with Ed Moses, of hurdling fame. And he is not a man to raise his voice without good reason.

Quickly he pushed past officials, respectfully skirted the mat and went straight to Jim Kojime, the Canadian IJF Director of Refereeing. Surrounded by the press and photographers, he reasoned with Kojime about the disputed winning point. Kojime was heard to agree with Yamashita, saying that he too thought it was a scoring point in favor of Shinohara but that nothing could now be done about the decision. Reluctantly Yamashita moved away and spent all of the next two hours being interviewed by Japanese journalists and TV interviewers.

At the end of the final day the men's heavyweight gold medal was awarded to Douillet and France. Although the record was clear cut, to those privileged to be present at such a contest of giants there were many who felt that there had been an injustice of major proportions. This was not a wrongly awarded *koka* or misapplied decision. A 'knock out blow' had been ignored!

Even the IJF Commission had immediately agreed that the refereeing decision had been controversial and prevented the official television rights holders from rerunning the disputed throw on the two gigantic screens in the hall. Throughout the seven days of judo this had only happened on one other occasion. That was when Yoshida of Japan in the 81 kg. division had broken his arm in several places in an attempt to avoid a quarter final winning point throw by Honorato of Brazil. At all other times the video screens had been used to rerun even the slightest score for the audience.

The refusal to allow the television rights holder to rerun controversial decisions stems from the 1997 Paris World Championships. There, during the men's 60 kg. division, there had been a refereeing decision of unimaginable incompetence when Kang of North Korea threw Revazishvili of Georgia for a minimum of half a winning point (*waza-ari*). The referee and two judges incorrectly awarded the score to the Georgian. Kang objected to the blatant error and refused to move from the spot. Consequently he was penalized and lost the contest through passivity. The television company repeated the throw on the large screens and it confirmed to all present that the score should have legitimately been awarded to the Korean. The crowd went mad, and pandemonium followed with many in the crowd throwing coins at the referee and judges.

The score was not reversed and at Paris Jim Kojima, IJF refereeing director, took the far reaching decision to protect his referees from their own incompetence by banning all future television reruns of controversial decisions. Referees can never be perfect. In the days before television it was not unreasonable for the referee to hold court and to have the last word on a contest. However, with television technology improving all the time, the IJF has its head in the sand.

This refusal to come to terms with the video recorder and to not use it to assist the referee and judges flies in the face of what is happening in other sports. In particular, wrestling uses video recorders specifically to aid referees, and it was so used at Sydney for the first time. Wrestling also has an appeals procedure that is almost instantaneous in its result. In the event that one side feels that there has been a wrong judgment they can appeal for a possible rerun of the match. However, they know that they have to put up a $1,000 security, and if they are proved wrong, then they will have to stump up the cash. Should they be proved right, then the match will be run again. It certainly prevents the frivolous appeals that are a common part of sport.

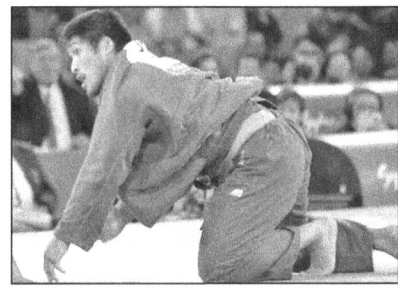

Shinohara on his hands and knees with a look of expectation on his face.

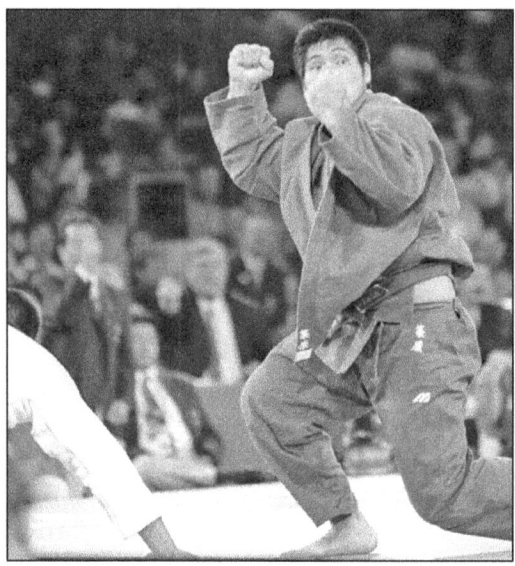

Shinohara turns towards the ecstatic Japanese crowd before the confused New Zealand referee indicates a perverse technical (*yuko*) score (5 points) to Douillet.

The Final Chapter

Following the completion of the Olympic judo competition, the All Japan Judo Federation wrote directly to the IJF on 29 September 2000, complaining about the inability of the referees to recognize Shinohara's uchi-mata-sukashi. On 9 October 2000 IJF President Park wrote back quoting the IJF rules and stating "All actions and decisions taken in accordance with the majority of three rule by the referee and judges shall be final and without appeal".

On 30 October the IJF Referee Commission chaired by Jim Kojime reported on the heavyweight final and the last line of their report read as follows: "... the IJF Referee Commission has come to the conclusion that neither contestant should be awarded a score since neither contestant had complete 'control' and a 'throw' was not executed."

If this was the true conclusion of the fight then the score would have been one technical point and a "small" scored point (*koka*) to Shinohara and a technical point to Douillet. But then the fight might very well have been played differently and perhaps more fairly if the referees were allowed to consult mat side video recorders.

In the All Japan Judo Federation letter of 29 September 2000 sent to the IJF, President Kano finished with the following: "In the event that no satisfactory decision is made, we will reluctantly be forced to file a more formal complaint in the Court of Arbitration for Sports (CAS)."

Perhaps Shinohara's silver medal will force the IJF to come to terms with modern video technology. It would certainly be better to decide a contest on the mat rather than at Lausanne through the Court of Arbitration in Sport.

▼▲▼

chapter 7

Judo and Character:
Moving from the Hard to the Gentle Way
by James Behrendt

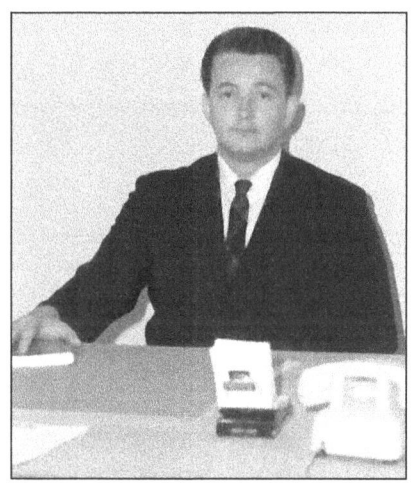
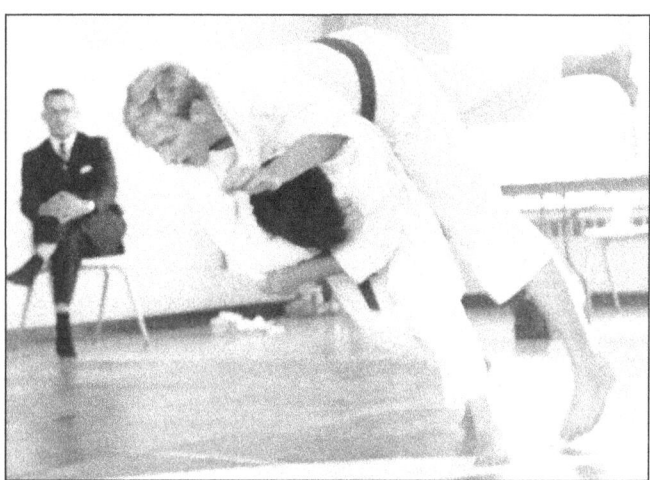

Left: James Behrendt in his judo school, October 1968.
Right: James Behrendt and the throw that won the
Iowa Amateur Athletic Union Grand Championship in 1968.

My philosophy of judo was learned the hard way. When I obtained my black belt in 1957, I was caught up in hard training and competition which became the center of my walk in the way. I was extremely fit and strong and I used those natural gifts to eventually defeat the purpose of the judo art. I had discipline but was lacking in spirituality and character. At that time I thought I would excel at the top if I were stronger and quicker than my opponents. I had aspirations of becoming a national or Olympic champion. I almost made it to the Olympics by winning the Iowa State Championships then the regional finals of the Pan Am Games. Those two wins qualified me to train with the Olympic candidates. An injury prevented me from finishing the training.

I won my berth at the nationals four times but never won at that level of competition; in fact the closest I came was placing fourth in Asbury Park, New Jersey. I missed the weight by 4 pounds and had to fight judo players 20 pounds heavier and stronger—players such as Iguchi Motohiko of Japan. Iguchi won the nationals in the heavyweight division. I prolonged my match with him almost to overtime and I thank God he finished me with only a wrenched knee.

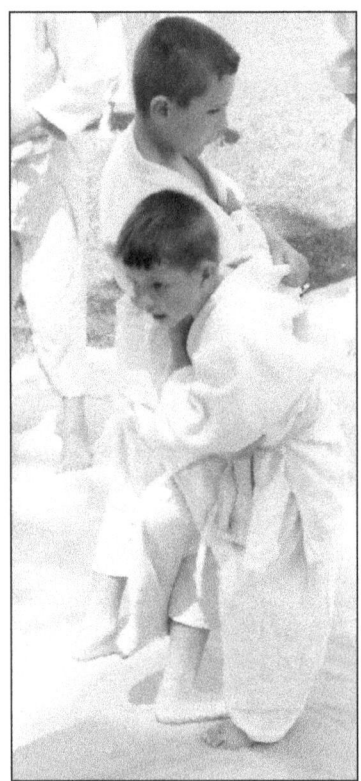 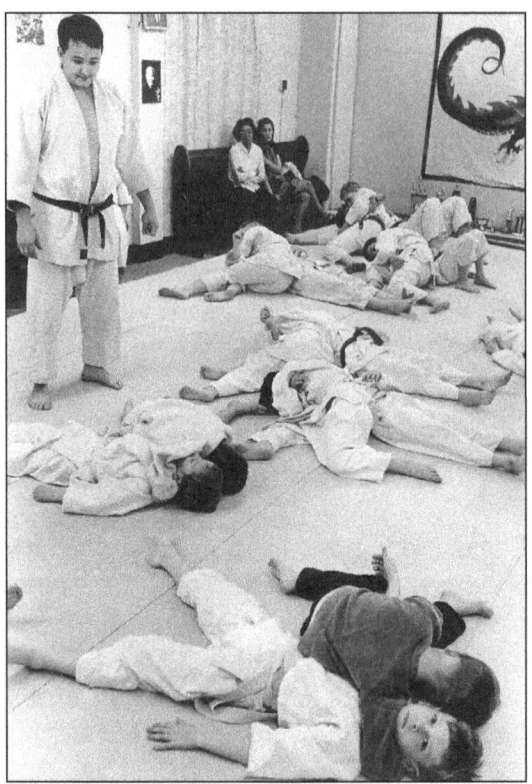

Left: Young students learning to leg sweep. The younger of the two is James Behrendt's son, Danny. Today, Danny is six feet tall, 200 pounds, and difficult to sweep! Right: James Behrendt teaching some groundwork with youngsters at his Rock Island Judo Training Center (1967).

I won dozens of local tournaments over a six-year period and that was not a good thing. I was unbeaten because my competition was weak and I loved the glory of the win. I was actually notorious everywhere in the country for being dangerous on the mat. My first devastating loss in years was when I drew a judo player named Leroy Abe. Abe looked like a slow, plodding, over weight, and out of shape Japanese. The match was in the later rounds and we munched and struggled with each other. With about thirty seconds left before the end of the match, I reminded myself that my strongest technique was on the floor. In desperation, I pulled Leroy upon me with brute strength, thinking that I would turn him over and pin him for thirty seconds for the winning point I thought I deserved. My teammates were aghast because they could only see a hand here and a foot there. It was like being crushed to death; never was I pinned so hard and defeated so badly. I wanted to perform harikiri after the match. I wouldn't have batted an eye if he had won by a decision or a throw, but to lose on the mat was like death. To lose that way was worse than death.

Some of the depression I was experiencing left at the restaurant at the Holiday Inn where we all were staying. I gasped as Leroy walked in with his team. I knew why I had lost. The man looked like a gorilla that had just come off the vine. He was huge; he had large biceps and wrists as big as most ankles; shoulders like coconuts and no neck. The man looked like a power lifter, not a judo player.

I learned my lesson well that day. Another match I lost on a decision was to a brown belt. For me, this was shocking. This brown belt attacked non-stop until time ran out. Being a black belt, I felt I would just defend and after four minutes, pull him to the mat and hold him for the win. The judge tossed the beanbag in and I was stunned. The bag was tossed three minutes into the match because brown belts, at that time, only fought three-minute rounds while black belts fought for five minutes.

That match was in Omaha, Nebraska, five hundred miles from my home in Illinois. Driving home on interstate 80, my car gave out. I asked my wife Marge and our four kids to get out of the car. As they stood by with their mouths wide open, I proceeded to push the four-year-old Mercury station wagon over the cliff. The car went through a barbed wire fence and made a "the the the" sound as it passed through the tall row of corn disappearing forever. A half hour later, my best friend and judo student came along and picked us up and drove us to the Greyhound station in Des Moines, Iowa, where we took the bus to Illinois. The kids loved the bus ride back. Poor Marge starred out the window in an almost catatonic stare into vast prairie and corn.

Pushing the car over the cliff exemplified the serious cracks in my character that I mentioned earlier: the strongest was hubris, the sickness of pride. Most religions of the world teach that pride is the deadliest of all sins, because when a person has hubris he is not teachable and never grows spiritually. He just keeps repeating his mistakes over and over without proper reflection or examination of conscience.

In 1992, my 16-year-old son Jimmy was training in a professional boxing stable with Orlin Norris and Jesus Salued, both world champions. Jimmy's coach, Jesse Valdez, had won a silver medal in the Olympics and was a champion in the professional ranks. He told me that young Jimmy had the tools to go all the way to the top in the boxing world because Jimmy out-trained everyone and could hit. Jimmy displayed knock-out power in both hands—a rare gift for a boxer.

Jimmy had another gift: common sense. One day he came home from training and said, "Dad, I'm in a very unique sport because the better I get, the more beat up I get." He made an evaluation: better skills, better opponents and a great chance of permanent brain damage. So he quit, joined a muscle grunt and groan gym, and went for a law degree. The kid is happy he never made it to the top and now boxes for fun, not for wins.

The point I'm making is, be humble enough to know your limitations and be able to accept your fate. Not everybody is a natural judo player. I have taught thousands of young men and women over the past 25 years and found only a small handful of people who had the tools go all the way. I knew of a girl here who was the world champion and when she weighed in she missed the weight by one more pound than I did at Asbury Park, and she was a lightweight. Figure that one out.

When I first came to California in 1969, I worked out in all the strong clubs in Los Angeles and was amazed by one very soft spoken judo player named Tosh Seino. He was a tall lightweight who was the national U.S. champion. An article in a judo magazine written by Kotani Sumiyuki from the Kodokan commented on Tosh. He was commenting on a big event in Chicago, where the All-Japan champions were here bouncing us all over the mats at will. Mentioning Tosh Seino, the commentator said to Kotani that "Tosh is not physically strong. He is just average, not really fast, and his technique is good but not great. How come this man beats everyone he competes against?" Without hesitating, Kotani quickly responded "*Stukeko* [timing]. The man has perfect timing. The man is gifted, period, and was actually born that way with perfect timing."

That gift must be complimented with humility and peace of emotions. To have perfect timing during attack, and especially defense, one must be free of negative emotions and not be over anxious. If you are over anxious, your reflexes will be exaggerated and slower, although strong. There is definitely something to the samurai who empties his mind when he pulls the sword and becomes the technique. If you have fear, you will tire quickly and be too defensive and eventually make a serious error. If you have anger, you will also tire quickly and be too slow and inaccurate and become a casualty.

I believe winning judo contests with strength and a strong will to win is not enough. In judo, one must be patient and persistent with humility. When a judo player takes on a new technique and tries to make it part of his offense in a match, it is not always successful at first due to the lack of maturity in that throw or counter. If a judo player is unsuccessful in that technique and loses because of failure to execute it due to the lack of character, the judo player tends to revert back to what worked before. He then chalks up that loss as a learning experience when all that he could learn is that he is pig-headed and not growing into a wholesome person.

I was blessed to have good instruction in judo. I just fell short in learning the virtues needed to be that great champion I lusted to be. In 1956, I was a young marine stationed in Opama, Japan. The Marines paid two Japanese instructors to come on the base to teach judo three times a week for a year. I never missed a class during that year. Instructor Ichinoe Maseo had love coming out of his ears and I eventually befriended him. Ichinoe loved mat work and we would sometimes grapple for two hours straight while the other instructor, Corporal Dame, worked on standing techniques.

Years later he came to visit me in Chicago. Ichinoe was about five foot six and 240 pounds and had huge wide feet that were impossible to move with any type of sweep. His technique was the spring hip throw (*hane goshi*) and when he came to Chicago he lined up twenty black belts and threw them at will with only the spring hip throw. I was spellbound and couldn't believe he could pull that off at fifty plus years of age.

My judo philosophy tells me, if we want to grow and someday resemble judo in a style or the great master Mifune Kyuzo, one must remove personal faults and replace them with virtues. If we were to uncover Mifune's spiritual walk, one would find a wealth of information that would enhance one spiritually and psychologically. Recently, I was watching a televised segment on Japanese Olympic champions. They asked a young man what his favorite part of judo was and he replied: "The hot baths and the fellowship." That was part of his judo. A judo player is more than just a machine. He is a wonderful balanced person. Yamashita of Japan, the greatest judo player of all time, said the same thing. His favorite thing in training was eating with the children and telling them jokes and stories. I experienced a similar thing at a big religious prayer meeting. The priest stated at the coffee and doughnut break that the fellowship at the break was just as important as what goes on in the prayer circle. In summation, character does count, big time. We are not the center of the universe. That spot is reserved for a greater being, however you wish to name it.

As you know, most judo throws are based on circles and you want to be in the center because that is where the power is. Move closer to the center because, in addition to power, peace is there too. Ride on the shirt tails of a power greater than yourself and you will have a Gentle Way.

chapter 8

Ulla Werbrouck: Olympic and European Judo Champion Retires
by David Finch

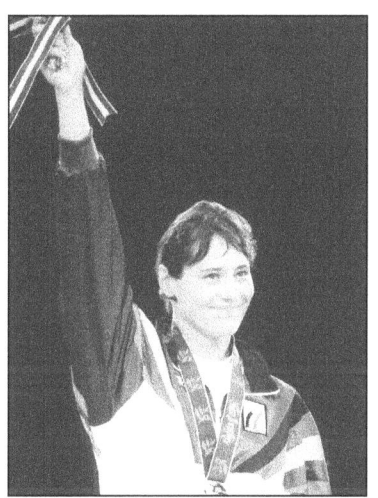

On the final day of the 2002 Wuppertal German World Open (23-24 February), 1996 Olympic champion Ulla Werbrouck of Belgium retired from competition judo. Her international career started in 1987 when she won a silver medal at the Junior German Open at Hamm and culminated in spectacular style with the 72 kgs (158.7 lbs.) Olympic title at Atlanta. She retires as the current 70 kgs (154 lbs.) European champion and since 1994 had accumulated seven European light heavyweight titles.

Ulla Werbrouck is not a stranger to North America: She reached seventh place in the Hamilton (Canada) 1993 World Championships, won the Atlanta Olympics 72 kgs (158.7 lbs.) gold medal, and won a gold medal at the 1998 US Open at Colorado Springs. She has even trained in Cuba, where her most serious opponents came from: Veranes, who beat her for the gold medal at the 1999 Birmingham World Championships, and Luna Castellano who took the 1995 World title from under her nose by a whisker. Over the past ten years, she has resoundly beaten her US competitors: Jiveden lost at the 1995 Tokyo Worlds; D'Anya Bierria lost at the 1997 Paris Worlds and the 1999 Munich World Masters; and Sandra Bacher lost at the 1999 Munich World Masters and 2001 Munich Worlds. So, Werbrouck's retirement will come as a relief to United States judo.

All photos courtesy of Judo Photos Unlimited,
Grove House Cross Dr., Chartway St. Sutton Valence, Kent ME17 3NP England
Tel/Fax: +44 (0) 1622.842240 Email: davidfinch@judophotos.com

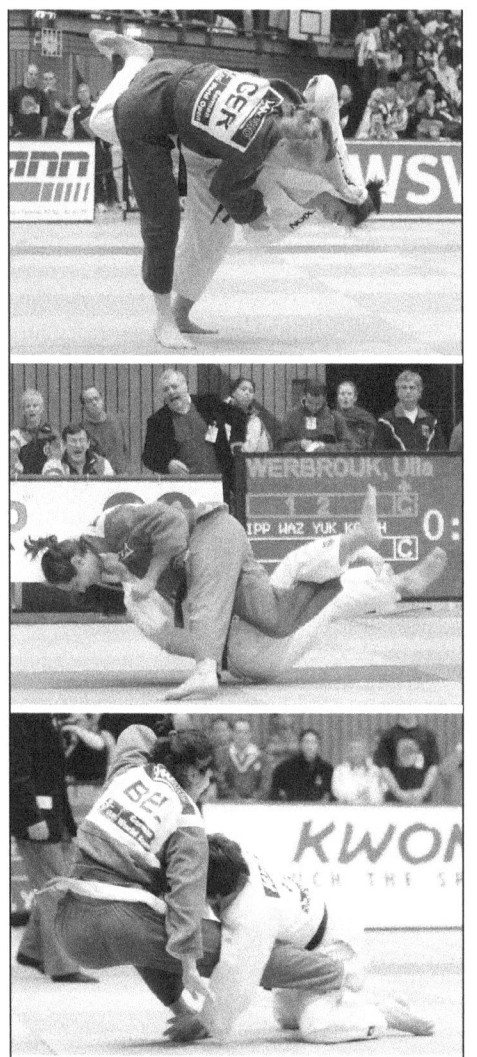

It was not a coincidence that Werbrouck's announcement that she would retire from competition at the German World Open followed her dismal display at the Tourni de Paris two weeks earlier and a few days after her thirtieth birthday. There, Werbrouck—one of the few 'big hitters' in women's judo and a national heroine in Belgium with the car license plate of JUDO 43—had lost in the first round by a "small advantage" (*koka*) and then a throw that lacked enough quality to score a full-point (*wazari*) in the repercharge (the repercharge is a tournament judo system where the contestants beaten by the four semi-finalists in each weight category fight each other to fight the loser of the semi-final contests. This contest is then known as the "bronze medal contest" and there are two bronze medals in judo.)

Coincidentally, the last time she had lost so badly was at the February 1998 Paris Tournament when she crashed out to a tremendous scoring point by an unrated rival and failed to make the repercharge. But the reasons then were very different. In her efforts to add the October 1997 world title to her Olympic crown, she had badly damaged her shoulder ligaments at a training camp in Cuba and could only manage a World bronze. It was the same nagging injury that started the 1998 season off so badly.

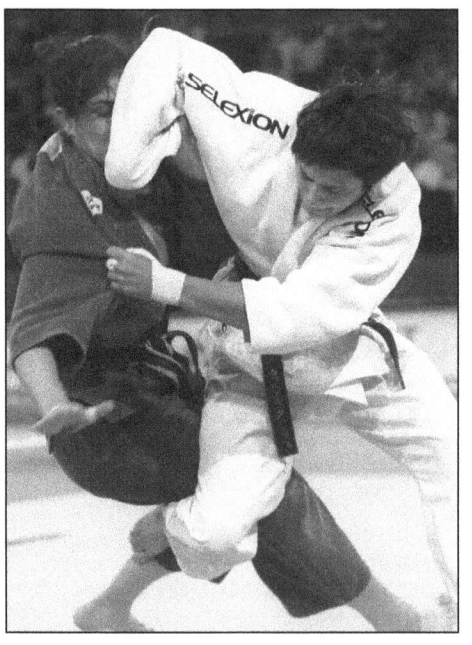
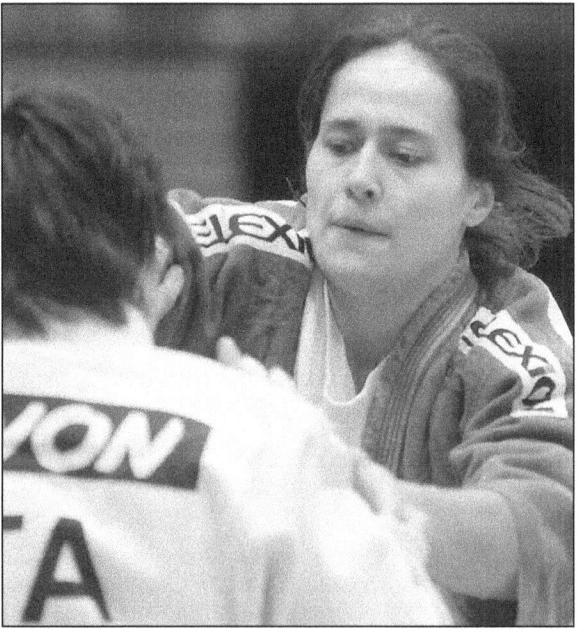

Ulla Werbrouck's next tournament was the Munich World Masters, two weeks later. There she reached the final, but for the first time in several meetings lost to 1996 Olympic bronze medalist Ylenia Scapin, an Italian fighter three years her junior. They met again in the final of the 1999 Wroclaw (Poland) Europeans, where Werbrouck returned to form and in an early flurry of action took both to the ground with Werbrouck in a dominant position on top. She systematically tied up Scapin with a "chest hold" (*mune-gatame*) and "cuddled the upstart" into submission. At the same time, Werbrouck set a European record as the first person to win six consecutive gold medals. Along with the rest of the Belgian team, she went wild and her longtime coach, Jean-Marie Dedecker, could not restrain his feelings, almost weeping with delight on her shoulder.

Werbrouck dominated further meetings with Scapin until they met in the third round of this year's Wuppertal German World Open. There, in front of over 400 yellow-shirted and "Werbrouck" chanting Belgian supporters, Scapin floored Werbrouck with a left major inner throw (*ouchi-gari*, see picture) for the only score of the match, a minor "small advantage." But the damage had been done and Werbrouck was prevented from retiring in style. She fought back through the repercharge with several spectacular throws and bowed out to her loyal and jubilant fans on the podium with a bronze medal.

All day, her mentor and coach, Jean-Marie Dedecker, had been at mat side, urging her on and sharing in the sadness of her farewell speech that afternoon. He had first spotted her as a 13-year-old Belgian junior champion in 1985. He quickly convinced her and her parents that she needed to train with the Belgian National Team. Four years later, she had won two European Junior 72 kgs (158.7 lbs.) titles and took the 66 kgs (145.5 lbs.) senior bronze medal at the Helsinki Europeans, where Belgian Ingrid Berghmans fought at the heavier weight. The following year, she won the Junior World 72 kgs gold medal, ideally placing her to take over the mantle of the Belgian heroine and world legend, Ingrid Berghmans, who was about to retire from competition.

There is nobody more responsible for the success of Ulla Werbrouck and Belgian judo than Jean-Marie Dedecker. Now an elected Belgian senator and astute businessman, he is consistently gaining the best sponsorship for Belgian judo; even now, he personally sponsors six judo fighters and athletes from other sports, including figure skating and the triathlon. But his first love is judo. In twenty years at the top, he has masterminded the winning of more than 130 Olympic, World, and European judo medals for one of the smaller countries of the world. His team even took six of the sixteen gold medals at the 1997 European Championships; an unprecedented feat.

At the 1996 Atlanta Olympics, Ulla Werbrouck reached the pinnacle of her career. This followed a particularly disappointing world silver medal the previous year at the Mukuhari (Japan) Worlds, when she lost on a referee's split decision. In fact, in six senior World Championships (earning her two silver and two bronze medals), this was the closest she ever came to winning the title that she craved, losing to Diadenis Luna Castellano of Cuba, whose hyperactive and persistent aggressiveness prevented Werbrouck from getting into position for a clean attack, relegating her to be considered the most passive of the two fighters. The defeat made her more determined and, luckily for Werbrouck, Luna Castellano was in the other pool at Atlanta, along with the two other front-runners for the title, Essombe of France and Yoko Tanabe of Japan. Tanabe emerged at the top of the other table following earlier point wins with her favorite left throw to the inner thigh. Werbrouck sailed through her half with a variety of holds and throws culminating with her favorite right uchi-mata throw for the winning point in the semi-final.

The final was to be dominated by the inner thigh throws of both women. Tanabe was six years older than Werbrouck and nearly the same height of 5 feet 8 inches (1.79m). She

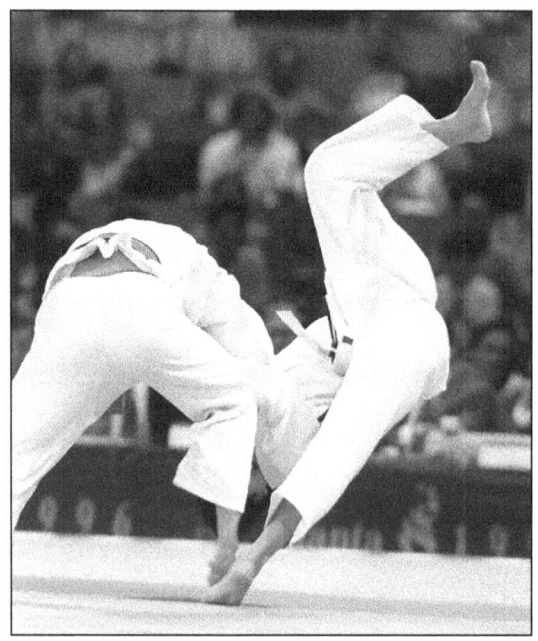
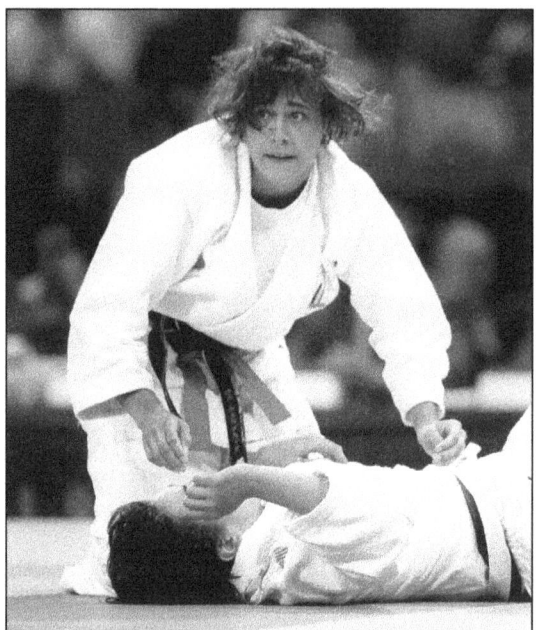

already had an Olympic silver and bronze medal to her credit and was determined to improve on that. She attacked first, with her left inner thigh throw and was easily pushed aside by Werbrouck as the attack lacked penetration. Werbrouck followed up with a left counter sweep and scored a technical point.

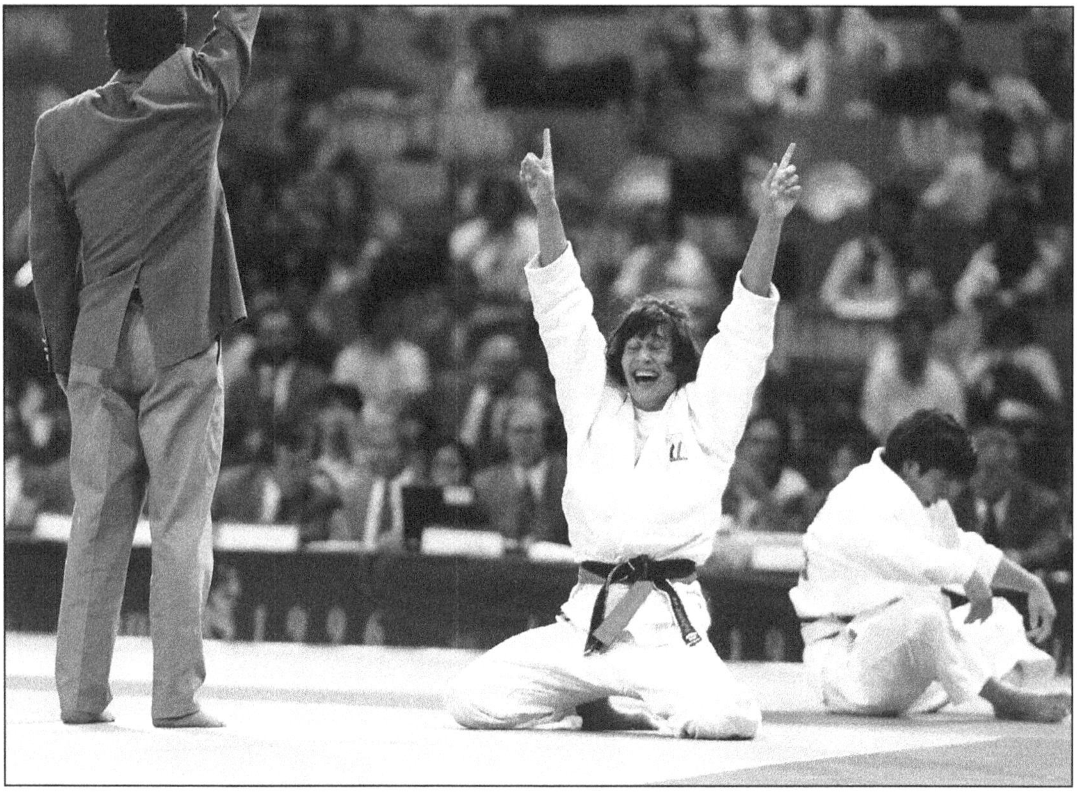

Troubled by the score, Tanabe again attacked with a fiercer left inner thigh throw, taking Werbrouck scorelessly to the mat. Then, hovering close to the red area, Werbrouck unleashed her right inner thigh throw, almost head diving into the mat but rolling over

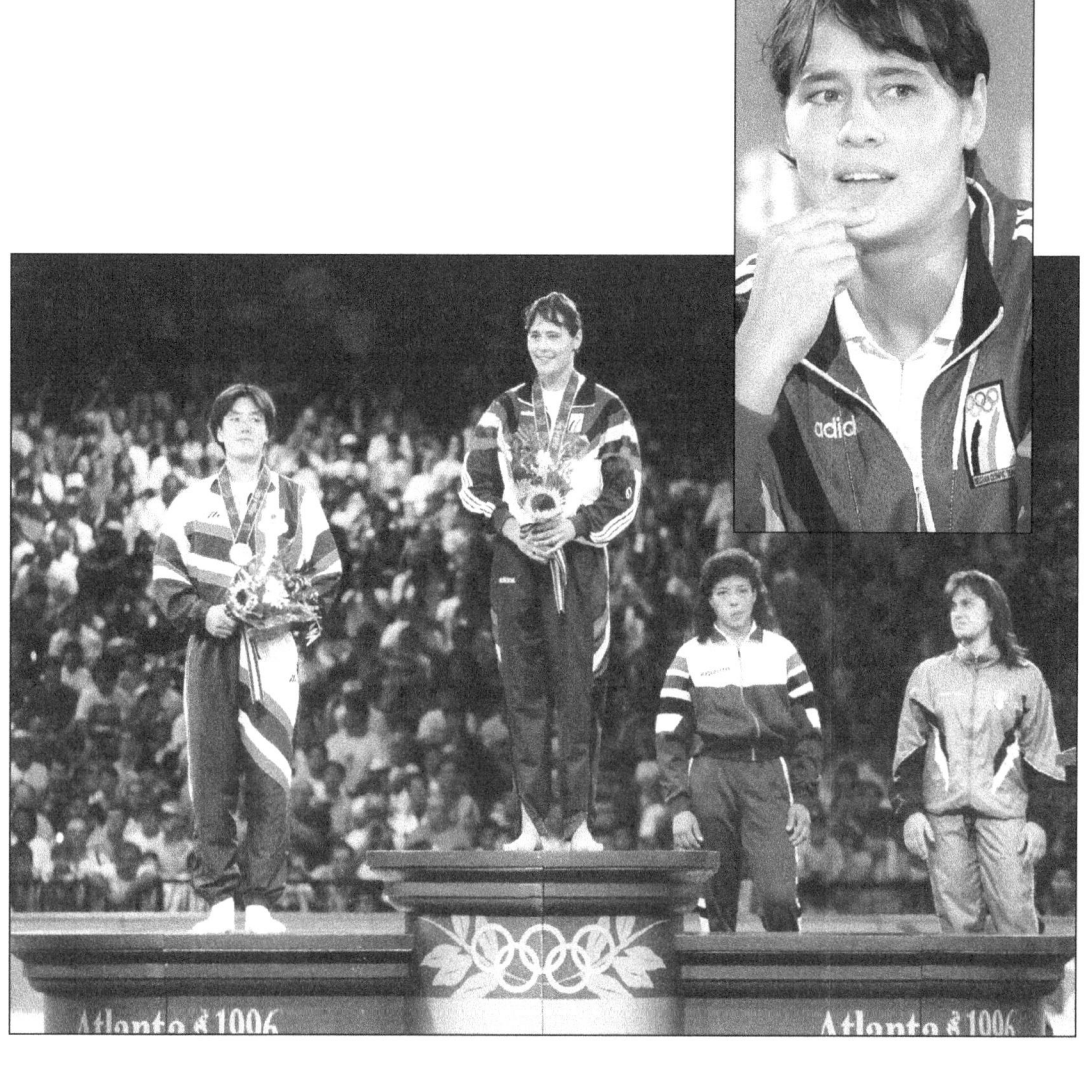

her right arm and elbow to prevent a penalty and putting Tanabe heavily on her side and another technical point on the board. Trailing by two five-point scores (*yuko*) and with only a few seconds of the contest left, out of exasperation, Tanabe came in for her third and even fiercer left inner thigh throw. By this time, Werbrouck aware of the pattern, sidestepped the furious attack and easily slipped her right leg over Tanabe's flying left. In an almost body drop like position (see photo), and with only two seconds left on the clock, she pivoted Tanabe over her own hands heavily onto the mat. The result was a perfect inner thigh sweep (*uchi-mata sukashi*) for a full point and the Olympic title, followed by a deliriously ecstatic Werbrouck (see photo).

Ulla Werbrouck, who enjoys wearing high heels to increase her height and feminine charms after judo training, married Dimitri Himpe in January 1998 and at the time said, "I have no plans for children until after the 2000 Sydney Olympics." With the Olympics nearly two years ago, are children now on her mind or is it even possible that her first child is on the way?

▼▲▼

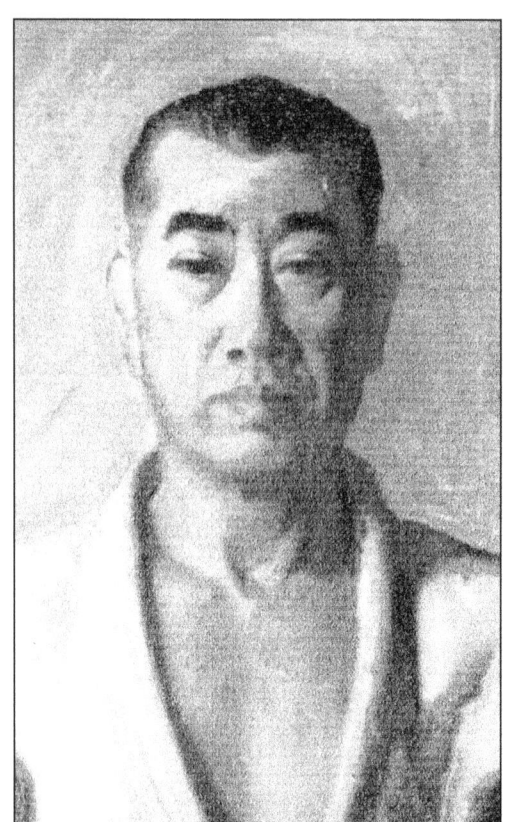 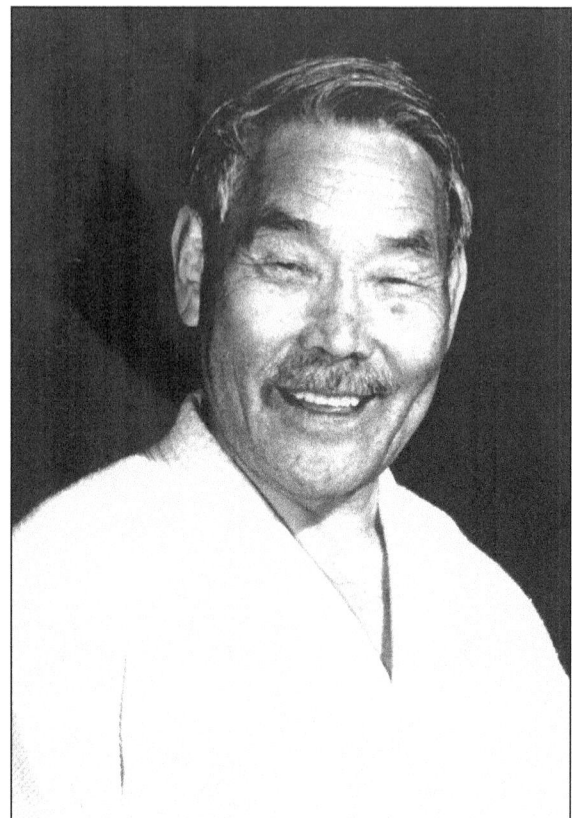

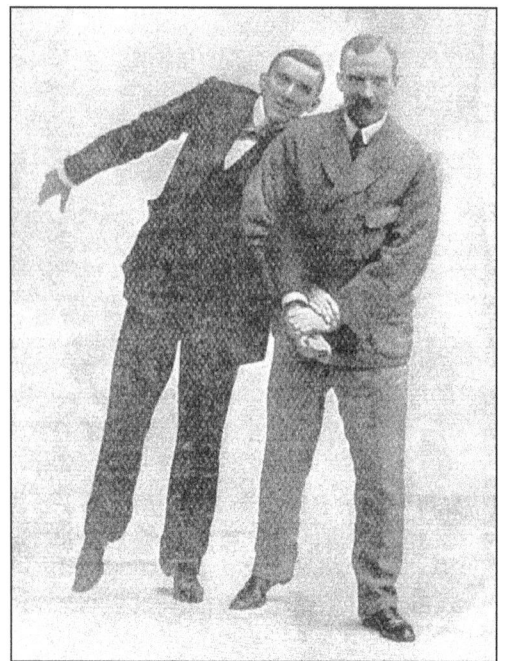 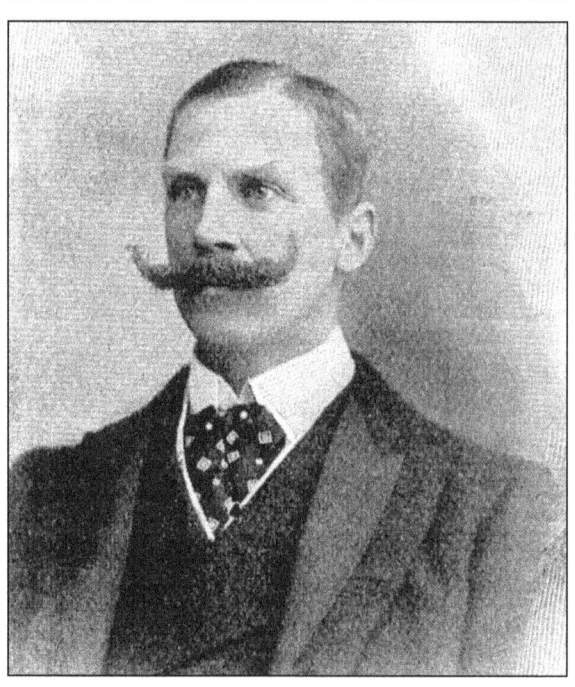

1) One of the prime movers of judo in England: Yukio Tani (1930's).
2) Another prime mover of judo in England: Gunji Koizumi (below, 1950's). Courtesy of Richard Bowen and the London Budokwai.
3-4) William Barton-Wright (1860–1951), studied Kodokan Judo in Japan. He was responsible for bringing Yukio Tani to England in 1900 to teach judo.

chapter 9

Sport, Industrialism, and the Japanese "Gentle Way": Judo in Late Victorian England
by Geoffrey Wingard, M.A.

On April 18, 1888, two men, one English and one Japanese, presented a lecture to the Asiatic Society of Japan in Yokohama entitled, "Jiujutsu [sic]: The Old Samurai Art of Fighting Without Weapons" (Lindsay and Kano, 1889). The lecture, in English, was delivered to a European audience. This event stands as the first recorded lecture delivered to a body of Western academics covering the history, methodology, and philosophy of Japanese unarmed fighting. Within the next twenty years, however, lectures and demonstrations of Japanese unarmed fighting methods grew in popularity. Talks and demonstrations on the subject were presented in London on at least three occasions during the late Victorian era and a number of books and articles were published in English.[1] During the same period, clubs and training halls opened throughout England to teach the Japanese methods of unarmed combat and eclectic methods of self-defense composed of English boxing, French savate (kick-boxing) and Japanese "wrestling."[2]

The growing interest among Westerners (especially among the English) in Japanese fighting systems was not simply another example of the Victorian penchant for collecting esoteria. The rapid introduction of Japanese combatives to England (and from England to the rest of the Euro-American world) was the result of broader trends both within English society and Japan's political and martial culture. For several unique reasons, the English at the end of the 19th century embraced an idealized characterization of Japanese society that predisposed them to accept the special combination of moral and physical practices that were promoted as the cornerstone of the Japanese martial arts. At the same time, the Japanese were anxious to showcase aspects of their culture on the world stage as they sought to rapidly modernize Japanese industry and to quell secession within Japan. The result of these complementary trends was the popular acceptance of the Japanese martial arts in Britain, especially the acceptance of judo and jujutsu. The integration of the Japanese martial arts into English society occurred rapidly. By the first decade of the 20th century, judo was being taught at Oxford University and other colleges and in the upper-class public school system. Public martial arts instruction was available in London and other urban centers (Miyake and Tani, 1906:9). By 1918, there was enough popular interest in judo for Japanese ex-patriot Gunji Koizumi to establish the Budokwai in London, an organization that continues to set the standard for judo instruction in Britain and which is now the oldest martial arts organization in England (Bowen, 1999). Judo was taught by both men and women to adults of both sexes (a radical development in the practice of Victorian sport) and to children. Significantly, the popularity of judo and other martial arts has only increased over time. As political scientist Max Skidmore (1995:129) has stated, "There is hardly a community of any size in Europe and the English-speaking lands in which there is no instruction available in one or more of the martial arts." Judo and other Japanese martial arts were clearly important in Victorian England and subsequently have made great inroads in Western society. Their historical popularity was hardly accidental. There were several reasons why the English showed such great interest in and enthusiasm for Japanese fighting methods, reasons that can only be understood in the broader context of Victorian class stratification and industrialization.

Of the several factors that coalesced to create an atmosphere hospitable to the introduction of Japanese martial arts in late Victorian England, Britain's role in the creation of modern sport weighed heavily. Modern sport and the sports ideal were disseminated from the upper and middle-classes to workers and the poor. At the same time, increasing urbanization and the concurrent rise in the fear of urban crime and ruffianism contributed to England's rapid acceptance of Japanese fighting methods. Finally, widespread disillusionment with the management and practice of traditional English fighting sports and a strong, anti-modern, nostalgic longing for the (largely mythic) pre-industrial past combined to make English society receptive to the introduction of the Asian martial arts, particularly Japanese judo and jujutsu. Examining the interconnected complex of these factors is the only way to explain why the Japanese martial arts were introduced and rapidly accepted in English society.

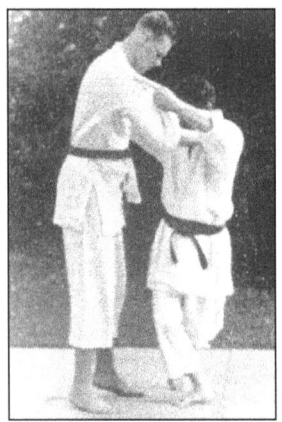 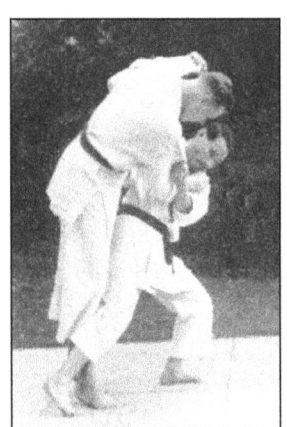 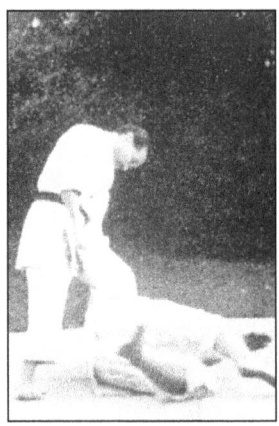

Gunji Koizumi (8th-dan), Father of the Budokwai,
does a body drop throw on Trevor Leggett.
Courtesy of Richard Bowen and the London Budokwai.

As the modern sport ethic developed in England, first within upper-class public school students and administrators and later among middle and working-class players, English attitudes toward sports underwent a radical transformation (Guttmann, 1978; Holt, 1989). Sports were transformed from celebratory, local, participatory events into codified, multi-local and national games that were supported by hierarchical institutions regulated at levels above those occupied by most players and spectators. An eventual result of this shift in the composition of English sport and the growth of modern athleticism was the development of a strange dichotomy among supporters of the athletic movement that pitted two views of sports against each other. On one hand, sports were seen as institutions bound by rules that limited participation and encouraged spectatorship (sowing the seeds of professionalism and commercialism). On the other hand, sports were ideally practiced for their own sake with the understanding that diligent practice and "good sportsmanship" would generate positive behavior and attributes among players off the field as well as on.

Primarily this last tenet, which held that sports were good for the soul as well as for the body, that encouraged sports proselytizers to cast their nets wide as they embraced games and game-players outside of the public-school milieu. The rise of the new sports ethic (and its proselytizing moral accompaniment, "Muscular Christianity") fostered a missionary desire to spread the sport message beyond its original school, class and national boundaries. Both Christian and athletic missionaries carried the sports message to the far corners of the English empire and consequently brought it into contact with games and attitudes alien to English upper and middle-class society. It was these missionary movements that initially introduced the Japanese martial arts (especially a new, "scientific" martial art called judo) to England.

Within England, one effect of the sports missionary movement was that groups of people who had little previous exposure to modern sports (although they may have been familiar with traditional games) were encouraged to participate as players or spectators. Middle and upper-class sports missionaries fully expected that the benefits of good sportsmanship, moral righteousness, Christian virtue, and good health would transfer to poor and working-class athletes. Victorian sportsmen felt that participation in athletics would not only change the behavior of the more "sordid" classes to which sports were introduced, but also that sport could change the moral character of participants. Sports were supposed to solve anachronistic problems of class and region that hindered expansion and industrial urbanization; in essence sport was intended to create new, moral, modern men. The physical and philosophical amalgam that Victorian sports missionaries found in the Japanese martial arts seemed perfectly suited to their moral/athletic mission.

Of primary concern of upper and middle-class English urban elites was the question of how to mitigate behaviors and attitudes among the poor and working-classes that seemed symptomatic of the deeper negative effects of city life. Working in factories rather than in shops and living in tenements rather than on farms had had the effect of weakening the social controls that had developed along with the strong British agricultural and artisan traditions. Changes in social structure and in class relations between workers and elites threatened the elite status quo. Members of the upper-class viewed these changes as the negative by-products of industrialism and urbanization and worried that they would jeopardize England's ability to bear the burden of maintaining industrial and political primacy.

These upper-class concerns contained at least a germ of substance. Once free of traditional social controls, the poor and working-classes began to rebel against authority and to organize in ways that threatened the established upper-classes. The upper-class response was to devalue liberal working-class mores and to accuse any working-class departure from the upper-class standard as sin. After nearly a hundred years of industrialization (and rebellion), the poor were routinely accused of engaging in a variety of vices. The upper classes believed (with at least a degree of accuracy) that gambling, drunkenness, prostitution, and thievery were endemic in poor and working-class neighborhoods and that they were, in fact, the natural consequences of poverty when allowed to proceed unconstrained by upper class morality (Thompson, 1963). The wealthier classes, who claimed to be concerned for the souls of the poor, were more likely concerned with the integrity of their social system and in some neighborhoods with the sanctity of their own skins. The upper-classes grasped at a variety of methods by which they could influence the social behavior of the poor and working classes. Their support for the moral sport movement was one such attempt to impose at least some nominal social controls upon the urban working-classes.

However, there were also real physical threats associated with inter-class discontent in Victorian England. The threat of "ruffianism" was a widely held concern among upper- and middle-class urban professionals, and there is some evidence that this fear may have been legitimate. While it is undoubtedly true that upper-class Victorians had a somewhat inflated sense of danger and an unsubstantiated fear of crime, there were undoubtedly dangers to living in the city (Englander, 1991). Drunkenness, prostitution, and lewd behavior threatened the integrity of moral institutions such as church societies upon which many facets of upper-class Victorian authority were based. Furthermore, governmental authorities could not guarantee individuals' safety outside of limited venues. There were real physical dangers inherent in 19th-century urban life to which city dwellers had to respond. One way that the Victorian elite used to fight back was through the practice of the traditional "manly arts," among which judo was rapidly integrated.

The specter of the physical threat to upper- and middle-class individuals from poor and working class hooligans in the streets could take different forms. Andrew Davies has examined one of the most prominent physical threats, a form of gang violence called "scuttling." Davies has analyzed the role played by "scuttlers" or youth gang members in violent crime in two late Victorian industrial cities, Manchester and Salford (Davies, 1998). He concluded that, although the most frequent targets of scuttlers were rival gang members, there was a real threat to any individual forced to travel in a gang area regardless of class, even among those who had no gang connections. Gang members were known to assault "local people who complained about a gang's activities, and occasionally, passers-by who strayed into territory to which a scuttling gang laid claim" (Davies, 1998). Though their fears may have been exaggerated, late Victorian elites shared attitudes about urban danger that had at least some basis in fact. Along with their need to assert social control, upper-class Victorians had need of a means of self-defense to respond to urban danger. Victorian urbanites uniquely combined their solutions to the dilemmas posed by both moral and physical threats. They synthesized physical methods of self-defense with a moral mission as they introduced the sport ethic into the "Satan's strongholds" inhabited by the working poor (Thompson, 1963). One way they did this was by adopting Japanese martial arts that, like judo, incorporated moral instruction along with physical practice into the English sports curriculum.

Some English sportsmen did try to refine traditional English fighting sports (primarily boxing and wrestling) to meet their moral and practical purposes. However, for a number of reasons, this option proved largely unacceptable in late Victorian, upper-class society. Boxing (pugilism or fisticuffs) and wrestling were hardly considered appropriate past-times for upper-class Britons. Pugilism and prize fighting, for example, although originally accepted and sponsored by the upper classes (Holt, 1989:19–20), had fallen into disrepute due to their association with gambling, drunkenness, and publicanism. Popular boxing had become the province of the lower classes as fisticuffs became "the poor man's version of dueling." Meanwhile, reforms to sport pugilism such as the introduction of gloves and timed rounds actually made it more dangerous and therefore less accessible to upper-class practitioners (Gray, 1897). Furthermore, wrestling was considered a coarse country sport and as such it held little appeal for the increasingly sophisticated urban crowd (at least among the upper-class English who composed the majority of sports proselytizers). Wrestling was associated with fairs, gambling, and drunkenness and seemed to glorify an anachronistic sense of regionalism. In Farkas and Corcoran's *The Overlook Martial Arts Dictionary*, the only indigenous English fighting system listed is "Corno-Breton" wrestling, a style of fighting relegated to the culturally and linguistically distinct Cornwall region. The limited characteristics attributed to this sport speak to the regional nature of wrestling sports in general in England and wrestling's limited appeal to upper and middle-class individuals in the urban setting (Farkas and Corcoran, 1983:50–51). Upper and middle-class sports enthusiasts, especially those seeking a socially acceptable means of self-defense that could double as a model modern sport, were therefore forced to look outside of the traditional English fighting sports milieu.

The place to which middle- and upper-class urban Britons looked for a solution then was not to their own backyard, but rather to their past. Upper-class Victorian men, born into a society steeped in traditions of duty, honor, and masculinity and raised on an intellectual diet of hero stories, were enthralled with the myth of idyllic militarism and impassioned by imperialism (Mangan, 1994). As the size of the standing army was decreased, the popularity of reserve and militia service blossomed among wealthy Victorians (Gray, 1897:59). Geoffrey Best states, "Soldiering ... appears to have been the hobby of the aristocracy and gentry" (Mangan 1994:13). Upper-class Britons (and emulative middle-class industrialists) rallied around the notion that all Englishmen, from the lowliest subaltern to the proudest brigadier should be "capable of pacifying a frontier, quelling a rebellion or improvising and administering an empire" (Mangan 1994:19). The English (first the elite and later the urbanized workforce seeking spiritual respite from the tyranny of the machine-age) romantically longed for a return to their idealized past where, they imagined, men were strong, brave, patriotic, and proud. The English, who had become urbanized, compartmentalized, and marginalized by industry and the social changes associated with industrialism at the end of the 19th century, sought an escape from the disharmony and squalor of the cities and the licentious and immoral behavior of "common" urban recreation.

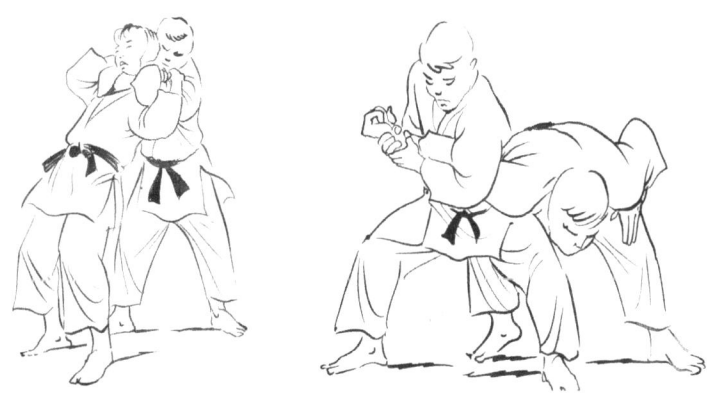

Illustrations by Oscar Ratti.
©1999 Courtesy of Futuro Designs and Publications.

In search of a solution to the problem posed by the lack of an acceptable, indigenous fighting sport in late Victorian society to combine with the new sports ethic, Victorian sportsmen were forced to look abroad.[3] They searched for a sport that would meet strict criteria and that would be able to mitigate at least the most outstanding aspects of English anti-industrialism. They looked for an activity that conformed to or was pliant enough to be molded to the template of modern sport; that had a certain utility to the English either in terms of imparting a useful skill or improving moral character; and that, at least nominally, fit a culturally acceptable form the English could understand or appropriate. At the periphery of their empire, the English discovered a sport that met these three criteria: judo.[4]

Judo was the modern synthesis of older Japanese unarmed fighting systems. It had been created in 1882 by Jigoro Kano (1860–1938), a Japanese university student and jujutsu expert. Kano had studied two older jujutsu styles, but, for a variety of reasons, had found them unsuited to the temperament of modern Japan and impractical for modern study. Kano, a professional educator, subsequently refined the old warrior arts discarding aspects that he felt were antiquated or too dangerous for modern use and organized a new systematic way of teaching the old samurai skills. Kano based his new system on two premises: that the practice of the sport had to be safe for its participants (unlike the older styles of jujutsu practice in which practitioners were often injured) and that the sport had to appeal to practitioners of all ability levels. To increase judo's appeal within both rational, industrial society and within conservative, anti-modern circles, Kano sought to integrate modern theories on training and competition (influenced by Japanese contact with the West) with neo-traditional warrior philosophies in his new style. Kano called his new sport judo, the "gentle way."[5]

Jujutsu was the first of many traditional Japanese martial arts to undergo this type of modern philosophical and sportive reformation. At the end of the 19th century, many feudal practices in Japan were adapted to satisfy the needs of the new pro-Western, industrial culture supported by the Meiji government. In 1868, the Meiji emperor overthrew the last of the Tokugawa shoguns and the military government, the Bakufu. To solidify his initially tenuous position and assert control over the conservative feudal aristocracy, the emperor embarked on a course of rapid modernization in both economic and social circles throughout Japan. As part of this modernization campaign, many trappings of the old regime were outlawed or fell into disuse. To regain popular acceptance and to compete with Western sports in the modern arena, many of the old martial arts changed their curricula to appeal to more popular audiences. Gichin Funakoshi, the "founder" of modern karate-do and a younger colleague of Jigoro Kano, summarized the feelings of some Victorian era martial arts reformers, "Times change, the world changes, and obviously the martial arts must change too" (Funakoshi, 1975:36).

Judo quite naturally met the criteria for modern sports that sport historian Alan Guttmann established in his seminal book, *From Ritual to Record*. These conditions encompass the sorts of changes that Victorian sports reformers had made to 19th-century sport. Guttmann's (and the Victorian's) criteria include secularism, equality of opportunity, a specialization of roles, rationalization, bureaucratic organization, quantification, and the quest for records (Guttmann, 1978:16). Judo has lately been examined according to Guttmann's precepts and found to meet most of the conditions necessary for characterization as a modern sport. Analyzed in Guttmann's terms, judo fails to qualify as a modern sport only in its relative inability to be "quantified." This, however, is a condition shared by many performance-oriented sports such as boxing, gymnastics, and competitive dance that suffer from subjective judging and standards and should not be seen as automatically disqualifying (Carr, 1993:185–187).

In addition to firmly fitting the mold of a modern sport, judo also had obvious utility to English city-dwellers. It was a system of self-defense or "wrestling" that theoretically did not require mass or strength to overcome opponents. It was comprised of a variety of techniques applicable under a wide variety of circumstances and could be augmented by Western fighting methods as necessary. It was reportedly safe to practice (Barton-Wright, 1902:77) and could be practiced easily in the limited space available in the city (Matsudaira, 1910:117). Furthermore, judo was an intentionally moral and philosophical sport (Lindsay and Kano, 1889:204–205; Carr, 1993:168). Jigoro Kano consciously included instruction in moral precepts as part of judo's curriculum. Drawn from traditional Japanese philosophy and the Japanese warrior's code (*bushido*), judo philosophy contained elements that appealed directly to both moral and anti-modern sport enthusiasts.

Judo's promise as an ethical and practical sport was lauded in late-19th century England. As an early exponent, Lafcadio Hearn declared, "it is a philosophical system, it is an ethical system ... and it is, above all, the expression of a racial genius." (Jones, 1943:9). The English saw parallels between the old feudal code of the samurai, upon which judo philosophy was partially based, and the legendary chivalry of English knights-errant.[6] While undeniably foreign, judo seemed to speak to a universal warrior sentiment, an idea that enjoyed widespread appeal among the popularly militarized English. Furthermore, judo and bushido's moral codes bore at least cursory similarities to the ethics championed by advocates of the modern sports movement. In the commentary to a lecture given to the Japan Society in 1910, Count Mutsu, a member of the Japanese Society offered, "our Bushido is your sportsmanship" (Matsudaira, 1910:133). In Nitobe's *Bushido* (1905:xiii), chapters three through nine are titled: "Rectitude or Justice," "Courage, The Spirit of Daring and Bearing," "Benevolence, The Feeling of Distress," "Politeness," "Veracity and Sincerity," "Honour," and "The Duty of Loyalty." These chapter titles bear striking similarities to the goals espoused by organizers of the modern sports establishment who sought to instill the virtues of honor, loyalty, good sportsmanship, and Christian charity in players and spectators.

Conclusion

Judo was accepted in England at the end of the 19th century because certain unique circumstances combined which allowed it to flourish. The rise of the modern sports movement, the response to the social upheaval that coincided with rapid urbanization, upper-class fears of urban crime, a disdain for traditional English fighting sports, and widespread anti-industrial sentiments encouraged English sport proselytizers to look outside England for a morally acceptable, and physically and intellectually accessible, martial sport. The answer to the Victorian's search for a sport that could meet their diverse criteria was found in the Japanese wrestling style called judo. Philosophically, judo embodied the virtues of honor, chivalry, and good sportsmanship in the form of (idealized) bushido. Physically, judo was safe to practice and was accessible to Europeans both in its unadulterated form and combined with European fighting systems. Judo also provided a degree of personal protection to combat street-crime and ruffianism, but was free of the sordid taints of gambling, drunkenness, regionality, and publicanism associated with the English sports of boxing and wrestling. Finally, judo provided an outlet for anti-modern and anti-industrial sentiments as it aesthetically provided its practitioners access to a pre-modern, idealized, warrior archetype. The Victorian judo player became, at least figuratively, the embodiment of the loyal Japanese feudal warrior, the fierce samurai, the moral yeoman, and the virtuous knight-errant.

NOTES

[1] Three early lectures on the subject were recorded in the Transactions and Proceedings of the Japan Society, London. They are: Shidachi (1893), Barton-Wright (1902), and Matsudaira (1910). Two examples of early monographs published in English on the subject are: Norman (1905) and Miyake and Tani (1906).

[2] While it is likely that some private judo instruction was offered prior to this period, it can be established that The Japanese School of Ju-Jitsu was actively promoting the art and offering public instruction in London by 1906 (Miyake and Tani, 1906:9). The most successful eclectic martial art in England at the time was "Bartitsu," taught by W. Barton-Wright, which combined English boxing, fencing, French savate, and judo (Noble, 1999).

[3] Anti-industrial sentiments in England were not limited to, and primarily did not consist of, efforts to find or create acceptable fighting sports. Anti-industrial feelings were most popularly expressed in the rambling movement. In the late 19th century, rambling became an accepted form of recreation whose purpose was not only exercise and sport, but the re-creation and re-discovery of an idealized pre-modern England. Mandler (1997:155–175) summarizes facets of both elite and popular responses to anti-industrialism through rambling in the chapter.

[4] The British, of course, had already encountered indigenous fighting styles in other parts of the empire. In the Far East, Chinese boxing provides perhaps the best example. However, despite a certain amount of technical diffusion between Chinese boxers and English sailors (Goodwin, 1986:39), Chinese boxing did not make great inroads into English society. This is largely because, unlike judo, the various Chinese boxing schools were not able to meet all the criteria necessary for acceptance into the English sports regime.

[5] Literally hundreds of histories of the establishment of judo have been published. Most paraphrase the account provided in Lindsay and Kano (1889:204–205). Recently, scholarly examinations of the early years of judo have been published with increasing frequency, including Carr (1993), Smith (1996), and Bowen (1999).

[6] It is important to note that the Japanese warrior ideal the English admired was a concept largely derived from Nitobe (1905) and by pamphlets published by Westerners residing for short periods in Japan (e.g. Norman, 1905:1–3). Nitobe, however, had been educated in English public schools and was a Christian. It is likely that his version of the samurai honor code was highly idealized if not specifically coordinated to appeal to an English audience. Similarly, the pamphleteers accounts must also be viewed critically as their motives were frequently commercial or evangelical.

BIBLIOGRAPHY

Bartlett, E. (1962). *Judo and self-defense*. New York: Arc Books.

Barton-Wright, E. (1902). Ju-jitsu and ju-do. *Transactions and Proceedings of the Japan Society*, 5:261–264.

Bowen, R. (1999). Origins of the British Judo Association, the European Judo Union and the International Judo Federation. *Journal of Asian Martial Arts*, 8(3):42–53.

Burgin, G. (October 1892). Japanese fighting (Self-defence by sleight of body). *The Idler*, 281–286.

Carr, K. (1993). Making way: War, philosophy and sport in Japanese judo. *Journal of Sport History*, 20(2):167–188.

Davies, A. (1998). Youth gangs, masculinity and violence in Late Victorian Manchester and Salford. *Journal of Social History*, 32(2):349–369.

Englander, D. (1992). Criminality upon and beneath the surface in Victorian England. *Criminal Justice History*, 12:235-239.

Farkas, E. and Corcoran, J. (1983). *The Overlook martial arts dictionary*. New York: The Overlook Press.

Funakoshi, G. (1975). *Karate-do: My way of life*. New York: Kodansha International.

Goodwin, K. (1986, June). In search of Wing Chun's roots: Did it evolve from Western boxing or the Shaolin Temple? *Blackbelt*, 39.

Gray, W. (1987). For whom the bell tolled: The decline of prize fighting in the Victorian Era. *Journal of Popular Culture*, 21(2):53-64.

Guttmann, A. (1978). *From ritual to record: The nature of modern sports*. New York: Columbia University Press.

Holt, R. (1989). *Sport and the British: A modern history*. Oxford: Clarendon Press.

Jones, H. (1943). *Judo, jiu-jitsu, and hand-to-hand fighting: A list of references*. Washington: Library of Congress Division of Bibliography.

Lindsay, T. and Kano, J. (1889). Jiujutsu the old samurai art of fighting without weapons. *Transactions of the Asiatic Society of Japan*, 16:192-205.

Lowry, D. (1995). *Sword and brush: The spirit of the martial arts*. Boston: Shambhala.

Mandler, P. (1997). Against Englishness: English culture and the limits to rural nostalgia, 1850-1940. *Transactions of the Royal Historical Society*, 7:155-175.

Mangan, J. (1995). Duty unto death: English masculinity and militarism in the age of the new imperialism. *International Journal of the History of Sport*, 12(2):10-38.

Matsudaira, T. (1910). Sports and physical training in modern Japan. *Transactions and Proceedings of the Japan Society*, 8:114-134.

Miyake, T. and Tani, Y. (1906). *The game of ju-jitsu for the use of schools and colleges*. London: Hazel, Watson, and Viney.

Nitobe, I. (1905). *Bushido: The soul of Japan*. New York: G.P. Putnam's Sons.

Noble, G. (1999). An introduction to W. Barton-Wright (1860-1951) and the eclectic art of Bartitsu. *Journal of Asian Martial Arts*, 8(2):50-61.

Norman, F. (1905). *The fighting man of Japan: The training and exercises of the samurai*. London: Archibald Constable.

Reid, H. and Croucher, M. (1983). *The way of the warrior*. New York: Simon and Schuster.

Shidachi T. (1905). Ju-jitsu: The ancient art of self-defence by sleight of body. *Transactions and Proceedings of the Japan Society*, 1:4-21.

Skidmore, M. (1991). Oriental contributions to Western popular culture: The martial arts. *Journal of Popular Culture*, 25(1):129-148.

Smith, R. (1996). The masters contest of 1926: An epiphany in judo history. *Journal of Asian Martial Arts*, 5(3):60-65.

Terry, T. (1902 February). Japanese self-defence without weapons. *The Idler*, 543-549.

Thompson, E. (1963). *The making of the English working class*. New York: Vintage Books.

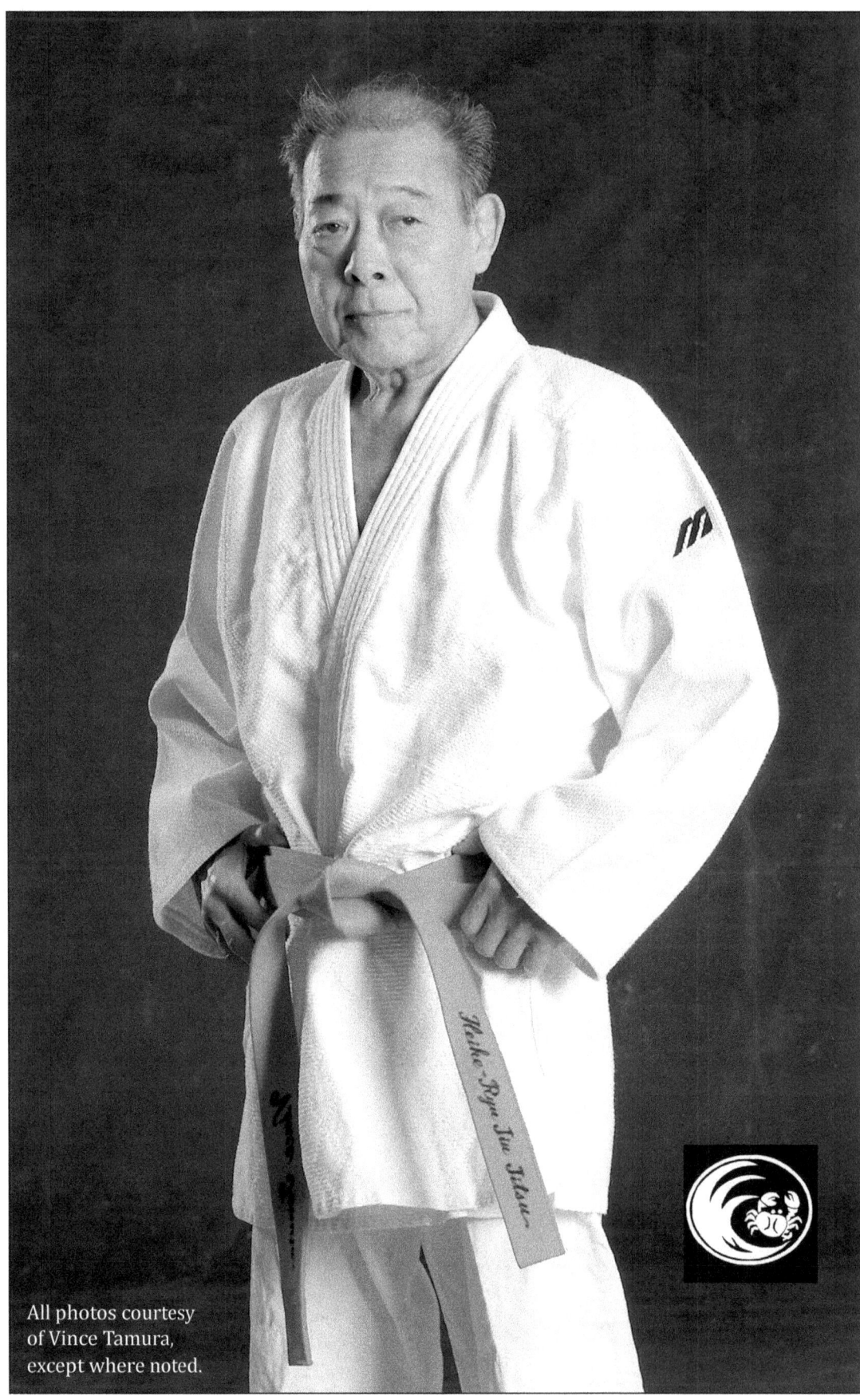

All photos courtesy of Vince Tamura, except where noted.

chapter 10

American Judo Pioneer
Vince Tamura and Heike-ryu Jujutsu
by James Webb, M.A.

Introduction

The name Vince Tamura is synonymous with the growth and establishment of judo in America. Among his firsts were his being chosen as the "A" player (a top player in the country) to represent the United States at the First World Championship of Judo (Tokyo, 1956) and his further being chosen to be a referee at the introduction of judo to the Olympic Games (Tokyo, 1964). The U.S. team was made up of Paul Maruyama, Jim Bregman (who took bronze), George Harris, and Ben Campbell.

Vince Tamura's legacy can be readily seen today through the many champions he has produced, a tournament that still draws the some of the toughest players in the world, and a revitalized jujutsu (sometimes written as "jiujitsu") system. His family story, going back hundreds of years, shows a strong lineage of people making an impact on history.

History of the Taira Clan

The roots of the Tamura family can be found in ancient Japan. The two most influential clans vying for control of Japan during the end of the Heian period (784–1184) were the Taira and Minamoto. Vince Tamura is a descendent of the Taira clan. Takami, the grandson of the Emperor Kammu, first adopted the name Taira. Emperor Kammu (r. 781–806) founded Kyoto.

"Genji" is the Sino-Japanese pronunciation of the written character that the Japanese read as "Minamoto." In the same way, the Taira are often referred to as the Heike. This has always resulted in some confusion to idle observers of Japanese history. For while the Taira went on to control Japan, the novel written by the famous author Eiji Yoshikawa describing the clans story was called *The Tale of the Heike*.

As the two clans rose in military strength and political influence, it became inevitable that they would clash. Unfortunately, throughout the Gempei War (1180–1185), the situation of the Taira clan grew progressively worse until the final battle of Dannoura, which marked the utter destruction of the Taira as they were driven into the sea. The most tragic event was enacted by Nii-no-Ama, the grandmother of the infant Emperor Antoku who, when confronted with the alternative of surrendering to the warriors of the Minamoto clan, clasped the child tightly in her arms and plunged into waves of the straits, followed by the other court ladies. So complete was the defeat that the name Taira temporarily disappeared from Japanese history, leaving the site to be more renown for ghost stories of fallen samurai bent on revenge.

The best known legend from the battle concerns the Heike crabs, which are said to contain within their shells the spirits of the dead samurai. Their shells do indeed bear the shape of a human face, when viewed with an active imagination.

Heike-ryu Jujutsu

Not all of the members of the Taira clan perished in the final series of battles. Those descendants of Taira Kiyomori that managed to survive the final wrath of the Minamoto fled to the hills. They would remain there perfecting their samurai skills for a day of revenge that would never surface. Vince's mother, a direct descendent of Taira Kiyomori, remained in Japan until her death in Yamaguchi-ken, Honshu Prefecture.

One of the skills that had been handed down through the family for generations was the Tamura family jujutsu style: Heike-ryu.

The symbol of Heike-ryu Jujutsu shows the Heike crab returning from the sea. Two American brothers, well-known in both judo and jujutsu circles, have surfaced from this tradition: Mas and Vince Tamura. While many modern coaches have abandoned the original roots of judo in pursuit of mastering the Olympic sport, the Tamura family has continually encouraged students to study jujutsu to master not only the self-defense aspects but also the roots of the martial art and the warrior spirit (*bushido*). It is important to note that the ancient style of Heike-ryu jujutsu had been dormant for many years until the brothers revitalized the art with modern techniques.

The style is called Heike-ryu Jujutsu mostly out of respect for the family history as it bears little resemblance to the jujutsu style of ancient Japan. The old Heike-ryu techniques were developed for the samurai to be used while in armor and on the field of battle. Modern techniques have been adapted from these roots to be practical in a more modern environment with street clothes.

While many of the throws and grappling techniques resemble those of Kodokan judo, an equally large number of techniques come from the more traditional jujutsu lineage—those techniques such as wrist locks and striking techniques that are illegal in judo competition but have been found to be effective in a modern hostile environment.

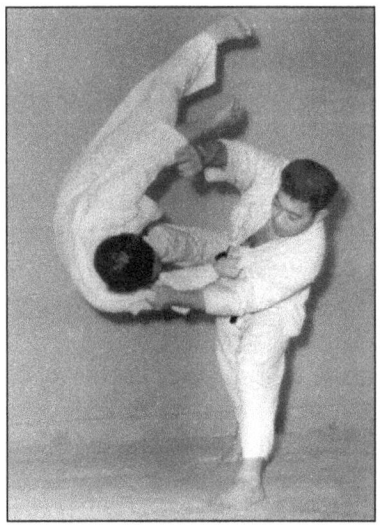 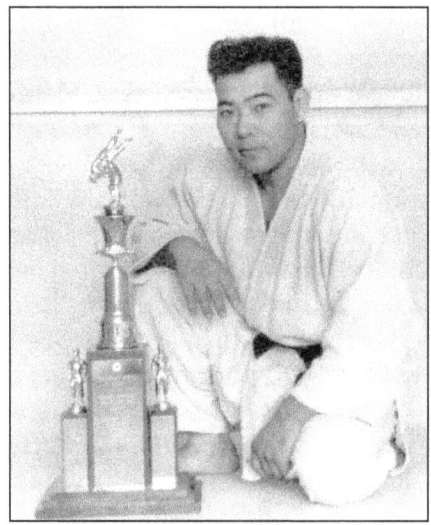

Left: Vince Tamura throwing brother Mas with "floating throw" (*uki otoshi*) (1957).
Right: He wins the 1957 Midwestern Championships in Detroit, Michigan.
He defeated the very tough and established John Osako in the final.

Vince Tamura's Role in the Growth of American Judo

Vince's older brother, Mas Tamura, grew into a formidable judo competitor in his hometown of Fife, Washington, under the direction of Iwakiri Ryochi. Iwakiri had a produce business but had learned judo in Japan and had volunteered this skill to the community. Kumagai Yasuyuki was also instrumental in molding this program as he was an instructor sent by the Kodokan.

In 1936, Professor Kano Jigoro (the founder of Kodokan Judo) saw Mas win the individual competition of a large tournament held in Seattle, Washington. Kano was so impressed with the abilities of the competitor that he personally promoted Mas Tamura to 3rd-degree black belt. Mas' success in judo had a profound effect upon his younger brother. To this day, Vince still greatly admires Mas.

The Fife Dojo was the result of the Japanese community building a school to ensure that their children captured their Japanese roots. At the far end of the school, a dojo was built, separated from the remainder of the school by a sliding door, and boasting the traditional mat fashioned from woven rice straw (*tatami*).

The youngest and seventh son, Vince remembers his early tournaments as his being "first up, first down." He started judo at a very young age, and, being the smallest, he started at the beginning of the traditional line-up tournaments (where competitors lined up along the side of the mat by size and skill and fought until they lost). Vince usually lost his first match to older and stronger competitors. His first judo match was in 1933 at the age of four.

With the outbreak of World War II, the Tamura family was relocated to the assembly center at Camp Harmony in Puyallup, Washington. Not all of the memories here were bitter; however, as many days spent practicing judo and sumo finally paid off for Vince as he won his first tournament—the award being a coveted pocketknife.

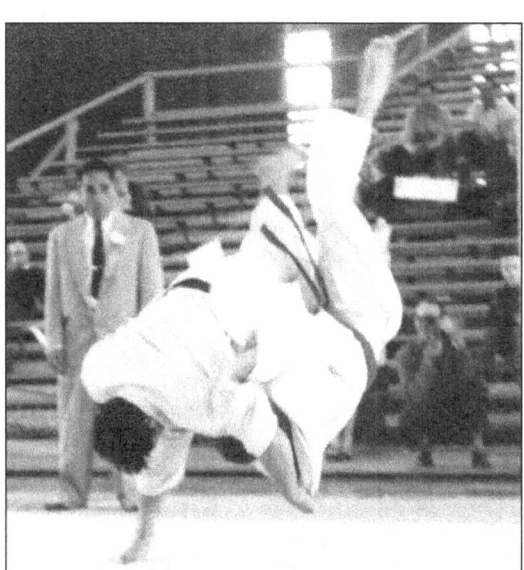 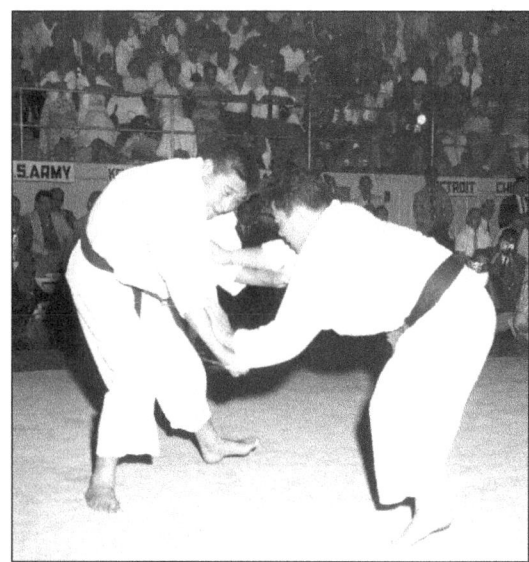

Left: Vince Tamura "attacking the inside of the thigh"
(*uchi-mata*) at the 1958 Nationals in Chicago.
Right: He squares off against Ken Hatae in the finals of the 1959
US National Championships in San Jose, California. Ken Hatae was a recent arrival from Japan, where he was the captain of his university judo team, and was training in San Jose. Vince won the match and the National Championship.

In 1941, Mas moved to Illinois to take over the reins of Chicago's Jiujitsu Institute. There he found a serious test in 1943 when the *Chicago Times* encouraged a match between the 216-pound international wrestler Karl Pojello and the 143-pound Tamura. The audience was primarily made up of the top athletic officers of the Armed Forces and notables such as Avery Bundage, the head of the Olympic Committee. Mas won the match in one minute twenty seconds by rendering Pojello unconscious. Mas taught in Chicago for thirty-one years and died in 1982.

Vince joined Mas in Chicago at the Jiujitsu Institute at the age of fourteen. Chicago area judo quickly grew as other instructors left the relocation camps for Chicago: John Osako (Chicago Judo Club), Henry Okamura (Lawson YMCA—usually where the competitions were held), and Hic Nagao (University of Chicago). Bill Kaufman migrated from the Jiujitsu Institute to start a club at the Evanston YMCA.

No longer "first up, first down," Vince entered one tournament in which eight black belts formed the black belt division (this was an unusually large number of black belts at the time) and Vince defeated them all to earn his 3rd-degree black belt.

The second US National Championships was held in San Francisco in 1954. Vince Tamura won the tournament. He went on to win the US Nationals three times. In the seven years of his active competition, he never failed to place in the top three.

It was little wonder that Vince Tamura was chosen to represent the United States at the First World Judo Championship in 1956. He made it to the semi-final, losing a close match to Anton Geesink, the future world champion from The Netherlands. The honor was noteworthy as there was only one division contested during that time. The "B" player from the United States, the more established Mitsuo Kimura, drew a tough Frenchman by the name of Cortine and went out in the first round.

The World Championships was Vince's second visit to Japan. On his first visit, he was returning from serving in the Korean war (where he received a Bronze Star for bravery in action) and stopped in Japan to visit his relatives in Honshu. He stopped by the Kodokan to work out and met Donn Draeger (whom he had known in Chicago) and one of his brother's friends, Tomonari. Through Tomonari, Mifune Kyuzo (1883–1965, one of the famous Kodokan 10th-degree black belts) had given Vince a judo uniform to take back to Mas as a gift. Mas was the president of the Chicago Yudanshakai (black belt association) at that time. At the end of a long, hard workout, Vince remembers that he could not walk up the few steps to his hotel room and had to crawl on his hands and knees.

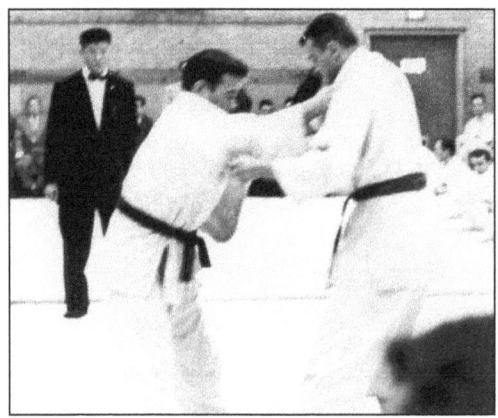

Action in Chicago in 1960. The competitor
on the left is Vince Tamura. The referee is John Osako.

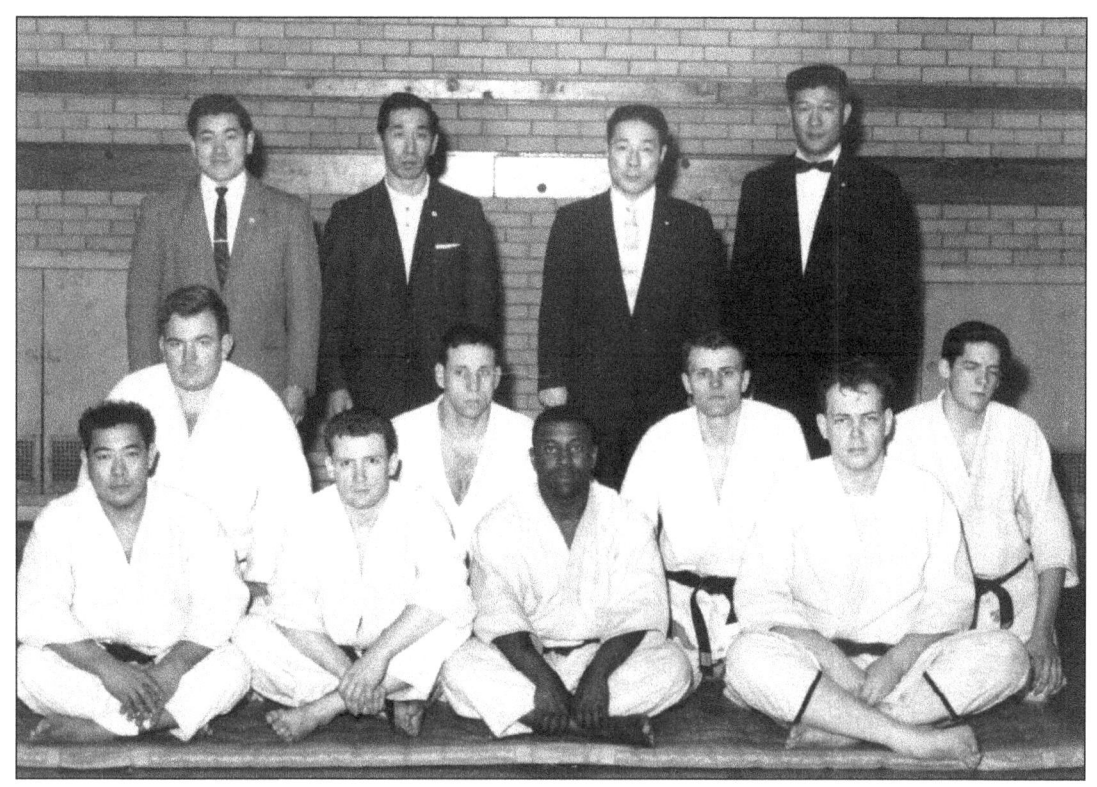

The Chicago Team attends the 1960 Nationals.
Front row (left to right): Vince Tamura, George Colgan, Curtis Belmont, Jim Colgan.
Second row: Fred Jorgensen, Bill Kaufman, Ed Ernst, Rhett Summerville.
Back row: Henry Okamura, Hik Nagao, Masato Tamura, and John Osako.

Vince returned to Chicago to live in an apartment complex and found Ms. Shiratori Yuri living in the same complex. Jim Colgan (now an 8th-degree black belt still living in Chicago) claims that Yuri was one of the most beautiful girls he had ever seen. Vince soon married her.

Vince's second visit to Japan, and the World Championship, found his introduction to Ms. Fukuda Keiko, who was contemplating a move to the United States at the time. She moved to California shortly thereafter and began to teach excellence in kata. Fukida is the granddaughter of Fukuda Hachinosuke. Kano Jigoro studied Tenshin Shinyo-ryu jujutsu under Hachinosuke before founding the Kodokan.

With the start of a family, Vince found that his two young boys (David and Bob) had trouble coping with the harsh Chicago winters and sought warmer climates. Finding themselves in Florida for the US National Championships, Vince and Yuri thought that would be great place to live—until a hurricane hit. They then headed west, enjoying the hospitality of Jaques LeGrand (a Frenchman who had fought Vince in several national championships) in New Orleans along the way. Eventually, they made it to Dallas, Texas, where one of the buildings downtown reminded Vince of Chicago. This became their new home, and Vince quickly opened a judo school.

His first school was located next to a bar called The Doll House. The bar owner learned to both love and hate having the judo school next door. On the one hand, some of his best customers were judo students. On the other hand, very often a student would be thrown into the common wall and glasses would be knocked over.

In the Texas Yudanshakai, Vince found some great company: Bill Nagase and Sam Numajiri were in Fort Worth, Fred Usui had come from Hawaii to open a club in the Dallas Downtown YMCA, Gail Stolzenburg was in Austin with Pop Moore, Karl Geis was in Houston, Eddie Elizalde was in San Antonio with Herb Bellamy, and Tim Joe was in Amarillo. Typically shunning political positions, Vince eventually agreed to become the chairman of the Texas Yudanshakai Board of Examiners—a position now held by Vince's longtime student, Jim Webb.

With 1964 came the Olympic Games in Tokyo and Vince's return to Japan to be a referee in the judo competition. While there, Olympic team members Jim Bregman and George Harris remarked on what a great help Vince was in helping them prepare for the Games. Jim Bregman captured the bronze medal.

TECHNICAL SECTION

Defense Against a Knife

The defender moves away from the direction of the knife lunge, while bringing his hands up to grab the attacker's right wrist. He then pushes the attacker's fingers back toward his elbow, forcing the attacker's hand to loosen its grip on the knife. Stepping back with the left foot, the defender twists the attacker's bent wrist to the outside to throw the attacker.

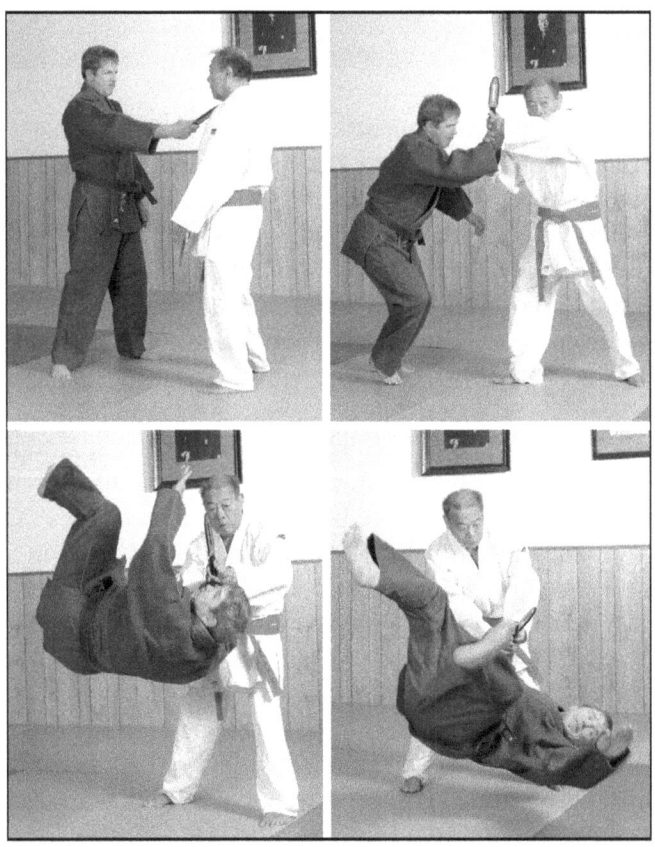

Note the focus remains on controlling the knife throughout the technique until the weapon is taken from the attacker or used to injure the attacker. James Webb acts as the attacker in this technical section, with Vince Tamura showing the defense techniques. Photography in this section courtesy of P. Robbins.

Defense Against a Gun from the Rear

Turn the body out of the line of fire while bringing the arm up to lock the attacker's elbow. Apply pressure to the attacker's elbow and drive him to the ground while maintaining control of the weapon at all times.

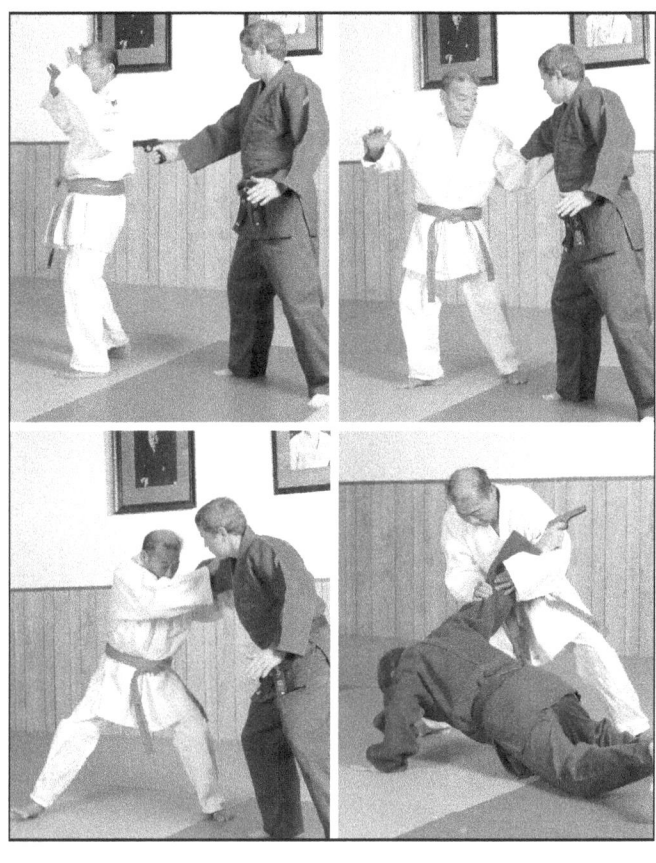

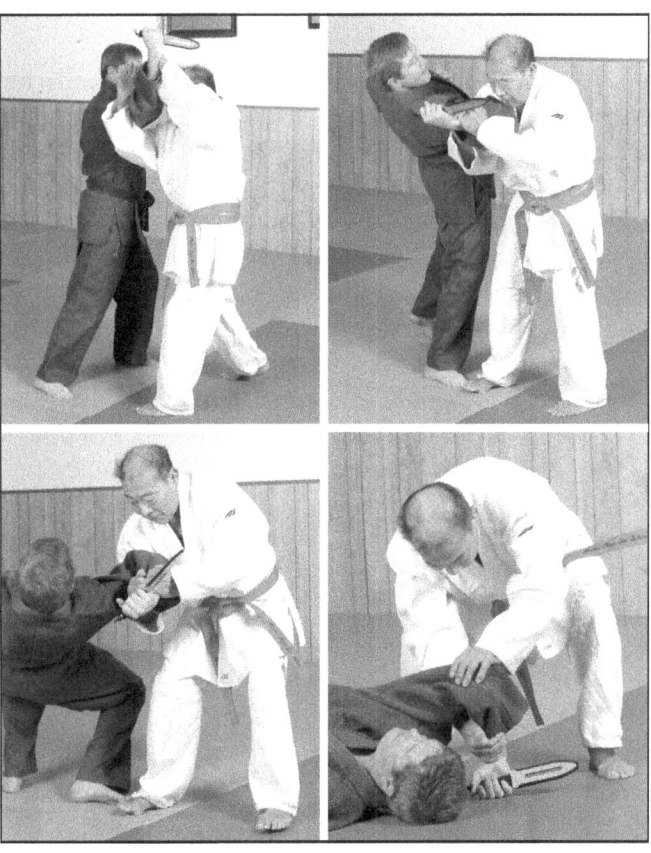

Defense Against an Overhand Knife Strike

The defender blocks with the left hand while bringing his right hand up behind the attacker's arm and around to the attacker's wrist. With the attacker's arm bent, the defender leverages the forearm to throw the attacker to the ground. The defender continues to apply pressure to the arm until the attacker releases the weapon.

Defense Against an Overhead Club Strike

The defender steps forward with the left foot while simultaneously blocking with his left hand. The right hand pushes the attacker's shoulder back and down while the right leg sweeps the attacker's leg, throwing him to the ground. The defender locks the attacking arm with a figure four arm bar until the attacker releases the weapon.

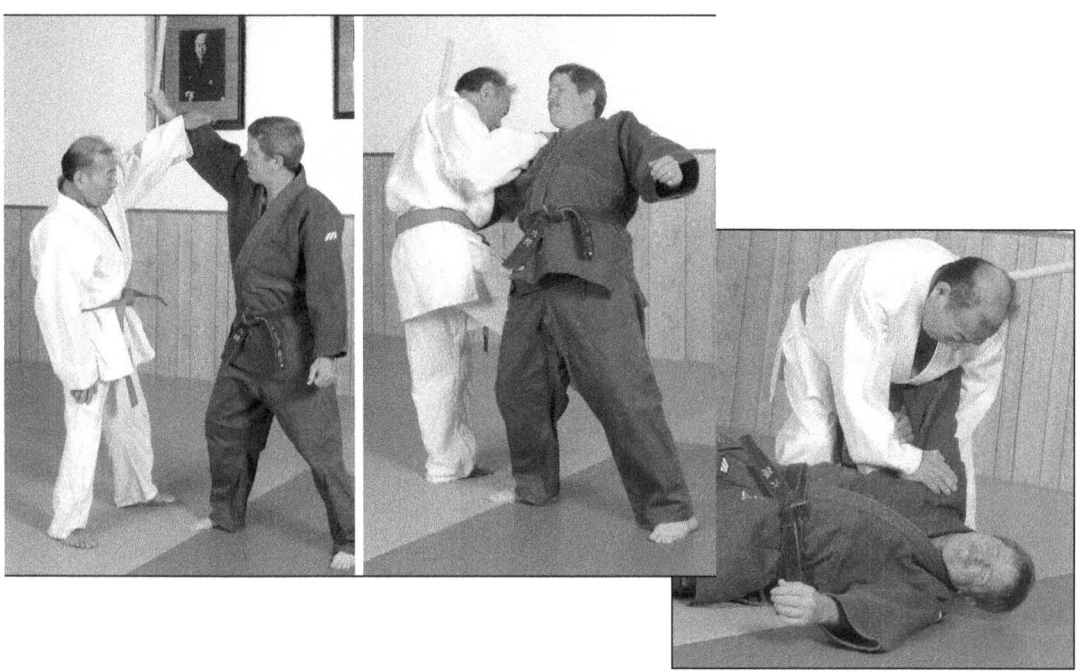

Conclusion

Since opening the dojo in Dallas, Vince won the National Masters Championship for fourteen consecutive years before retiring from competition. He also founded and oversaw the Dallas Invitational Judo Championship that just held its 37th annual event and has risen to become one of the toughest elite athlete competitions in the country. He has also produced many national and international champions. Most recently, longtime students Ryan and Reno Reser (who are currently on scholarship at the Olympic Training Center) are starting to accumulate such titles as US Senior National Champion, US Open Champion, and Pacific Rim Champion, Swedish Open Champion, and British Open Champion.

Vince Tamura has come a long way since his "first up, first down" days in Fife, Washington. Years of training and love of his art has produced numerous championship titles, a plethora of students who are national and international champions, the legacy of one of the toughest tournaments in the USA, and the revitalization of a jujutsu style.

BIBLIOGRAPHY

Svinth, J. (1999). Masato Tamura, Ryoichi Iwakiri, and the Fife Judo Dojo, 1923–1942. *Journal of Asian Martial Arts*, 8(1):30–43.
Tamura, V. Personal interviews.
Tamura, Y. Personal interviews.
Turnbull, S. (1977). *The samurai: A military history*. Oxford, England: Osprey Publishing.
Yoshikawa, E. (1956). *The Heike story*. Boston: Charles E. Tuttle.

chapter 11

Isao Okano's Impact on Judo
Since the Lausanne World Championships
by David Finch

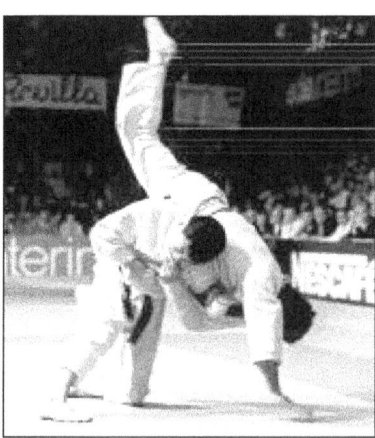 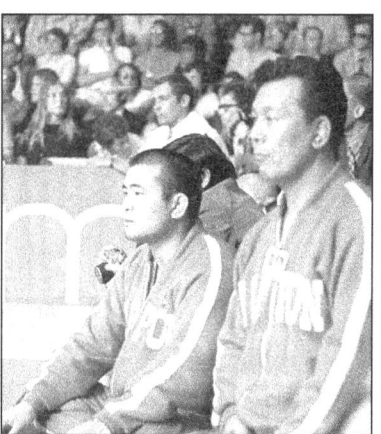

Left: In the semi-finals lightweight division, Yoshiharu Minami (Japan) throws Schangeli Pitskhelauri (RUS) for ippon in 10 seconds to reach the final. Right: During the Lausanne World Championship finals, Japanese teach coach Isao Okano (right) quietly watches the finals with former All-Japan champion Toshiro Daigo. All photos courtesy of Judo Photos Unlimited.

At the 1972 Munich Olympic Games, Japan failed dismally to stamp its authority on world judo, mustering gold in only the three lightest weights. At the 1973 Lausanne World Judo Championships, Japanese judo regained its soul when Japan ruthlessly swept the board taking all six world titles. In 1973, it all came down to one man, the extraordinarily brilliant 1964 Olympic middleweight champion, Isao Okano.

Weeks after the Munich Olympics failure, Okano was "parachuted in" as team manager to restore Japanese judo pride. One commentator said that before Munich, the Japanese team "was slapped around and told how useless they were." When Okano took over, they were told "how brilliant they were. And they believed it."

Okano also encouraged the team to believe that if a foreigner beat them it was a "complete fluke." While generous enough to accept a loss as a "fluke," Okano was not prepared to tolerate many losses, ensuring that the failing team member was thoroughly tested to exhaustion at the next line-up of his renowned True Meaning (*Seiku-Juku*) training camp, a tempering experience that was meant to hurt more than the contest loss.

In fact, Okano was such a disciplinarian that when his own protégé, Kasuhiro Ninomiya, was forty-five minutes late for bed, he was immediately sent on a fifteen-mile run to make sure that he was tired enough for sleep. Such discipline produced the desired result: Ninomiya won the Lausanne Open title by brutally throwing Klaus Glahn of Germany for the winning point in eight seconds. At the time, Glahn was an Olympic silver medalist, twice former European Champion, and one of the most favored contestants in the category.

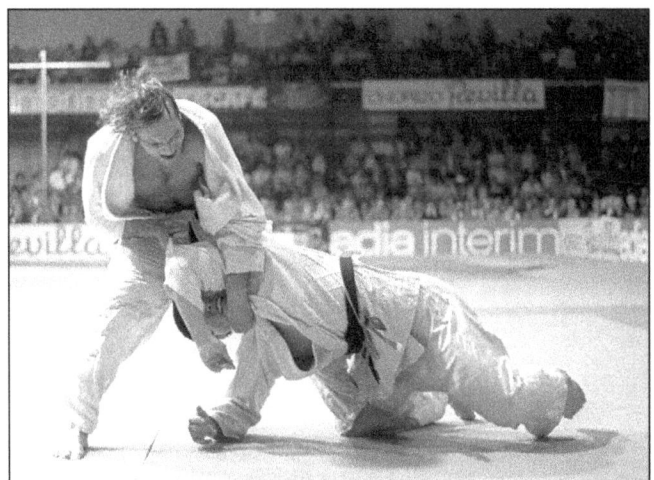 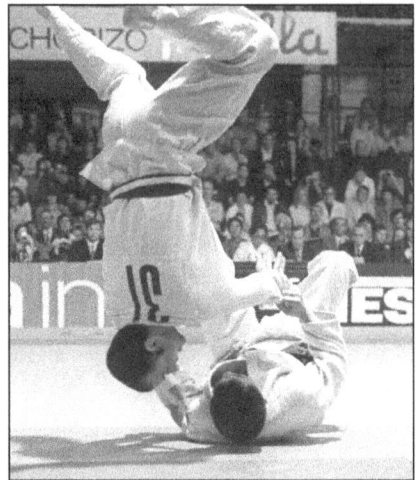

Left: European heavyweight champion Klaus Glahn (Germany) gives Haruki Uemura (Japan) a hard time during the Lausanne Worlds semi-finals.
Right: During the eliminations, Takao Kawaguchi (Japan) throws Gueorgiu Guerguiev (Bulgaria) with a circle throw (*tomoe-nage*).

At 29, the squatly built Okano was barely older than most of his team at the 1973 Worlds and considerably shorter than most. But he possessed an exceptional track record that included two All-Japan titles as the lightest winner ever and the 1965 World middleweight title. That was in addition to his 1964 Olympic gold when he was only 21. He was therefore well qualified to lead from the front, get on the mat, and work over a few team members including heavyweights, before taking them aside for special instruction, something almost unknown in previous managers.

With the intellectual 47-year-old Toshiro Daigo (vastly experienced and twice All-Japan champion) at his side, Okano, in a matter of months, turned the Japanese team into a force that firmly reversed the advancing European judo movement that had started so well with the fortunes of Olympic champions Anton Geesink and Wilhelm Ruska of Holland in the sixties and early seventies.

Japan's twelve entries, with two in each weight division, led to twelve medals with the loss of only two finalists to the European countries of East Germany (Dietmar Hoetger) and the Soviet Union (Ramaz Nijeradze). In the case of Nijeradze, he comprehensively beat Takagi during the quarterfinals and then lost to him in the final under the old repercharge system,[1] which was later substantially modified to prevent such anomalies. The Japanese dominance of world judo encouraged the European-led International Judo Federation to eventually restrict the world championships, starting at Paris in 1979 (the 1977 Worlds was cancelled for political reasons), to one national entry for each weight category in line with the Olympic Games.

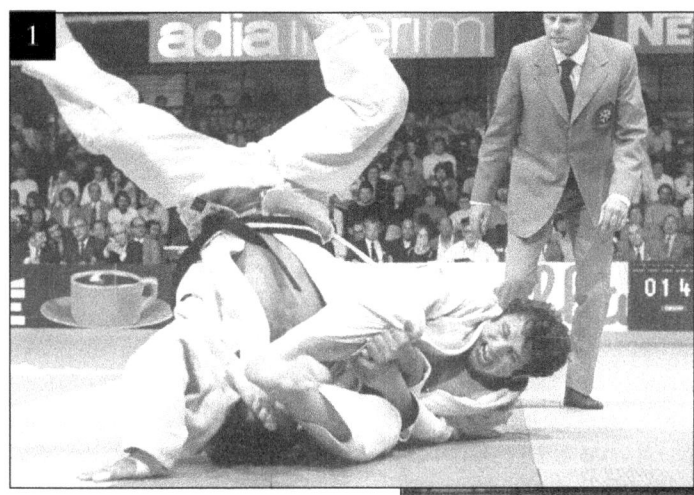
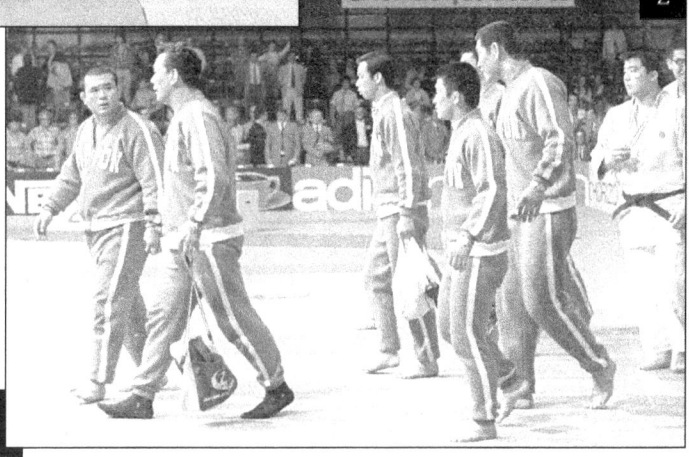
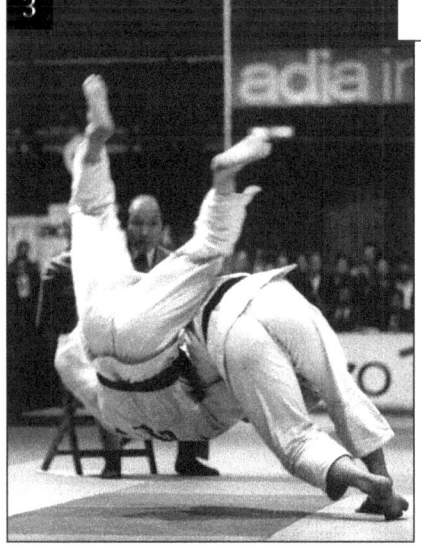
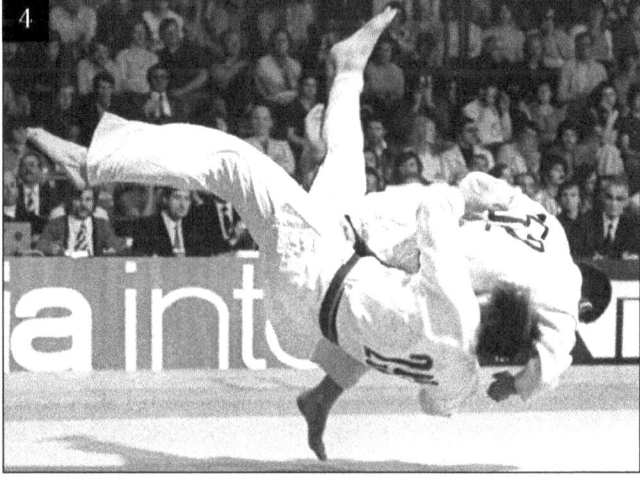

1) Ramaz Nijeradze (URS) fiercely attacks Takagi Chonosuke (Japan) defeating him in the heavyweight division quarter final.
2) The Japanese gold medalists follow Isao Okano and Toshiro Daigo across the mat.
3) Nomura Toyokazu (Japan) throws K. Yoshimura (Japan) to reach the light middle weight final.
4) Kasuhiro Ninomiya (Japan) throws Klaus Glahn (Germany) with a major outer reap (*osoto-gari*).

World judo did not have to wait until 1979 to see the decline of Japanese superiority. It started in 1975 following the relegation of Isao Okano to the "judo wilderness" when he was "overlooked" as team manager for the Vienna World Championships. Okano, although a firm disciplinarian and traditionalist, was aware that some liberal Western views could benefit world judo. However, instead of arguing for change behind closed doors, he made the fatal mistake of offending the Kodokan by appearing, in the spring of 1975, on the front cover of the French *Judo Magazine* with Anton Geesink wearing red and blue judo outfits. Okano and Geesink were twenty years before their time and Okano and Japanese judo paid the price.

The Kodokan concluded that Jigaro Kano was so offended he turned over in his grave and immediately appointed twice world champion Sato Nobuyuki team manager over Okano. Okano remained in Japan sidelined by his error of judgment while Sato, who should have been on the mat instead of in charge of the team, tried to reverse the now inevitable decline of Japanese judo superiority. With three quarters of the gold medals at the 2001 Munich World Championships held by non-Japanese nations, it is improbable that Japan will ever regain the 100-percent dominance that it had at Lausanne.

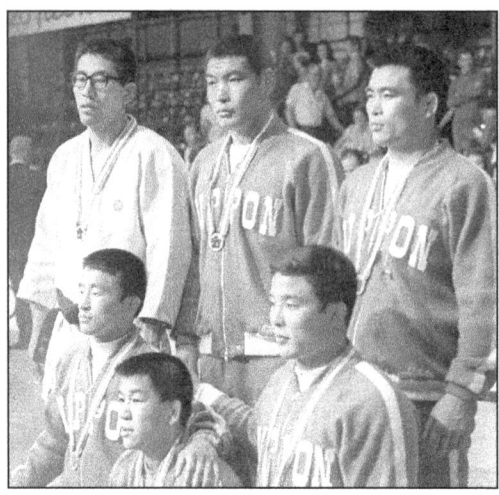

Japan's gold medal winners at the 1974 Lausanne World Championships.
Back row: Ninomiya, Tagaki, and Sato. Front row: Nomura, Minami, and Fujii.

This September, the World Judo Championships return to Japan at Osaka, not far from the seaside town of Mikage where the founder of judo, Jigoro Kano, was born. I suspect that he would be quietly pleased to see how much the world appreciates his judo and how it has progressed from the first Kodokan in Tokyo in 1882 of twelve mats and nine students to the worldwide movement, sport, and way of life that it is now for so many people, men and women. Kano might even have approved of Okano wearing a colored judo jacket so that the uninitiated watching judo might find it a little easier to follow.

▼▲▼

[1] The repercharge is a tournament judo system where the contestants beaten by the four semi-finalists in each weight category fight each other to fight the loser of the semi-final contests. This contest is then known as the "bronze medal contest" and there are two bronze medals in judo.

chapter 12

Jujutsu's Image in Spain's Wrestling Shows: A Historic Review
by Carlos Gutiérrez, Ph.D., and Julián Espartero, Ph.D.
Translated from Spanish by Dave and Sonia Katz

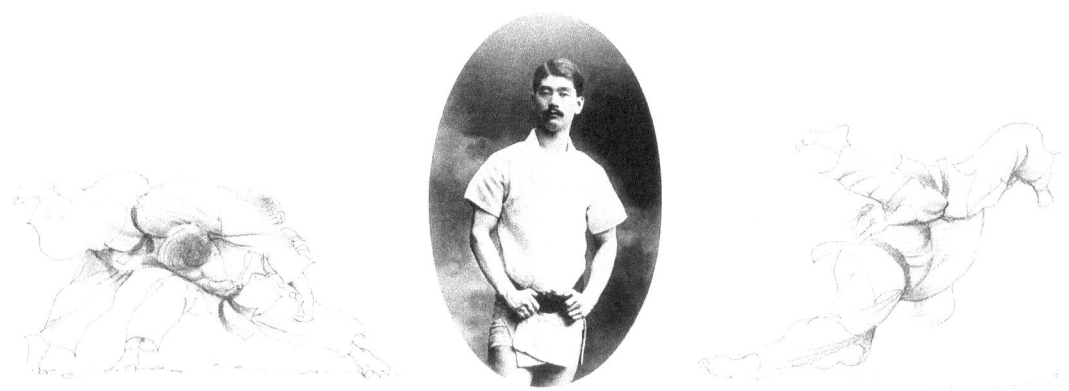

Center, Uyenishi portrait (cir. 1908). (Archivo General de
la Administración, Cultural Section, box F/397, envelope 31).
Illustrations by Oscar Ratti. © 2004 Futuro Designs & Publications.

Introduction

The Tivoli Theater—Barcelona, Spain, 1 November, 1907. On that Friday afternoon, a small Japanese man, smartly attired in a tuxedo, introduced a form of fighting to the public that was, until that time, practically unknown in Spain. Sadakazu Uyenishi, known simply as "Raku," began his presentation of jujutsu with an exhibition of the characteristics and possibilities of the fighting style as both a means of personal defense and as a gymnastic sport. Raku and his assistant, Etaro "Deko" Deguchi, demonstrated various responses to armed and unarmed attacks. Afterwards, they presented the technical possibilities of jujutsu: punches, throws, strangulations, dislocations and body-strengthening exercises. This was followed by a simulated fight between Raku and Deko in the "Japanese Style." Finally, the presentation concluded with the moment everyone had been waiting for: the challenge that made Raku famous throughout all of Spain. Raku offered five hundred pesetas—a fortune at the time—to anyone who could either defeat him or last fifteen minutes in combat with him under the rules of jujutsu.

Some days later, the Barcelona newspapers began to announce matches between Raku and various strongmen/professional fighters. The best known were touted for their immense size, like the 245 lb. Englishman Ted Milles, or for a dubious international title holder like Otto Brandt, trumpeted as the reigning German wrestling champion. These bouts successfully forged a relationship between Japanese wrestling and other methods of combat found at that time in theater or circuses. Each afternoon the public filled the theater, anxious to see the diminutive 5'5" tall, 128 lb. Japanese man destroy all the wrestlers he encountered. *El Mundo Deportivo* (The Sporting World) reported, "one couldn't find a ticket window that remained open, only a 'sold out' sign for tickets that were being sold for the fortune of five pesetas! (The normal entry price was half a peseta). These prices are a testament to the interest and passion that these fights have stirred up, even though Raku's inevitable triumph is a foregone conclusion" ("El jujutsu," 1907:3).

Jujutsu's introduction to the Barcelonan public is illustrative of its introduction to other Spanish capitals like Madrid, Valencia, Bilbao, San Sebastian and Zaragoza (Gutiérrez, 2003:108–26). More so than through any other means, Japanese wrestling was introduced to Spain through the world of spectacle in the theaters, circuses, and music halls of the period. This was echoed in other European countries, with relative frequency from the beginning of the 20th century up until the First World War (Brousse, 2000:184–8; Brousse and Matsumoto, 1999:92–4; Noble, 2001).

Understanding how jujutsu fits into the world of entertainment and its corresponding symbiotic relationship with other forms of self-defense is of interest for three principal reasons. First, it allows us to gain an appreciation for the sport's social repercussions. The theaters and circuses of the age were gathering points for the top aristocrats and leaders of society as well as for the more humble working classes. As a result, jujutsu became known to all social classes instead of being targeted to a restricted group as would have been the case had it been introduced through sport or the military.

Second, it helps to illustrate how the imagery of jujutsu was formed and perpetuated through its entertainment origins. The theaters and circuses have always been places prone to exaggeration and myth; Japanese wrestling participated in these exaggerations, and became known as an infallible combat method with which, thanks to its "scientific principles" and "technical secrets", even the most feeble person could defeat the colossal giants of combat. Finally, it elucidates the sport's symbiotic relationship with other forms of self-defense, many of which enhanced their own presentation by utilizing the technical resources and imagery associated with jujutsu, and later with judo.

This chapter will show the symbiotic influences that jujutsu, judo, and other theater arena fighting styles practiced in Spain have historically had on each other. These influences, also seen in other countries, have created and strengthened a large part of the imagery that has defined jujutsu and judo during most of the 20th century up until the present day. Likewise, other martial arts styles born in the Far East have both benefited from and enriched jujutsu and judo's technical repertoire, making them more efficient and spectacular.

Greco-Roman Wrestling

In true Spanish fashion, Madrid launched a massive celebration to mark the May 1906 marriage of Alfonso XIII, King of Spain, to Victoria Eugenia of Battenberg, niece of Edward VII of England. Hoping to benefit from the festive atmosphere and numerous people present in the capital, a troupe of wrestlers arrived in Madrid to put on the Criterium Internacional de Lucha, Spain's first Greco-Roman wrestling tournament.

Backed by the Parisian newspaper, *L'Auto*, and directed by several-time world professional fighting champion, Paul Pons, the troupe consisted of 12 fighters: Pons (French), Le Boucher (French), Vervet (French), Lemousin (French), Shakman (German), Plikplank (Austrian), Clement (Swiss), Van Beber (Dutch), Milo (Italian), Chomiakin (Russian), Amathou (Senegalese), and Ortola (Spanish). For the Spanish public, who were unfamiliar with-the fighting style, the athletes' power and physiques were astonishing. Pons weighed in at an imposing 260 pounds and stood 6'5" tall, startling to a relatively diminutive Spaniard. The fighters' massive presence conveyed an image of wrestling as a sport reserved for the hefty and strong. The rules of Roman wrestling furthered this perception. Touching an opponent below the waist or utilizing a leg hold was prohibited. Without doubt, these rules greatly limited the technical possibilities of the sport, leaving weight and strength as the determining factors in a wrestler's ultimate success. As Rimet (1996:77-78) indicated, the combatants preferred a static opposition, a slow attack based on force.

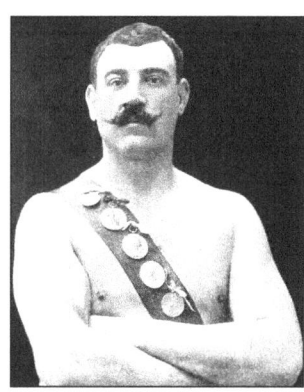

Frenchman Paul Pons, several times professional
World Greco-Roman Wrestling Champion (Pons, 1915:8).

It was precisely these restrictive rules that allowed wrestling to be praised as a noble and gentlemanly sport. As one journalist wrote in one of the most widely read Madrid newspapers, "There is no lack of those who consider the spectacle disagreeable, who consider it pointless to attend a conflict between men who mutually wish to assert themselves by force; but it must be said that, with its sensible rules prohibiting violence, tricks and tripping, there is a great deal that is noble in this fight between two strong men" ("Las luchas en la Zarzuela," 1913:3).

Nevertheless, this observation corresponded more to the theory than to the reality of the spectacle. There were numerous reasons to doubt the true character of this first Madrid championship, not the least of which were the accusations that frequently appeared in the newspapers during the 26 May to 20 June tournament. In an article entitled "The Fight Scam," journalist L. Zosaya (1906:3) stated, "Paul Pons ... had dedicated himself to moving a troupe of athletes from one place to another, hiring them out in France's regional capitals for fantastic wrestling tournaments and championships, but on the sole condition that none of his companions defeat him." The tournament finale, as described below, proved Zosaya's suppositions correct: "the International Criterion and its prizes were a joke, an exhibition of wrestlers reduced to a hired circus" ("El campeón vencido," 1906:1).

Further evidence of the lack of sportsmanship in the championship can be found in the composition of the troupe and the behavior of its wrestlers. To make the competition as interesting as possible, the troupe consisted of an assortment of fighter roles: Paul Pons, the champion to beat; Raoul le Boucher, the upstart; Ortola, the representative of the Spanish people; Amathou, the exotic and agile black Sengalese; Shackman, the violent and unsportsmanlike wrestler; and so on. Similar to modern American professional wrestling, the troupe's exhibitions followed a script. For example, Paul Pons and le Boucher remained undefeated until the grand finale, in which they were pitted against each other to determine the strongest wrestler; Shackman taunted the audience and utilized prohibited techniques on his opponents; and Ortola, despite losing, would always show the bravery and courage of the Spanish people. As Díaz-Cañabate (1943:4) noted years later, "It is known that in these professional Greco-Roman wrestling tournaments, the promoter took care in the selection of his wrestlers. The essential ingredients were the lovable rogue; the despicable rule breaker; the wretch with a frightened face and a body much thinner than the rest of his companions who all exceeded one hundred kilograms (220 pounds); the indispensable black man; the wrestler who would occasionally yell at and argue with the referee; and the wrestler who always smiled, even when imprisoned by his opponent in an inescapable hold."

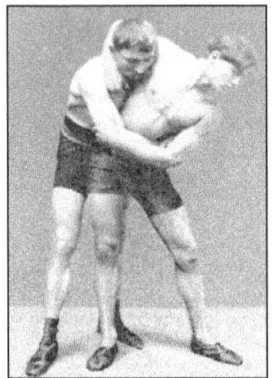 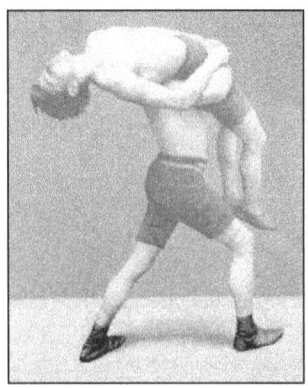 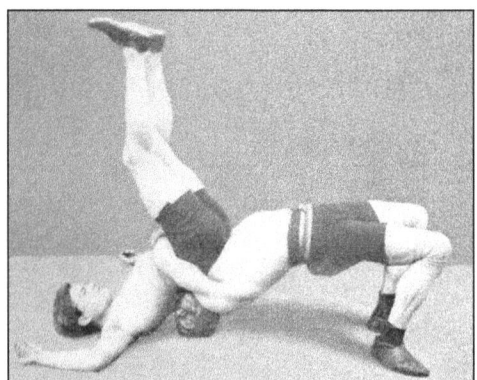

Greco-Roman wrestling
techniques (Pons, 1909: 15, 16, 21).

The peculiar and questionable manner in which the Criterium closed highlights the true nature of the competition. The final match between Pons and le Boucher finished in a tie forcing the spectators to return the next day, but only after having bought a new ticket. The consolation for their purchase? The knowledge that the second contest would be conclusive as it was an untimed match. But it was not conclusive. During the second contest, Pons injured his clavicle and could not continue. Faced with yet another postponement and another ticket to buy, the spectators caused such a brouhaha that the troupe was forced to declare le Boucher the tournament champion, contrary to the outcome desired by both Pons and, ironically, by le Boucher himself.

From the above, it is obvious that by 1906, the wrestling tournament was already a well-rehearsed show. Fifty years after the 1848 establishment of the rules of Greco-Roman wrestling by Frenchman Innocent Truquettil (Le Floc'hmoan, 1965:193), the first professional Greco-Roman World Wrestling Championship took place in Paris in 1898.

This period was Europe's "Golden Age" of professional wrestling (Noble, 2001), but it also marked the beginning of the sport's perversion as, after that, wrestling was constantly refined to attract a wider audience, or, more specifically, the money in their pockets. A key element in this metamorphosis was the media, who began to act as an unofficial promoter of the show, amplifying the effect of the already ubiquitous theater and circus fliers. By characterizing the wrestlers, exaggerating their skills and their defects, the media emphasized the social appeal of the sport. Fair play and sincerity, more frequently than not, ended up as forgotten victims of show business. After all, at times it made sense for two wrestlers to tie; at other times, the public was purposefully angered by unsportsmanlike gestures or referee errors; sometimes the wrestlers would gain admiration through their noble behavior; and the hometown wrestler always, but always, won. Of course, these roles did not mean that all matches were a farce. But in wrestling tournaments that could last longer than a month, a show based purely on fair play would not have had the sufficient pull to fill the theater every afternoon.

All of these entertainment elements, including extensive media coverage, were particularly evident in the 1912 and 1913 Madrid World Wrestling Championships. Organized and sponsored by the newspaper, *Heraldo de Madrid*, and the Parisian magazine, *La Culture Physique*, the 1912 World Wrestling Championship took place between 20 July and 29 August. Beginning on 9 July, the *Heraldo de Madrid* published daily reports on the tournament wrestlers (see Table 1), extolling their measurements, their titles, their knowledge, and their nicknames. The newspaper also published the competition's rules and the wrestlers' expectations and opinions of the tournament and of their rivals.

Beginning with the opening of the championship on 20 July, the *Heraldo de Madrid* dedicated generous coverage to the previous day's tournament results. Although in less detail, other papers also covered the championship. Now, anyone who wished to know the fighters' stories or to live the drama of the matches no longer had to buy an expensive theater ticket; they could simply buy a newspaper.

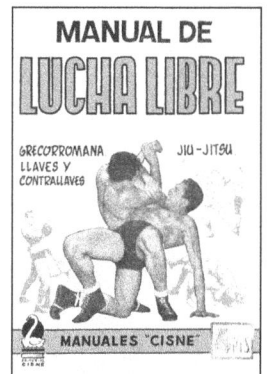

A jujutsu technique (*ude garami*) in the cover of the book *Lucha Libre, Grecorromana y Jiu-jitsu* (Del Cuadernal, n.d).

TABLE 1:
Participants in the 1912 Madrid World Wrestling Championship (*Heraldo de Madrid*).

NAME	COUNTRY	WEIGHT	HEIGHT
Anastase Anglio	Martinique	132 kg. (291 lb.)	1.88 m. (6'2")
Crouzas	Holland	122 kg. (269 lb.)	1.92 m. (6'4")
Maurice de Riaz	Switzerland	90 kg. (198 lb.)	1.70 m. (5'7")
Dérona	Luxembourg	100 kg. (221 lb.)	unknown
Eltzecondo	Spain	125 kg. (276 lb.)	unknown
Jimmy Esson	Scotland	120 kg. (265 lb.)	2.05 m. (6'9")
Galby	Italy	105 kg. (232 lb.)	unknown
S. Ch. Ivanhoff	Russia	100 kg. (220 lb.)	1.80 m. (5'11")
Raoul le Bayonnais	France	96 kg. (212 lb.)	1.76 m. (5'9")
Noel le Bordelais	France	112 kg. (247 lb.)	1.80 m. (5'11")
Javier Ochoa	Spain	106 kg. (234 lb.)	1.75 m. (5'9")
José Salvador	Spain	105 kg. (231 lb.)	1.83 m. (6'0")
Maurice Vance	Belgium	100 kg. (220 lb.)	1.80 m. (5'11")
Emile Vervet	France	120 kg. (265 lb.)	1.73 m. (5'8")
Ernest Von Roeber	USA	110 kg. (243 lb.)	1.77 m. (5'7")
Wilson	USA	100 kg. (220 lb.)	1.80 m. (5'11")

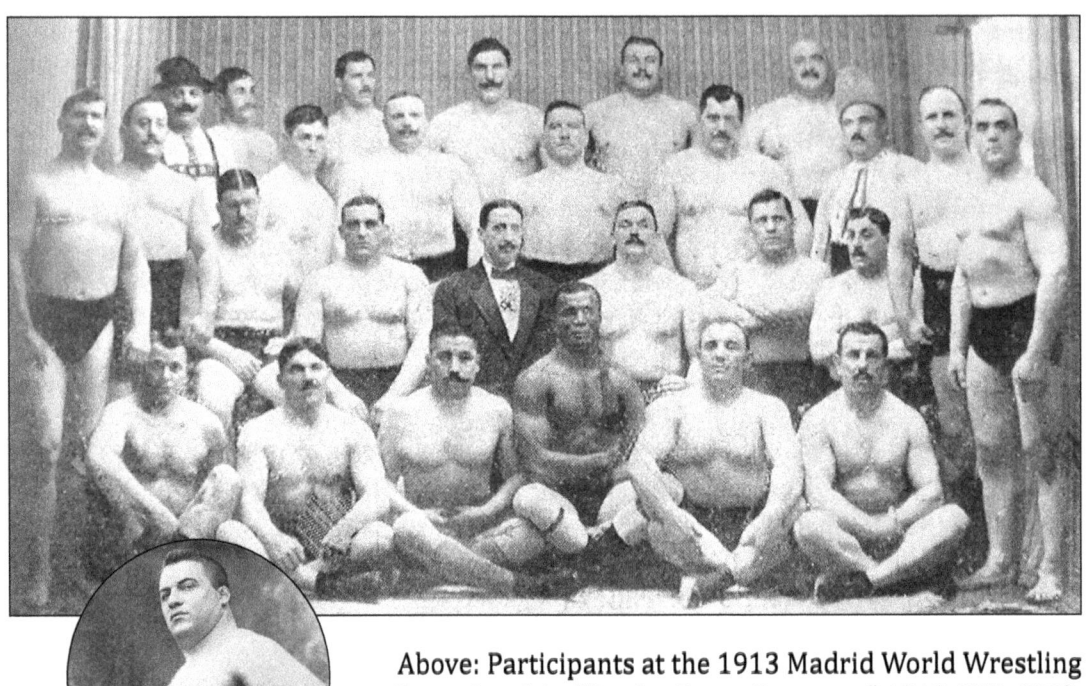

Above: Participants at the 1913 Madrid World Wrestling Championship ("Lucha Greco-Romanas," 1913:233–239). Left: Spaniard Javier Ochoa "The Navarrese Lion" ("Lucha Greco-Romanas," 1913:233–239).

For those who followed the championship, it did not lack interesting stories. The most significant of which was, without doubt, the entrance of "the Navarrese Lion," the Spaniard, Javier Ochoa. Ochoa entered the championship more than ten days after it had begun. This entry, by all measures, was a violation of tournament rules. Seventy matches had already been fought, with numerous wrestlers having been eliminated from title contention, but Ochoa was tall, strong, handsome and Spanish. In other words, he was the perfect hook with which to improve attendance, much more so than the rough, somewhat hairy Basque, Eltzecondo, or the Catalanonian, José Salvador. Ochoa succeeded in delivering more spectators to the theater and survived until the end of the championship where in a match attended by an estimated 6,000 spectators, he fought against the Swiss, Maurice de Riaz. Although Ochoa lost to de Riaz, he managed to hold him off for an epic 50 minutes and 47 seconds, thrilling the public. Ricardo Ruiz (1912:4), one of the best-known Spanish sport journalists of the time, commented: "for one moment—and it was an hour long—the Spanish flag waved honorably in an international contest." Beginning then, and for a long time thereafter, Javier Ochoa was the Spanish star of Greco-Roman wrestling, making the sport triumph through his presence alone.

In Madrid, 1913 was characterized by public "fever" and "delirium" for Greco-Roman wrestling (de Rivero, 1913:201). Between 8 and 30 March, in Madrid's Central Jai Alai Courts the International Sumo and Greco-Roman Wrestling Championship was held (described later). Then from 20 June until 6 July, the International Greco-Roman Wrestling Championship was held in the famous La Zarzuela Theater. In this tournament, Javier Ochoa remained undefeated in all of his matches, taking home the ultimate tournament title. Finally, between 10 July and 1 September 1913, the World Wrestling Championship was held in Madrid in the Ciudad Lineal development, brilliantly closing the Madrid wrestling season.

TABLE 2:
Participants in the 1913 Madrid World Wrestling Championship (El Liberal).

NAME	COUNTRY	WEIGHT	HEIGHT
Frank Crozier	Jamaica	92 kg. (203 lb.)	1.77 m. (5'10")
Juan Pedro Darrigol	Spain	104 kg. (230 lb.)	1.78 m. (5'10")
Raoul de Rouen	France	114 kg. (252 lb.)	1.88 m. (6'2")
Maurice De Riaz	Switzerland	94 kg. (208 lb.)	1.7 m. (5'7")
Jimmy Esson	Scotland	112 kg. (247 lb.)	2.05 m. (6'9")
Ferrari	Italy	106 kg. (234 lb.)	1.72 m. (5'8")
Max Gelhard	Netherlands	110 kg. (243 lb.)	1.78 m. (5'10")
Carl Grunewald	Germany	105 kg. (232 lb.)	1.82 m. (5'12")
Grave	France	100 kg. (220 lb.)	1.82 m. (5'12")
Hansen	Hungary	110 kg. (243 lb.)	1.85 m. (6'1")
S. Ch. Ivanhoff	Russia	100 kg. (220 lb.)	1.8 m. (5'11")
Gaumont Le Frappeur	France	95 kg. (210 lb.)	1.74 m. (5'9")
Camile Le Terrasier	Belgium	102 kg. (225 lb.)	1.76 m. (5'9")
Louis Lemaire	France	99 kg. (219 lb.)	1.72 m. (5'8")
Maierhanz	Luxembourg	100 kg. (220 lb.)	1.82 m. (5'12")
Celestin Moret	France	90 kg. (199 lb.)	1.75 m. (5'9")
Jess Petersen	Denmark	115 kg. (254 lb.)	1.78 m. (5'10")
Pickardt	Germany	134 kg. (296 lb.)	1.85 m. (6'1")
Charles Poirée	France	100 kg. (220 lb.)	1.75 m. (5'9")
Herman Reglin	Germany	108 kg. (238 lb.)	1.85 m. (6'1")
Röld	Austria	105 kg. (232 lb.)	1.74 m. (5'9")
Van Rothen	Netherlands	105 kg. (232 lb.)	1.76 m. (5'9")
Carl Saft	Germany	123 kg. (271 lb.)	1.77 m. (5'10")
Spoul	Russia	110 kg. (243 lb.)	1.75 m. (5'9")
Tarkowsky	Russia	132 kg. (291 lb.)	1.78 m. (5'10")
Bayard Wallon	Belgium	108 kg. (238 lb.)	1.8 m. (5'11")
Zarakiki	Manchuria	96 kg. (212 lb.)	1.78 m. (5'10")

Sponsored and organized by the Madrid newspapers, *El Liberal* and *El Mundo*, and the Parisian newspaper, *L'Auto*, the 1913 World Wrestling Championship brought together 28 fighters from 15 nations (see Table 2). Particularly noteworthy fighters included Maurice de Riaz, 1912 world champion; Frank Crozier, world middleweight freestyle wrestling champion in 1909; and the ultimate victor, Jess Petersen, prior world wrestling champion in 1908 and 1910. Proof of the tournament's success can be seen in its mammoth 54-session length.

After this "fever" year for Greco-Roman wrestling, the First World War broke out, dramatically interrupting the sport's development. In spite of Spain's neutrality in the conflict, international wrestling troupes disappeared from the country, and only isolated challenges took place. Wrestlers performing in Spain during the war included Maurice de

Riaz, Frank Crozier, Antoine de Bone (middleweight 1910 world freestyle wrestling champion), and Spaniards Javier Ochoa, José Ardevol and Heliodoro Ruiz.

After the Armistice, several years passed before Greco-Roman tournaments started up again and even when they did, they never achieved the splendor of the past. The most reputable international tournaments continued to be held annually in Madrid in the Circo Parish (later in the Circo Price), under the name *Cinturón de Madrid* (Belt of Madrid) or *Cinturón de Oro de Madrid* (Golden Belt of Madrid). The first Cinturón de Madrid was held in 1920, while the last (in the Greco-Roman wrestling style) was held in 1932. It is noteworthy how the wrestling exhibition and its associated images grew and changed in these post-war tournaments. Although the fighters continued to be athletes of Herculean strength and Greco-Roman wrestling continued to be a sport based in great measure on force with a rather limited technical repertoire, the tournaments began to include other combat styles, adding more variety to the wrestling exhibitions. Styles, like "Canary" wrestling—a sport indigenous to the Canary Islands—and jujutsu, were introduced into the circus amphitheater during these years (see jujutsu, below).

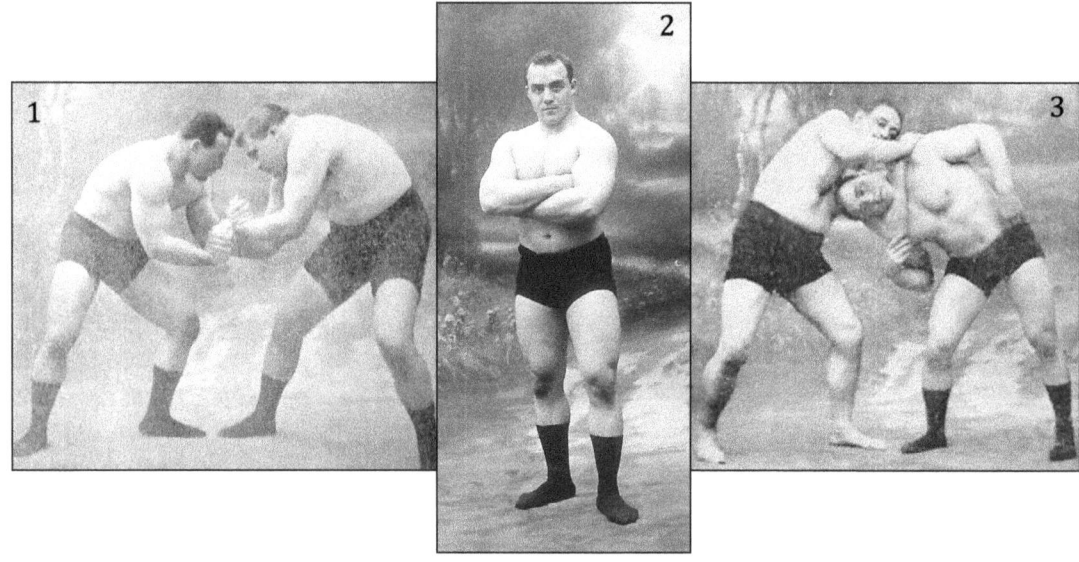

1) Javier Ochoa (right) and Maurice de Riaz, the two finalists at the 1912 Madrid World Greco-Roman Championship (González, 1912:239–242).
2) Maurice de Riaz, 1912 World Wrestling Champion. (Archivo General de la Administración, Culture section, box F/397, envelope 31).
3) Maurice de Riaz and Emile Vervet (González, 1912:239–242).

Despite the inclusion of other styles of wrestling, the Greco-Roman wrestling spectacle steadily declined in popularity. Authors like Badenas (1934:94) and Diem (1966:274) identified diminishing honor among the combatants and over-marketing of the sport as leading factors in its decline. In the same vein, Valsera (1944:384) affirmed: "the popularity that wrestling exhibitions enjoyed at the beginning of the century decreased until it disappeared completely as a result of the fraudulence of the majority of the matches and their associated degeneration into parody." Is this the true cause of the decay of Greco-Roman wrestling? The hypothesis must be questioned given that (as discussed later) the styles of wrestling that took Greco-Roman wrestling's place (principally Pancrase and Catch-As-Catch-Can) are not characterized by a reversion to a display of wrestling in its purest form.

Jujutsu

Raku defined jujutsu as "the victor establishing the superiority of leverage and balance, two soft, delicate qualities, over the harder, rougher ones of strength and force" (Uyenishi, 1905:12). Certainly, the concept of "soft" perfectly describes a practice that was quickly characterized by science, esotericism, elegance, and invincibility (Brousse, 2000: 138–52, Gutiérrez, 2003:92–101). This characterization originated in great measure from the comparison between jujutsu and pre-existing Western styles of combat like Greco-Roman wrestling, freestyle wrestling, and boxing. The nature of its competitors, the extraordinary variety of its techniques, and even its elegant uniforms, soon marked a sharp contrast between jujutsu and these other styles of fighting.

However, jujutsu was not above the influences of the public. Generally unimpressed by exercises demonstrating strength building or self-defense techniques, the Spanish public demanded challenges in which Japanese wrestlers faced off against a diverse set of rivals. These challenges were driven by the ultimate aim of attracting the greatest number of spectators possible to the circus or to the theater. Catering to this aim led the sport to suffer similar corruption to its integrity as had Greco-Roman wrestling.

These corrupting influences were clearly visible in Raku's continued Spanish exploits. Sponsored by the entrepreneur, William Parish, proprietor of the Circus Variety Agency and of Circo de Parish, Raku travelled to Madrid to perform in the Circo de Parish between 25 May and 29 June 1908. In his performances, Raku continued the pattern of demonstrations and duels discussed earlier with the same successful results as he had previously experienced. *Nuevo Mundo* commented: "Great enthusiasm and interest has been awoken in the sporting world and in the public at large by the presentation in the Circo de Parish of the notable Japanese 'jiu-jitsu' professor, Mr. Raku.... It is astonishing to actually behold Mr. Raku, of diminutive stature, wrapped up in his impeccable gentleman's attire, smiling, kind, his small oblique eyes shining behind golden spectacles, seemingly harmless, and then to see him toss himself with immeasurable speed into the ring, crouching, jumping above his opponent, and in brief seconds demolishing (his opponent)... without resorting to any weapon, only formidable oriental wrestling, based on anatomic knowledge" (Anteo, 1908).

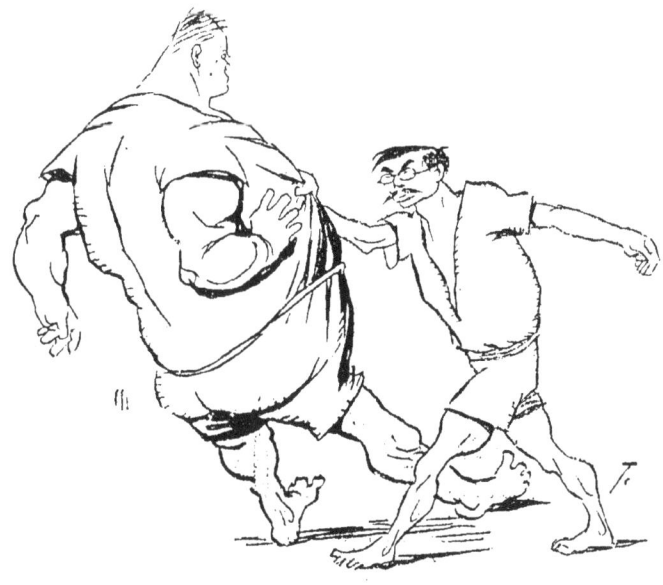

Raku caricature (del Campillo, 1908).

Nevertheless, the success heralded by the *Nuevo Mundo* article should be qualified by the difficulties that Raku's show first encountered. First, despite the 500-peseta prize offer (approximately $5,000 in today's money), no one showed up to fight Raku, and, second, the exhibitions barely received any mention in the press. In fact, between 8 and 15 June the press only gave notices of upcoming matches. Reacting to this scanty coverage, professional wrestler Ted Miles was brought in as a "hook" to revitalize the exhibition (del Campillo, 1908). The ploy succeeded. The match between Raku and Miles held on 17 June received extensive coverage.

Raku won, but the audience claimed his victory was due to his advantageous dress. As such, the fight was to be repeated on 19 June without Raku's jujutsu uniform, but at the time of the match, Raku again wrestled in his uniform, claiming it undignified to wrestle while "nude." After the resulting hullabaloo, Raku capitulated and fought on 20 June without his uniform. Raku's third consecutive win was not nearly as impressive as was the way three matches had so successfully been milked from one.

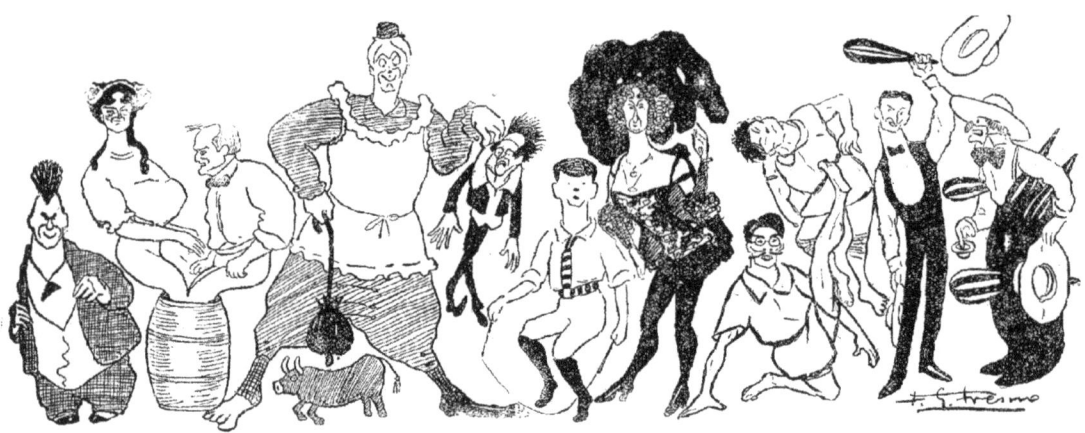

Parish Circus Caricature (1908), includes Raku ("Un rato," 1908:13).

After the matches, a tongue-in-cheek article by journalist Félix Méndez (1908) described Raku's increasing popularity: "The intelligent say ... that (Raku) has completed a special study of the human body, and that when he touches his adversaries in a sensitive point, a secret that he alone possesses ... they fall to the floor as if struck by lightening." In addition to mocking Raku, the article wryly illustrates the growing imagery associated with jujutsu as well as the "theories" that abounded about the superiority of that wrestling style.

When Raku returned to Barcelona to perform between 19 and 28 July 1908, things had changed in the city; jujutsu was no longer the raw novelty that it had been when he had left. Between 23 June and 7 July 1908, an Anglo-Japanese troupe of four wrestlers headed by Taro Miyake (80 kg. / 176 lb.) performed in the Teatro Tivoli. Miyake, another of the most famous early 20th century jujutsu wrestlers, offered 1,000 British pounds (approximately $100,000 in today's money) to any professional that could beat him. He also publicly challenged Raku to a match that, as far as we know, never took place. When Raku debuted in Barcelona on 19 July, he only faced European fighters, offering them the familiar 500 pesetas for a successful fifteen-minute match.

Demanding a fight between two true specialists, the fans of jujutsu attempted to arrange a match between Raku and another of the better known Japanese wrestlers of the time: Mitsuyo Maeda, also known as "Conde Koma" (Count Koma [sic]). However, Raku did not accept the challenge, stating that the Japanese consul to Spain had asked him not to fight another Japanese (Cárcamo, 1908:1). In the face of this refusal, classified as a "fiasco" by the sporting press, the fans organized a three day jujutsu championship between two Japanese fighters: Mitsuyo Maeda (76 kg. / 166 lb.) and Akitaro Ohno (95 kg. / 209 lb.). Held on 20, 21 and 22 July, the tournament was a great public success. After a predictable beginning in which each wrestler won one match, the tournament was resolved in the third match when Maeda triumphed over Ohno. The following day, both Maeda and Ohno, attired in traditional kimonos, attended an extraordinary function in the Teatro Tivoli to honor Maeda's victory.

A few days later, on 31 July, another jujutsu exhibition was held in which Maeda was joined by the diminutive Japanese wrestler, Yuzo Hirano (145 cm./57 inches, 50 kg./110 lb.) and by Miss Roberts (Svinth, 2001). The exhibition permitted the Barcelona public to see how, thanks to the "omnipotent" skills of jujutsu (Almasqué, 1908:1), a man of so small a stature and weight like Hirano could hold his own against anyone. The public also saw how jujutsu's techniques enabled a woman to defend herself against any type of attack. Jujutsu's usefulness for the feminine sex was also illustrated in the Teatro Principal by Raku and the famous variety artist, Consuelo Portela "Chelito."

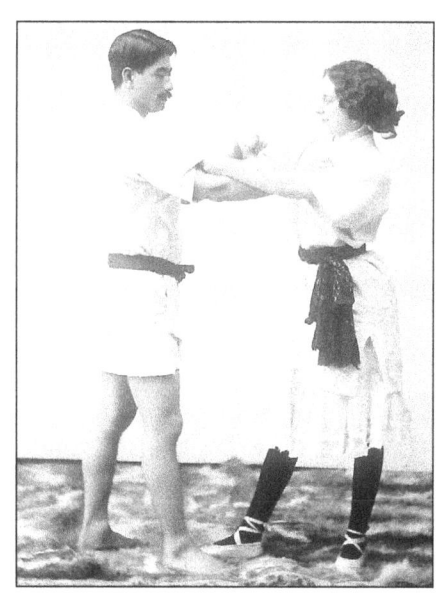

Raku and the famous variety artist Consuelo Portela "Chelito" (1908). (Archivo General de la Administración, Cultural Section, box F/397, envelope 31).

After Raku and Chelito's exhibitions, which took place concurrently with the championship matches between Maeda and Ohno, a surprising notice was published: Raku had accepted a match with Akitaro Ohno. The clash took place on 25 July and ended in a tie. Was the match a singular exception to Raku's agreement with the Japanese consul not to fight a fellow Japanese? The facts illustrate the contrary. Raku and Ohno fought again in Santander on 6 August, and in Bilbao on 30 and 31 August. Raku's promises not to fight another Japanese wrestler can therefore be considered as just another part of the showmanship that defined jujutsu. This turnabout, first refusing to fight another Japanese wrestler, then sacrificing "the rules" in the face of popular demand was, in fact, a well-managed guarantee of performance success. Similar showmanship was patent in Raku's 22-31 August Bilbao stay.

Raku was introduced in Bilbao as the star of the Circo del Ensanche. He lived up to his star billing, gaining such success in his initial performances that he began to be known throughout all of Spain. As always, his normal fifteen minute challenge, announced in papers like *El Nervión, El Porvenir Vasco* and *El Noticiero Bilbaíno*, was directed exclusively to Europeans. However, on 28 August, *El Noticiero Bilbaíno*, published the following note:

> Raku is no champion. Encountering the so-called jujutsu wrestling Champion of the World in this town, I privately challenged him to a match he did not accept. So that the public of this noble city are not deceived, I Aksihima Onoro (Akitaro Onho) will go to the Circo del Ensanche on the night of the 28th of this month to publicly challenge him. — "Raku no es campeón," 1908:1

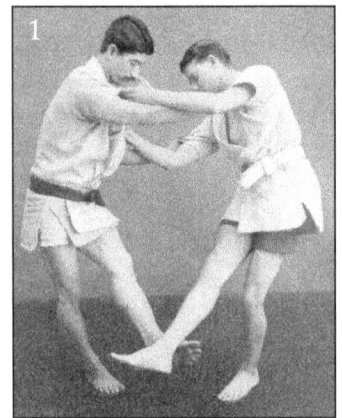 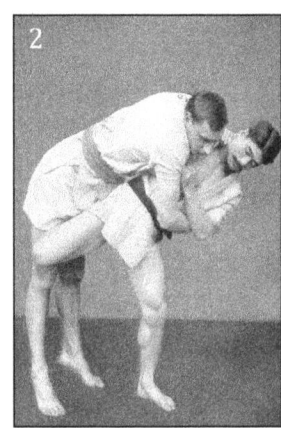 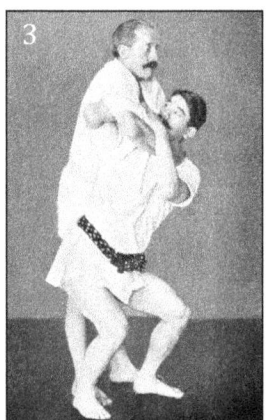

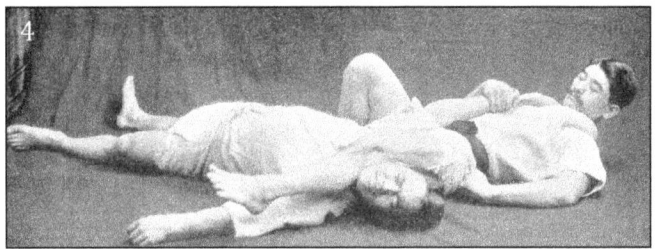

1) Ankle thow, 2) spring hip throw, 3) shoulder throw, and 4) arm lock (Uyenishi, 1905:47, 59, 65, 82).

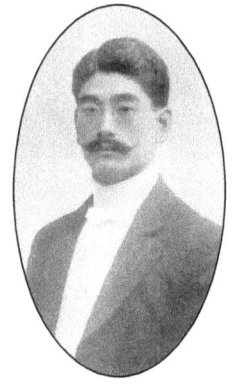 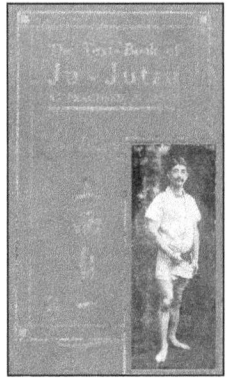

Sadakazu Uyenishi "Raku" portrait and book cover (Uyenishi, 1905: n.p.).

The article stated that upon being asked by journalists about this challenge, Raku had responded that he did not want to accept it as he could not defeat a rival that weighed so much more than he. But Raku left the door open, indicating that if Ohno's threat was published—as came to pass—he would respond immediately. That same day, Ohno's manager showed up at the circus stating that his wrestler wanted to fight that very night against Raku. Raku declined, producing an uproar in the circus so large that the police had to intervene. Thanks to this controversy, the following night a huge number of people went to the Circo del Ensanche. After his exhibition, Raku announced that the following day a twenty-minute match would be held between Ohno and himself. On 30 August, the match *took place, with an attendance so large, as noted* El Noticiero Bilbaíno, "to define the times and make the owner happy" ("De teatros," 1909:4). This first encounter finished in a tie, angering the public who believed it to have been a prearranged outcome. The following day, a definitive combat was held between the two wrestlers, with ten minute rounds followed by five minute breaks, until Raku finally achieved victory after twenty-six minutes. Fewer spectators attended this fight than attended the previous one. As noted by the journalists of the time, a large portion of the public now considered the matches as little more than staged combat.

After this match, despite the economic success of their collaboration, Raku and Ohno did not work together again. With his corpulence, his arrogance in challenging Raku, and his bad manners in refusing to shake Raku's hand after their first match, Ohno had played the villain. Raku, on the other hand, had gained the sympathy and admiration of the public as the small and simple jujutsu teacher. Furthermore, the careful marketing that surrounded the duels had made the conflicts a popular event commented on by the press and by the Bilbao public. But this staging had left a certain "bad taste in the mouth" in Bilbao that was reflected in the newspaper stories. This manifested itself during Raku's second stay in Bilbao, between 5 and 9 November 1909. By this point, certain sectors of society already considered the jujutsu show as false and lowbrow:

> Raku debuted last night in this theater and his performance contained no novelty, not even in the scandals that accompanied it... A foreigner threatened Raku and the public became divided with some declaring the challenge a farce and others claiming it was real... The theater seemed like a bullring until the curtain dropped and the performance was called off... We call these events to the attention of the appropriate authorities so that they can investigate the matter and avoid the repetition of such vulgar scenes.
> — "De teatros," 1909:4

After the Bilbao performance of 1908, Raku's tour continued in cities like Valladolid, Tolosa, San Sebastián, Zaragoza, Logroño, Valencia and Alicante. In these cities, the show's success was assured by using the same formula. Before the first performance, Raku was presented as the famous jujutsu champion and his previous successes were described in detail. If there were no rivals in the city to fight against Raku, which was the case more often than not, Raku fought against wrestlers or artists from within the circus company. Some of these artists after putting up a grand fight against Raku, were defeated with "strange techniques" (ie. strangulation techniques). For one reason or another, these defeats worked the spectators up to the point where the circus was "forced" to schedule "rematches." Likewise, when there were locals willing to take part in the show, as in Valladolid, Tolosa, San Sebastián and Valencia, the locals were utilized as a means of garnering public interest and ensuring a wide public turnout for the circus shows.

For his ultimate Spanish appearance, Raku returned to the Circo de Parish in Madrid. Performing between 21 June and 3 July 1910, Raku used the Swiss, Maurice De Ríaz to put a new face on his old wrestling exhibition routine. On 27 June, in his first match against De Ríaz, Raku emerged victorious after applying a strangle hold that left the Swiss wrestler unconscious. After reawakening, De Ríaz worked himself and the audience up into a furious anger. This tried and tested formula of creating an audience antagonist—De Ríaz in this case—again proved successful. The show received expanded press coverage and Circo de Parish sold-out all of its performances. Then, on 3 July, during the circus' last performance in Madrid, Raku–De Ríaz's match ended after ten minutes of combat with a totally unexpected outcome: a tie. This tie was the first and only time that Raku did not defeat a non-Japanese fighter in a Spanish match. After the match, as far as we know, Raku did not perform again in Spain.

From 1909 to the First World War, a number of other wrestlers gave diverse jujutsu exhibitions throughout Spain. Eido and his female assistant, Nelli, gave an exhibition of "jujutsu-based dance" in the Circo de Parish, between 19 and 27 June 1909. After Madrid, they moved to Valladolid's Teatro Zorrilla. Performing there between 5 and 11 July, the artists received good reviews, but in neither location did their show achieve the same success as had Raku's. Doubtless, this was due to their reliance on "dance" (in actuality, the dances were likely to have been katas) instead of the more familiar challenge and match arrangement that had previously been employed by Raku, Miyake, and Maeda. Two years later, between 3 and 17 October 1911, Yukio Tani (57 kg./126 lb.), the first Japanese wrestler to introduce jujutsu to Europe (Noble, 2000), performed in the Teatro Tivoli in Barcelona. Tani, known as "the pocket Hercules" filled his shows by using Raku's challenge and match format. Almost a year later, between 17 June and 1 July 1912, Tani and Miyake performed together in the Circo de Parish. In these performances, Miyake, touted as the "Champion of Champions," confronted Mr. Ito, a Belgian introduced as the European champion, and Maurice De Ríaz who, as described earlier in the article, followed this match up with a victory in his 1912 Madrid World Wrestling Championship.

On 8 March 1913 sumo wrestling was introduced to Spain in the "International Wrestling Tournament" held in Madrid's Central Jai Alai Courts. Sponsored by *L'Auto* and the *Heraldo de Madrid* newspapers, the championship brought together eight Japanese and fourteen European wrestlers (including well known personalities like former World Champions Paul Pons and Apollon) in a competition for 22,500 pesetas in prizes. Even though sumo wrestling was presented as the tournament's principal attraction, Greco-Roman wrestling and jujutsu exhibitions were also held. Despite the novelty of the sport, sumo wrestling failed to capture the public's interest, at least with the same degree of success as had Greco-Roman wrestling. In fact, on 17 March, the tournament organizers announced that, due to the withdrawal of six of the eight Japanese wrestlers (officially for "health reasons"), the championship would continue as a Greco-Roman wrestling championship. Paul Pons walked away with the title.

After the previous description of jujutsu's introduction into Spain, one can appreciate how jujutsu surprised Spanish society with its exoticism, the elegance of its wrestlers, the richness of its techniques, and its extreme efficiency. This efficiency was especially evident in the matches seen in Spain's theaters and circuses, where Raku and his countrymen systematically destroyed the middle-rank of European wrestlers (choosing as described above, not to fight against the best that the West had to offer). However, jujutsu's visceral and technical marvels were not sufficient to ensure its long-term popularity. Beginning several years before World War I, the jujutsu show began a quick decline that would result in its disappearance from the Spanish theaters.

This decline was due to several factors. First, beginning at the end of 1905, the French began to question and even reject the sport (Brousse, 2000:189–192). Then in 1908, two Parisian tournaments saw the defeat of jujutsu experts (the first of Frenchman, Regnier, by Russian wrestler, Padoubny, and the second of alleged World jujutsu Champion, Matsuda Tano by Californian boxer Sam McVey). The Spanish press covered these upsets extensively, questioning the theretofore-accepted superiority of the Japanese combat method over Western methods. Second, from the point of view of showmanship, jujutsu could not continually offer the novelties that the public demanded. The exclusion of Japanese wrestlers from Greco-Roman wrestling tournaments by the powerful professional wrestlers of the period (Brousse, 2000:189) left the Japanese wrestlers in a hopeless situation. Furthermore, the number of Japanese wrestlers in the country was not sufficient to enable them to compete with the immensely popular Greco-Roman wrestling tournaments. The lack of public exposure of jujutsu led to the loss of the following that it had developed in Spain and the development of a reputation as an "out-dated" fighting method. Some years later, when jujutsu reappeared in wrestling shows, it played second fiddle to other fighting methods, but the positive imagery of the Japanese method had been consolidated into wrestling shows and used to strengthen their popularity.

Onishiko, a Japanese jujutsu wrestler, performed in the 1925–1928 Cinturón de Madrid Greco-Roman wrestling championships. In these tournaments, Onishiko did not compete, but instead fought against tournament participants in exhibition matches held under jujutsu rules. From the beginning, Onishiko was compared to Raku. As a journalist of the day poeticized:

> "(Onishiko), a little man of feeble constitution and sharp, slippery, agile, feline features, ...vulpine eyes and a malicious smile" faced "spare-tire laden, pinkish, fat-necked, wide-backed, iron-biceped . . . slow, phlegmatic (wrestlers with) windmill-blade hands and sausage fingers" in front of whom he "crouched down like a spring, launched himself like a rabbit, and turned his fingers into hooks upon leaping onto the bull-like necks of the Greco-Roman wrestlers."
> — de la Peña, 1928

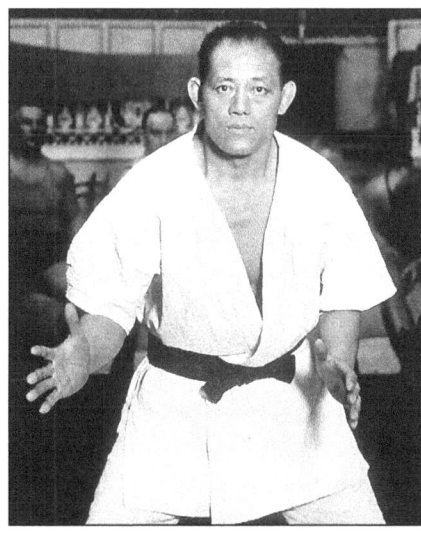

Jujutsu expert Onishiko (cir. 1925)
(Archivo General de la administración, Cultural Section, box F/429, envelope 89).

The resemblance to Raku was further strengthened by Onishiko's 500 peseta offer—the same amount as Raku had offered—to any wrestler that could either defeat Onishiko or simply survive three five minute rounds. The matches were presented as a competition: science, skill, and cunning versus strength. After consistently winning these early matches, Onishiko cemented the similarity with his predecessor by his self-aggrandizing adoption of the moniker "invincible."

Following Onishiko's exhibitions, a Portuguese jujutsu expert, known simply as "Grilo," performed in the 1930-1932 Cinturón de Madrid tournaments. Grilo was presented in the newspapers as the "mouse" who continued Raku and Onishiko's legacy by easily triumphing over the "lions" of Greco-Roman wrestling. These fighter's performances and their continual presence in Spanish fighting illustrates the clear and indisputable manner in which wrestlers used the images that had grown to define jujutsu since the beginning of the century: the weak against the strong, intelligence versus brawn, the Japanese cunning against the Western nobility, the uniqueness of the Japanese combat method, its scientific nature, etc. Likewise, public and press reaction to these shows, demonstrates the firm place the images held in the collective consciousness of the middle-class, who made up most of the audience for the wrestling exhibitions.

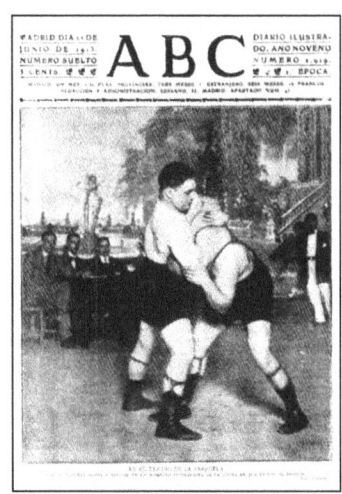

Wrestlers Javier Ochoa and Müller on the cover of *ABC Newspaper* (11 June 1913).

Pancrase and Freestyle American Wrestling (Catch-as-Catch-Can)

Greco-Roman wrestling exhibitions definitively fell out of favor in Spain at the beginning of the 1930s. In the author's opinion, the foremost reason was the monotony and lack of visual appeal that characterized the Greco-Roman wrestling of that period more than the lack of integrity of its tournaments. As previously commented, the sport was static and based predominantly on force. The sport's visual deficiency was observed as early as 1913, when the *ABC* newspaper made the following comment after the completion of that year's World Championship:

> These matches in which the gladiators have shown off their 100-odd kilos of fat and exhibited their abundant sweat and out-of-shape physiques can not be . . . the wrestling of the Roman arena or Greek gymnasium. . . . In athletics, the names of Greece and Rome are always associated with art, grace and elegance. These spectacles of two fat, sweaty, halfway-nude, malodorous men tumbling about over a mat like toads on the grass, seem more appropriate for the floor of a Chicago sausage factory . . . — "Las luchas grecorromanas," 1913:4

To survive, wrestling exhibitions urgently needed a profound renovation. In 1933, Pancrase was introduced as an alternative to the now passé Greco-Roman wrestling. A heterodox style of wrestling imported from the United States, Pancrase allowed a large number of techniques banned in other forms of wrestling. In an article titled "Do you want to tell me what 'Pancrase' is," Carlos Rodríguez (1933:8) observed:

> A new sport on the horizon? We know 'Pancrase' from the reports that have arrived from abroad, principally from North America, reports that show all the signs of a spectacular sensation. Freestyle wrestling? Japanese wrestling? Boxing-wrestling?... We believe we have found a little bit of each of these in this sport that has arrived in Spain through movie reels and American press cuttings... The (sport's only) prohibitions are biting; scratching; nose, ear or mouth twisting; kicking; face clawing; throwing the opponent outside the ring in a manner that prevents him from grabbing the ropes; head-butting; kneeing and elbowing; choking; twisting sexual areas; and poking the eyes of an opponent.

Thanks to these rules, Pancrase wrestling was a great deal more dynamic, varied, agile, acrobatic, violent, and emotional—in sum, more spectacular—than was Greco-Roman wrestling. The contrast between the two types of wrestling was extreme. The 1st International Championship of Pancrase, held in Madrid between 24 May and 14 June 1933, shocked the public with the sport's violence. In reaction, the government banned the new sport. So, the following year, Pancrase was replaced by another style of wrestling: freestyle American wrestling or Catch-As-Catch-Can.

Through an assimilation of the techniques of other wrestling styles and a relaxation of the rules for these styles, Catch-As-Catch-Can, or simply Catch, had evolved towards the extravagant and spectacular. Nevertheless, in theory, it did not exhibit the extreme violence inherent in Pancrase. Hence, upon its importation into Spain from the United States, it was accepted by the authorities and enthusiastically embraced by Spain's middle classes who made it one of the country's favorite pastimes up through the 1970s.

The first Catch tournaments held in Spain, took place in Madrid and Barcelona in the period prior to the Spanish Civil War (1936–1939). Following that conflict, wrestling exhibitions did not start again until 1943. Capitalizing on public interest even greater than that for boxing, by 1945 three Madrid firms (Circo Price, Bullring [Plaza de Toros] and Joyous Jai-Alai Court [Frontón Fiesta Alegre]) and one Barcelona firm (Gran Price) organized weekly and semi-weekly Catch exhibitions. The public thirst for Catch was so widespread that by the end of the 1940s, exhibitions were commonplace in many major Spanish cities. Madrid, Barcelona, Valencia, Bilbao, Zaragoza, Palma de Mallorca and Alicante all had well-established firms dedicated to the organization of Catch exhibitions. As Barbosa (1952) noted "The seat of the professional freestyle wrestling exhibition is in our country" as evidenced by the 632 Catch exhibitions in 1950 alone and the regular participation in these events by nearly 35 foreign wrestlers. Without doubt, in this era, the holy triumvirate of Spanish sport was soccer, boxing and Catch-As-Catch-Can.

Despite, or perhaps in order to earn and preserve, this success, Catch did not return to the "noble" matches of yesteryear as claimed by purists. On the contrary, the "sport" embraced the most theatrical and exaggerated aspects of wrestling. Coronado's (1935) critical observations clearly characterize the quality of the matches:

> As is to be expected, the Spaniards did the best. Things would have been

different, if the tournament had been held in France or Switzerland.... In these shows, there is always a terrible man that hits the referee and confronts the audience ... it is not a wrestling style that lends itself to a sincere attempt to organize seventeen participants for a tournament of more than five weeks in duration...within three to four days the entire troupe would be 'destroyed'... The conduct of the coordinators and the participants is worthy of praise: the exhibition finishes every night at the same time, no matter the number or the quality of the combatants ... the spectator that would like to see a more convincing fight has to do nothing more than drop a 5-peseta coin onto a streetcar platform.

But Catch-As-Catch-Can was a show, a "sport" typified by its acrobatics: various jumps and spins that would have been impossible to use in a real fight. Furthermore, many of Catch's techniques, if unaltered, were exceptionally dangerous and, therefore, had to be softened to avoid causing serious injury to one's opponent. In turn, the opponent had to pretend that the softened or feigned techniques had actually been effective. This obliged Catch wrestlers, even more than Greco-Roman wrestlers, to stage their matches, meaning that the wrestlers already knew what their opponents would do and how they would respond.

Catch, as an amalgamation of other wrestling styles, owes a great deal to the characteristics and imagery of jujutsu. Specifically, Catch adopted diverse, and, on occasion, fantastic techniques from this "lethal" Japanese method—throws, hold downs, joint locks, chokes, strikes, etc.—techniques that, at the time, did not exist in other wrestling styles. Jujutsu's contributions helped Catch to liberate the public from the monotony that characterized Greco-Roman wrestling. Even to the eyes of the uninformed spectator attending the June 1934 Catch-As-Catch-Can tournament held in Madrid's Circo Price, jujutsu's influence was apparent, with Catch appearing like "jujutsu without a kimono, pure freestyle wrestling" (Soriano, 1934:6). Likewise, it was noted that the rules of the International Catch-As-Catch-Can tournament held in Circo Price between 18 February and 7 April 1936, allowed "all the blows and attacks of boxing, Greco-Roman wrestling, Japanese jujutsu and any other technique the wrestler can invent inside the ring" ("Reglamento por el que," 1936:4). Jujutsu's influence on Catch can also be seen in the techniques used by the winner of the 1934 and 1935 Cinturón de Madrid. Soroa, a Brazilian of Spanish descent, won these tournaments through his jujutsu knowledge and his utilization of dislocation techniques, garnering him a comparison to the aforementioned Raku.

Further examining the relationship between Catch and jujutsu, it is interesting to see how the exaggerations of the former served to reinforce the exotic imagery, mysteriousness, and invincibility already associated with the latter. This reinforcement was especially evident in Spain at the end of the 1940s, when judo, despite already being practiced in other European countries like France or England, was practically unknown in Spain. Exploiting this imagery during judo's introduction, various wrestlers used the "secret" techniques of Japanese wrestling to intimidate and defeat their opponents.

Notable examples include Loozen, a Belgian who specialized in the application of Japanese wrestling's "mysterious pressure points" ("Mañana," 1947:10). Max Looder, a wrestler from the Belgian Congo, possessed an extensive repertoire of "laughing holds" and various joint locking techniques that he used to escape from his rivals' holds and to subsequently beat them (García, 1950:1; "Flaviano venció," 1948:3). The small Texan wrestler, Dom Carver, touted as "the Man of Inconceivable Skills," employed the "secrets of Nippon wrestling" on his opponents, causing them to suffer "Saint Vitus' dance (convulsions) upon expertly striking their nerve centers" ("El jujutsu de Dom," 1948; "Dom Carver," 1948: 2; "Dos revanchas," 1948:10).

Likewise, the Belgian Lambert Grailet, known as "the Strangler"—due to his domination of *shime-waza* (choking techniques)—exhibited a certificate that accredited him as a Professor of jujutsu at the Centre Sportif des Bains de la Sauvenière in Liège, Belgium ("Flaviano tiene," 1948:3). Another wrestler who exploited his "credentials" to create an atmosphere of fear was the Frenchman, Gen Tilly, presented as European Champion of jujutsu—a title that he said he had obtained in London. Tilly was also presented as one of only two people on the continent who had obtained a black belt, a rank that he had achieved after winning thirty consecutive combats. Thanks to his scientific knowledge of jujutsu, Gen Tilly "defeated his opponents by attacking their tendons in the point where they met the bone, or by driving his fingers into his opponent's nerve centers, putting (his opponents) at his mercy, as if they were a simple toy" ("Tarrés," 1949:1; "Presentación," 1949:1; "Gen Tilly," 1950:1).

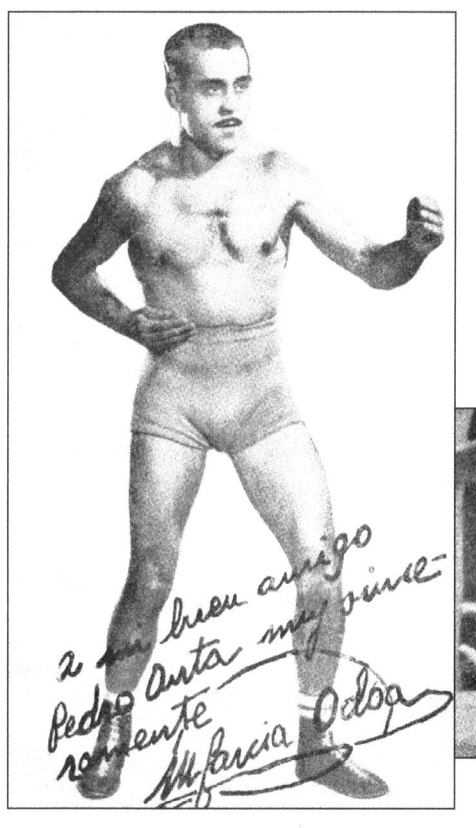
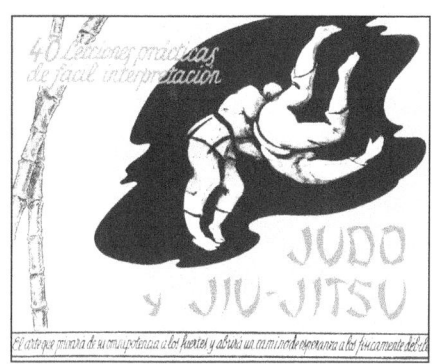
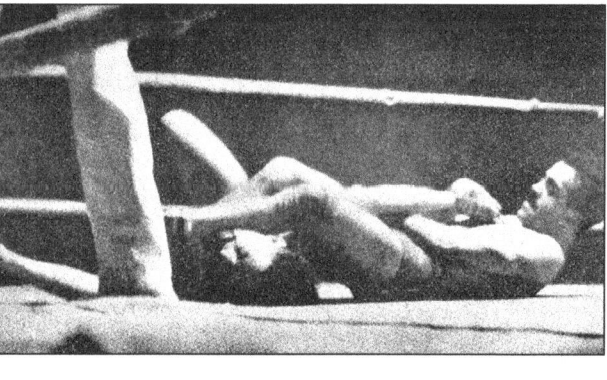

Left: Mariano García Ochoa portrait (Anta, c. 1947:26). Top right: Cover of one of the first Spanish judo books: *Judo and Jujitsu— 40 Easily Interpreted Practical Lessons* (c. 1952). Bottom right: The "atomica" (*ude hisigui juji gatame*) by Mariano García Ochoa (Anta, c. 1947:52).

There were also some Spanish wrestlers who were familiar with Japanese wrestling. Mariano García Ochoa, several time champion of Spain and one of the country's most famous Catch wrestlers, was well-known for his devastating "Atomic" hold. Despite García Ochoa's claim that the hold was his own invention (Anta, ca. 1947:51), it was in fact the judo technique known as ude *hisigi juji gatame* (forearm break with a cross-hold).

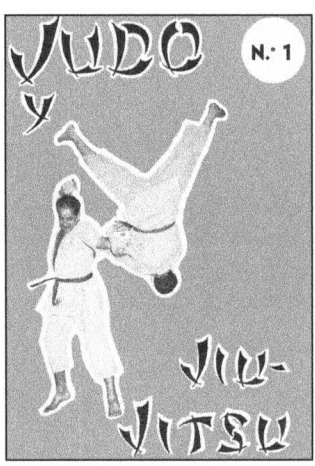

One of the first Spanish judo books:
Judo and Jujitsu, Volume 1 (1954).

Cinci, another well-known wrestler, noted the Atomic was "simply a Japanese wrestling hold, but certainly one of the most dangerous in that if it were applied with force it could break the strongest arm" ("Font," 1947:1). This appreciation of the danger of jujutsu's more hazardous moves was not uncommon. José Trapiella "Suin," for his part, responded to the question of whether he was familiar with Japanese wrestling:

"Yes ... but I barely use it, because its attacks are dangerous ... I know how to twist every joint. For example, I can twist the elbow joint using *kwansetsu waza* (joint-locking techniques), but in doing so, the forearm or the arm can easily break. Nor do I use *ashiate*, which is an attack to the vital points of the foot. I prefer to attack the ears or the nose ... But by breaking a bone, one can rob one's adversary of his livelihood, and that is something I will not do" (K., 1948:6).

Another famous Spanish catch wrestler, Lambán, was known as "The Spanish Strangler" due to his application of a "demolishing torsion hold to the cervical vertebrae." The Aragonese wrestler had learned the move "from a foreign jujutsu instructor (and had applied it) for the first time on the Italian, Brosatti ... The effect of the new technique was such that Brosatti had to be hospitalized" (K.O., 1950:2).

All of these examples serve to illustrate the halo of mystery that continued to surround Japanese wrestling in Spain, shaping the Spanish middle-class' impression of the sport as an infallible combat method composed of an infinite variety of strange and brutal techniques that permitted one to easily triumph over one's opponent.

Epilogue

In 1950, the Asociación Española de Judo y Jiu-Jitsu was founded in Madrid. The establishment of this club, the first Spanish club dedicated to the promotion of judo as a sport, was followed a year later by the inauguration in Barcelona of the Academia de Judo y Jiu-Jitsu de España and in Zaragoza of the Yudo y Jiu-Jitsu Club. These years also saw the publication of the first Spanish judo books, carrying titles like: *Defensa Personal – Judo, Jiu-Jitsu, Boxeo* (Personal Defense – Judo, Jujutsu, Boxing) (Valle, 1950); *Judo y Jiu-Jutsu – 40 Lecciones prácticas de fácil interpretación* (Judo and Jujutsu – 40 Easily Interpreted

Practical Lessons) (Ungría, ca. 1952); and *Judo y Jiu-Jitsu* (Judo and Jujutsu) (Franco, 1954).

In Spain, since its introduction, judo has been inextricably linked to jujutsu. Wishing to introduce it through something familiar, the pioneers of Spanish judo, introduced the unknown sport to the public through the use of jujutsu's imagery. Sergio Madrigal, one of the first Spanish judo wrestlers, stated that the majority of wrestlers "were more comfortable supporting themselves with the exotic myth and its associated stereotypes" (Gutiérrez, 2003:181). Jujutsu's imagery and prestige was the tool that pulled people into the gymnasiums, people wanting to learn to "kill with just one finger," to know the "pressure points" of the human body, or to know how to defend themselves against "any type" of attack. Where had these people gotten this impression of judo? In large part, it was the legacy of the theater, circus, and music hall shows of the last half-century, where the "great colossals" of wrestling had performed together with jujutsu's intelligent Japanese representatives.

▼▲▼

BIBLIOGRAPHY

Almasqué, A. (1908, Sep. 24). Jujutsu. *El Mundo Deportivo*, 1.

Anta, P. (ca. 1947). *Mariano García Ochoa*. Madrid: Gráficas A. Carrasco.

Anteo, El Gigante. (1908, June 4). El 'jiu-jitsu' en Madrid. *Nuevo Mundo*, n.p.

Badenas, J. (1934). *Deportes de combate: Tomo I.* Toledo: Establecimiento Tipográfico de Rafael G.-Menor.

Barbosa, R. (1952, Mar. 15). Panorama del deporte de la lucha en España. *Antorcha*, n.p.

Brousse, M. (2000). Les origines du judo en France: De la fin du XIX siècle aux années 1950 – Historie d'une culture sportive. Unpublished doctoral dissertation. Université Bordeaux, France.

Brousse, M., and Matsumoto, D. (1999). *Judo: A sport and a way of life.* Seoul: International Judo Federation.

Cárcamo. (1908, Nov. 10). Habla Raku. *La Rioja*, 1.

Coronado, R. (1935). Lucha. Un poco de historia y unos comentarios de actualidad. *Campeón*, 118, n.p.

de la Peña, H.R. (1928, July 6). El 'jiu-jitsu' y las luchas grecorromanas. La araña de acero y los atletas de cuello de toro. *Nuevo Mundo*, n.p.

de Rivero, Ricardo. (1913, July). Lucha Greco-romana. *Gran Vida*, 201.

De teatros. (1909, Nov. 6). *El Noticiero Bilbaíno*, 4.

del Campillo, El Sastre. (1908, June 27). Cosas del otro jueves. *La Semana Ilustrada*, n.p.

Díaz-Cañabate, A. (1943, Jan. 7). ¡¡Aquella luchas grecorromanas!! *Marca*, 4.

Diem, C. (1966). *Historia de los deportes: Volumen II.* Barcelona: Luis de Caralt.

Dom Carver forzó unas tablas al tigre Americano. (1948, Aug. 7). *Marca*, p. 2.

Dos revanchas decisivas entre Joe Luis y Marcel Manuel y Mike Brendel y Dom Carver. (1948, Aug. 12). *Marca*, 10.

El campeón vencido. (1906, June 21). *Heraldo de Madrid*, 1.

El jujutsu. (1907, Dec. 26). *El Mundo Deportivo*, 3.

El jujutsu de Dom Carver puede restar posibilidades al Tigre Americano. (1948, Aug. 6). *Marca*, 1+.

Flaviano tiene un encuentro decisivo con el belga Grailet. (1948, July 18). *Marca*, 3.

Flaviano venció a Loozen por golpe bajo. (1948, Apr. 18). *Marca*, 3.

Font y Victorio Ochoa se disputan hoy, en Price, el título nacional. (1947, Mar. 26). *Marca*, 1+.

Franco, F. (1954). *Judo y jiu-jitsu* (five volumes). Madrid: Imprenta Fernando Franco.

García, C. (n.d.). *Boxeo y lucha libre*. n.p.

Gen Tilly, un formidable campeón de lucha Japonesa. (1950, July 26). *El Mundo Deportivo*, 1.

Gutiérrez, C. (2003). Introducción y desarrollo del judo en España (de principios del siglo XX a 1965): El proceso de implantación de un método educativo y de combate importado de Japón. Unpublished doctoral dissertation. Universidad de León, Spain.

K. (1948, Aug. 26). Para Suin la mejor presa es la ballesta Japonesa. *Marca*, 6.

K.O. (1950, Jan. 5). Un año de lucha libre. *El Mundo Deportivo*, 1–2.

Las luchas en la Zarzuela. (1906, May 28). *Heraldo de Madrid*, 3.

Las luchas grecorromanas. (1913, Sep. 1). *ABC*, 4.

Le Floc'hmoan, J. (1965). *La génesis de los deportes*. Barcelona: Labor.

Mañana, en Price, Bamala-José Luis y Loozen-Dom Carver. (1947, Dec. 22). *Marca*, 10.

Méndez, F. (1908, June 25). Todo titiriteros. *Nuevo Mundo*, n.p.

Noble, G. (2000, Oct.). The Odyssey of Yukio Tani. *InYo: Journal of Alternate Perspectives*. [On-line serial]. Available: <http://ejmas.com/jalt/jaltart_Noble_1000.htm>.

Noble, G. (2001, May). The life and dead the terrible turk. *Journal of Manly Arts*. [On-line]. Available: <http://ejmas.com/jmanlyart_noble0501.htm>.

Presentación del francés Gen Tilly, campeón del cinturón negro de judo. (1949, Nov. 16). *Marca*, p. 1.

Raku no es campeón. (1908, Aug. 28). *El Noticiero Bilbaíno*, 1.

Reglamento por el que ha de regirse el campeonato internacional de 'catch as catch can' que comienza esta noche en Price." (1936, Feb. 18). *Heraldo de Madrid*, 4.

Rimet, D. (1996). La lutte libre olympique. Une histoire contemporaine et ses apports didactiques. In P. Goirand and J. Metzler (Eds.), *Une histoire culturelle du sport*. París: Revue EPS, 69-97.

Rodríguez, C. (1933, May 17). Quiere vd contarme... Qué es el 'pancrace'? *Heraldo de Madrid*, 8.

Ruiz, R. (1912, Aug. 30). El campeonato de lucha. *Heraldo de Madrid*, 4.

Soriano, J. (1934, June 18). Una figura hispana en la moderna lucha 'catch-as-catch-can', AS, 6.

Svinth, J. (2001, Feb.). The evolution of women's judo, 1900–1945. *InYo: Journal of Alternative Perspectives*. [On-line]. Available: <http://ejmas.com/jalt/jaltframe.htm>.

Tarrés ante el duro Pirock y la presentación de Gen-Tilly mañana en Price. (1949, Oct. 27). *El Mundo Deportivo*: 1.

Ungría, B. (ca. 1952). *Judo y jiu-jitsu – 40 lecciones prácticas de fácil interpretación*. Madrid: Gráficas Express.

Uyenishi, S. ("Raku"). (1905). *The text-book of jujutsu as practised in Japan – Being a simple treatise on the Japanese method of self-defence*. London: Athletic Publications Ltd.

Valle, F. Vicente del. (1950). *Defensa personal – Judo, jiu-jitsu, boxeo)*. Madrid: Imprenta Fernando Franco.

Valserra, F. (1944). *Historia del deporte*. Madrid: Plus Ultra.

Zosaya, L. (1906, June 12). El timo de las luchas. *Heraldo de Madrid*: 3.

chapter 13

Haragatame: Judo's Rare Stomach Armlock
by David Finch

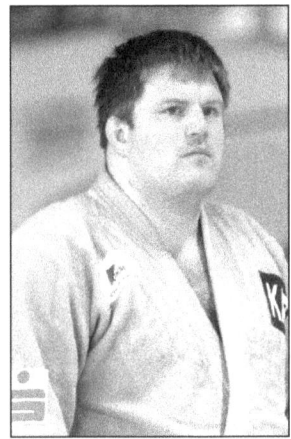
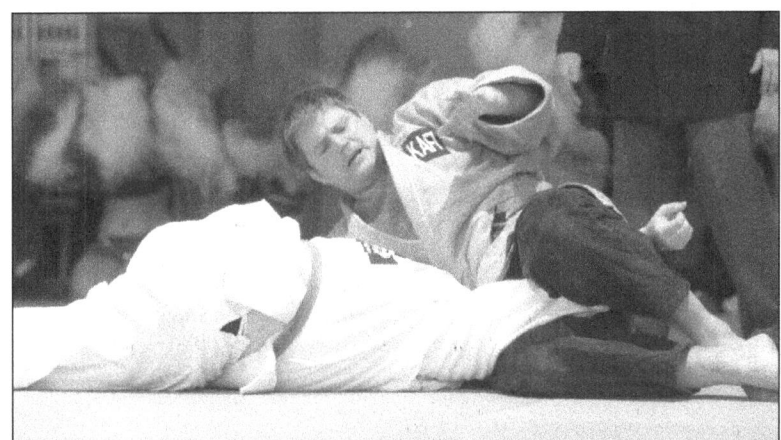

Ben Sonnemans beat Pascale Pauke by 10 points with an unusual armlock.
All photos courtesy of Judo Photos Unlimited.

Introduction
One of the fascinations of judo is the incredible array of arm locks that, if taken to the extreme, can immediately disable an opponent. Two such examples, used in competition and leading to submission, are illustrated here.

Example One (see next page)
The first was taken recently at the Budesliga match (German teams are allowing to use foreign fighters in the domestic league matches) between the Eberswalde Judo Club and the Hattingen Judo and Ju-Jitsu Club. Ben Sonnemanns, the 1997 Dutch heavyweight European Champion (-95 kgs), was fighting for Eberswalde as a super heavyweight (+100 kgs). His opportunity came two and half minutes into the fight when both were on the ground with Pascale Pauke face down underneath Sonnemanns. The Dutchman was unsighted but he trapped Pauke's right arm with his left leg, entangling his ankles to prevent escape.

Once trapped, the arm was straightened by Sonnemanns pressing heavily down on Pauke to flatten his body. At the same time, he revolved his body to the right putting pressure on the arm with his locked legs leading to immediate submission. One photo shows Sonnemanns looking at the arm for the first time to make sure he did not go too far.

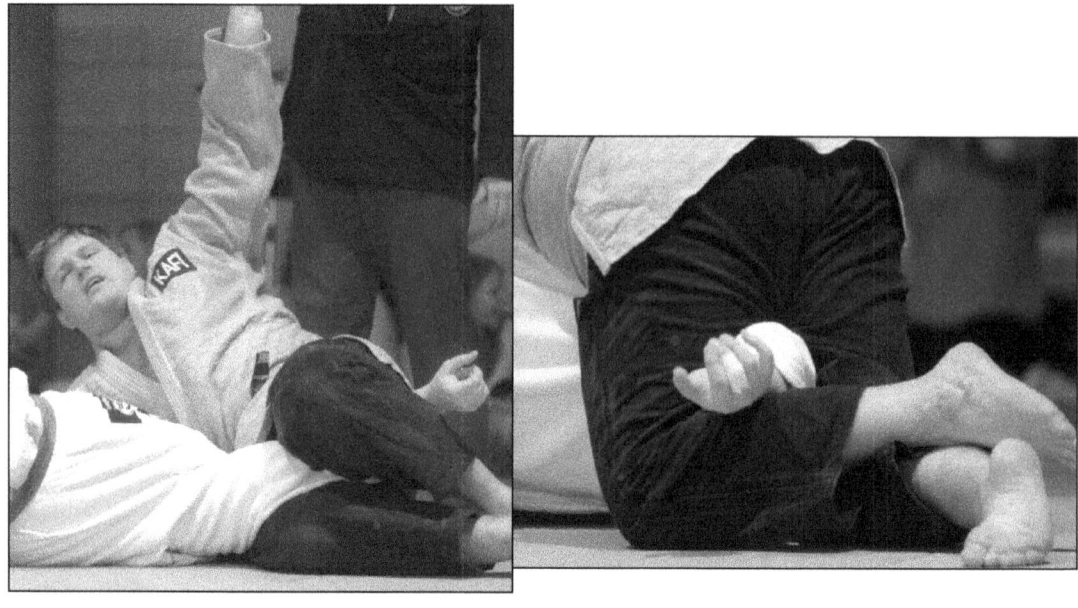

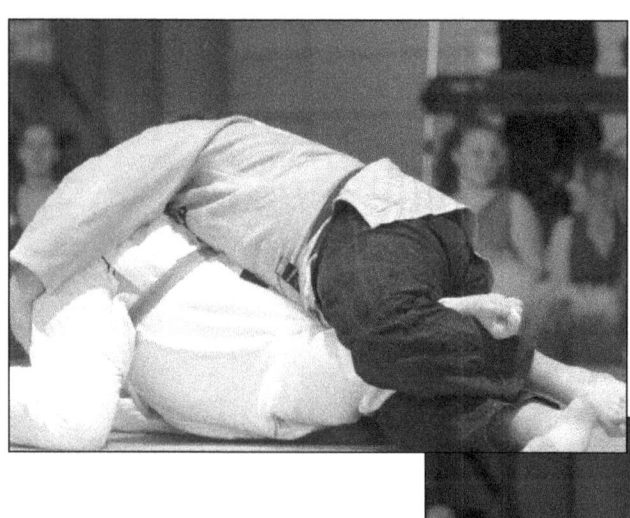

Example Two

The second example, from the 1985 Seoul World Championships, shows Hitoshi Saito of Japan armlocking Steve Cohen of the USA. The technique, on the same right arm with the American face down, starts similarly except that Saito, again unsighted, hooks the arm with his right leg rather than his left. This leads to Saito rolling his body leftwards but only after controlling Cohen with the weight of his stomach and then locking the half folded arm and putting dangerous pressure on Cohen's shoulder.

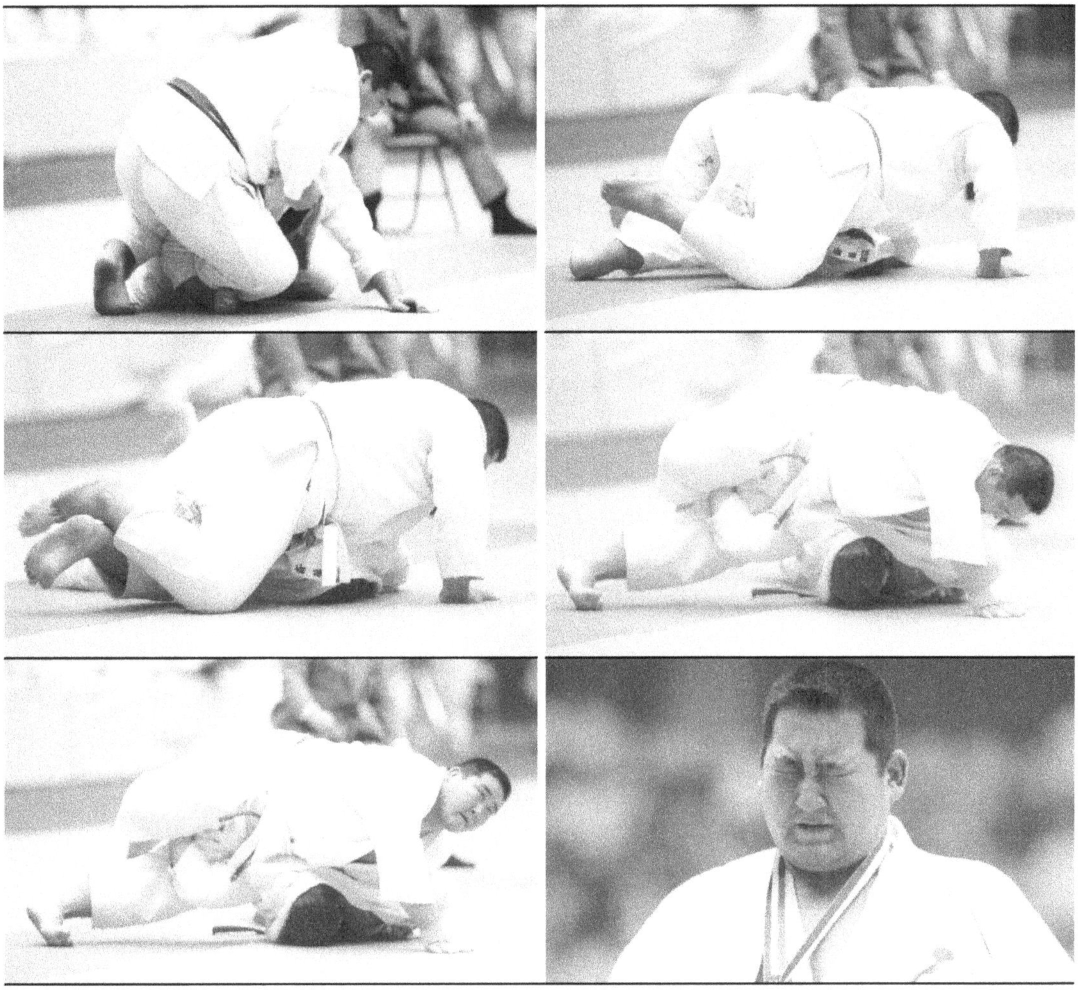

Hitoshi Saito (Japan) armlocks Cohen (USA).
Bottom right: Saito in pain during the medal ceremony
following the standing armlock applied by Cho (Korea).

Interestingly Saito—one of the best heavyweights at the time—met his match in the final when Yong-Chul Cho of Korea sneakily snapped on a standing armlock in the opening few seconds. True samurai-like warrior that he was, Saito tried to fight on after a few minutes of medical attention, but the damage from when he refused to submit was so severe, that he had to retire to the delight of the home crowd.

Without an intimate knowledge of the Japanese language it would be easy to categorize these techniques alongside existing widely known arm locks such as *waki-gatame* (armbar on elbow) and *ude-garami* (elbow lock). However, according to the Kodansha book *Kodakan Judo* (1986), they would both fall into the category of *haragatame* (stomach armlock) where the stomach of the opponent on top is used to create the initial overpowering control.

REFERENCE
Kano, J. (1986). *Kodokan judo*. Tokyo: Kodansha.

chapter 14

Kataguruma: Judo's Spectacular Shoulder Wheel Throw
by David Finch

One of the more spectacular throws in judo, the shoulder wheel throw (*kata-guruma*) is a technique that has become particularly associated with East European judo. At the December 2003 European Team Finals held in London, two very competent exponents of the technique, Gennadi Bilodid of the Ukraine and Zurab Zviabuari of Georgia, graphically demonstrated the throw's effectiveness, but from different directions.

Gennadi Bilodid was the 2003 73-kg European champion. He also won the title at the 2001 Paris European Championships. His sequence involves the "cack-handed," left-sided grip that easily confuses the majority of right-handed fighters. If fast enough, the shoulder wheel throw invariably surprises the opponent. In this case, Bilodid dives low to the left in preference to lifting his opponent, grips the left leg to prevent the instinctive retreat, and causes his opponent to do a "forward roll" onto his back and instant defeat.

Gennadiy Bilodid (Ukraine) beats Ian Francis (Great Britain).
All photos courtesy of Judo Photos Unlimited.

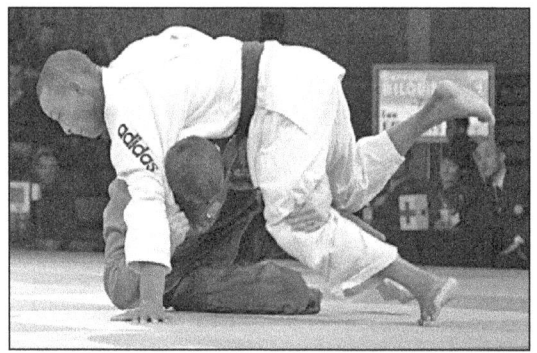
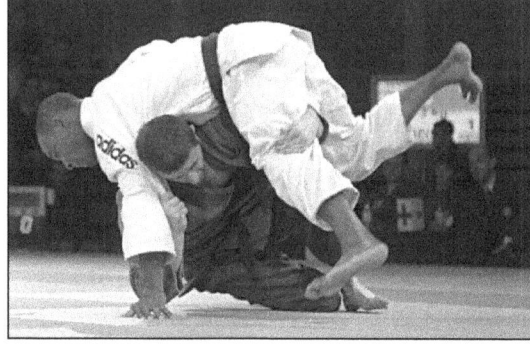
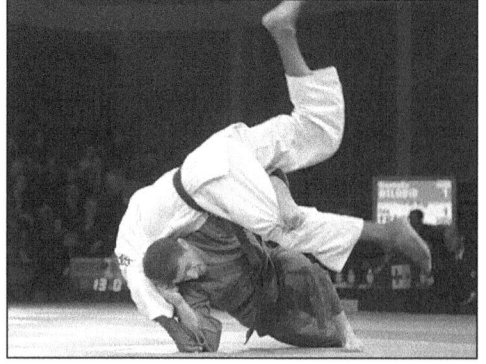

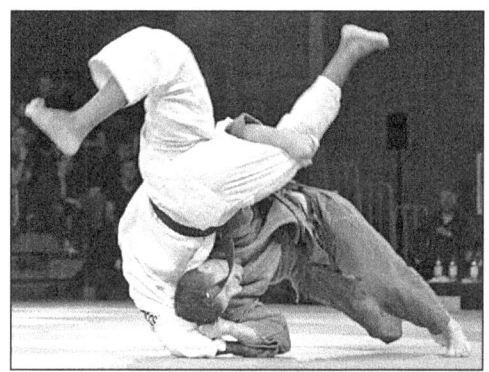

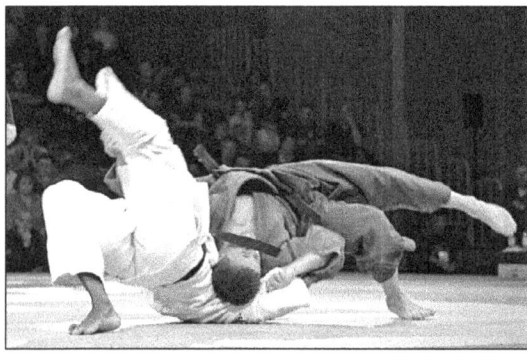
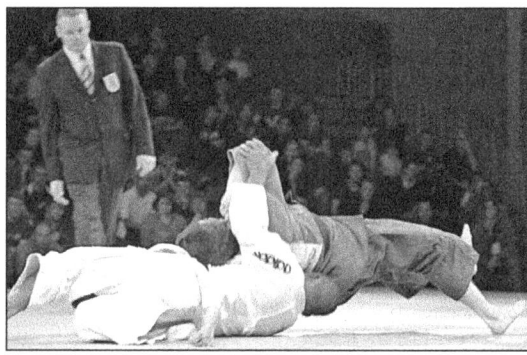

At the Osaka World Championships, Zurab Zviabuari used the same diving shoulder wheel throw attack in the finals of the 90-kgs division against Hwang Hee-tae of South Korea. Although it worked, he was only awarded minor points, leaving the Korean enough time to win the contest with a hold. It was Zviabuari's second World silver, his first being at Munich in 2001.

Zviabuari's right-handed sequence of photos starts with a shot from the final of the Osaka 90-kg division. You can see quite clearly that Zviabuari starts the attack by slipping his left leg across Hwang's advancing right foot and at the same time dropping beneath him. In the first photo of the London Team Finals sequence, Zviabuari uses his left leg to the same effect, but this time dropping on his extended knee because he was closer to his opponent. The result is the same with his Spanish opponent falling cleanly across the Georgian's shoulders, but extending his arms in a desperate attempt to frustrate the attack.

Zurab Zviabuari (Georgia) scores a full point
on David Alarza (Spain) to put Georgia ahead.

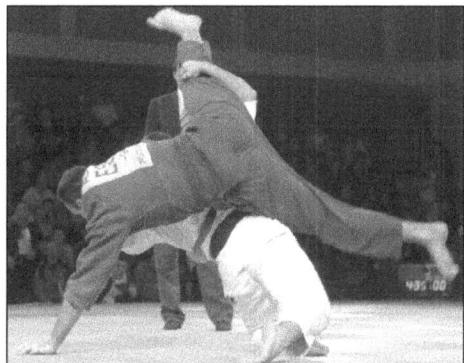
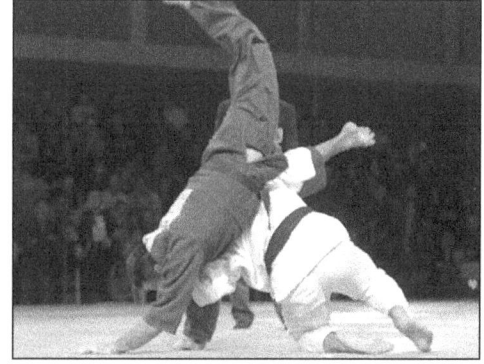

Feeling the resistance, and in complete control of the situation because his left hand is on the back of the right arm, Zviabuari pivots on his left knee and flips the Spaniard over his head and the propping right arm cleanly onto his back for a winning point.

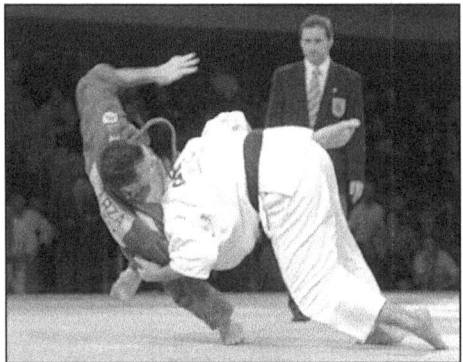 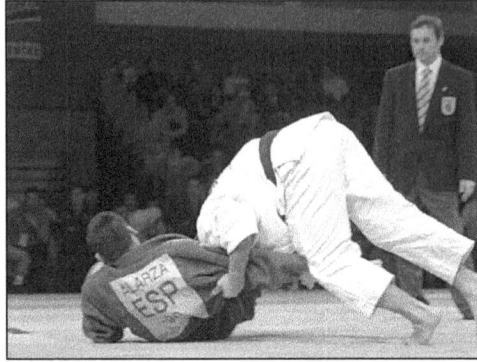

The shoulder wheel throw, in all its forms, is not an exercise in strength but a very technical move reliant on skill, good timing, and a change of direction that puts the opponent irresistibly across the attacker's shoulders. The two sequences here clearly demonstrate that.

chapter 15

Competition, Kata, and the Art of Judo
by Llyr C. Jones, Ph.D.

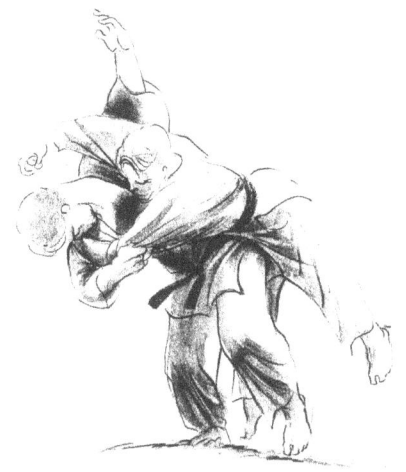

Illustration by Oscar Ratti.
© 2001 Futuro Designs & Publications.

Introduction

The word "judo" comes from a combination of two Japanese words—*ju* meaning gentle or supple and *do* meaning path or way. This literally defines judo as the "gentle way."

At the level of first principles, the essence of Kodokan* judo is turning an opponent's strength against himself and overcoming the opponent through skill rather than sheer strength (Kano, 1986). This theory is captured by the Japanese expression *ju yoku go o seisu*—usually translated as "softness overcomes hardness," "flexibility overcomes stiffness," "gentleness controls strength," or "win by yielding."

Watching the seemingly effortless combination of grace, technique, and power of a true judo expert in action, it would be very easy (but very wrong) to underestimate the intense physical and mental demands that judo makes upon its exponents. Achieving excellence in judo demands considerable single mindedness. Achieving mastery of all of the throwing, grappling, and striking techniques that makes up the system demands intensive and demanding training over an extended period of time under the guidance of an experienced and knowledgeable teacher.

---

* *Kodokan*: The headquarters of judo, originally founded in 1882 by Kano Jigoro who himself had established judo.

Judo has been well established in the West since the early 1900's and is now practiced in almost every country in the world. The aim of this chapter, however, is to question the direction that judo has taken in the West (especially in the United Kingdom) and to challenge whether a significant re-orientation is now required. Where specific statistics or statements are used to support an argument, data and examples from the British Judo Association (BJA)—the national governing body for the Olympic sport of judo in the United Kingdom—are used.

The State of Judo Today

As a starting point, it is worthwhile stating the definition of judo as provided by the *Kodokan New Japanese-English Dictionary of Judo* (Kawamura and Daigo, 2000): *"Judo*: A martial art formulated by Jigoro Kano based on his reformulation and adaptation of several classical jujutsu systems as well as his own philosophical ideals."

Such a definition may not resonate well with the image of judo promoted by the official accredited national governing bodies—i.e., those belonging to the International Judo Federation (IJF)—the majority of whom seem to be actively encouraging the distancing of judo from its martial arts origins. In these early years of the 21st century, it is difficult to challenge the view that in the West (and in the United Kingdom in particular) judo is promoted one dimensionally, as a combat sport—organized around championships and competition—often for competition's sake. To reinforce this sporting dimension, the competitive style of judo is often referred to as *Olympic Judo or Performance Judo* (a style in its own right).

A direct consequence of the leadership and policies of the accredited judo governing bodies is that, for the majority of judo practitioners, judo is now just about medals and prizes. These bodies measure the health of their country's judo simply in terms of results at major championships and accordingly focus their investment only on the handful of elite athletes who have the potential to be World or Olympic medalists. Bethers (n.d.) recognizes this issue:

> It seems that some modern judo leaders have narrowed the objective of judo to only "Contest Proficiency." For many, world-wide judo has become equated with contest proficiency. Although this belief is today wide-spread, it is the very thing that Dr. Kano warned against throughout his life. Dr. Kano stated, "Judo should only be a means to the end of skill and principles for higher self-development, and any 'drift' toward 'contest' judo as the 'sole' interpretation of judo should be carefully regulated." This "drift" has become a major focus among many well intended *judoka* [practitioners], but in the minds of many *sensei* [teachers], technique has suffered and judo has become (more often than not) a sport in which "win at all costs" is the underlying objective.

It is evident that the strategy of focusing on Performance Judo must now be challenged, as judo today is an activity in decline. In the United Kingdom, this is manifested by decreasing adult membership of the British Judo Association—75% of the BJA membership is under the age of 16 (British Judo Association, n.d.)—and the continuing lack of consistent and substantial success of British judo players in international competition despite all the effort directed to this end.

It is a matter of additional concern that the governing bodies have overwhelmingly biased their rank promotion structures (i.e. grading) toward accelerating the grade advancement of those who are successful in competition, with often only lip service being plaid to the breadth and depth of an individual's technical judo knowledge. Again, Bethers (n.d.) writes:

> This emphasis on "Contest Proficiency" has caused the true meaning or purpose of judo to be unclear and somewhat out of proportion to what was intended by Dr. Kano. This problem is surfaced nowhere more clearly than in "notion" that contest victories are rewarded with rapid rank promotions.

Currently there is little prospect for grade advancement for those who (through age, physical condition, or personal preference) wish to practice judo as an art as opposed to a sport. This is, of course, with the notable exception of the promotions that governing body officials and administrators seem to receive as a matter of course. The risk one runs with such a policy is a resultant judo hierarchy that is both one-dimensional in its knowledge and skewed in its priorities.

It is especially disappointing that those judo players who prefer to focus their study on the more traditional and technical aspects of judo (e.g. forms or *kata*) have become tagged with the label recreational players—implying that they are somehow inferior to contest players and not worthy of attention or recognition.

Back to Basics

This author and other writers (Watanabe, 2003; Burkland, 1998) advocate the thesis that judo in the West has lost its way and that there is a real need for it to return to its martial art roots. In doing so, the author's aim for this paper is not to decry the considerable merits of Performance Judo— indeed success in contest over several traditional jujutsu schools was key in establishing Kodokan judo as an effective combat system (Kano, 1986). Rather, it is to argue that judo based solely on sport is not judo *in toto* and that the original and arguably truer meaning of the art lies elsewhere.

Elementary research will reveal that the underlying concept of judo as envisioned by Kano was that it was to be a means of (cooperative) physical and social education—in simple terms, a training for life. Kano captured this principle of mutual welfare and prosperity via the maxim: you and I shining together (*jita kyo ei*, mutual welfare and prosperity) (Kano, 1986).

Indeed, with the overwhelming majority of those now practicing Performance Judo, it is reasonable to conclude that mainstream contemporary judo has now deviated significantly (and quite possibly permanently) from Kano's original ideas. Smith (1999: 221) notes:

> The popularization and spread of judo has weakened Kano's base so greatly, I see no chance of it ever recovering. Judo is now merely a jacketed wrestling sport. The competitive has ousted the cooperative.

Bates (n.d.) argues that judo has two essential components—martial and art. The martial component of judo can be related to combat through the way of the warrior (*budo*)—the contemporary representation of which is competition (*shiai*). In preparation for contest, the modern judo player focuses on the development of physical conditioning and fitness, motivation, tactics, and technique for the sole purpose of securing victory. Conversely, art can be defined as technical excellence and understanding of techniques developed through repeated practice (*uchi-komi* and *nage-komi*), free-practice (*randori*), and kata.

Judo is, of course, both martial and art, but today the concept most people have of judo is martial. Martial represents but one small element of judo, yet almost without exception, most judo teachers focus on developing their students' contest prowess and many believe it unnecessary to practice or even know any kata.

Rediscovering Kata

In the most general sense, any cooperative judo training between partners—e.g. a sequence of combinations or counters etc.—can be considered kata. However, a greater degree of focus is provided in a dictionary of judo (Kawamura and Daigo, 2000), which defines kata as follows:

> **Kata:** Formal movement pattern exercises containing idealized model movements illustrating specific combative principles.

Kata is not unique to judo—it is recognized as a valuable training drill in most Japanese martial arts. The exact nature of kata training, however, varies from art to art. For example, karate kata is a solo form (like shadow boxing), whereas the judo kata are usually performed with partner—each partner having a specific role and performance objective depending on the kata. In judo, there are kata for throwing techniques, ground-work techniques, self-defense, as well as others that illustrate the fundamental principles of judo (Kano, 1986; Otaki and Draeger, 1983; Leggett and Kano, 1982; Kawaishihi, 1982; Fromm and Soames, 1982; Ohlenkamp, 2005).

For completeness, a comprehensive list of the kata practiced in judo follows, together with a summary description of each (Ohlenkamp, 2005). Illustrations of techniques from the seven most common kata are provided in Figures 1 to 7.

Note that not all of these kata were created by Kano or at the Kodokan and, as such, some are not official Kodokan kata. Note also that the last six kata in the list are seldom practiced outside Japan and, even in Japan, few judo players would be familiar with them.

- **Nage-no-kata:** The kata of throws. Includes examples of hand, hip, leg, and sacrifice throws (Figure 1).
- **Katame-no-kata:** The kata of grappling. Includes examples of holds, strangles, and chokes and joint locks (Figure 2).

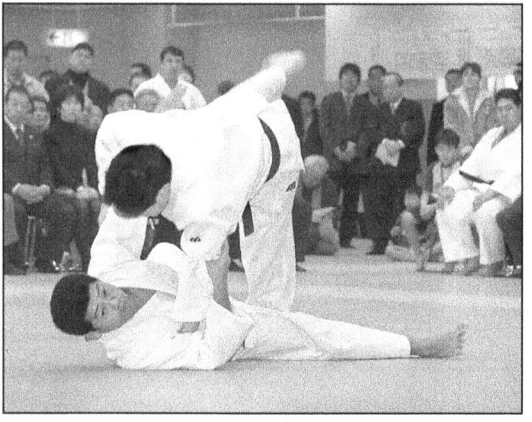 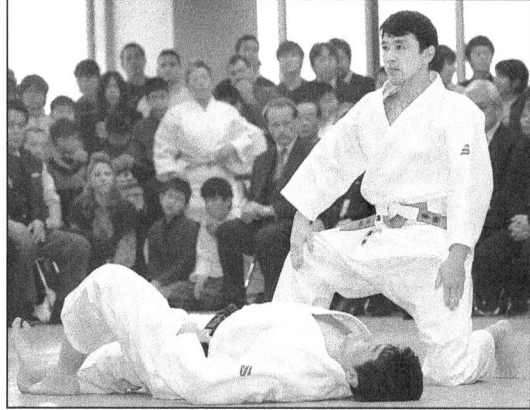

Figure 1: Nage-no-kata　　　　　**Figure 2:** Katame-no-kata

© Photography by Bob Willingham. bob@twoj.org

- **Kime-no-kata:** The kata of decision. This is the traditional judo self-defense kata. It includes both standing and kneeling defense against empty handed, knife, and sword attacks using strikes, chokes, joint locks, and throws (Figure 3). Kime-no-kata is also known as Shinken Shobu-no-kata (combat forms).
- **Kodokan Goshin-jutsu:** The modern Kodokan self-defense kata (Figure 4). It includes defense against empty hand, knife, stick (*jo*), and pistol attacks using strikes, joint locks, and throws.
- **Ju-no-kata:** The kata of gentleness. It includes a number of attacks and defenses demonstrating the efficient redirection of force and movement (Figure 5).
- **Itsutsu-no-kata:** The kata of five principles. This kata is intended for the demonstration and practice of body movement (*tai-sabaki*) and for the application and redirection of energy as in nature (Figure 6).

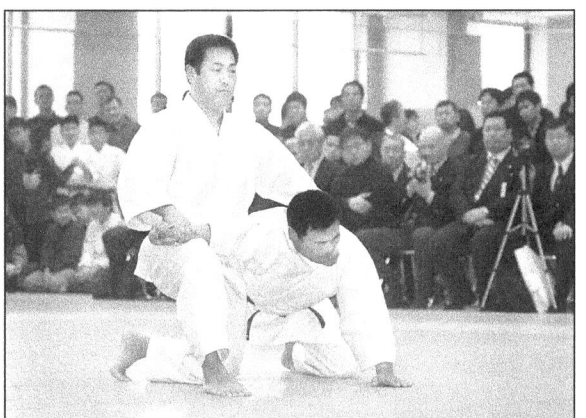

Figure 3: Kime-no-kata.

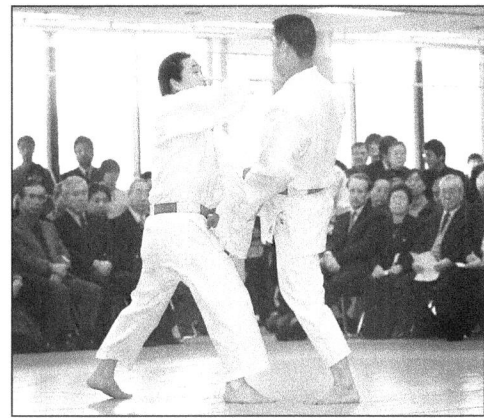

Figure 4: Kodokan Goshin-jutsu.

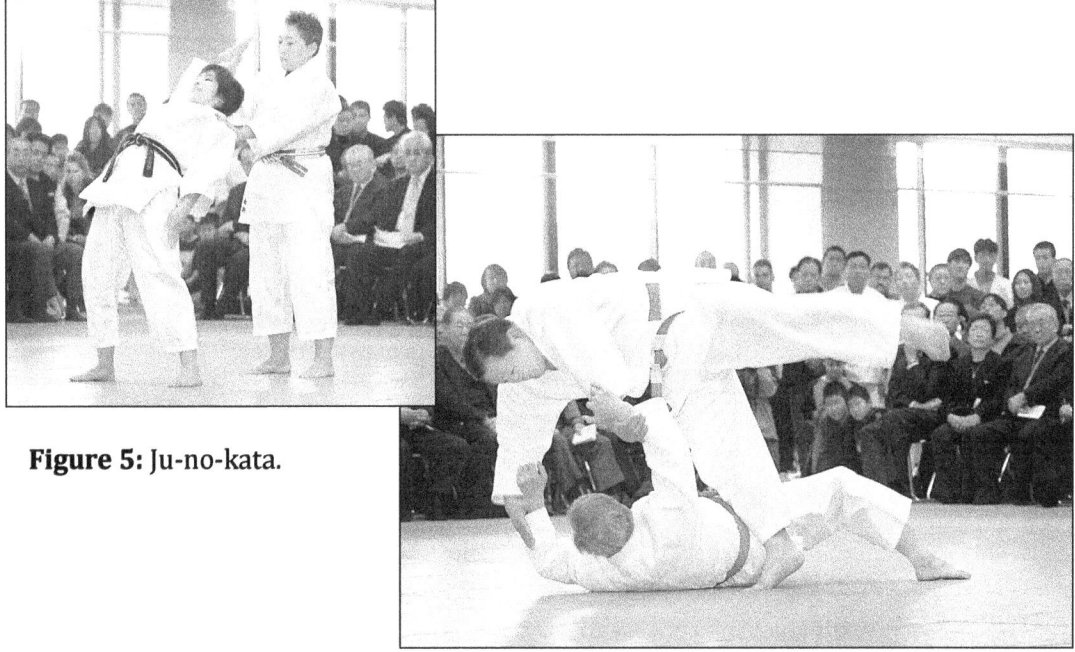

Figure 5: Ju-no-kata.

Figure 6: Itsutsu-no-kata.

- **Koshiki-no-kata**: The ancient kata. This kata has its origins in Kito-ryu Jujutsu and demonstrates the techniques of fighting while wearing armor (*kumiuchi*), and is intended to illustrate the ancient origins of judo techniques (Figure 7).

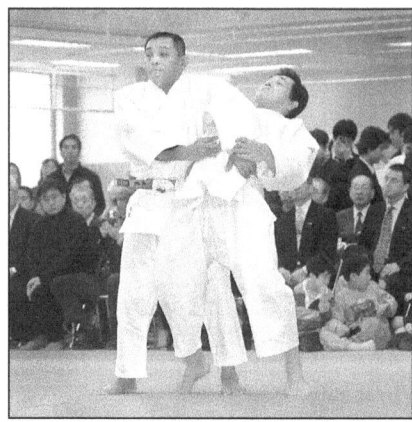

Figure 7: Koshiki-no-kata.

- **Go no Sen-no-kata:** The kata of counters. This kata includes counter throws for a number of common techniques.
- **Kaeshi-no-kata:** An alternative kata of counters.
- **Seiryoku Zenyo Kokumin Taiiku:** The national exercise based on the principles of maximum efficiency. This kata is atypical of judo in being a completely solo kata and comprises a variety of striking and kicking techniques.
- **Kodokan Joshi Goshin-Ho:** The Kodokan's women's self-defense kata. This kata includes a number of escapes from holds and grabs, some basic striking techniques, and one throw.
- **Renkoho**: The kata of arresting techniques. This kata includes a number of control and submission holds useful in restraining criminals.
- **Kimi Shiki:** The kata of decision. This kata emphasizes the use of body movement in responding to attacks and includes both kneeling and standing defenses against empty hand, knife, and sword attacks.
- **Shobu-no-kata:** The kata of attack or contest.
- **Go-no-kata:** The kata of the proper use of force. This kata is the complement to the Ju-no-ata and dates back to the earliest days of the Kodokan where it was used as a training drill.

In nearly all martial art styles, forms are used as training tools from the novice stage upwards. In judo, however, its significance has long been under-emphasized and kata practice is now largely confined to very high grades or those who are not contest-inclined. It is a tragedy of modern judo that, in the headlong rush into Olympic-type competition, most ranked black belt holders regard forms as an anachronism of little relevance to competition that should be discarded. The late Charles Palmer (then BJA president) anticipated this situation when he wrote his 1982 foreword to Leggett and Kano's kata text (Leggett and Kano, 1982):

> ... too much emphasis is being placed on winning at all costs. Not enough time is being spent by judo players on acquiring the vital self-discipline necessary to proper performance of the sport, and the ability to continue enjoying it later in life after the ability to win contests has decreased.

It was particularly insightful of Palmer to recognize that Performance Judo is age limited. Such sport judo is the domain of the young, whereas Kodokan judo (especially kata) can be done up until a very advanced age.

A direct consequence of kata not being part of the normal activity of most judo clubs is that the availability of people with the required knowledge and teaching skills is very limited. Today some of the better known judo forms are in serious danger of becoming extinct.

For the reader's interest, teaching sequences for two techniques from *Kodokan Goshin-jutsu*—two-hand hold (*ryote dori*) and uppercut (*ago tsuki*)—are provided in Figures 8 and 9. Similarly, teaching sequences for two techniques from the Koshiki no Kata—strength dodging (*ryokuhi*) and water wheel (*mizu guruma*)—are provided in Figures 10 and 11. These sequences were performed under the technical direction of world masters international kata judge Bob Thomas.

Two-Hand Hold

8a Bob Thomas (right) and Eddie Cassidy approach each other.
8b The attacker steps with his left foot forward into the proper distance to simultaneously grab the defender's wrists and tries to strike with his right knee to the groin.
8c The defender bends his right arm hard toward his chest to free it and,
8d continues his motion to strike the attacker's right temple with the knife-edge of his right hand.
8e The defender grabs the attacker's right wrist from the top with his right hand and applies an armlock (*kote hineri*). He steps back with his right foot and opens his body to his right. The defender clamps the attacker's right arm under his left arm and twists the attacker's wrist. The attacker is forced to submit, or have his arm broken.

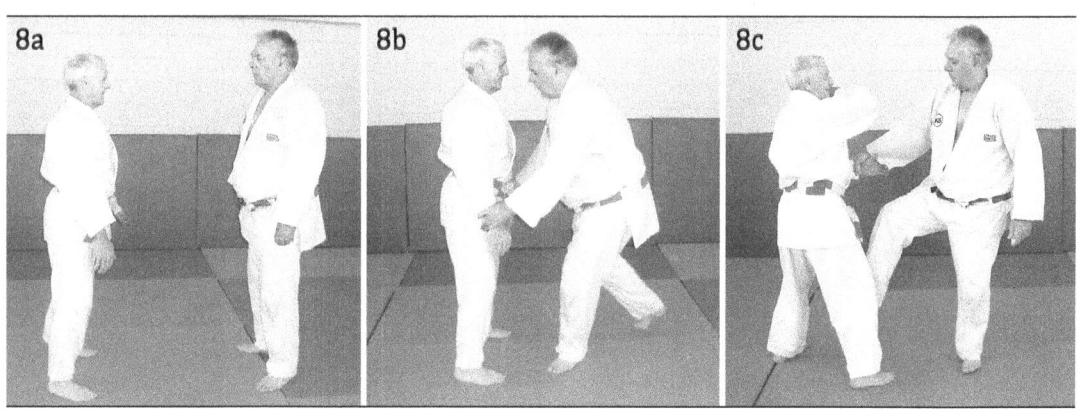

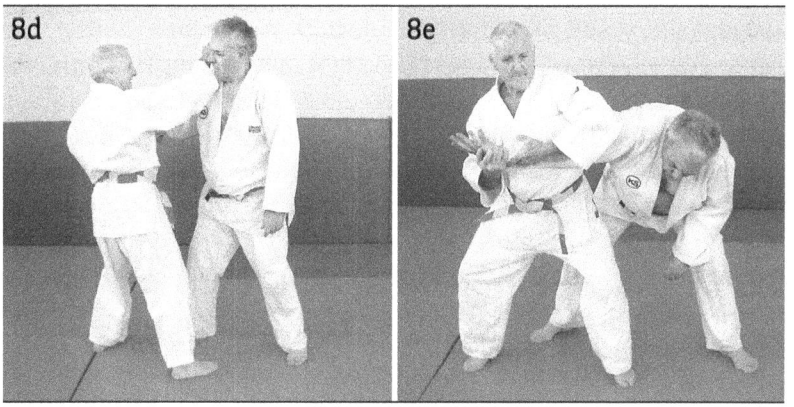

Uppercut

9a Eddie Cassidy (right) and Bob Thomas approach each other.

9b The attacker steps with his right foot forward into the proper distance to simultaneously throw a right uppercut. The defender steps slightly back with his left foot and deflects the attacker's uppercut from below with his right hand.

9c Immediately, the defender grabs the attacker's right wrist with his right hand, thumb down, and the attacker's elbow with his left hand. He twists the attacker's wrist away from him and pushed the attacker's elbow toward his face.

9d While keeping his arm extended and locking the attacker's elbow, the defender takes a big step forward with his left foot and throws the attacker forward.

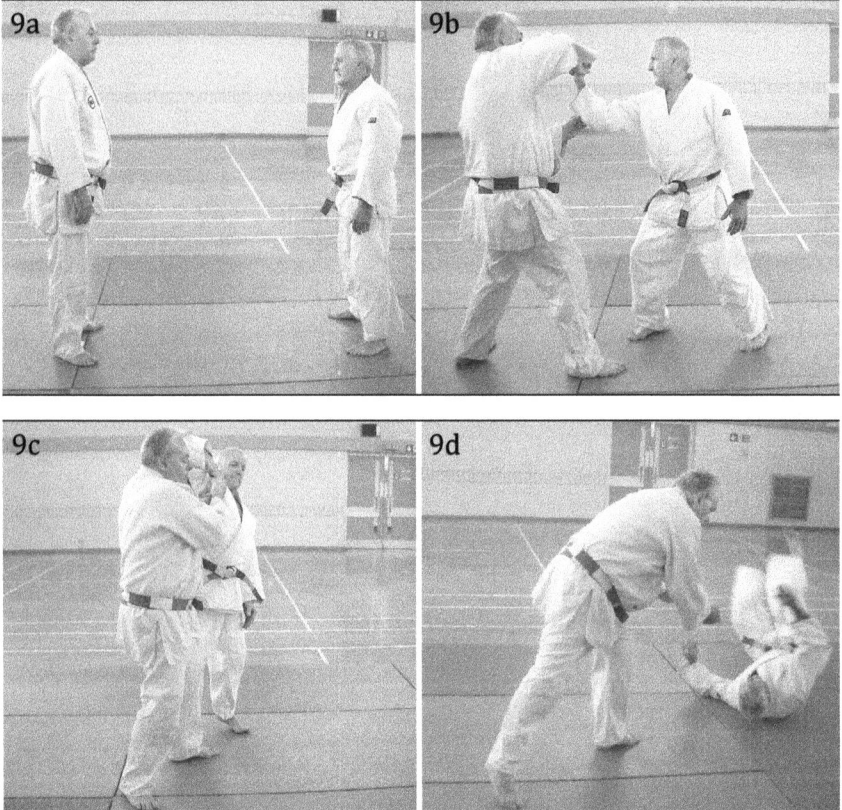

Strength Dodging

10a Eddie Cassidy (right) and Bob Thomas approach each other.

10b The attacker steps forward, left foot then right, and attempts to grab the defender's belt with a cross grip—right hand upper-most. The defender simultaneously pulls the attacker's right arm forward.

10c The defender pulls the attacker forward to his right side, while placing himself behind the attacker. He holds the attacker's elbow bringing the arm upwards while holding the attacker's upper left arm.

10d The defender pulls the attacker backward to the right side while dropping to his left knee as the attacker falls to the ground.

10e As the defender kneels, the attacker sits up, keeping his legs spread with straight legs, toes up.

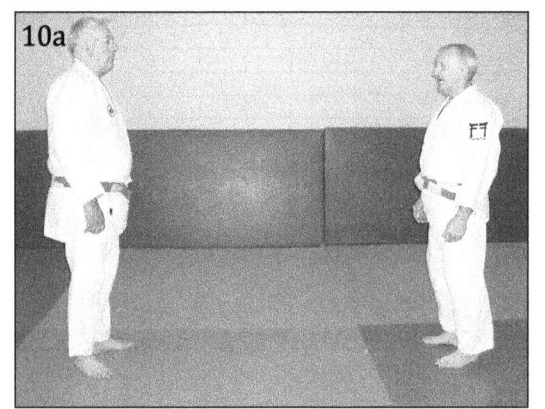
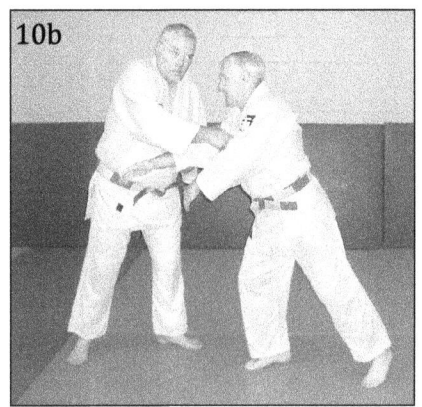
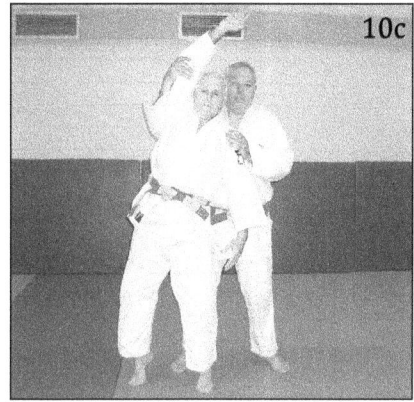
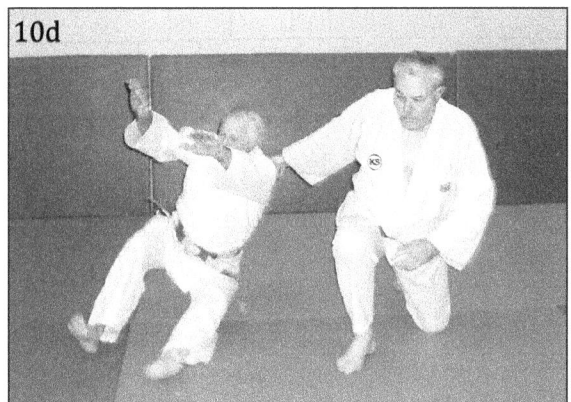
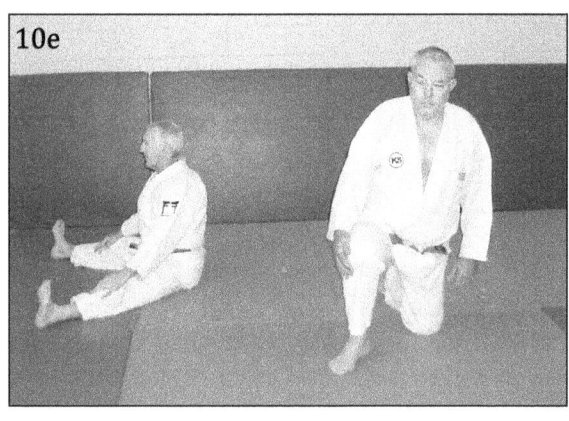

Water Wheel

11a Eddie Cassidy (right) and Bob Thomas approach each other.

11b The attacker steps forward with his left foot then right, and attempts to seize the defender's belt with a cross grip—right hand uppermost. The defender simultaneously pulls the attacker's right arm forward.

11c The attacker resists by pulling backward. The defender responds by changing his direction of movement, lifting the attacker's right arm, and presses it toward the attacker's forehead.

11d The defender moves in closer and unbalances the attacker by bending the attacker at the waist with his left hand and pressing the attacker's right arm against his own forehead with his right hand. This makes it easy to push to attacker backward.

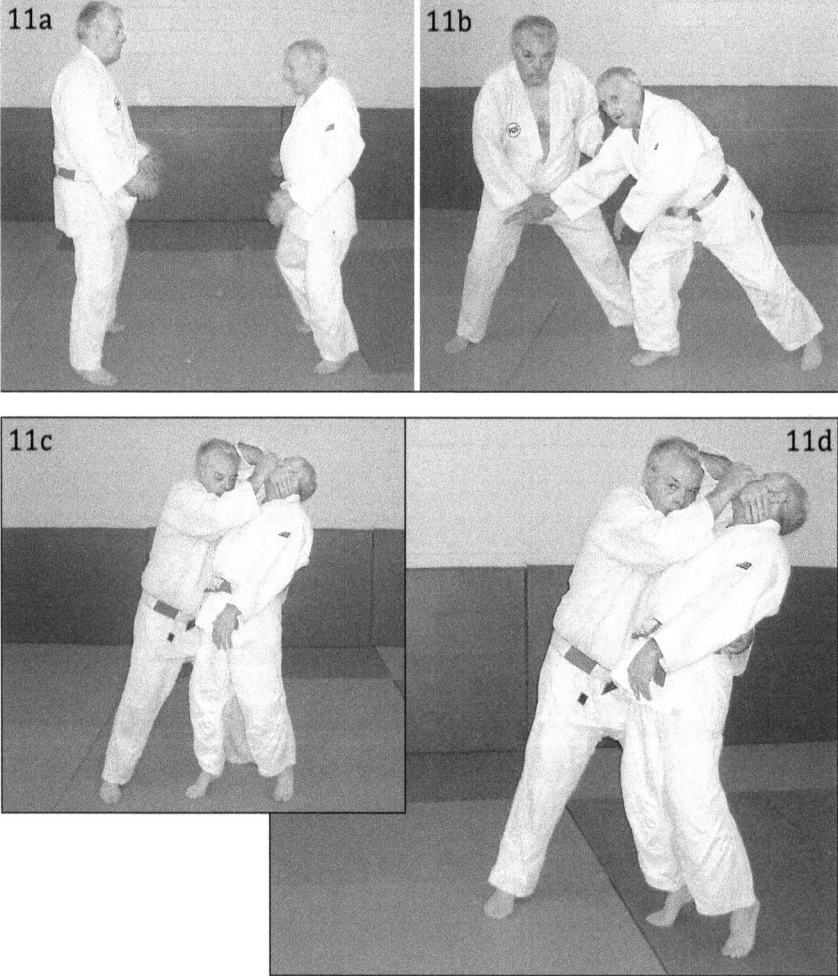

11e The defender bends the attacker backward and the attacker responds by resisting and straightening up and inclining forward a little. The defender then takes advantage of the attacker's forward inclination and changes his grip. He also adjusts the position of his feet.

11f The defender then falls backward and executes a sacrifice throw.

11g The attacker rolls over the defender in mid-air.

11h The attacker comes onto his feet and the defender remains on his back with legs and hands spread for about three seconds. This concludes the action.

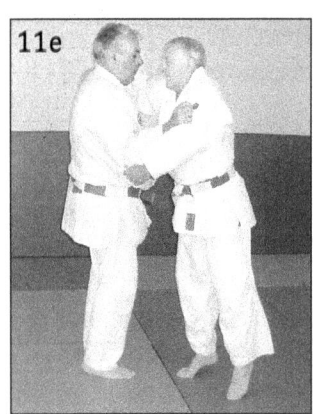
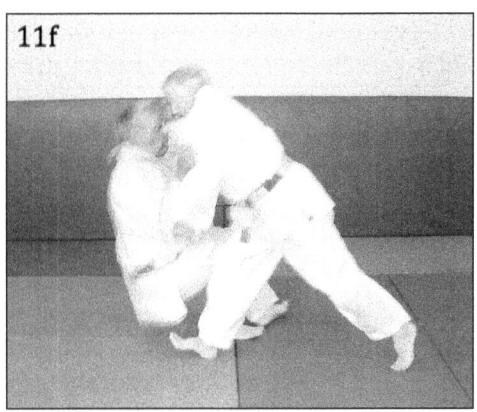
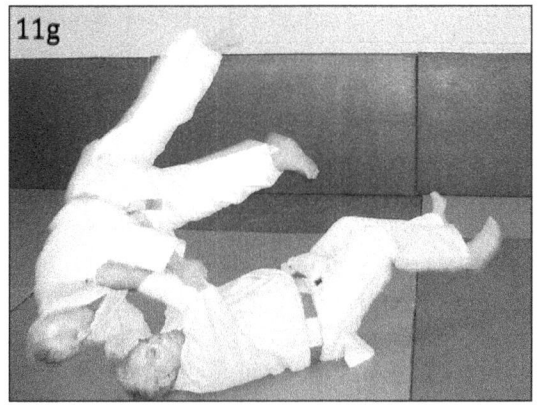
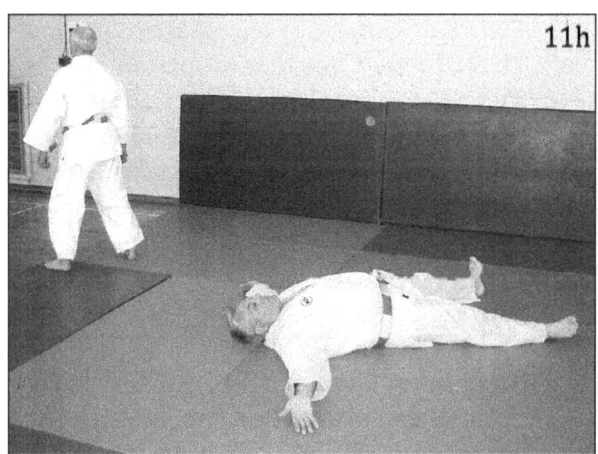

The Importance of Kata

To gain a true understanding of judo as envisioned by Kano, it is necessary to look beyond competition to kata. This author believes that the link between judo's past and future is embodied in the accurate teaching of kata for it is only in kata that the totality of judo has been preserved— especially the traditional and more dangerous self-defense techniques that are also present in judo.

Kano identified two types of training for judo—forms and free-practice—and held the firm belief that these two training systems had to co-exist in parallel. Kano envisaged kata being the laboratory for judo development and free-practice as the testing ground (Otaki and Draeger, 1983).

In particular, Kano developed kata to demonstrate the principles of judo and to provide a type of training in which students could examine techniques under ideal circumstances—thus penetrating their very essence.

Through repeated practice, the techniques of the various forms can be performed without thinking and, in the extreme, kata can unify mind, body and spirit—arguably the purest goal of a martial art. Indeed, many judo practitioners claim to have experienced moments of enlightenment and insight as a result of a perfect kata performance. Notwithstanding the subjective spiritual dimension, it is certainly true that all judo players involved can derive a great deal of self-satisfaction from a high-quality kata performance and the associated focus, awareness, attention to detail, and self-discipline demanded. Furthermore, students and teachers should also not overlook the significance of forms as purely a part of general instruction: kata teaches movement, timing, and coordination. Kata was, and remains, the basis of judo, and provides the vehicle for perfecting many throws, holds, and other techniques in a finer way than individual technical instruction or general free-practice.

Critics of kata argue that forms bear very little resemblance to competition in that the techniques are performed at a standard pace with a predetermined outcome in an overly symbolized style. It is not widely known that most high-grade Japanese teachers still emphasize the importance of kata for a judo practitioner's development and that many consider the study of the *Randori no Kata* (*Nage-no-kata* and *Katame-no-kata*) in particular to be an essential part of training for the highest level of contest success (Watanabe, 2003; Otaki and Draeger, 1983; Kawaishihi, 1982).

In their seminal text *Judo Formal Techniques*, Otaki and Draeger (1983) state:

Sufficient kata study and practice impose a well-defined technical discipline on the judoist, one that is unattainable by only *randori* and contest methods. This discipline, instead of hampering the judoist, actually frees him from undue restrictions, liberates his bodily expression in movement, and teaches him economy of mental and physical energy. This process can only be understood through experience, and only through kata performance can judoist come to appreciate judo in its fullest sense.

Kawaishi (1982) reinforces the point:

The kata will temper the combative ardor of the young performer and will undoubtedly also enable him to discover the reason for certain errors he commits in competition ... Thus the kata is a valuable source of technical progress.

Accordingly, the contest player should consider kata as part of his training for physical, mental, and contest proficiency in an identical fashion to free-practice and conditioning work, etc.

Concluding Remarks

Given the substantial decline in the number of adults practicing judo, it can be argued that there is a real need to re-examine the value system associated with judo. A way must be found to retain and ideally attract more adults into judo. As part of this exercise, the emphasis between the martial and art strands of judo should be examined simultaneously because the strands should not be separated. In doing so, one would be well served to note Burkland's (1998) conclusions:

Judo must focus on its heritage as a traditional martial way by emphasising *randori* [free-practice] and kata as the primary training vehicles for the development.... *Shiai* [competition] must be returned to its proper perspective and cannot be allowed to dominate our thinking and our efforts.

Gleeson (1976) showed that there was a close connection between the three dimensions of judo and argued that free-practice, competition, and forms were all essential to each other. Gleeson recognized that, through ignorance and neglect, artificial boundaries had been built between the dimensions, preventing people from moving easily from one to another. Gleeson also acknowledged the need to deconstruct these boundaries for judo to prosper.

A similar idea has been expressed metaphorically by relating judo to a three-legged stool—the three legs being free-practice, competition, and forms (Kin Ryu Judo, n.d.). The metaphor proceeds to argue that if any one leg is removed, the stool falls over. Therefore, without equal emphasis on all three elements, judo will be flawed. The interested reader requiring a further perspective on Kodokan judo—including the introduction of a concept of four overlapping areas for study (i.e. physical education, sport, unarmed combat, and philosophy) is also directed to Anderson (n.d.).

Additionally implicit in the re-evaluation of judo's value structure is a real need to reassess and reformulate the promotion system. In doing so, a fundamental tenet of Kano's philosophy should be at the fore:

> It's not that you are better than someone else that's important,
> but that you are better than you were yesterday.
> – British Judo Association, 2004

The principles expounded in this chapter are already starting to come to the fore with the emergence of a number of bodies dedicated to the preservation of the traditional techniques and values of judo as a martial art. Such bodies could provide a more natural home for the judo purist than the official sport-orientated governing bodies.

Judo today faces a crisis no different than that facing Kano Jigoro in 1882 when he founded judo from jujutsu. In evolving judo from jujutsu, Kano endeavored to preserve jujutsu's fundamental elements unless they be lost forever. In the West, similar radical steps are needed to re-establish and preserve the heritage, traditions, and forms of judo that were Kano's true genius.

BIBLIOGRAPHY

Anderson, V. (n.d.). The four pillars of judo. *Fightingarts.com.* http://www.fightingarts.com/reading/article.php?id=146

Bates, A. (n.d.). Classical judo—Time to realise. In *Tokushima Budo Council Official Bulletin*, No. 79.

Bethers, B. (n.d.). Training in Kodokan judo—"One perspective." *Martial Arts International Federation (MAIF) Traditional Kodokan Judo Program.* http://www.maintlfed.org/resources/kodokan.html

British Judo Association. (2004). *One of Britain's most senior judoka inspires soucoast youngsters.* http://www.britishjudo.org.uk/home/percysekine.php\

British Judo Association. (n.d.). *British judo facts and figures.* http://www.britishjudo.org.uk/media/documents/BritishJudo-Facts_000.pdf

Burkland, R. (1998, Spring). Judo: Martial way or modern sport. *Shudokan Martial Arts Association Newsletter.* http://www.michionline.org/smaa/articles/burkland_judo.html

Fromm, A. and Soames, N. (1982). *Judo: The gentle way.* London: Routledge and Kegan Paul.

Gleeson, G. (1976). *The complete book of judo.* Toronto: Coles Publishing.

Kano, J. (1986). *Kodokan judo.* Tokyo: Kodansha International.

Kawaisihi, M. (1982). *The complete 7 katas of judo.* Woodstock, New York: The Overlook Press.

Kawamura, T. and Daigo, T. (2000). *Kodokan new Japanese-English dictionary of judo.* Tokyo: Kodokan Institute.

Kin Ryu Judo Club. (n.d.). *The basics of judo.* http://www.kinryu.org.uk/judobasics.htm

Leggett, T. and Kano, J. (1982). *Kata judo.* Slough, Berkshire, UK: W. Foulsham and Co.

Ohlenkamp, N. (2005 February 3). Forms of judo (kata). *Judo Information Site.* http://judoinfo.com/katamenu.htm

Otaki, T. and Draeger, D. (1983). *Judo formal techniques.* Tokyo: Charles E. Tuttle Co.

Smith, R. (1999). *Martial musings: A portrayal of martial arts in the 20th century.* Erie, Pennsylvania: Via Media Publishing.

Watanabe, K. (2003). *World masters judo championship kata booklet.* Richmond Hill, Ontario: World Master Judo Association.

chapter 16

North Korean Kye Sun Hui: An Extraordinary Olympic Judo Player
by David Finch

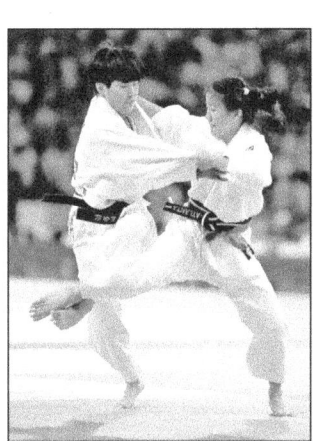
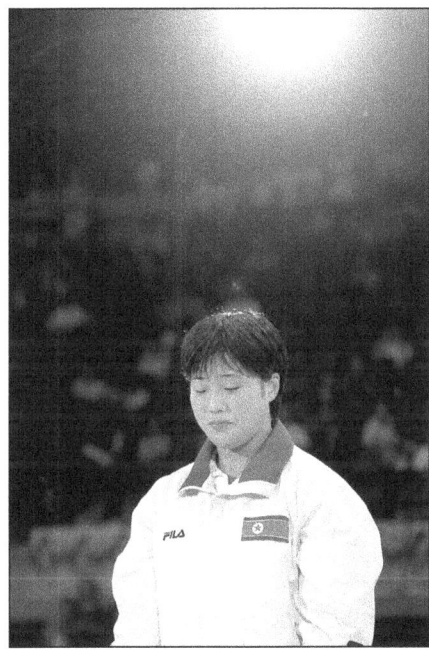
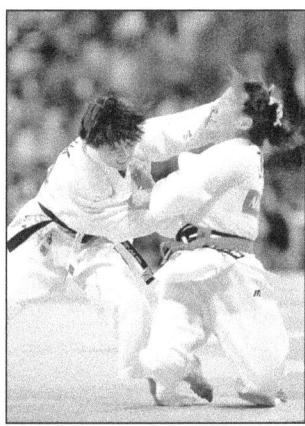

Kye defeats Japan's Tamura Ryoko at the 1996 Atlanta Olympics.
All photos courtesy of Judo Photos Unlimited.

At the 1996 Atlanta Olympics, North Korean Kye Sun Hui became the youngest gold medallist in Olympic Judo history at the age of sixteen. As a 'wild card' chosen by the International Judo Federation (IJF), she astonishingly defeated Japan's Tamura Ryoko (Tani) with a sweeping hip counter (*harai-goshi-gaeshi*). Afterwards Kye cheekily said: "It is easier to fight in international tournaments abroad than it is to fight at home," referring to the strong domestic opposition.

Until her defeat in Atlanta, Tamura had been unbeaten in 84 contests and was universally expected to take the title. In fact, until Atlanta, Kye had never fought outside North Korea, was entirely unknown, and didn't even know who Tamura was until the day they met. That proved to be a distinct psychological advantage to the North Korean who later stood on the podium draped in the North Korean flag.

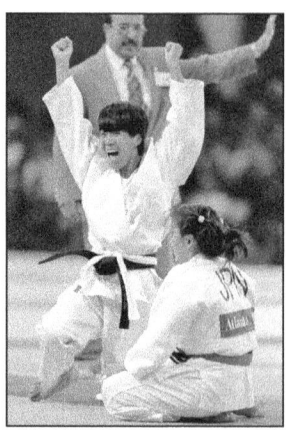

By the time of the Paris World Judo Championships a year later in 1997, she was at a weight heavier class (52 kgs, or 115 lbs) and won the silver medal, losing to France's Marie-Claire Restoux. Kye lost momentum at the 1999 Birmingham World Judo Championships and could only manage a bronze medal, repeating this at the Sydney Olympics where she lost the semi-final to Cuba's Legna Verdecia, the eventual gold medalist. At the age of twenty, Kye appeared to be fading rapidly. However, the 2001 Munich Worlds Championships re-established her reputation when she defeated Germany's Rafaella Imbriani in the final, again in the 52 kgs (115 lbs) class.

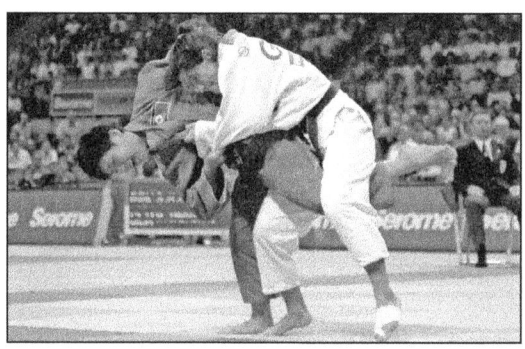

Germany's Rafaella Imbriani gets defeated by Kye in the final Munich World Championships, 2001.

Two years later at the Osaka World Championships in 2003, she moved up to the 57 kgs (125.4 lbs) weight class. There she stormed through the opposition winning every contest by *ippon* (equivalent to a knockout), including the final against Germany's Yvonne Boenisch. In response, her opponents could only manage minor technical points against her—such was the intensity of her style. In the final, Kye led Boenisch by a strong lead in points until fifteen seconds from the bell. Then Kye unleashed an explosive major hip throw (*ogoshi*) that resulted in a winning ippon. Trying to avoid the score with an outstretched arm, Boenisch dislocated her elbow. But not a scream came from her even though she was in great pain.

Nearly a year later in 2004, Kye and Boenisch met again in the 57kgs (125.4 lbs) final of the Athens Olympics. Boenisch was better prepared and this time turned the tables on Kye. She had fought Kye earlier in the year at the final of the Warsaw 'A' tournament where she had defeated her. Now, fully aware of Kye's style, Boenisch proved too awkward for her, never giving her time to settle into the fight, thus ensuring that Kye could not use her favorite grip. Boenisch comprehensively outwitted her and then scored with an inner-thigh throw (*uchi-mata*) while Kye was warned for passivity, resulting in a particularly satisfying tactical victory for Boenisch.

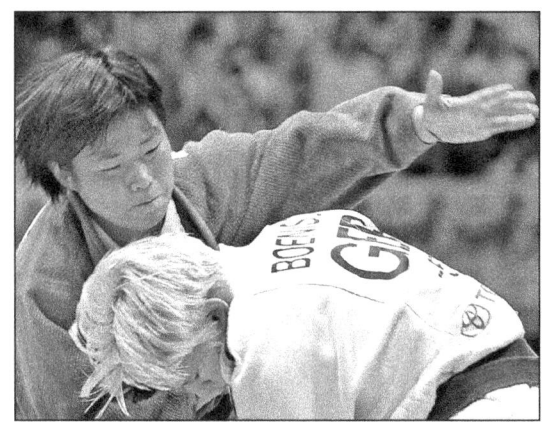
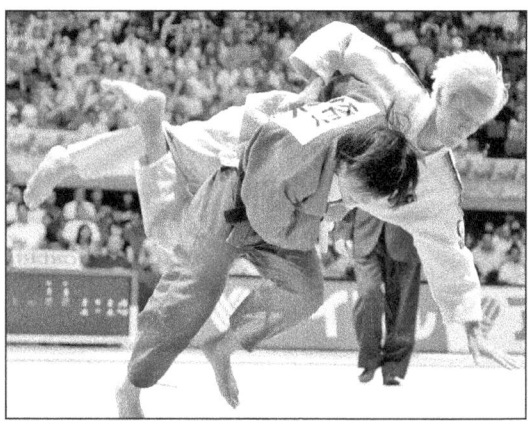
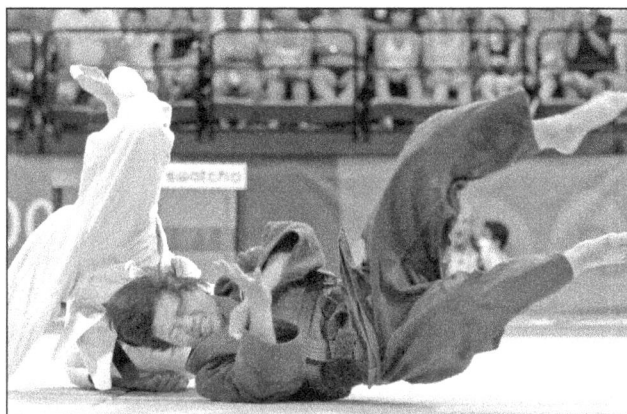

Kye employs a major hip throw (*ogoshi*) to defeat Germany's Yvonne Boenisch in the finals of the Osaka World Championships, 2003.

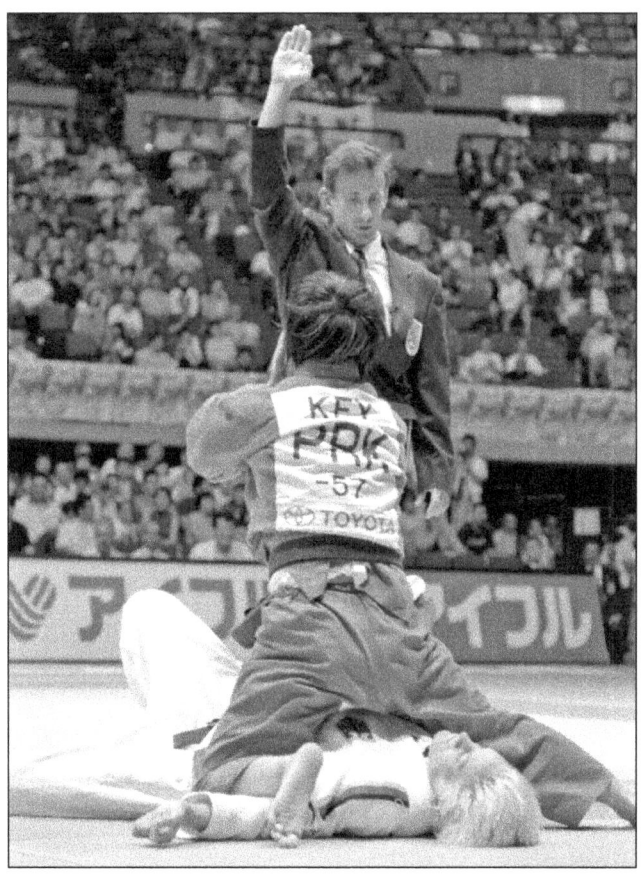

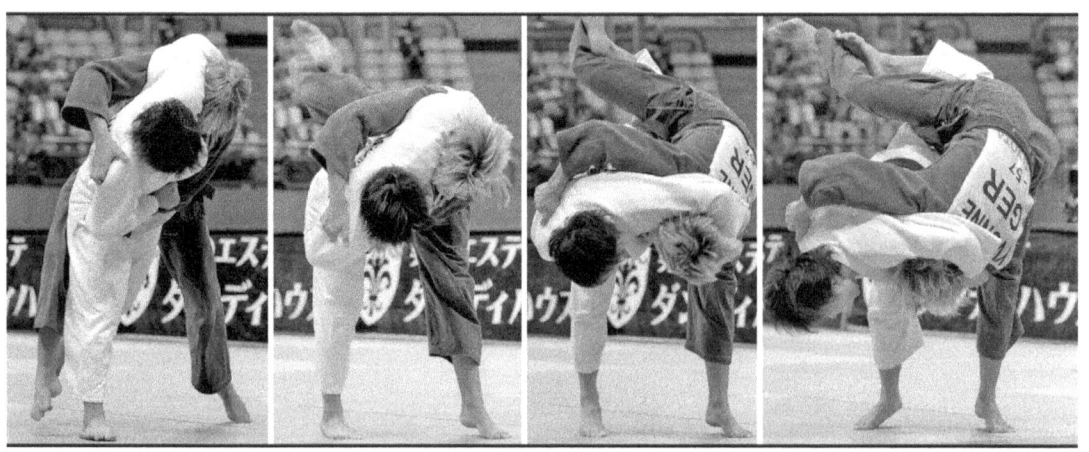
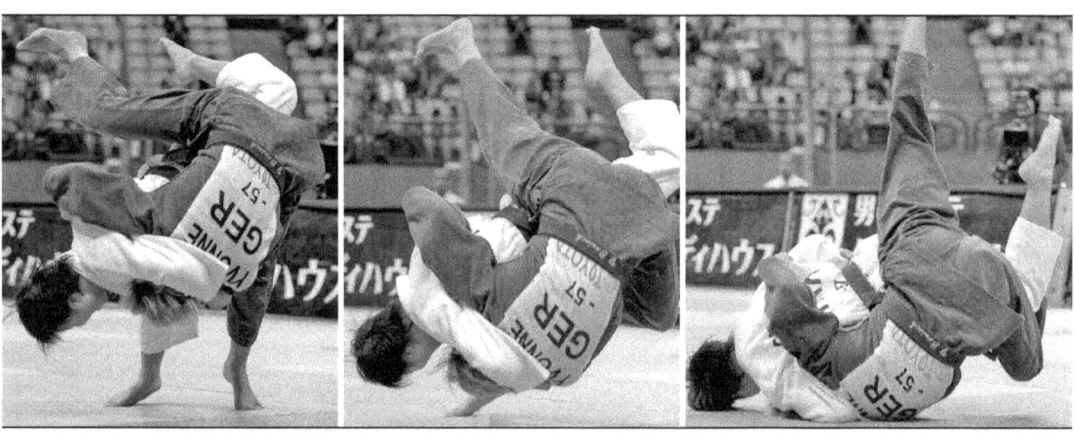
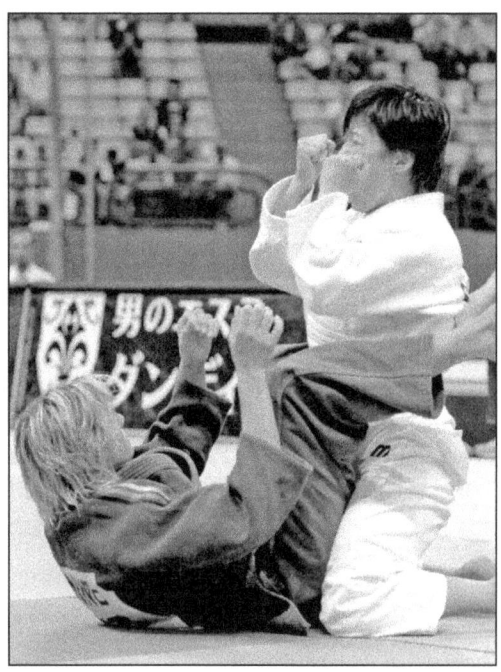

With extreme precision, Kye caught Boenisch with an inner-thigh throw to claim her third world title in just 38 seconds at the Cairo World Championships, 2005.

At the recent Cairo World Championships, held in September of 2005, both Kye and Boenisch were destined to meet again for their third major finals confrontation. Unlike the Osaka World Championships, Kye reached the final having finished only one contest with an ippon inside the five minutes. That is until she met Cuba's Yurisle Lupetey in the semi-final.

Leading by five points, Kye unleashed a determined attack that resulted in Lupetey being carried off in a stretcher with a broken elbow just like Boenisch's at Osaka. One spectator who saw the throw at close quarters, Rusty Kanokogi of the IJF, said: "When force met force, something had to give. Kye was determined to throw Lupetey through the mat, but the Cuban was not going to give away a score resulting in her elbow giving way while attempting to avoid an ippon loss." The break was so painful that the Cuban was unable to stop screaming while receiving attention.

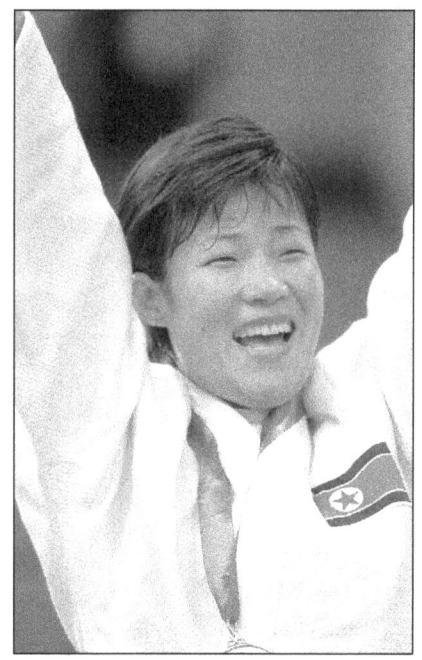

The final was not a repetition of what happened in Osaka. This was a far more convincing win for Kye against Boenisch. Now firing on all cylinders, Kye attacked with an inner-thigh throw (*uchi-mata*). Boenisch resisted the threat, but not the next. With extreme precision, Kye caught Boenisch perfectly with a second inner-thigh throw to claim her third world title in just 38 seconds. The win caused the small gathering of North Korean spectators to go wild with joy.

In North Korea, Kye is the "People's Athlete" and has been given the title of a "Labor Heroine of the Democratic People's Republic of Korea." She was also given a special award by the late Kim Il Sung, founder of that state.

When Kye returned from Cairo, North Korean Television reported that about 100,000 people turned out to welcome her with bouquets, slogan boards, drums, cymbals, and confetti, reminiscent of a New York "ticker tape" welcome. The television station reported that she had said that current leader Kim Jong Il had given her "strength, courage, matchless guts, and resolution," attributing her success to what she called Kim's "unbounded love and trust." In a freer society, such gifts are more likely to be attributed to God than a politician. But certainly she is highly gifted and, at 26-years of age, still has time to receive more judo titles, and sporting accolades from leader Kim Jong Il.

Judo Weight Classes

Extra lightweight:
Men -60kg,   Women -48kg

Half lightweight:
Men -66kg,   Women -52kg

Lightweight:
Men -73kg,   Women -57kg

Half-middleweight:
Men -81kg,   Women -63kg

Middleweight:
Men -90kg,   Women -70kg

Half-heavyweight:
Men -100kg,   Women -78kg

Heavyweight:
Men +100kg,   Women +78kg

chapter 17

Competition Versus Tradition in Kodokan Judo
by S. Biron Ebell, M.A.

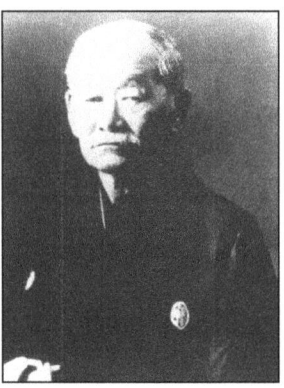

Jigoro Kano (1860–1938),
founder of judo.

Introduction

Practitioners of oriental martial arts are sometimes surprised to find that katas (formal prearranged form [Otaki and Draeger, 1983:441]) are actually part of Kodokan Judo. This belief seems to be based on the opinion—probably also shared by the general public—that judo is a sport; plain and simple (Nurse, 2004). A belief further reinforced by the fact that judo is an Olympic sport. Today, however, most people generally do not consider it to be a martial art and, some senior judo practitioners would rather not have the term "martial art" be applied to judo at all (Sadej, 1999:2–3; Schell, 1999:2-3); despite judo's obvious historic connection to the Japanese martial traditions. This view, I feel, may be turned on its head when the history and stated purpose of judo is taken into account. In fact, when considered in detail, judo is actually a modern *budo* or martial way (Draeger, 1974), whose purpose far exceeds sport or competition. Therefore, this short chapter will briefly touch on several important topics including:

- The historical foundation of judo
- The learning and practice of judo
- How the current focus on competitive judo is narrowing its purpose and eroding principles and practices espoused by its founder
- How economic priorities are driving judo's evolution away from the interests of its majority participants

Judo History and Purpose

Judo, or Kodokan Judo, as it is more properly known, is a synthesis of several styles of jujutsu by the 19th century Japanese visionary and educator Jigoro Kano (1860–1938). Kano was born October 28, in Mikage, which is now part of Kobe city. In 1874, he entered the Tokyo School of Foreign Languages, where he mastered English to the point that all of his personal notes and later, his budo journals, were written in that language (Stevens, 1995:11–12). Ironically, his journals have been published in Japanese, but not English!

In 1877 he became a student at Tokyo University and fell victim to "bullies" and "ruffians." It was about this time that he began his study of Tenshin Shin'yo-ryu jujutsu under the tutelage of Hashinosuke Fukuda (1829–1880). This he did in spite of being admonished by his family and colleagues to forget jujutsu because "…times have changed and such things are no longer useful" (Stevens, 1995:14–15). By this time in history, jujutsu had fallen into disrepute for a number of reasons, not the least of which was because it had become a means of public spectacle and bravado—losing the honor that it and other martial arts had enjoyed for many centuries in Japan (Kano, 2005:20-21). However, Tenshin Shin'yo-ryu jujutsu was comparatively new but had a reputation of being an effective means of self-defense (Draeger, 1974:113). It specialized in *atemi waza* (techniques for striking anatomically weak points of the body) and *katame* or *ne-waza* (grappling techniques).

Within the first year of Kano's training, his teacher died, but he continued his study under the direction of Masamoto Iso (1818–1881), the son of the school's founder. Following Iso's death in 1881, Kano began studying Kito-ryu jujutsu under Tsunetoshi Iikubo (1835–1889). An extremely esoteric and philosophical art, Kito-ryu specialized in *nage-waza* (throwing or projecting techniques) (Kano, 2005:22–23; Draeger, 1974:113). In 1883, Iikubo awarded Kano a Kito-ryu teaching license.

In 1882, after five years of diligent study, Jigoro Kano established his own martial art he called "Kodokan Judo," synthesized primarily from Tenshin Shin'yo-ryu jujutsu, Kito-ryu jujutsu, and others. Kodokan usually is translated as "school for studying the way" (Kano et. al., 1986:16). He adopted the term "judo" to differentiate his martial art from jujutsu (Kano, 2005:18–22). *Ju*, implies flexibility or adaptability, as it did with jujutsu, but the suffix "do," suggests a more sophisticated purpose for the art. "Do" is an esoteric term generally implying a way of life, a way of thinking, and/or a way of living (Kano, 2005).

But judo did not, by any means, spring from Kano's head fully formed. It progressed slowly from the original concepts of the jutsu forms he studied, and continues to evolve to this day. One of his greatest innovations was devising a curriculum—an organized, graded sequence of study that insured both safety and structure for students (Donohue, 2005: 26) and an efficient means of learning that differed from that used in jujutsu (Kano, 2005: 33–34). As Nurse (2004) points out: "Perhaps his [Kano's] greatest innovation was (sic) the teaching of *ukemi*, or 'break-falling,' before a new student begins the study of technique. This ensures that when a novice is thrown, he or she has already learned how to land safely and efficiently on the mats without danger. This was a significant departure from many of the jujutsu systems Kano had examined previously, where students were thrown—sometimes having their limbs deliberately wrenched in the bargain—and had to land as best they could."

Kano's Raison D'etre for Judo

Kodokan Judo Principles and Aims (Kano et. al., 1986:20–25), state clearly the primary objectives of judo are physical fitness, studying attack and defense, and moral training. Kano (2005:23) states: "…I divided it [judo] into three parts: its use as a fighting method (martial art), as a training method (physical education), and as a method of mental training (including the development of the intellect and morals and the application of judo to everyday life ...)."

The ultimate aim of physical fitness and physical education, Kano states, is to "make the body strong, useful and healthy while building character through mental and moral discipline, ... making efficient use of mental and physical energy ... (while progressing) ...toward the goal of promoting health, strength and usefulness" (Kano et. al., 1986:20). He also observed that sports are competitive in nature and as such, overemphasize a less than balanced physical development to accomplish their particular ends, while doing little or nothing for the moral discipline of their participants.

Kano emphasized training the whole body as well as mind and moral fibre, for the good of society. He saw the means to accomplish this while learning the arts of attack and defense. To do so safely, judo players require the cooperation of their training partners. And in order to continue to have training partners, they must consider each other's well being. Doing so instills a sense of responsibility for ones training partners and by extension, ones fellow man. This important concept was distilled in Kano's dictum of "*jita kyoei*" or Mutual Benefit and Well-being, which advocates "... perfecting one's self and benefiting the world (Brousse and Matsumoto 1999: 84; Kano, 2005). So, Kano envisioned the use of judo as a means of achieving a healthy body, a moral sense of mutual respect and responsibility, and the ability to apply self-defense techniques should they be required in day-to-day life using modified techniques of attack and defense from jujutsu.

Another, but nonetheless important dictum of Kano was, "*seiryoku zenyo,*" which translates to mean "putting your energy to work most efficiently," or "maximum efficiency," directs the physical execution and understanding of judo technique. This dictum advocates "that no matter what the goal, in order to achieve it, you must put your mental and physical energy to work in the most effective manner" (Kano, 2005:43). In other words, in all endeavors, whether in judo or daily life, efficiency in action and thought are sought as an ideal.

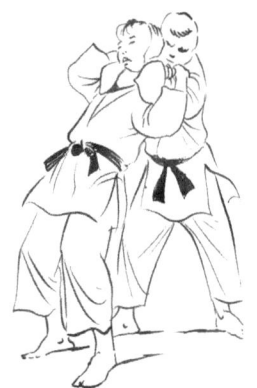 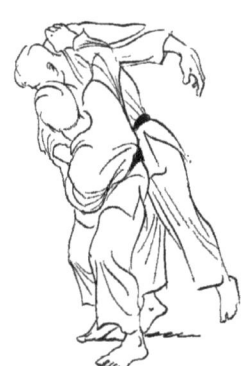 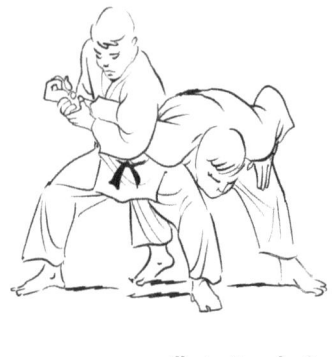

Illustrations by Oscar Ratti.
©Futuro Designs & Publications.

Judo as Sport

Referring to the modern Japanese sword art of kendo, Kiyota (2002:1) identifies sport as "a structured human activity carried out in leisure time for the purpose of recreating the human personality." Further, he directs us to a statement by Joseph W. Elder, who says sports include three components: competition (with an opponent), physical activity, and established rules. If these definitions are accepted, then for the most part, much of judo is truly practiced as a sport, but the overarching philosophical and moral priorities advocated by Kano, significantly differentiate it from other sports.

Learning Judo — Randori, Kata and Shiai

Judo is normally practiced in three ways. Foremost, there is *randori*. Originally, both Kito-ryu and Tenshin Shin'yo-ryu jujutsu used randori, in which "the two players did not compete with each other, but rather trained together to improve their art. This was permitted only after proficiency was attained in kata" (Kano, et. al., 1986:141). And, it was in the concept of randori that Kano's genius shown. Most *shin budo* (modern martial ways) even today are practiced primarily as kata. Kano significantly broke with tradition when he made randori a priority in judo study.

Randori is a form of sparing or free exercise, where judo players are at liberty to freely practice their judo skills against a resisting opponent. The objective is to develop both attack and defense tactics, but within judo's rules of engagement. In order for students to be able to freely engage each other, Kano found it necessary to select and modify jujutsu techniques (*waza*) so they could be safely practiced in this manner. So it was in 1895 when the Kodokan established a graded curriculum of throwing techniques (*nage-waza*) known as the Gokyu-no-wza. This was revised in 1920 and today 67 throwing techniques are recognized by the Kodokan (Daigo, 2005:9).

Ideally there are no winners or losers in randori! This is where spirit and fighting skills are developed and honed. As Kano et. al. (1986:142) state: "The ultimate goal of randori is to develop the ability to rapidly cope with changing circumstances, to build a strong and supple body, and to prepare mind and body for competition. Unfortunately, in many dojo today randori is not practiced as it should be. One reason is the stress on training for competition. . . . The resulting contest-style judo is far from ideal."

With randori, judo players practice their techniques without restraint, seeing directly and without doubt, the full effect of their techniques. In fact randori differentiates judo from most other modern martial arts where the full effects of techniques must be restrained for safety reasons.

Second, judo is practiced as kata. Most things Japanese are learned as *shikata* or "the way of doing things" (De Mente, 2003:1). This is a practice "that had been ritualized or sanctified over the centuries" (De Mente, 2004:73). Traditionally, all day-to-day activities are initially learned in a kata-like manner by rote or repetitive practice. As De Mente (2003: 4) states: "the Japanese kata-ized their whole existence. Practically nothing was left to chance or personal inclination. The kata factor applied to everything."

With kata a formal presence in most Japanese behavior, it is not surprising to find katas in their martial arts. In this regard, katas are forms to be followed assuring that a precise body of knowledge is transferred from teacher to student. It is a kind of template to be followed both in learning and performance. Judo is no exception, as katas are an important aspect of learning and practice.

Judo katas are formal, prearranged forms of attack and defense including techniques such as striking techniques that are not allowed in randori. It is in these katas that the martial art aspect of judo is learned and practiced. This aspect of judo is not sport. Further, as judo players are not in competition in kata study, the katas provide the opportunity to continue practicing judo well into old age (Kano, 2005:141–142). In judo, then, katas function to: direct the correct performance of technique; provide a controlled, predictable environment wherein techniques may be practiced and perfected; allow the study and practice of techniques that have practical self-defense application; maintain physical fitness after competition training is no longer feasible. And by striving for the perfection of technique, discipline and patience are honed. But in the strictest sense, *uchi-komi* (practice drills) are katas as well (Otaki and Draeger 1983:40, 428). It is by doing uchi-komi that the basic technical details of techniques are learned. Under a teacher's strict supervision, the rote, sometimes monotonous repetition of techniques embed the motor skills that are necessary for judo practitioners to properly execute judo's techniques. Often during a training session, a technique may be repeated hundreds of times. Because judo players cooperate in this form of practice, and actions are pre-arranged, agreed upon and repetitive, this learning process is a form of kata.

To understand judo as a Japanese art requires that its katas be studied. If judo is considered to be a tiny thread in Japan's cultural tapestry, a tapestry learned as shi-kata, then to know and understand judo in the Japanese context, one should know and understand its katas. In western dojos (training halls), katas are usually perceived as an inconvenient hurdle necessary for promotion. De Mente (2003:14) points out that there is an interesting dichotomy between Japanese and Western attitude toward katas: "The Japanese were traditionally conditioned to get their pleasure from conforming to kata, from doing things in the prescribed manner. One of the affects of this conditioning was to make the Japanese process-oriented instead of result-oriented."

Western society hurries toward clearly defined end results that symbolically mark the completion of a body of work, such as a university diploma or black belt. But, for most things Japanese, the process of learning takes priority over the final product: in the case of judo, diligent, ongoing study and practice takes priority (at least in theory) over achievement of rank or competitive success. Whether this continues to be so in Japanese society today is a moot point.

Third, there is *shiai*. It is competition that includes referees, adherence to rules, etc. The rules themselves are rather complex. Like most modern combat sports, winning is symbolic. In judo, a contest is decided when a contestant successfully throws an opponent from a standing position mostly on their back with speed, force, and impetus. For this he or she receives an *ippon* or single point that ends the contest. If the contest moves to the ground, an ippon may be scored by controlling the opponent on their back for 25 seconds, or by obtaining a submission using an effectively applied choke or arm-lock, all within a rather concise set of rules.

The ippon is awarded for techniques achieved in contest that would presumably incapacitate or injure an assailant in an uncontrolled combat situation. Like many other martial arts, judo's techniques were considered to be effective in real combat. The ability to produce an *ippon* or *wazari* (almost ippon) in contest translates to being able to develop an effective attack, or defend one's self, if needed—an important historic component of Kano's concept of judo (Kano, 2005:23).

Prior to 1972, only ippon and wazari, were awarded. To achieve an ippon in competition required tremendous determination and spirit. It's not easy to throw or immobilize a less than willing opponent. To receive ippon, it was all or nothing. Today, not only have the criteria for ippon been reduced—requiring less force and less speed—but two other scores lower than wazari are now awarded. Of course, competitors have adapted to these new scoring options by designing their techniques to achieve these lower scores and still win their matches, a fact decried by some (Takahashi, 2005:20). In fact, the new scoring regime has reduced the emphasis on "ippon judo." As Daigo Toshiro (2003:151), observes, today you can be a winner without ever "taking ippon." Likewise, Kano (2005:133) observes: "in competition or in fighting, feeling proud of yourself after winning by inconveniencing your opponent does not fulfill the spirit of judo. If you do not win by using waza superior to those of your opponent or by turning his waza against him, this cannot be said to be a true victory."

With the reduced emphasis in contest on "taking ippon" and winning by "inconveniencing your opponent," one can only imagine what might happen if such techniques are attempted in an uncontrolled adversarial situation. Without "speed, force and impetus," a genuinely dangerous situation may ensue. The adversary may merely recover from momentary embarrassment to retaliate to the serious detriment of the judo player. It follows from this that reducing the criteria necessary to win a shiai contest, also reduces the inherent skills of the practicing judo player that may be required in real combat. True enough, Kodokan Judo historically is already four or more times removed from the reality of the battlefield, but to condone a reduction in requirements for winning contests continues to erode its already reduced potency as a means of attack and defense.

Shiai and the Championship

It is in shiai that judo players apply all their skills in an effort to defeat an opponent. Shiai is traditionally a tool used to test a judo player's progress and expertise against others of similar skill. As such, shiai provides an opportunity for personal and private assessment of progress: one that is not usually concerned with public acknowledgment. The only person with a vested interest in shiai success, other than the judo player, is his or her instructor. The shiai was, and still is, an occasion for teachers to evaluate students' technique, spirit, and sportsmanship. In fact, a successful shiai sometimes results in a judo player being awarded immediate grade advancement, known as *batsugun*.

But, call the shiai a "championship," and competitive rational changes. A "championship" sets the scene for the public acknowledgment of achieved prowess over others. Competition, then, becomes an affirmation of superiority among peers and is no longer only a self-evaluation tool of progress in skill. The change is subtle, but significant, moving from an opportunity for self-evaluation, as found in shiai, to one of self-aggrandizement as an acclaimed, recognized champion (Bowen, 1999:53). Though the objective of both shiai and championship is to win, the public celebration of winning changes the emphasis from personal, private success, to public acknowledgment, adulation, and fame. And, human vanity being what it is seems to favor fame over self-satisfaction.

Sport Heroes and Social Status

Saul (1992:506) mentions that seeking "excellence" in sport is an endeavor to move up the class system "with the king of the best on top." It is a seeking of celebrity, and our society seems to "give power to the stars themselves" as a result of public notoriety, no matter however it was received, achieved, or perceived. With respect to sports excellence, Saul (ibid.) observes "we have taken to celebrating competition as a self-evident value." What Saul seems to be saying is that sporting excellence is an excepted way of achieving perceived celebrity so as to move upward in a fictitious social system. The reality is that with almost all amateur sports—judo included—there is little or no financial or social benefit derived from competitive success. This is particularly true of Kodokan Judo where few (if any) professional opportunities exist post-heroism, and where public memory of competitive success, if understood at all, is transitory in the extreme. Occupying the pedestal of heroism merely creates the inherent challenge of those who follow to knock the hero from his/her prominent place; something that is bound to happen given time, age, and the challenge of youth.

Competitive priority has driven judo to evolve inexorably. The administrative focus of the International Judo Federation (IJF), the governing body of world judo, has, and continues to sharpen in the area of competition. One need only glance at their web site to infer that competition, competitive results, and elite competitors are their priority.

This priority is further reflected by contest rules that have increased in complexity over time and the continuing need to more clearly articulate how contests are conducted.

Compare, for example, the rather brief 1953 Kodokan rules preserved by Koizumi (1960: 157–165), and Kobayashi and Sharp (1956:99–102); the 1961 rules (Ishikawa and Draeger, 1962:291–298); the 1967 Contest Rules (IJF 1967:20–22); and the 63 page, 14,500-word, "Refereeing Rules" of 2003, as they are now called (IJF, 2003). One of the reasons contest rules have become increasingly more complex is because of the need to assure "equality of chances" in competition (Brousse and Matsumoto, 1999: 42).

Take for example the relatively simple description of judo uniform found in earlier rules which describes the general size and make-up of the jacket, pants, and belt (Koizumi, 1960:157–165). Contrast this with current regulations where detail includes such minutiae as to how it should fit, amount of overlap of the lapel, length of sleeve relative to contestants arm length, etc. Such detail reflects the inherent struggle among judo players to obtain a small competitive advantage over their opponents, and the rules that attempt to assure the contestants' "equality of chance."

Judo and the Olympics

Judo and the International Olympic Committee (IOC) have enjoyed a long association. As Nurse (2004) states: "... in London in 1933, Dr. Kano spoke of his desire for a world judo federation and the dissemination of Kodokan Judo teachings throughout the world as a means of aiding in achievement of world peace. Already he had become Japan's first representative on the International Olympic Committee (1909), as well as the first president of the newly formed Japanese Amateur Sports Association (1911)." One may easily understand why Kano wanted judo to become part of the Olympic movement considering their similar objectives. The Olympic Charter established by Pierre de Coubertin states:

> ... the goal of the Olympic Movement is to contribute to building a peaceful and better world by educating youth through sport practiced without discrimination of any kind and in the Olympic spirit, which requires mutual understanding with a spirit of friendship, solidarity and fair play. Olympism is a philosophy of life, exalting and combining in a balanced whole the qualities of body, will and mind. Blending sport with culture and education, Olympism seeks to create a way of life based on the joy found in effort, the educational value of good example and respect for universal fundamental ethical principles.

Both of these statements essentially duplicate the high moral intent of Kodokan Judo and the wishes expressed by Kano that judo function to promote world peace and benefit the world (Brousse and Matsumoto, 1999:84; Kano, 2005).

Kano's dream that judo become part of the Olympic Games was realized in 1964 when the Olympics were held in Tokyo. Thus began a relationship that has been a mixed blessing to Kodokan Judo. As Holme (1995:38) points out: "Just after the Munich Olympics there were major changes in the rules. The powers that be had realized that, to attract sponsors, television viewers had to be appeased."

Regarding the role of advertising revenue, the IOC (2005) itself observes: "Television is the engine that has driven the growth of the Olympic Movement. Increases in broadcast revenue over the past two decades have provided the Olympic Movement and sport with an unprecedented financial base. TV rights fees continue to account for approximately 50 percent of Olympic revenue."

Regarding participant Olympic sports, the IOC (2005) states: "While conserving their independence and autonomy in the administration of their sports, International Sports

Federations seeking IOC recognition must ensure that their statutes, practice and activities conform with the Olympic Charter."

The International Sports Federation concerned with judo is the IJF. From the above, rather contradictory statement by the IOC, the IJF is expected to meet certain criterion in order to comply with Olympic needs. Further one of the IJF's aims is "To support and maintain the ideals and objectives of the Olympic Movement" (IJF, Mission Statement: Aims 2006).

From the above statements, it follows that one of these criteria is to assure television viewer interest and sponsor endorsement. Many of the rule changes mentioned before are the result of the need to make judo more viewer-friendly and increase "spectator appeal" (Takahashi et. al., 2005:7, 15, 17). The IJF has gone to great lengths to accommodate this (Takahashi et. al., 2005:7). For instance, traditionally, contestants wore a white or red sash over their belts to aid referees in tracking who scored what. Now, contestants wear either white or blue judo uniforms. This innovation was introduced by the IJF to make it easier to differentiate the contestants on TV, much to the chagrin of traditional Japanese judo practitioners (Takahashi, 2005:15). On the positive side, the contrasting colors also make refereeing easier. Though not thought to have serious consequence to contest, contestants wearing the blue judo uniform seem to be statistically winners more often than those wearing the traditional white one (IJF, 2006/05/04). The reason for this is still being debated.

Though the IJF, not the IOC, determines the rules of the game, it seems that the rules change all too frequently. This makes it difficult not only for the competitors themselves to know what are appropriate tactics and techniques, but even referees find it difficult to keep abreast of changes (Holme, 1995:37–45).

The emphasis currently placed on competitive excellence and result has caused judo to divide into two different camps—"recreational" judo and "Olympic-style or Performance" judo. This conceptual and practical dichotomy is having great impact on judo practice (Jones, 2005). This is perhaps a natural consequence of the need to win in the Olympic arena, causing a change in training priority, method and focus. As a result, athletes train extremely hard in a limited number of judo and related techniques that provide the best opportunity to win, while eschewing most of judo's 67 or so techniques. Though this extreme training results in a low general knowledge of judo, frequent injury, early retirement, etc., contemporary judo has, indeed, switched its emphasis from the learning process to achieving an end (De Mente, 2003:14). This is causing a not too subtle schism between competitors and recreational judo players that is reflected in the priorities of judo's governing bodies. As Jones (2005: 75) points out, recreational judo is demeaned as somewhat inferior and, "...judo players who prefer to focus their study on the more traditional and technical aspects of judo (e.g. forms or kata) have become tagged with the label recreational players—implying that they are somehow inferior to contest players and not worthy of attention or recognition."

However, the vast majority of practicing judo players are involved in recreational activity. In terms of philosophy, recreational judo would seem best equated with the tradition of ongoing learning, physical fitness, and the moral ideals espoused by Kano (2005).

The competitive priority of "Olympic Judo," leaves the unfortunate impression in the public eye that in order to participate in judo, one must engage in elite competition. It is viewed as another competitive sport and that seems to be where it is ultimately headed. However, the competitive imperative deflects focus from judo's primary objectives established by Kano in the late 19th and early 20th centuries. Yes, by normal process, it has evolved to be somewhat different than it was over a century ago. But as mentioned before, judo is a component of world culture. Unlike organic species that are born into the world with only their genes to prepare them for the vagaries that the environment presents and their ultimate evolution or extinction, judo's "genes" are its participants. These "genes" have the benefit of a collective memory and purpose and, unlike organic species, its evolution can be directed by knowledge of the past and a perception of what judo should be in the future. So instead of bowing to the needs of a disinterested minority TV public and in turn, the profits of advertisers, judo must remain the property all judo practitioners—competitors, recreational judo players, and their teachers. All should play a role in determining how judo should evolve.

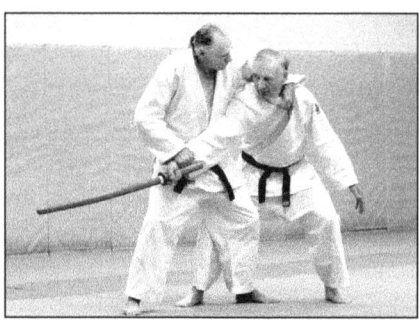

The final position of *kiri-oroshi* (downward cut), one of the *kata* (form) found in Kodokan Judo's *Kime-no-kata* (forms of decision). Also known as Shinken Shobu-no-kata (combat forms), this kata incorporates attack and defense techniques, such as striking techniques and counters to weapon attacks, as shown here. Competitive Olympic judo does not permit the use of striking or weapons. The complete Kodokan curriculum may only be experienced if kata are included as part of regular judo practice. Biron Ebell and Milton Jones (*uke*) demonstrating. Photography by Brook Jones.

With changes in rules to accommodate spectator understanding and IOC sponsors, the nationally driven need to win, and the loss of historic purpose, judo is in danger of coming full-circle and becoming what jujutsu was in the 19th century. Without intervention by judo's governing bodies and instructors, it stands the chance of assuming the same low status that Kano found jujutsu in 19th century Japan (Kano, 2005: 136). In fact, the use of the term "martial art" in the "ground and pound" cage wrestling of so called "mixed martial arts (MMA)" demeans the higher purpose, not only of judo, but of other budo usually included in the martial art genre. Keep in mind that the term, martial art, has been misappropriated and is not legitimately affiliated with the kind of demeaning public display found in the MMA cage sports.

On the contrary, Kodokan Judo should cling tenaciously to any, or all of the terms: martial art, martial way, or budo in reference to itself. All these terms reflect a glorious tradition and greater goals than found solely in sport. As Jhoon Rhee (1998), the father of American Taekwondo, states unequivocally, "I call martial arts without philosophy, street fighting." Oriental martial arts are generally grounded in moral and ethical codes that abhor violence, shun public titillation and display, and are somewhat offended or entertained by the self-aggrandizement of so called masters or cage-match winners. As Donohue (1998:27) observes " the real purpose of the martial arts is to forge spirit." And so it was, is, and should continue to be for Kodokan Judo!

ACKNOWLEDGMENT

The author extends special thanks to Milton Jones (3rd-dan) and Henry Epp (6th-dan) who read and commented on earlier drafts of this manuscript.

REFERENCES

Brousse, M. and Matsumoto, D. (1999). *Judo: A sport and a way of life*. Seoul: International Judo Federation.
Daigo, T. (2005). *Kodokan Judo throwing techniques*. Tokyo: Kodansha International.
DeMente, B. (2003). *Kata: The key to understanding and dealing with the Japanese!* Boston: Tuttle.
DeMente, B. (2004). *The Japanese samurai code: Classic strategies for success*. Boston: Tuttle.
Donohue, J. (1998). *Herding the ox: The martial arts as moral metaphor*. Wethersfield, CT: Turtle Press.
Donohue, J. (2005). Modern educational theories and traditional Japanese martial arts training methods. *Journal of Asian Martial Arts, 14*(2): 8–29.
Draeger, D. (1974). *Modern bujutsu and budo. The martial arts and ways of Japan: Volume 3*. New York: Weatherhill.
Holme, P. (1996). Get to grips with judo. Dorset, England: Blandford. International Judo Federation (2006, April 21). International Judo Federation,
Mission Statement http://www.ijf.org/rule/rule_role_mission.php#4 International Judo Federation (2006, May 4). The color of judogis: Wear blue if you have the choice. http://www.ijf.org/board/board_view.php?Page=1&SearchSelc=&SearchText=&Idx=293
International Olympic Committee (2005, Dec., 28). The International Olympic Charter. http://www.olympic.org/uk/organisation/missions/charter_uk.asp
Jones, L. (2005). Competition, kata and the art of judo. *Journal of Asian Martial Arts, 8*(3): 72–85.
Kano, J. (2005). *Mind over muscle: Writings from the founder of judo*. Tokyo: Kodansha.
Kano, J., et. al. (1986). *Kodokan Judo*. Tokyo: Kodansha.
Kiyota, M. (2002). *The Shambhala guide to kendo*. Boston: Shambhala.
Nurse, P. (2004, November 12). The beginnings of Kodokan Judo, 1882–1938. http:\\www.fightingarts.com/reading/article.php?id=53
Otaki, T. and Draeger, D. (1994). *Judo formal techniques: A complete guide to Kodokan Randori no Kata*. Boston: Tuttle.
Rhee, J. (1998). *The mystic origins of the martial arts*. A&E Home Video. A&E Television Networks.
Sadej, A. (1999). Should we promote judo as a martial art? Commentary in: *Yudansha Journal: Official Publication of Judo Canada, 5*(1):2–3.
Saul, J. (1992). *Voltaire's bastards: The dictatorship of reason in the west*. New York: Penguin Books.
Schell, C. (1999). Commentary in: *Yudansha Journal: Official Publication of Judo Canada, 5*(2):2–3.
Sidney, J. (Ed.) (2003). *The warrior's path: Wisdom from contemporary martial arts masters*. Boston: Shambhala.
Stevens, J. (1995). *Three budo masters*. Tokyo: Kodansha.
Takahashi, M. and Family. (2005). *Mastering judo*. Champaign, IL: Human Kinetics.

chapter 18

The First Kodokan Judo International Competition and Its Katas
by W. Lance Gatling, M.A., M.P.S.

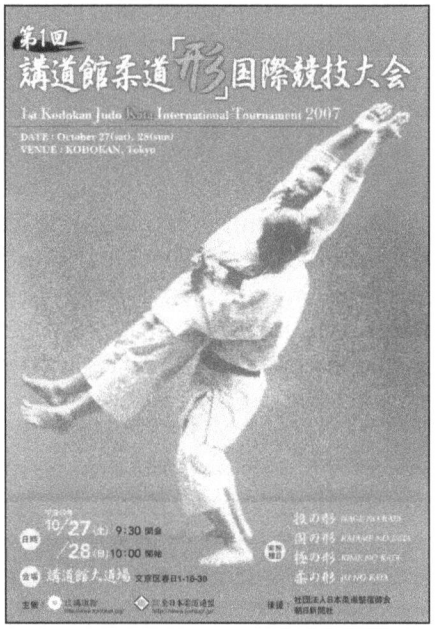

First Kodokan Judo Kata International Tournament program showing
Jigoro Kano, the founder of Kodokan judo, demonstrating Ju-no-kata.
All photographs © 2007 Lance Gatling.

The first world judo kata competition was held on Saturday and Sunday, October 27 and 28, 2007 in Tokyo, Japan, at the Kodokan, the headquarters of worldwide judo. There, 78 judo players from seventeen different countries, representing hundreds of years of judo experience, participated. Thirty-nine teams competed in four different forms (katas, or prearranged formal exercises) performed before five-member panels of twenty expert judges from thirteen different countries. Those teams were either seeded by regional international judo associations or were winners from regional competitions over the past year in the Pan-Am, European, African, and Asian Judo Unions. Eight teams from Japan, two competing in each kata, were chosen from top performers in the All-Japan Judo Federation's All-Japan Judo Kata Competition earlier in 2007. Like some judo competitions, there was no age or weight discrimination. Unlike other judo competitions, judo kata competitions were not segregated by sex.

But what role do the katas play in judo, and why are they important today?

Judo is comprised of relatively modern adaptations of selected techniques from numerous traditional styles of Japanese jujutsu combined with newer techniques. Since establishing the Kodokan in 1882, Professor Jigoro Kano, the founder of judo, and his technical instructors modified traditional jujutsu techniques into a sporting, competitive, rule-defined, modern martial way (*budo*). While originally constructed to help teach a total way of life, judo continued to evolve. Today, in most countries, competition plays the largest role in judo, much larger than originally envisioned, and partially as a result, today's judo is different from the original judo of 120 years ago.

Therefore, arguably the purest form of the early judo and its jujutsu origins are preserved not in the competition, but rather in its oldest katas. Perhaps the purest presentation of these forms worldwide is during the annual Kodokan kata national contest in Japan, so everyone knew the competition was tough for international competitors.

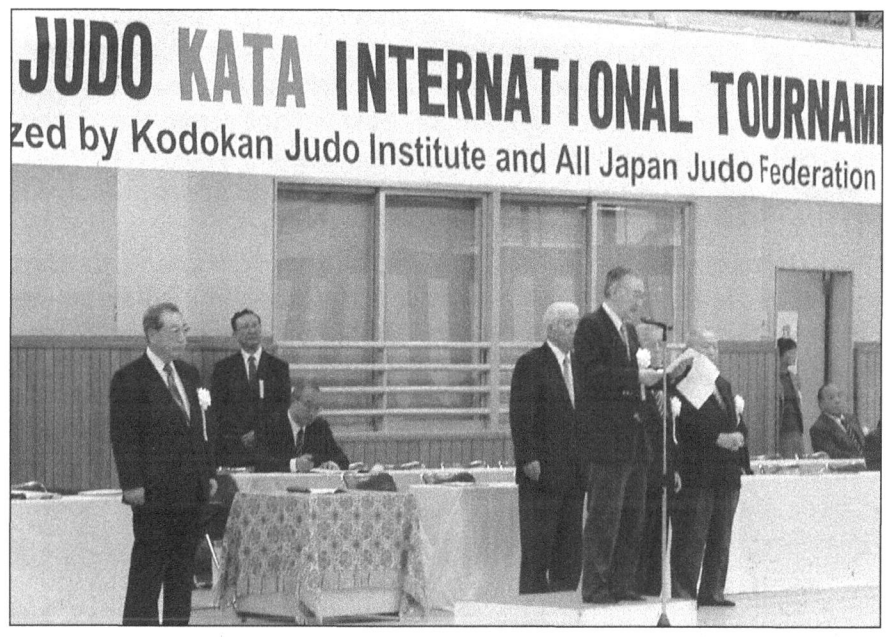

Opening address by Kodokan President Yukimitsu Kano.

In his opening speech, Yukimitsu Kano, president of both the Kodokan and the All-Japan Judo Federation, and grandson of Jigoro Kano, noted that the founder stressed that judo must be studied through both free sparring (*randori*) and kata, comparing them to the grammar and composition of judo. He congratulated the contestants on their interest, skills, and long hours of practice. He also noted growing interest in judo katas worldwide.

Modern judo primarily trains via basic technique practice and free sparring, as well as periodic competitions (*shiai*). Unfortunately, in the view of judo purists and traditionalists, most dojo typically seldom practice katas. While modern judo techniques are safe enough to practice via free sparring or competition; traditionally, jujutsu's more dangerous techniques were and are still practiced in pre-arranged katas, not via randori or shiai. This is because the traditional no-holds-barred jujutsu techniques still practiced in the judo katas are incapacitating if not lethal—including knife-edged hand slashes ("chops"); chokes; joint breaks; head-first body slams; eye gouges; stomps; kicks; and club, knife, and sword attacks. This may be judo's greatest innovation: the modification of these dangerous jujutsu techniques to enable safe, competitive free practice of a deadly art; in fact, taught and performed correctly, judo is statistically one of the world's safest contact sports.

For this competition, four of the main Kodokan katas were chosen; Nage-no-kata (throwing form), Katame-no-kata (grappling form), Kime-no-kata (decision form), and Ju-no-kata (flexible form).

Nage-no-kata is typically shown in every kata competition because it demonstrates the core of modern judo, with samples of all the main throwing techniques. Every Japanese judo practitioner from 1st-degree (dan) black belt is required to demonstrate increasing proficiency and depth in this kata, which was compiled around 1884. Kano was an advanced practitioner of both Tenshin Shinyo-ryu and Kito-ryu jujutsu, which provided many techniques to the Kodokan judo repertoire.

The original Nage-no-kata was later modified and expanded, largely by adding more rapid, agile moves afforded by the wear of modern, lightweight judo clothing (*judogi*) rather than the traditional, top-heavy cumbersome moves of armored warriors. The attacker of the technique (*uke*, "giver") strikes, grasps, and shoves, ever modifying the attacks to adjust to the previous defense. The defender (*tori*, "taker," "receiver") responds with hand, hip, foot, sacrifice, and side sacrifice throws. They repeat all fifteen techniques from both left and right sides for a total of thirty throws (and thirty jarring falls for uke).

The Japanese teams in the Nage-no-kata were the winners in the annual Kodokan Kata Taikai national competition earlier in 2007. Japanese teams from across the country, winners of a series of regional competitions, performed four different katas.

Kime-no-kata (decision form) is a combative kata from 1888. Appropriately for the early Meiji era (1868–1912) when it was established, it starts with eight armed and unarmed attacks from the formal, seated position (*seiza*), and ends with twelve standing attacks using holds, fists, a wooden knife, and a wooden sword (*bokken*). Judo's jujutsu roots are evident in this kata, in which tori uses strikes, joint locks, strangles, and throws to defeat the attacker.

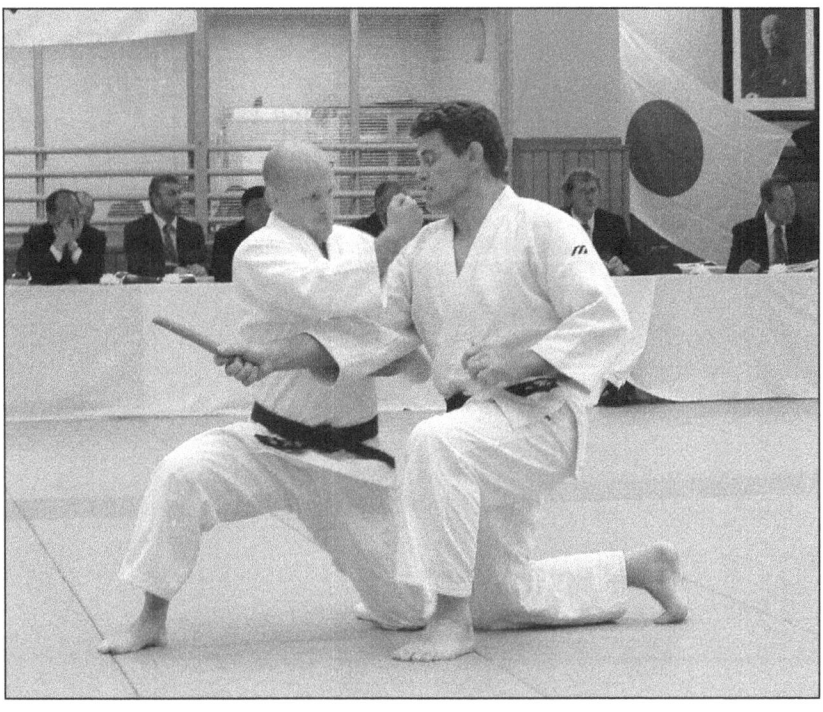

Robert Ivers and Robert Maurency (Australia) showing
Kime-no-kata defense against a knife attack.

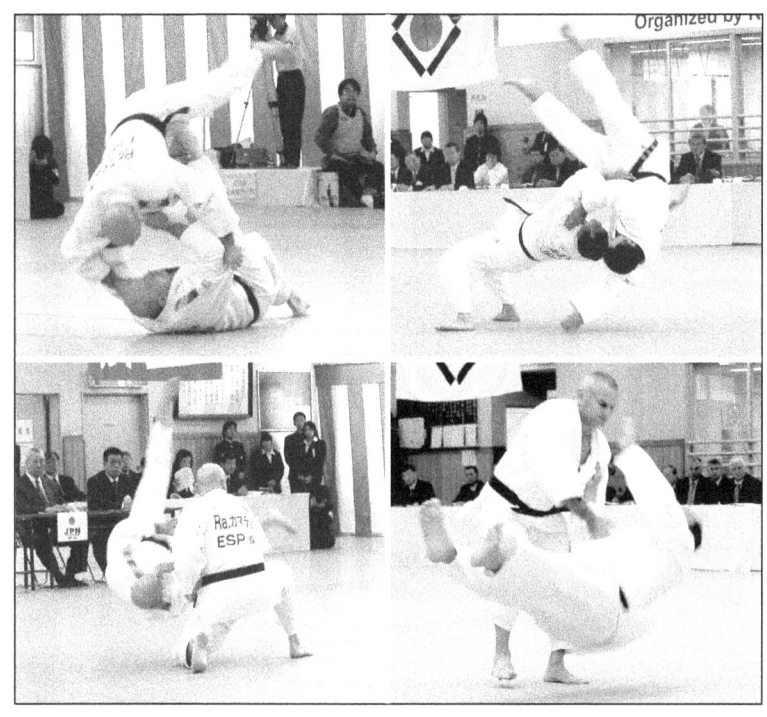

Nage no Kata teams from Japan, Spain, and Italy.

Katame-no-kata (grappling form) was compiled between 1884 to 1887, and was largely influenced by Tenshin Shin-yo-ryu jujutsu. It can be difficult for the layman to follow because the action is all floor grappling: tori demonstrates pins, joint locks, and chokes to immobilize the supine uke, who then attempts various escapes.

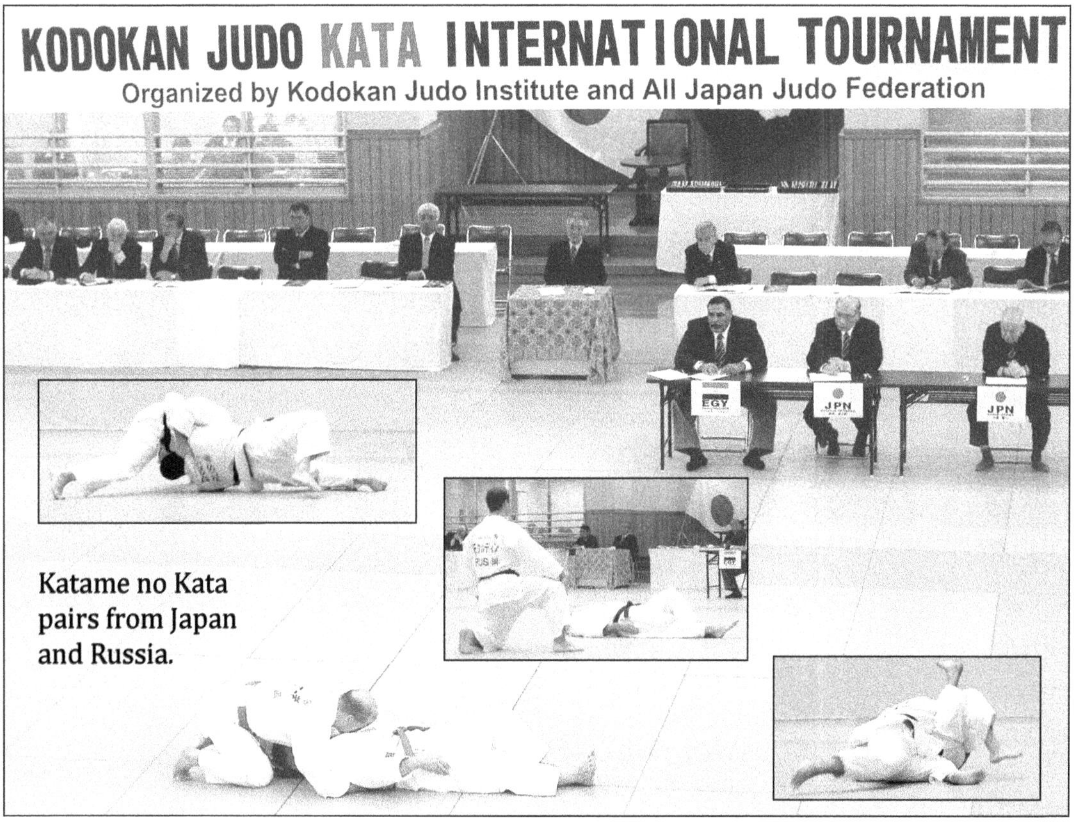

Katame no Kata pairs from Japan and Russia.

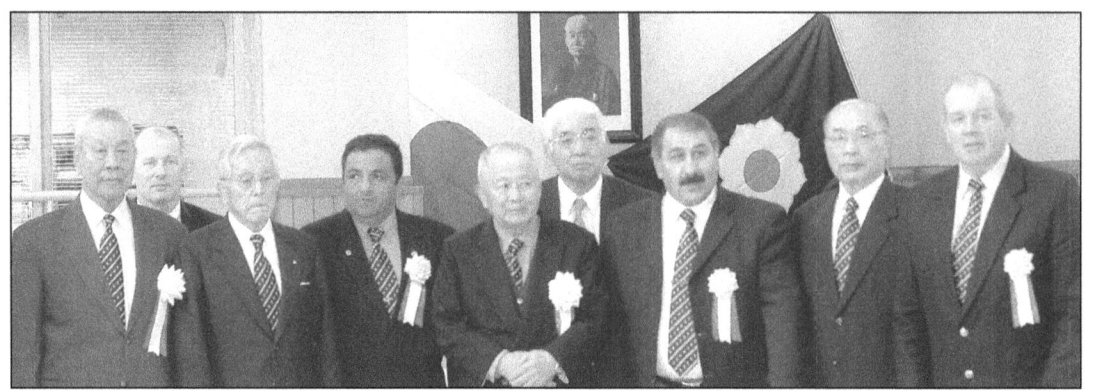

INTERNATIONAL JUDGES AND SOME OF THE HIGHEST RANKING MEMBERS OF THE KODOKAN
Left to right: Toshiro Daigo, 10th-dan (Japan); Raymond de Clerq (Belgium); Ichiro Abe, 10th-dan (Japan); Jose Gerardo Serna Norena (Columbia); Yoshima Osawa, 10th-dan (Japan); Saburo Matsushita, 8th-dan (Japan); Yassin Al-Ayoubi (Syra); Eihachio Okamoto, 8th-dan (Japan); Ivor Endicott-Davies (Australia). Background is the formal alcove with Jigoro Kano's portrait, displayed with Japanese and Kodokan flags, in the main dojo.

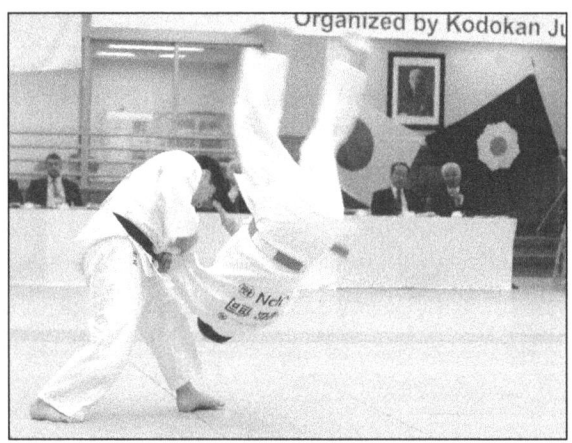

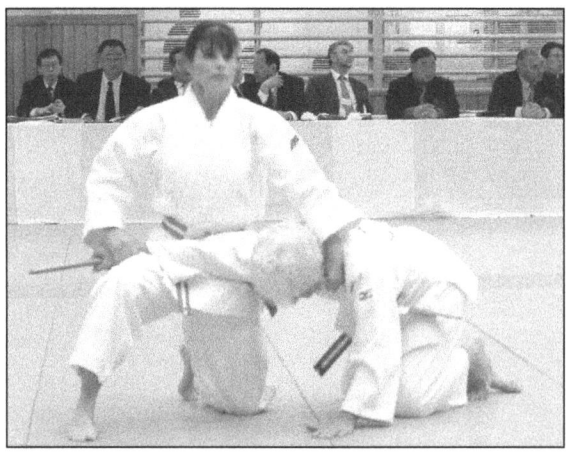

Above: Kenji Takeishi (L) and Koji Uematsu (Japan), the top Kime-no-kata pair. Below: Monette La Blanc (L) blocks Gesele Grave's (Canada) knife attack in Kime-no-kata.

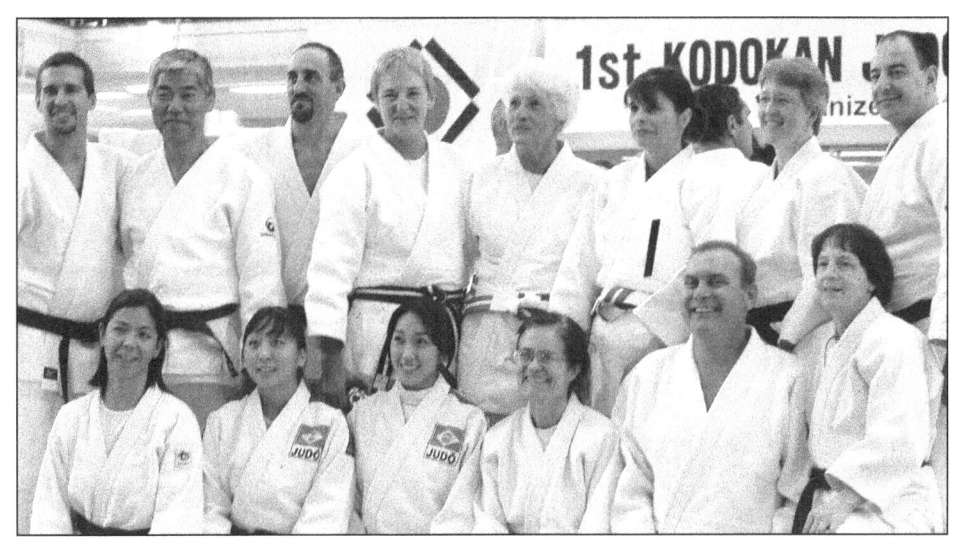

FRIENDS AND COMPETITORS FROM THE PANAM JUDO UNION
Front row, from left: Diane Jackson (USA), Suzi Yamamoto (Brazil), Kelly Yamamoto (Brazil), Karen Whilden (USA), Ryan O'Connor (USA), and Jan Moss (USA). Back row, from left: Heiko Rommelmann (USA), Rioti Uchida (Brazil), Jeff Giunta (USA), Frances Glaze (USA), Gesel Gravel (Canada), Montette LeBlanc (USA), Barbara Houston-Shimizi (USA), and Luis dos Santos (Brazil).

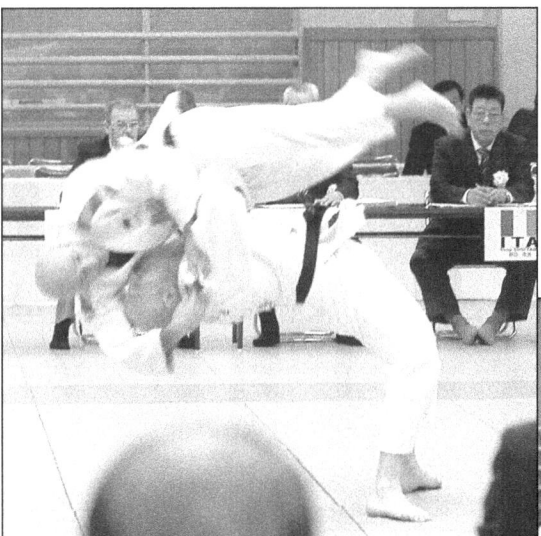

Left: Third place Nage no Kata team of Raul Camacho and Roberto Camacho (Spain).

Right: Alberto Grandi (L) throws Nicola Grandi (Italy) in Nage no Kata while winning the Secretary General's honorable mention award. The strong Italian pairs placed fourth in all four events.

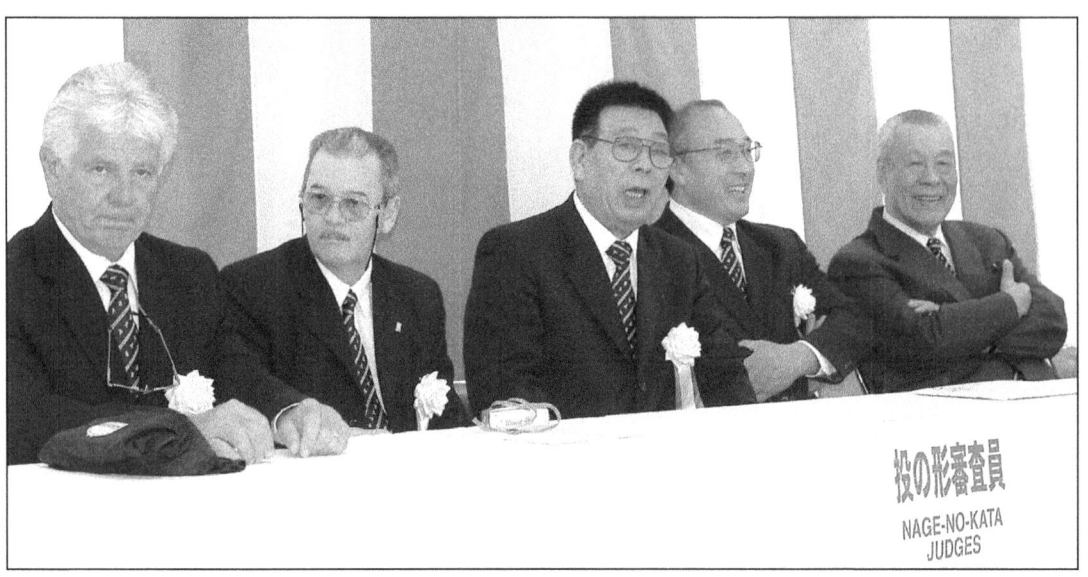

Nage no Kata judges during a break in the action (left to right),
Michael Job (S. Africa), Miguel A. Russo (Argentina), Shoji Sugiyama (Italy),
Koshi Onozawa (Japan) and Toshiro Daigo (Japan).

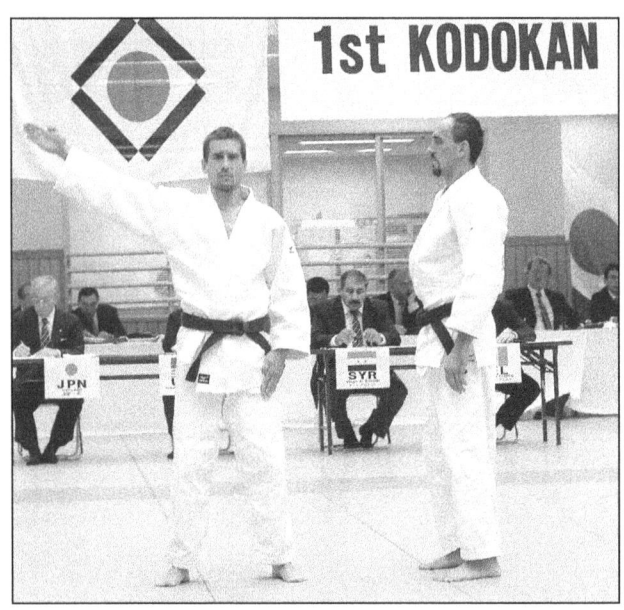

Ju no Kata team of Heiko Rommelmann (l.)
and Jeff Giunta (USA) perform before judges
from Japan, Belgium, U.S., and Syria.

Ju no Kata was invented in 1887 to develop strength, balance, and flexibility in female judo neophytes. This kata sometimes resembles paired gymnastics because the players move in graceful cooperation without throws or falls, rather than in attack and defense sequences. Even today, women often fill the Ju no Kata teams at competitions, but senior male judo players are required to demonstrate proficiency as well. Three of the ten teams were male, including one from the U.S., and the eventual third place Spanish team.

Regardless of the kata, proficiency at this level of competition does not come easily. The Japanese Nage-no-kata winners of the 2007 Kodokan All-Japan Kata Competition practiced together two hours a day for months in their police gym before the competition. Also, competent kata instruction can often be difficult to find; Mr. Heiko Rommelmann and Mr. Jeff Giunta, senior Pan-Am Judo Union competitors, and the sole U.S. pair in the Ju no Kata competition, described their difficulty in finding kata instruction: for years they drove hours one way to practice with their instructor, Mr. Tony Owed (now deceased) of Toledo, Ohio. As in previous Japanese national competitions, the Japanese police had a very strong showing; the police, particularly the Tokyo Metropolitan Police, have very strong judo training and kata programs.

In the end, the Japanese teams swept both first and second in all four events, and the Spanish teams took third in all four events; the Italian teams all placed very highly, too. Italian teams won the secretary general's prize.

There seemed to be little controversy despite the Japanese teams sweeping all top eight positions; the level of competition in Japan is clearly very high and very competitive, and Italy and Spain have dominated European kata competitions. The results did of course engender discussion of the relative levels of kata instruction in Japan, Europe, and the rest of the world, but plenty of foreign players vowed to study hard and return to do better. Some competitors praised the administration afterward, saying it was the best-organized tournament they had ever attended. Several of the foreign players had studied at the Kodokan or at overseas Kodokan seminars in preparation; the two Laotian teams studied there for days immediately prior to the event, and had made remarkable progress, according to one of their training partners.

In a post-competition interview, the Nage no Kata team of Toshimitsu Takahashi and Fumikazu Yoda described how they had focused on competition early in their judo careers, but came to believe that understanding the katas was key to their further development as well-rounded judoka and competitors. Policemen from Nagano City on the western side of Honshu, they started kata practice in the fall of 2006 and spent hours a day studying Nage no Kata. Their practice ended in a top three finish at the All-Japan competition, and second place in this first global competition.

Kodokan Museum Curator Naoki Murata, the general secretary of the event, and a judo 7th-dan, said in his closing address that while the katas' primary purpose is physical education and combat skills, certain katas were practiced primarily as cultural studies of judo's ancient jujutsu roots. In a later interview, he said that the main purpose of the competition was to highlight the katas' role in judo. Randori is now overly emphasized in judo training, he said, and this tournament is part of an effort by the Kodokan to return kata training to its proper place of importance. Unfortunately, because of the preparation required for the judo events in the upcoming Beijing 2008 Olympics and the need to have the All-Japan Judo Kata Competition in 2008, the Kodokan does not plan an international event in 2008, but perhaps in 2009.

Asked to comment on rumors that Japan may try to get acceptance of judo katas as an Olympic event, perhaps in time for Tokyo's bid to host the 2016 Summer Games, Mr. Murata noted that the trend in the Olympics has been to reduce judo events, not increase them, since the inclusion of women's events doubled the number of judo events. He also cited the success of the Pan-American and European Judo Unions' kata competitions, and said that the Kodokan leadership hopes that the other regional judo unions, the Asian, Oceania, and African Judo Unions, will take the lead in fostering interest in the katas through more instruction and competition. The Kodokan supports such efforts, he said, and hopes to help foster technical kata instruction worldwide.

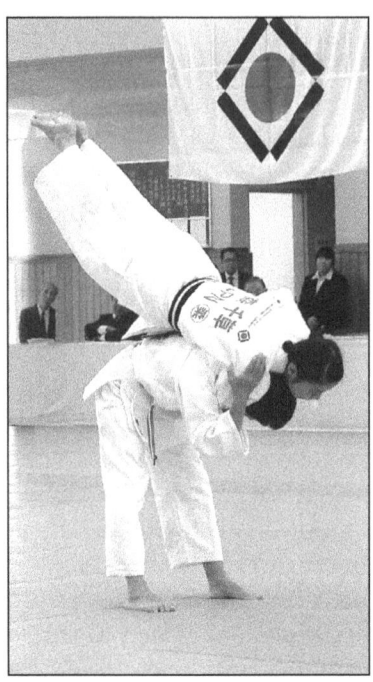

Ju no Kata winning team of
Estuko Yokoyama and Chigusa Omori (Japan).

To that end, there was an extensive kata seminar for international judges and participants after the competition, led by the Kodokan's chief instructor, Toshiro Daigo, one of the world's most famous judoka and one of only seventeen 10th-dans, the highest rank in judo. He provided detailed insights into the katas' historic origins and the principles behind each move in an effort to increase the general level of competence.

By preserving and demonstrating the ancient jujutsu techniques and practical applications of judo, the practice of katas and events like the First Kodokan Judo Kata International Tournament provide great insights into the heritage of this modern, global martial art.

BIBLIOGRAPHY

Kano, J. (1986). *Kodokan Judo*. Tokyo: Kodansha.

Kodokan. Kodokan judo kata series. Tokyo: Kodokan, various years. The Kodokan recently published a series of small, introductory books for each kata, but only in Japanese. See http://www.hint.co.jp/cgi-bin/kshop/kshop_j.pl/page=book_fr_j.html

Kotani, S. and Otaki, T. (1971). *Judo no kata: Zen.* (Judo kata: Complete.) Tokyo: Fumaido.

Mifune, K. (2004). *The canon of judo: Classic teachings on principles and techniques*. Tokyo: Kodansha International.

Otaki, T., and Draeger, D. (1983). *Judo formal techniques: A complete guide to Kodokan randori no kata*. Tokyo: Tuttle.

Shinagawa Judo Association (1984). *Miru, manabu, oshieru: Irasu judo no kata* (See, learn, teach: Illustrated judo kata). Tokyo: Shinagawa Judo Association.

chapter 19

Building Men on the Mat:
Traditional Manly Arts and the Asian Martial Arts in America
by Geoffrey Wingard, M.Ed.

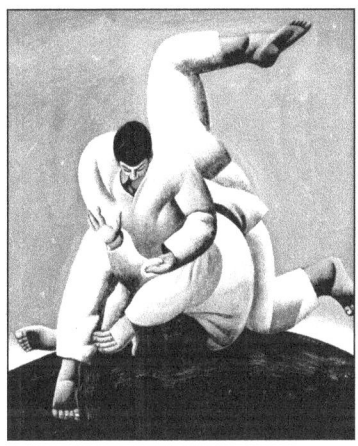

Painting by Curtis Parker. www.curtisparker.com

Introduction

In the post-World War II era, the commodification and dissemination of martial sports based upon traditional Asian fighting methodologies has become a prevalent feature of American culture. The institution and popularization of these martial activities at all levels of society—and the prevailing opinion that they are legitimate forms of recreation and physical and moral education for children and adults—is commonly seen as an example of the development of a new institution in American society. This phenomenon is either an outgrowth of cultural globalism or a corollary to America's appropriation of the traditions and cultures of occupied and colonized peoples. However, the adaptation of Asian martial arts into American society is not a break with American tradition, nor is it an example of a recently developed institution in America. Rather, the popularization of martial arts and combative sports based upon anachronistic Asian fighting methodologies should be viewed as the continuation of a long-standing American process of adapting various traditional, often elite, martial methodologies into American popular culture. The American appropriation and dissemination of martial methodologies from a variety of nations at various times and the publicization of diverse forms of violent recreation, self-protection and militaristic character education is a trend that may be observed not only today, but throughout American history.

While the development of practical fighting skills has certainly been important to Americans for a variety of reasons, the expansion of opportunities to practice martial arts in America in the past half-century seems unprecedented. As sociologist Max Skidmore states, "There is hardly a community of any size in Europe and the English-speaking lands in which there is no instruction available in one or more of the martial arts" (Skidmore, 1995:129).

However, the practice of all sorts of fighting styles, sports, and techniques has a long history in America. Italian and French fencing schools proliferated at times in early American urban areas (Nadi, 1943:22). Instruction in English fencing, notably instruction in the English small-sword, was extant in North America from the colonial period at least through the end of the 18th century (Blackwell, 1734). Truly American fighting methods developed unique characteristics based upon regional norms and practices throughout much of the 19th century (Gorn, 1985:18–43). The apparent difference between the traditional practice of the exercises and rituals of the manly arts, including fencing and other militaristic combat skills in the pre-World War II era, and the practice of Asian martial arts in America today seems, upon closer inspection, to be one of trappings, terminology, and mythology rather than one of any significant difference in availability of instruction or technical efficacy.

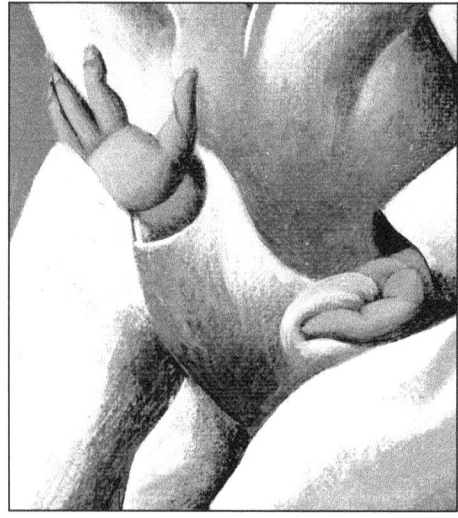

Detail of painting
by Curtis Parker.

The difference then is one of appearance rather than substance. The imagery surrounding the martial arts has changed, but their substance and practice in America has not. This imaginary change has occurred for a number of reasons and is not solely, or even primarily, the result of American hegemony in the Pacific following World War II. In fact, the appropriation and Americanization of Asian martial arts began well before Japanese and American military conflict in the Pacific.

It began during the first intensive period of East-West state interaction at the end of the 19th century and early in the 20th century. This was a time when Western public culture, particularly American culture, was engaged in a self-conscious attempt to modernize; yet still relied heavily on traditional institutions. It occurred at a time when the American elite articulated a conscious desire for industrial development and a need to reinforce strong moral and social values in boys and men. At the same time, upper-class social reformers sought to do away with practices and traditions of character education that they felt were embarrassing and anachronistic, so they looked abroad for alternative pedagogical modalities.

One traditional educational venue for the development of courage, strength, and loyalty American boys and men had been through the practice of the manly arts, a compendium of exercises that included games involving the risk of physical trauma or death to foster personal courage and loyalty to the group among participants. However, around the turn of the 20th century, the traditional manly arts, which included practices such as fencing, cudgel fighting, wrestling, and bare-knuckle boxing, had fallen out of public favor and new, modern sports practices had yet to completely fill the void. Modern sports were a new kind of social institution, a complex of behaviors and attitudes that complemented and were completed by industrialism in America while they drew on themes and practices made popular through pre-modern games. In the late 19th and early 20th centuries, amateur and professional sports, as opposed to participatory games, had yet to find universal acceptance.[1] At that time, Western sports proselytizers, Muscular Christians, and physical culture advocates looked abroad for practices they felt could be integrated into the Western masculine milieu and adapted to fill the void left by many elites' (and subsequently the public's) repudiation of the traditional manly arts. They found, developed, and adapted a variety of martial practices from around the world to meet their needs, notably including the new, "scientific" martial art imported from Japan (partially via England) known as judo. Quickly adopted by Victorian dilettantes and Orientalists, judo subsequently became the first of a series of updated and Westernized Asian martial sports to gain widespread popularity in the West.[2]

The study of the appropriation and dissemination of judo in America around the turn of the century reveals a lot about social and cultural developments occurring throughout the country at that time. It has been noted that "how men fight—who participates, who observes, which rules are followed, what is at stake, what tactics are allowed—reveals much about past cultures and societies" (Gorn, 1985:18). The study of sports in general and the study of physical practices, which, like many martial arts and particularly judo, contain both aspects of traditional masculine contest and modern sport (despite their participants consciously avoiding most types of professional competition), can tell much about the beliefs and ideals of participants and observers. Since modern sport, as defined by sports historian Alan Guttman, can only exist when there is both participation and observation or patronization, the study of modern sports involves the study of people across the social spectrum (Guttman, 1978). The study of sport is not just the study of frequently poor or under-class players, of frequently wealthy patrons, or of working-class and middle-class fans and observers, it is the study of all these groups and, most importantly, it is the analysis of their interactions. Because of the relatively early date of its introduction to the West and because it is a fighting system that was intentionally molded to fit the requirements of a modern sport from its inception, judo is particularly useful to study (Carr, 1993: 169). The study of the introduction and popularization of judo in America can therefore shed light on many issues of concern to social historians, particularly those interested in the complex set of rules and behaviors surrounding violence, social control, and the perpetuation of militaristic education in American society.

The "Manly Arts" in America

Prior to the introduction of judo to the United States at the end of the 19th century, strenuous and frequently violent recreation was subsumed within a category of athletic practices that were popularly known as the "manly arts." The traditional manly arts in America included a variety of public and private practices and games involving the cultivation of strength and spirit. The manly arts as understood by their participants from the late 18th through the early 20th centuries included boxing; wrestling; fencing; stick, staff, and cudgel fighting; gymnastics; and calisthenics, derived from or used to augment military exercises. The manly arts, "the combative arts of the late 1700's through to the early decades of the last century" (Wolf, 2000:1), were widespread in America as both elites and working-class people sought to strengthen their bodies, compete for prizes and prestige and to emotionally connect with a glorified and virile, although largely mythological, Anglo-Saxon archetype.

Prior to the rise of the professional sports movement in the late 19th and early 20th centuries, there was much less codification of sports and games than exists today and there is a particular dearth of recorded material on the rough and tumble games played by people as recreation from manual, agricultural, and industrial labor. However, these types of pastimes did exist and many people participated in them as sponsors, observers, or players. While the actual number of participants is impossible to determine, the variety of contests and practices and the varied and complex sets of rules and norms applied to combative recreation prior to the advent of the organized sports movement in the late 19th century speaks to the popularity of the manly arts for people of various classes, regions, ethnic, and social backgrounds throughout the United States.

While it may seem absurd to 21st-century observers that the practice of violent forms of recreation would be seen as useful for any purpose other than possible military preparation or popular entertainment, in the 18th and 19th centuries, the cultivation of martial skills were seen as part of the fundamental education of all gentlemen. In America, where an atmosphere of egalitarianism prevailed (at least among a segment of the republican faithful), the idea that there was value in the practice of ritualized violence quickly passed out of elite hands into the public domain. The manly arts and martial recreation became popular, public, and commercial.

This process had already begun by the early 18th century. In 1734, Edward Blackwell, an English immigrant to the American colonies, published a treatise on English fencing with the small sword. In England, small-sword fencing had been the province of gentlemen. The small sword had developed as a weapon for military officers and gentlemen out of the direct line of fire; it was a weapon for personal defense in situations when a saber or firearm would not have been close at hand. In America, however, small-sword fencing was not only the practice of the elite (although elites certainly patronized fencing masters in the 18th century), but quickly became available to the general public. Blackwell published his text on small-sword fencing for the American populace when he found that teaching fencing to the rarified few was neither an acceptable nor very lucrative career in the Colonies. As Blackwell states,

> Having, in my small practice in sundry parts of America, met with much Difficulty in Introducing the ART of the Small-Sword, I almost despaired of success, and that due Esteem which so ingenious an Art deserves.
> – Blackwell, 1734:A3

Not only were wealthy students scarce, but apparently a segment of the American public felt that upper-class fencing was of little use and possibly socially disruptive to an egalitarian citizenry. In an attempt to popularize his style of fighting, Blackwell responded by outlining a six-point argument in favor of fencing, culminating in the assertion,

> But was a Man never to fight with his Sword, no Exercise is more wholesome, and delightful to the Learner, than this Fencing: For, by working all the Parts of the Body, it strengthens the Limbs, opens the Chest, gives good Air, and handsome Deportment to the Body, a majestick Tread; and makes him active, vigorous and lively; and also enables him to serve his Friend, and Country.
> – Blackwell, 1734:ix

The public apparently responded favorably to Blackwell's arguments as various masters in many seaboard cities established fencing schools in the colonial era. By the 19th century, uniquely American styles of fighting had developed and the cultivation of martiality as a measure of masculinity was common. Some of these American combat systems, like American-rules singlestick fighting, were based on Old World models. Others, however, were more thoroughly American. Gorn relates that in the antebellum south, where fighting was common, "gouging" or fighting with the intent of removing an opponent's eye as a symbol of victory was prevalent. To distinguish themselves from boxers and wrestlers, Southern fighters intentionally labeled their style of combat "rough and tumble" or "gouging." Gouging became a practice that was so widespread and accepted that it developed its own folklore and popular mythology (Gorn, 1985:20–28). In other parts of the nation and among other classes, different rules of combat applied. In the "north woods," for example, "stomping" or knocking one's opponent down until he was susceptible to an attack with hob-nailed logging boots was far more prevalent and socially acceptable than gouging. In the mid-west, wrestling remained far more prominent than other forms of combative recreation leading to the development of the catch-as-catch-can style popularized by the successes of mid-western wrestlers such as a pre-presidential Abraham Lincoln (winner of a bout with the Louisiana state champion in New Salem, Louisiana in 1831) and Martin "Farmer" Burns (1861–1937), one of the first individuals to make instruction in wrestling commercially viable as a mail-order enterprise in the early part of the 20th century. Throughout the 18th and 19th centuries, as American identity was tied to the idea of the American frontier, the assertion that, "the early settlers of the frontier were the best wrestlers" became an almost self-fulfilling prophecy (although it is important to note that wrestling matches and other displays of manly arts took place at town meetings and in colleges, too) (Holliman, 1975:149).

The American elite continued to sponsor and participate in the manly arts. Fencing and singlestick, a method of wooden sword fencing, were practiced by cadets at nearly every secondary and post-secondary military academy in the country throughout the 19th century. Theodore Roosevelt, champion of the strenuous life, advocated the practice of the manly arts for all American boys and men. As president, Roosevelt had American and Japanese instructors of wrestling, boxing, judo, and singlestick visit and practice with him at the White House. Roosevelt encouraged the practice of the traditional manly arts alongside their newer, modern athletic counterparts.[3]

By the end the 19th century, however, Americans' perceptions of the manly arts had begun to change. While the cultivation of masculinity and strength was still admired, the practice of the traditional fighting arts had begun to decline. One reason had to do with the restrictions placed on fighting in urban areas. As America became an urban nation, the behavioral excesses, eccentricities, and violence previously permitted in rural communities, accepted among male work groups such as riverboat, mining, and logging crews and even allowed within small ethnic urban communities characterized by strong social solidarity, became restricted. In urban areas, poor and working class people were confronted by elite culture, religious practices, and commercial expectations that differed significantly from their previous experience. Unable to compete materially with elites they used social behavior including dress, etiquette, and reputation to normalize relationships with supervisors, landlords, and urban officials. Practices that brought to light class and regional differences, such as participation in gouging or stomping matches, were discouraged. Furthermore, in cities with modern court systems and police forces, the recourse to personal violence to mitigate affronts was severely restricted. The editor of the online publication Journal of Manly Arts, Tony Wolf explains (2000:1),

> This period [the first half of the 19th century] saw the decline of military swordplay, archery, and so-forth, concomitant with the inexorable advances of firearms and explosives. The age-old traditions of the duel of honour declined as well, and duels were eventually banned in most "civilised" countries. Towards the end of this period, many nations had established professional police forces, theoretically relieving their citizens of the need to openly carry weapons.

Other beliefs affected the practice and prevalence of the manly arts in America, as well. New theories on hygiene and disease exacerbated the decline in the practice of violent recreation. Physical contact came to be viewed as a vehicle for the transmission of disease. Contact with bodily fluids, such as blood and perspiration in the context of recreation, was particularly distasteful to many elite Americans in the Victorian-era. Elite participation and sponsorship of most traditional manly arts declined.

Fencing was the only of the archetypal manly arts that elites continued to patronize in large numbers. This was probably due to the association of fencing with a mythical Anglo-Saxon ideal and because the fencing accoutrements reasserted elites material and social primacy (Jackson-Lears, 1981:107–140). Aldo Nadi, an Italian fencing master credited with maintaining classical martial ideals in the modern sportive era, has described fencing as unique among all contact sports stating, "Fencing is a contact sport—a contact of steel, not of fists or bodies" (Nadi, 1943:13). In the same essay, Nadi compares fencing with boxing, concluding that fencing is physically, intellectually, and morally superior. As urbanization and the rule of law continued to discourage violent recreation in early industrial America, socially sensitive members of other classes followed the elites' lead and the appeal of bloody boxing, singlestick, and other fighting matches declined.

Nativist Americans looked askance at any form of recreation that seemed to celebrate foreign heritage. Fencing manuals, guides to the most cosmopolitan of the manly arts, were eventually rewritten to systematize and Americanize the various European fencing styles.[4] Participation in wrestling styles and boxing systems that seemed to celebrate one's immigrant heritage too strongly were seen as evidence that the practitioner was not sufficiently American. Even American styles of fighting such as catch-as-catch-can wrestling suffered as a result of their rural and regional character and their technical affinity with the Anglo-Gaelic wrestling traditions of Lancashire and Cornwall.[5]

Of the several factors that coalesced to create an atmosphere inhospitable to the practice of the traditional manly arts and favorable to the introduction of new martial sports based on the Asian martial arts in industrial-era America, the creation of modern sport weighed heavily. Modern sport and the sports ideal were disseminated from the upper and middle-classes to workers and the poor. At the same time, increasing urbanization and the concurrent rise in the fear of urban crime created a backlash against the sanitized modern sports that contributed to Americans' rapid acceptance of Asian fighting methods. Finally, widespread disillusionment with the management and practice of traditional fighting sports turned supporters of martial recreation away from the traditional manly arts even though many still had a preference for martial games, forcing them to look for new venues in which to participate in martial recreation. Concurrently, a popular, anti-modernist, nostalgic longing for the (largely mythic) pre-industrial past made American society receptive to the introduction of the Asian martial arts, particularly Japanese jujutsu and judo, which seemed to promise a sort of symbolic initiation into a universal warrior ethos. Examining the interconnected complex of these factors is the only way to explain why the Japanese martial arts were introduced, commercialized, and rapidly accepted in American society.

As the modern sport ethic developed, first among elites and Christian reformers and later among middle and working-class players, popular attitudes toward sports underwent a radical transformation.[6] Sports were transformed from celebratory, local, participatory events into codified, multi-local, and national games that were supported by hierarchical institutions regulated at levels above those occupied by most players and spectators. By the early 20th century, modern sports, as opposed to participatory games and contests, had become "the most universal aspect of popular culture" (Miller, et al., 2001:1). One eventual result of this shift in the composition of American sport and the growth of modern athleticism was the development of a strange dichotomy among supporters of the athletic movement that pitted two views of sport against each other. On one hand, sports were seen as institutions bound by rules that limited participation and encouraged spectatorship (sowing the seeds of professionalism and commercialism). On the other hand, sports were (ideally) practiced for their own sake with the understanding that diligent practice and good sportsmanship would generate positive behavior and attributes among players off the field as well as on.

It was primarily the latter tenet, which held that sports were good for the soul as well as for the body, that encouraged sports proselytizers to cast their nets wide as they embraced games and game players outside of their upper-class circle. The rise of the new sport ethic (and its proselytizing moral accompaniment, Muscular Christianity) fostered a missionary desire to spread the sport message beyond its original race, class, and national boundaries. Both Christian and athletic missionaries carried the sports message to the far corners of the rapidly industrializing world and consequently brought it into contact with games and attitudes alien to Western upper and middle-class society. These missionary movements initially introduced the Japanese martial arts (especially a new, "scientific" martial art called judo) to the West.

By the end of the 19th century, a crisis in American sport had become apparent. Sports that were acceptable on their face to modernist athletic and Christian associations (such as the YMCA) often held little appeal for the masses that had been raised on a diet of blood sports. Those who pursued modern sports were seen as elitist and effeminate by fighting sports advocates. At the same time though, the moral justification for participating in fighting sports was usurped by sports ethicists. Therefore, those who pursued fighting sports in the tradition of the manly arts were subject to ridicule for supporting an anti-social anachronistic tradition. An unstable position prevailed in which modern athletes appeared effeminate to a significant segment of the public by their refusal to participate in martial recreation, while those who participated in fighting arts were portrayed as morally deficient. Some sports advocates worked diligently to resolve this situation by devising a sport that met modern moral criteria while it appealed to traditional, base motivations, but it was not an easily resolved issue. As late as 1946, when British boxing champion Bruce Woodcock was felled by American Tami Mauriello, sports commentator Red Smith wrote, "[Woodcock fought] like someone who learned boxing out of a book and still believes it is a manly art" (Smith, 1996:61).

In the late 19th and early 20th centuries, participation in basketball, track and field, and bicycling flourished, but spectator patronage of those sports remained weak. At the same time, traditional bare-knuckle fighting was increasingly coming under legal censure and wrestling was beginning to show signs of becoming more show than contest. However, the public continued to patronize local (occasionally illegal) martial contests. Clearly, the manly arts still held some resonance for the American populace. Just as clearly, however, they were not going to receive the sponsorship or support that more sanitized sports enjoyed.

Asian Martial Arts Take Their Place in the U.S.A.

Sports advocates looked around the world for an activity that would meet a new set of criteria. They felt they needed an activity that held the appeal of traditional manly arts, but was free of the sordid history of boxing, free of the rural caricature that wrestling had become, and free of the elite class boundaries of fencing. They also required an activity that was modern in its approach, one that embodied the characteristics of modern sport such as regular record keeping, standardized rules, uniform entrance requirements, and norms of the industrial age (Guttman, 1978:16). Finally, the ideal sport had to appeal not only to sports enthusiasts, but also to the general population. That meant the activity had to respond to some perceived public need such as health maintenance, the enhancement of physical appearance, or, relevant to any discussion of the manly arts, the need for self-defense. At the periphery of the Western industrial world, these sports reformers discovered a sport that met these three criteria. They discovered the Japanese grappling style called judo.

Judo was a modern synthesis of older Japanese unarmed fighting systems (*jujutsu*) created in 1882 by Japanese physical education specialist and jujutsu expert, Kano Jigoro. Kano had studied classical jujutsu styles but had found them unsuitable for the temperament of modern Japan and impractical for modern study.[7] Kano, a professional educator, subsequently refined the old warrior arts and organized a new systematic way of teaching the old samurai skills. Kano based his new system on two premises: that the practice of the sport had to be safe for its participants (unlike the older jujutsu styles in which practitioners were often injured) and that the sport had to appeal to practitioners of all ability levels and social classes. To increase judo's appeal within both rational, industrial society and within conservative, anti-modern circles, Kano sought to integrate modern theories on training and competition (influenced by Japanese contact with the West) with neo-traditional warrior philosophies. According to Donn Draeger and Robert Smith, "Judo tuned itself toward physical education and culture" (1980:139). Kano even consciously planned the name of his new martial art to reflect the moral and physical characteristics he felt would popularize it as both a modern sport and a manly art. He formally called his new system Nippon Den Kodokan Judo, "an expression that implies 'the best budo of Japan'" (Draeger, 1996:118). It should be noted, however, that not all of the changes initiated by Kano and his contemporaries met with unadulterated success. In *Modern Bujutsu and Budo: The Martial Ways of Japan*, one of the first rigorous reviews of the Japanese martial arts in English, the author is critical of judo and its derivatives stating, "The grappling systems are the descendants of the polytypic series of tactics that had its beginnings in the martially ineffective styles of classical jujutsu of the late Edo period" (Draeger, 1996:60). Other martial arts, notably various styles of karate, have also been criticized for their modern emphasis on contests and the standardization of practice.[8]

From its inception, judo met the criteria that Western sports advocates sought. Judo also met most of the seven characteristics that historian Alan Guttman has stated must be present for an activity to be considered a modern sport. These characteristics encompass the sorts of changes that sports reformers had made to 19th-century Western sports such as various kinds of football and bicycle racing, characteristics that were also apparent in judo. Guttmann's criteria include secularism, equality of opportunity, the specialization of roles, rationalization, bureaucratic organization, quantification, and the quest for records (Guttman, 1978:16). Judo has been examined in Guttmann's terms and found to meet most of these conditions. Carr determined that judo fails to qualify as a modern sport only in its relative inability to be "quantified." This, however, is a condition shared by many performance-oriented sports such as figure skating, gymnastics, and competitive dance, which suffer from subjective judging and standards and should not be seen as automatically disqualifying (Carr, 1993:185–187).

In addition to sitting firmly in the mold of modern sport, judo also had obvious utility to urban Americans. It was a self-defense system that, theoretically at least, did not require a proponent to possess overwhelming mass or strength to overcome an opponent. It was comprised of a variety of techniques applicable under a wide variety of circumstances and could be augmented by Western fighting methods as necessary. It was reportedly safe for men, women, and children to practice and, from the outset, judo instruction in England and the United States was offered to both males and females.[9]

Judo could also be practiced easily in the limited space available in crowded industrial cities (Matsudaira, 1910:117). Finally, judo was an intentionally moral and philosophical sport (Lindsay and Kano, 1889:204–205; Carr, 1993:168). Kano Jigoro consciously included instruction in moral precepts as part of the judo curriculum. Drawn from traditional Japanese philosophy and the Japanese warrior's code (*bushido*), judo philosophy contained elements that appealed directly to moral sports enthusiasts.

Those who advocated for the expansion of sporting opportunities on the basis that they contributed to moral development through the ethics of good sportsmanship and fair play observed that respect for one's opponent and self-control were cornerstones of judo practice. As a later observer noted, 19th-century sports enthusiasts believed that, "In the martial arts of Asia, conflict appears very rigid, yet consideration of the opponent is very high" (Luschen, 1981:201). Even many Western anti-modernists, who were at best skeptical of the modern sports movement, begrudgingly accepted judo as they drew parallels between the old feudal samurai code (*bushido*) upon which judo philosophy was partially based and the legendary chivalry of English knights errant.[10]

In Japan, judo was considered one of the new-era martial ways (*shin budo*). These arts were seen as distinct from and superior to mere fighting systems because they explicitly contained a moral component. The 19th-century Japanese philosopher Aizawa Yasushi (1781–1863) stated, "To know etiquette and honor, to preserve the way of the gentleman, to strive for frugality, and thus become a bulwark of the state, is budo" (Friday, 1997:7). While undeniably foreign to Western sports proselytizers, judo seemed to speak to a universal warrior sentiment, an idea that enjoyed widespread appeal among expansionist Americans. Furthermore, the moral codes of judo and bushido bore at least cursory similarities to the ethics championed by modern sports movement advocates. In the commentary to a lecture given to the Japan Society in 1910, Count Mutsu, a member of the Meiji government and the British Japanese Society, offered, "Our Bushido is your sportsmanship" (Matsudaira, 1910:133). In Nitobe's *Bushido*, the 1905 English language guide to Japanese culture through its philosophical warrior tradition, chapters three through nine are titled:

    III. Rectitude or Justice
    IV. Courage, The Spirit of Daring and Bearing
    V. Benevolence, The Feeling of Distress
    VI. Politeness
    VII. Veracity and Sincerity
    VIII. Honour
    IX. The Duty of Loyalty

These chapter titles bear striking similarities to the goals espoused by organizers of the modern sports establishment who sought to instill the virtues of courage, honor, loyalty, good sportsmanship, and Christian charity in players and spectators. Early judo enthusiasts would likely have agreed with Yuasa Yasuo's (1925-2005) comment that, "Training in sports aims at developing the body's capacity.... On the other hand, the original goal in the *bushi* [warrior] way is to develop mental (or spiritual) capacity" (1993:32).

Although never popular enough to rival "American" sports like football, baseball, or even resurrected (gloved) prizefighting in the early 20th century, judo did set the stage for the introduction of other martial sports to America. From the early 20th century onward, successive "waves" of immigration of various fighting sports from around the world became nearly instantly popular only to vanish from the American public consciousness almost as quickly. Since the 1950's, East Asian martial sports with esoteric names such as Wing Chun, kempo (kenpo), ninjutsu, Muay Thai, and the syncretic martial art called Brazilian jujitsu have successively achieved popularity and commercial success in the American martial sports marketplace. American styles of fighting and American "masters" benefited from these successive waves of popularity even as they celebrated their competing martial systems as a foil to new or foreign "tricks" (Burns, 1913).

This process of acquisition, commercialization, and dissemination, begun early in American history with fencing and American styles of fighting, is characteristic of a variety of American cultural interactions. Furthermore, it addresses the situation in which "[w]e find ourselves perplexed as we try to balance winning with fair play, aggressiveness with control, freedom with technique, and the individual with community" (Hardy, 1990:77).

Cultural historians, as well as historians of the martial arts and sport, can take a lesson from the history of the changing practice of the manly arts in America. The continual process of adaptation and popularization apparent in the evolution of martial recreation in America from one of manly arts to modern martial sports seems to share many similarities with the American penchant for acquiring and "Americanizing" cultural institutions from around the world. Fencing, gouging, judo, and modern martial arts exist in a continuum as they integrate with and complement other aspects of American popular culture.

▼▲▼

ENDNOTES

[1] The two classical arguments among sports historians can be found in the works of Mandell and Sansone. Mandell (1984) argues that sport is a cultural complement to industrialism. Sansone (1988) maintains that sports are the modern expression of the universal human struggle with contest and cooperation.

[2] Most of the hundreds of summaries of judo history available paraphrase the account provided in Lindsay and Kano (1889:192-205). Judo's history and development have been treated at length in a variety of sources, notably in English in Draeger (1974/1996: 112-123). The integration of judo into British popular culture is described in Wingard

(2003:16–25).
3. The most thorough description of Roosevelt's martial activities is found in Donovan (1909). For a more complete analysis of the implications of Roosevelt's participation in martial sports on the man and the arts in America see Burdick (1999:22–54).
4. See Cass (1930:17–18), for an example of a consciously Americanized fencing manual.
5. For an example of the continuing dissemination and adaptation of Anglo-Gaelic wrestling in 20th-century U.S.A., see Pittman (1999:48–57), specifically pp. 49 and 57.
6. Guttmann (1978) and Holt (1989) treats the rise of modern sports in great detail.
7. In 1868, the Meiji emperor wrested control of Japan away from the last Tokugawa shogun. To solidify his position and assert control over conservative samurai, the emperor embarked on a course to rapidly modernize Japan. Many trappings of the old regime were outlawed and others quickly fell into disuse. Some martial arts changed their curricula to appeal to more popular audiences. An archetypal discussion of the symbolic character and implication of these changes to Japanese martial culture is included in Funakoshi Gichin's memoir (1975:1–7).
8. Recently, scholarly examinations of judo's early years of have been published with increasing frequency, including Gray Carr (1993:167–188), Smith (1996:60–65), and Bowen (1999:43–53).
9. Barton-Wright (1902: 261–264) and Norman (1905) both exalt the suitability of judo and related exercises across class, race, and gender boundaries.
10. It is important to note that the Japanese warrior ideal the English admired was a concept largely derived from Nitobe (1905) and by pamphlets published by Westerners residing for short periods in Japan (e.g. Norman (1905:1–3). Nitobe had been educated in English public schools and was Christian. It is likely that his version of the samurai honor code was highly idealized, if not specifically coordinated to appeal to an English audience. Similarly the pamphleteers' accounts must also be viewed critically as their motives were frequently commercial or evangelical.

REFERENCES

Barton-Wright, E.W. (1902). Ju-jitsu and Ju-do. *Transactions and proceedings of the Japan Society*, London 5:261–264.

Blackwell, E. (1734). *A complete system of fencing: Or, the art of defence.* Williamsburg: William Parks.

Bowen, R. (1999). Origins of the British Judo Association, the European Judo Union and the International Judo Federation. *Journal of Asian Martial Arts, 8*(3):43–53.

Burdick, D. (1999). The American way of fighting: Unarmed defense in the United States, 1845–1945. Ph.D. Dissertation, University of Indiana.

Burns, M. (1913). *Jiu Jitsu–Self defense and their relation to wrestling: Lesson XII* (Book VI). Omaha: Farmer Burns School of Wrestling.

Carr, K. (1993). Making way: War, philosophy and sport in Japanese judo. *Journal of Sport History, 20*(2):167–188.

Cass, E. (1930). *The book of fencing.* Boston: Lothrop, Lee and Shepard, Co.

Donovan, M. (1909). *The Roosevelt that I know: Ten years of boxing with the president – and other memories of famous men.* New York: B.W. Dodge and Co.

Draeger, D. (1996). *Modern bujutsu and budo: The martial arts and ways of Japan.* New York: Weatherhill.

Draeger, D. and R. Smith. (1980). *Comprehensive Asian fighting arts.* New York: Kodansha International.

Dykhuizen, J. (2000): Culture, training and perception of the martial arts: Aikido's example.

Journal of Asian Martial Arts, 9(3):9–31.
Friday, K. (1997). *Legacies of the sword: The Kashima-Shinryu and samurai martial culture.* Honolulu: University of Hawai'i Press.
Funakoshi, G. (1975). *Karate-do, my way of life.* New York: Kodansha International.
Gorn, E. (1985). Gouge and bite, pull hair and scratch: The social significance of fighting in the southern backcountry. *American Historical Quarterly,* 90(1):18–43.
Gray, W. (1987). For whom the bell tolled: The decline of British prize fighting in the Victorian era. *Journal of Popular Culture,* 21(2):53–64.
Guttmann, A. (1978). *From ritual to record: The nature of modern sports.* New York: Columbia University Press.
Holliman, J. (1975). American sports 1785–1835. No. 34 of *Perspectives in American History.* Philadelphia: Porcupine Press.
Holt, R. (1989). *Sport and the British: A modern history.* Oxford: Clarendon Press.
Hardy, S. (1990). Entrepreneurs, structures and sportgeist. In *Essays on Sport History and Sport Mythology,* edited by D. Kyle and G. Stark. College Station: Texas A&M University Press.
Jackson-Lears, T. (1981). *No place of grace: Anti-modernism and the transformation of American culture 1880–1920.* New York: Pantheon Books.
Jones, H. (1943). *Judo, jiu-jitsu, and hand-to-hand fighting: A list of references.* Washington, D.C.: The Library of Congress Division of Bibliography.
Lindsay, T. and J. Kano (1889). Jiujutsu the old samurai art of fighting without weapons, *Transactions of the Asiatic Society of Japan,* 16:192–205.
Luschen, G. (1981). The system of sport—Problems of methodology, conflict and social stratification. In *Handbook of the Social Science of Sport,* edited by Gunther Luschen and George Sage. Champaign, IL: Stipes Publishing Co.
Mandell, R. (1984). *Sport: A cultural history.* New York: Columbia University Press.
Matsudaira, T. (1910). Sports and physical training in modern Japan. *Transactions and proceedings of the Japan Society,* London, 8:114–134.
Miller, T., G. Lawrence, J. McCay and D. Rowe. (2001). *Globalization and sport: Playing the world.* London: Sage Publications.
Nadi, A. (1943). *On fencing.* New York: G.P Putnam's Son.
Nitobe, I. (1905). *Bushido.* New York: G.P. Putnam's Sons.
Norman, F. (1905). *The fighting man of Japan: the training and exercises of the samurai.* London: Archibald Constable and Co. Ltd.
Pittman, A. (1999). Combat wrestling: Geoghan's blend from East and West. *Journal of Asian Martial Arts,* 8(4):48–57.
Sansone, D. (1988). *Greek athletics and the genesis of sport.* Berkeley: University of California Press.
Sidmore, M. (1995). Oriental contributions to Western popular culture: The martial arts. *Journal of Popular Culture,* 25(1):129–148.
Smith, R. (1996). The masters contest of 1926: An epiphany in judo history. *Journal of Asian Martial Arts,* 5(3):60–65.
Wingard, G. (2003). Sport, industrialism and the Japanese gentle way: Judo in late Victorian England. *Journal of Asian Martial Arts,* 12(2):16–25.
Wolf, T. (2000). An introduction to the Journal of Manly Arts. *Electronic Journals of Martial Arts and Sciences: Journal of Manly Arts,* http://ejmas.com/jmanly/jmanlymission.htm (17 February, 2003).
Yuasa, Y. (1993). *The body, self-cultivation, and ki energy.* New York: State University of New York Press.

chapter 20

Judo Comes to California:
Judo vs. Wrestling in the American West, 1900–1920
by Matt Hlinak, M.A., J.D.

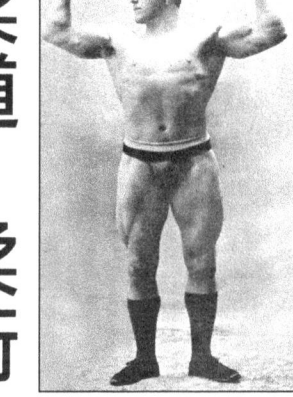

Left side: kanji script for "judo" and "jujutsu". Photograph of Georg Hackenschmidt (1878–1968), the first recognized World Heavyweight Wrestling Champion in 1905.

Introduction

This essay analyzes Japanese-American immigration into the American West through the prism of athletics, specifically by examining a series of contests between Japanese-American *judoka* (practitioners of judo) and European-American wrestlers from 1900 to 1920 in California. The popularity of these matches demonstrates the complex relationship between Japanese-Americans and the dominant European-American culture of the western states during this period.

This complexity will be shown first by looking at the way in which martial arts are closely linked to national and ethnic identity. During the latter half of the 1800s, the western martial arts of boxing and wrestling began the trend toward internationalization of sport which led to the first modern Olympic Games in 1896. Nationalism in sport followed almost immediately behind. The American style of "catch wrestling" evolved from European wrestling styles shaped by nineteenth-century notions of fair play and the manly arts. Significantly, early catch wrestlers honed their craft traveling with carnivals throughout the country, cultivating a backwoods sense of competition and masculinity. While professional wrestling has devolved into "muscular theater" today, wrestlers in the fin de siècle West were viewed as paragons of rough-and-tumble frontier masculinity.

Similarly, judo held an important position in Japanese society. Unlike American catch wrestling, with its origins in various European folk wrestling styles, judo is an entirely indigenous Japanese martial art. In an effort to prove the effectiveness of their art, a handful of skilled judoka traveled around the world, challenging (and often defeating) local wrestlers; these successes led many Japanese to equate judo with Japan's recent rise in global political and economic stature. Similarly, many westerners saw the mysterious art of judo as an explanation for Japan's seemingly inexplicable military victory over Russia in the Russo-Japanese War (1904–05). Japanese immigrants to the western United States brought judo with them and the sport quickly gained popularity with European-Americans.

Not all of the responses were positive, however. Many westerners simply dismissed judo based on perceptions of racial inferiority of Japanese. Others criticized judo's tactics, finding them inconsistent with the evolving ideals of western sportsmanship. But many European-American admired the way in which a skilled judoka could defeat a significantly larger opponent, and a few even attributed mystical or supernatural abilities to athletes of Japanese origin.

A strong barnstorming tradition existed in both judo and catch wrestling, so conflict between the two was inevitable. Matches pitting judoka against wrestlers almost always earned higher billing than matches featuring two competitors of the same style. They also spawned numerous essays in western newspapers comparing the two martial arts.

This chapter will conclude with a discussion of why these matches were so appealing to European-Americans in the western states. One reason was a simple interest in Japanese culture. But European-Americans also enjoyed the way in which these matches reinforced stereotypes about Japanese-Americans. For example, a judoka's ability to defeat a larger opponent emphasized the supposed smaller physical stature of Japanese people. Judoka were also portrayed as excessively polite, in contrast to the rugged western wrestlers, which presented contrasting notions of masculinity. Similarly, judo techniques that would be illegal in a western wrestling match were viewed as dirty tactics inconsistent with gentlemanly sporting traditions. In the eyes of European-Americans, judo, like the Japanese themselves, was an alien concept to be alternatively ridiculed and feared.

Much of the European-American interest in these matches arose out of anxiety over the larger socio-political context. Westerners felt threatened by Asian immigration as well as Japan's increasing military and economic power. These matches allowed them to vicariously act out their anxiety. For this reason, we continue to see racial match-ups in professional wrestling to this day. Indeed, legitimate sports today are contested in an atmosphere of subtle and not-so-subtle nationalism and even outright racism. By understanding the historical basis for the darker elements of athletics, modern competitors and fans may be able to conquer these elements and simply enjoy the match.

Announcement of bout between Adolph "Ad" Santal (above) and jujutsu expert Tarra Mikania. *Los Angeles Times* (7 April 1915).

A Note on Terminology

Throughout this work, the terms "judo" and "jujutsu" will be used interchangeably, although they are not synonymous. As will be discussed in greater detail in Part I, judo evolved from jujutsu, a process which began with the formation of Kano Jigaro Kodokan academy in 1882 and culminated in judo's debut as an Olympic sport at the 1964 Summer Games in Tokyo. During this transitional period, judo was often viewed simply as the particularly effective form of jujutsu practiced by Kano and his students, but not as a distinct martial art. The majority of *jujutsuka* (practitioners of jujutsu) discussed herein trace their martial arts lineage back to Kano, so it is not inaccurate to refer to them as judoka. More importantly, however, the rather ill-defined distinction between judo and jujutsu would not have been understood by the European-American journalists who produced much of the primary source material relied upon here. No attempt will therefore be made to attempt to discern whether a particular athlete considered himself a student of judo or jujutsu (Burdick, 1999; Carr, 1993; Shun, 1998).

While "judo" and "jujutsu" will be used more broadly than would be accurate, the term "wrestling" will be used more narrowly than it is often construed. The *American Heritage Dictionary* defines wrestling as, "[a] sport in which two competitors attempt to throw or immobilize each other by grappling," which would include both judo and jujutsu. In this work, "wrestling" will refer only to European-based grappling styles in which the goal is to pin the opponent's shoulders to the mat, rather than to cause the opponent to concede the match ("submit") by means of chokeholds or joint manipulation as in jujutsu-inspired martial arts. Western wrestling styles satisfying this definition will also be discussed in greater detail in Part I.

I. Martial Arts and National Identity

Wrestling and American Culture

Wrestling in the United States evolved from a number of European-based wrestling styles, particularly those of British origin. In the Cumberland and Westmorland style, competitors locked their arms around one another (a position known to modern wrestlers as "the clinch") and the loser was the first to break his grip. Wrestlers in the Cornish-style wore jackets, which were held in order to gain an advantage as in modern judo. Devonshire-style wrestling was similar to Cornish-style except it also allowed kicking to the shins. One of the most influential styles was Irish collar-and-elbow wrestling, in which competitors began by gripping one another by the collar and elbow; this form spread rapidly through the Northern states during the Civil War due to the large numbers of Irish immigrants in the Union armies. French, German, Dutch, African, and Native American wrestling styles further influenced the development of a uniquely American wrestling style (Archer and Svinth, 2005; Gorn, 1985; Morton and O'Brien, 1985; Pope, 1997; Savenga, 1995).

Wrestling played an important role in American culture in the nineteenth century. The sport found its way into "American folklore from the early days of Republic up to the Civil War" through "tales of the wrestling prowess of its men" (Morton and O'Brien 1985: 19–20). George Washington and Abraham Lincoln both garnered considerable acclaim for their grappling skills, while wrestlers featured prominently in the works of Mark Twain. Competitions between soldiers during the Civil War followed by post-war urbanization led to standardizing rules and techniques—with some resistance (see Guttmann, 1994)—into a style known as "catch-as-catch-can" or catch wrestling, which made it possible to pit champions from one locality against one another. This standardization, coupled with a strong interest in betting on matches, allowed wrestlers to evolve from rural strongmen into the nation's first professional athletes. While baseball would grow to become the national pastime, its development as a professional sport lagged significantly behind wrestling in the latter decades of the 1800s. At the peak of wrestling's popularity in 1911, more than 35,000 fans packed into Chicago's Comiskey Park to watch the rematch between Frank Gotch (1878-1917)—"one of America's earliest athletic superstars" (Hewitt, 2005:13-14)—and Georg Hackenschmidt (1878-1968); the live gate for the bout came to $87,000, or over 1.8 million in today's dollars (Betts, 1974; Fielding, 1975; Fielding, 1977; Hewitt, 2005; Rickard, 1999).

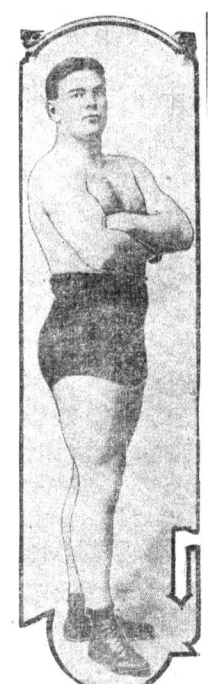

Frank Gotch, two-time victor over G. Hackenschmidt in 1908 and 1911.

But wrestling was not merely popular in the United States; it was a distinctly American endeavor, one that resonated with the frontier culture of the western states. A number of commentators have described the sport in this time period using the language of the borderlands. Morton and O'Brien (1985:9, 20) note that "[r]ecords of American westward expansion are replete with descriptions of one-eyed brawlers, earless innkeepers, and others who bore scars from pankration ['a no-holds barred combination of boxing and wrestling'] bouts". Hewitt (2005:1-2) describes a "rough-and-tumble fighting tradition long associated with the frontier [in which] [b]ackwoodsmen regularly engaged in anything-goes brawling . . .". Archer and Svinth (2005) place wrestlers at home in the quintessentially borderlands environs of "saloons, Wild West shows and circuses, and vaudeville."

Contemporary writers similarly viewed wrestling as an endeavor closely tied to American culture. Journalists of the pre-World War I era routinely made reference to the "All American" sport of wrestling (LAT, December 18, 1914), "the American method of catch-as-catch-can" (OT, August 29, 1905), or "the Yankee plan" of self-defense (LAT, March 4, 1905). The "American method" was a popular and thoroughly western sport in the United States at the dawn of the twentieth century.

Judo and Japanese Culture

All cultures in the world have participated in some form of grappling since before recorded history, and the Japanese are no exception. The precursors to jujutsu developed in the medieval period as a means of combat for samurai who found themselves without their swords. Because the striking techniques found in other Asian martial arts would be ineffective against a heavily-armored opponent, the samurai created a fighting style which would allow them to immobilize an opponent with limited use of punches or kicks. A style which would be recognizable to a modern jujutsuka took shape in the 1600s. While jujutsu's origins can be traced to the battlefield, it was a prolonged period of peace in the seventeenth and eighteenth centuries which caused the martial art to flourish. In the absence of war, jujutsu became the sole means by which members of the warrior class could demonstrate their masculinity, particularly as the government steadily eroded the privileges once held by the samurai. As jujutsu became increasingly divorced from its battlefield origins, the style abandoned many practical techniques in favor of those which were aesthetically pleasing (Burdick, 1997; Carr, 1993).

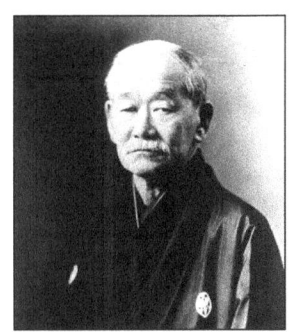

Founder of judo, Kano Jigoro (1860-1938). Photo from the Kodokan.

During this era of peace, the Tokugawa government kept Japan largely isolated from the rest of the world. In 1853, Commodore Matthew Perry of the United States Navy threatened Japan with military intervention if it did not open its ports to American merchant vessels. The humiliating 1858 Treaty of Amity and Commerce put an end to Japanese isolationism. This abrupt "opening" of the island nation shook Japanese society, causing simultaneous and contradictory pushes towards both tradition and modernity. Many Japanese clung to their traditional social customs, like jujutsu, in the face of American and European cultural invasion, while also striving to adopt the western military and economic systems which had made the influx of foreigners possible. It was against this socio-political backdrop that Kano Jigoro founded the Kodokan, his jujutsu academy in Tokyo (Burdick, 1997; Guttmann, 1994; Guttmann and Thompson, 2001; Rosenblum, 1981).

Kano very much typified the modernist/traditionalist dichotomy of late nineteenth century Japan. Born two years after the Treaty of Amity and Commerce, Kano was a student of western philosophers like John Stuart Mill and Herbert Spencer, as well as traditional Japanese jujutsu. Many martial arts schools at this time were, in Kano's view, overly reliant on ritual and aesthetics with insufficient emphasis on practical techniques, while other schools gave jujutsu a bad name by training ruffians who studied the art to make themselves more proficient street-fighters and muggers. His goal was to make jujutsu both more practical and more gentlemanly. In effect, he wanted to create a sport, which he did by gathering together those traditions he found useful and by abandoning those he found lacking (Burdick, 1997; Carr, 1993; Guttmann, 1994; Guttmann and Thompson, 2001; Kiku, 2004; Shun, 1998; Svinth, 2003).

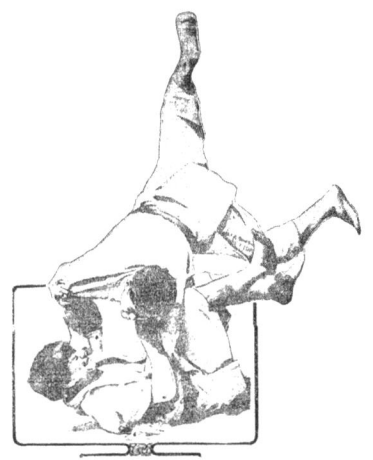

"Jap Jiu Jitsu" experts to appear at the Los Angeles Athletic Club in 1913. Illustration from the *Los Angeles Times* (7 April 1913).

Kano called his style Kodokan judo to distinguish his methods from other forms of jujutsu. The Tokyo Metropolitan Police Bureau periodically held jujutsu competitions in part to select instructors for training officers. As the Kodokan consistently defeated representatives from other schools, the resulting publicity caused Kano's student body to grow from ten students in 1884, to nearly 500 in 1887, to an astounding 2,755 in 1892. As Kano's students founded their own schools throughout Japan and the world, the practice of judo spread exponentially (Burdick, 1999; Carr, 1993; Shun, 1998).

The rise of judo did not occur in a vacuum, however. A strong nationalist movement was also taking hold in Japan. While Kano himself was not particularly conservative, his philosophy of fusing modernity and tradition struck a chord with the ruling élite who wanted to use modern western methods to bring traditional Japanese culture onto the world stage. In an effort to distance himself from some of the rougher elements which had been associated with jujutsu, Kano enforced a code of conduct which mirrored the bushido of the samurai. At the same time, the Japanese government was attempting to revive elements of samurai culture in order to restore national pride after the Treaty of Amity and Commerce. Judo quickly earned government support due to the combination of its effectiveness against other art forms and its seeming shared values with nationalist politics. By 1911, the Japanese Ministry of Education added judo to the national physical education curriculum. Many Japanese felt that judo was the institution that best represented Japan's rise from humiliation to power in the latter half of the nineteenth century (Burdick, 1999; Guttmann and Thompson, 2001; Shun, 1998).

While judo played a significant role in Japanese society during this period, many European-Americans viewed it as a virtually essential element of the culture. Contemporary American accounts were full exaggerated claims. One author proclaimed the entire nation of Japan, "from the emperor down to the humblest coolie," practiced judo (CRH, July 21, 1904). Even among immigrants, it was felt, "[t]here is not a Japanese in Los Angeles who doesn't know enough about the art to defend himself more than successfully against any man not of his own race" (LAT, February 18, 1918). Another rather bizarre article claims "the hardy little Jap, who is the embodiment of 'wiriness' and who seems incapable of fatigue, though his sustenance is only a few grains of rice," attains this superhuman endurance from the study of jujutsu, which requires such "daily habits" as bathing twice a day "if [the jujutsuka] would imitate his Japanese teachers" and drinking "a gallon of pure water" (SFC, March 27, 1904). While there was a good bit of journalistic exaggeration taking place in these articles, the sport enjoyed great popularity with Japanese-Americans as both participants and spectators (Svinth, 2003).

European-American Views of Judo

Due to an influx of Japanese immigrants from 1884–1907, European-Americans gained an interest in Japanese culture. Newspapers in this era spent much time explaining the mysterious art of judo to white audiences. These early accounts tended to fall into two extreme categories, dismissal and admiration. The most laughable of the former category simply argued that European-Americans were culturally and physiologically superior to Japanese-Americans, therefore American sports like wrestling and boxing must be superior to judo. In one representative account, an editorial in the *Oakland Tribune* argued, "a finished catch-as-catch can artist would be more than a match for any Jiu Jitsu enthusiasts for the reason that his science embraces the art of protection, which in conjunction with his native American aggressiveness, would be practically invulnerable" (OT, August 29, 1905). A writer for *Harper's Weekly* opined, "the Japanese temperament is uncertain and changeful... given to sudden flights and sudden flagging," and felt Japanese athletes possessed, "that notable deficiency of all Orientals, the lack of steadfastness and perseverance" (HW, February 12, 1898). The *Los Angeles Times* declared, "it would not take the average man very long to guess that a good boxer would make the best judo wrestler look like 20 cents worth of dog meat" (LAT, December 26, 1909). Another article described "jew-joot" as "a humbug the American people should be ashamed to fool with, and that any ordinary white man can make the brown chap lie down" (LAT, May 7, 1905). Spelling the first syllable of the word jujutsu as "jew" was fairly common in articles criticizing the Japanese style (see, e.g., MAB, June 1905); this was likely an attempt to denigrate Asian culture by appealing to existing anti-Semitic sentiment in the United States (Burdick, 1999; Wilson, 2000).

Other writers in the dismissal camp at least based their opinions on actual contests in which European-Americans defeated judoka. In these cases, headlines emphasized the race of the competitors rather than their fighting styles, such as, "Cadets Down the 'Jap'" (NYT, February 21, 1905) and "American Floors Victorious Jap" (LAT, March 4, 1905).

Some European-Americans continued to dismiss judo even when judoka defeated American wrestlers. As western sports standardized in the late nineteenth century, boxing and wrestling adopted rules to prevent injury and to help "civilize" the European immigrants who practiced these sports (Burdick, 1999). Judo allowed the use of chokes and joint-locks which were not permitted in western wrestling styles, such that "[m]any of the tricks employed by the little brown man would be scorned as 'foul' by our exponents of the manly art" (SFC, October 16, 1904). The *Los Angeles Times* described, "Judo or third degree business" as "'rough stuff' pure and simple" (LAT, December 26, 1909). One commentator summarized the criticism of judo techniques by declaring "[a]ny audience fond of fair play would brand them as fouls, and after their first appearance they would be ruled as unfair advantages" (Terry, 1902, quoted in Burdick, 1999).

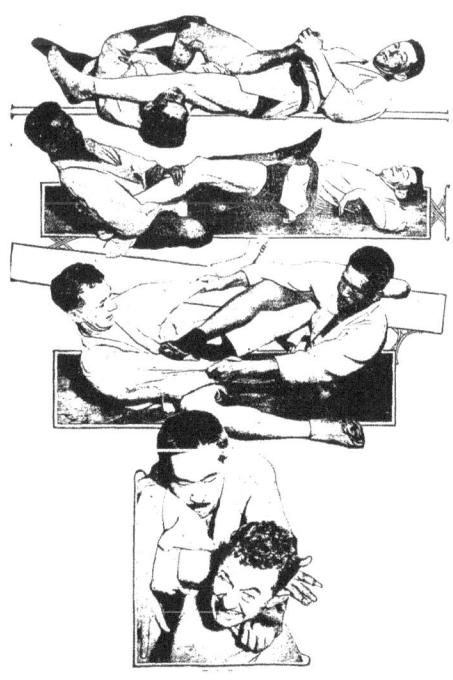

Pat Higgins and Ito Tokugoro at practice. *Los Angeles Times* (24 October 1916).

Other European-Americans, including President Theodore Roosevelt, were great admirers of judo (Burdick, 1999). Of particular interest to western audiences was the way in which judo could be used by a smaller man, or even a woman (see Svinth, 2000b; Svinth, 2001), to defeat a larger opponent. The *Salt Lake Herald* noted "a small Jap versed in [judo's] mysteries can easily overcome the largest athletes trained only in wrestling or boxing" (SLH, February 5, 1906). Indeed, "[t]he science of Jiu jitsu teaches the athlete to make the other man use his strength against himself, and once a little man gets a hold his larger opponent inflicts greater punishment upon himself by resisting because of his great size" (SFC, December 17, 1907). This ability was attributed to "the well-known mechanical principle of the lever" along with "the obvious result of the application of mechanical laws and strategic means" (LAT, September 4, 1904).

Other commentators attributed judo's efficacy to the quasi-supernatural abilities of its practitioners. Judoka were reported to be able to use "vital touches" against an opponent's "death points," the location of which were closely-guarded secrets, in order to cause "a temporary paralysis of the arm to the complete suspension of vital processes and instant death" (LAT, September 4, 1904). One judoka was "credited with a way of looking at an opponent that causes all the symptoms of painter's colic and some of his great victories have been won via mental grapevine" (LAT, April 3, 1919). There was even a fear that those Japanese-Americans who opened judo schools hid from their European-American students certain mysterious techniques which would come into play in some future conflict between Japan and the United States (Burdick, 1999).

II. The Barnstormers

As Japanese immigrants integrated into American society, contests between Japanese-American judoka and European-American wrestlers were inevitable. Both sports had strong barnstorming traditions. Professional wrestlers of this era were often carnival employees who took on local champions as the circus traveled from town to town. Wrestlers were therefore predisposed towards challenging athletes from other localities in order to prove their skills. Similarly, judo's popularity in Japan arose out of Kano Jigoro's desire to prove his style superior to other schools of jujutsu. It is no surprise that his students engaged in similar contests after immigrating to the United States (Burdick, 1999; Carr, 1993; Hewitt, 2005; Morton and O'Brien, 1985; Shun, 1998).

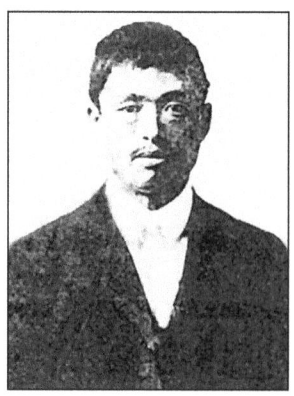

Ito Tokugoro, jujutsu wrestler extraordinaire. Images from the *Seattle Post-Intelligencer*, (6 November 6, 1909).

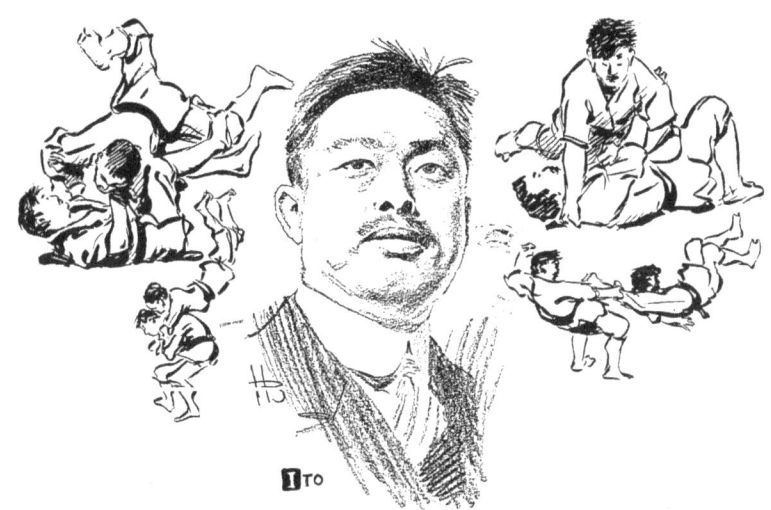

Ito Tokugoro, "the worlds greatest jiu-jitsu and judo expert, who threw Ad Santel and is the idol of his countrymen." *Los Angeles Times* (1 February 1917).

The earliest bouts were more or less inconclusive as the wrestler was generally able to take down and pin his opponent while the judoka was likewise able to throw and submit his; the result was therefore dependent upon which sport's rules were applied. Later bouts were contested under hybrid rules systems, which effectively leveled the playing field. There were at least forty major judoka/wrestler bouts that took place between 1904 and 1920, and almost three-quarters of these took place west of the Mississippi River. San Francisco catch wrestler Adolph "Ad" Santel (1887–1966) ran up a number of victories over judoka which led him to proclaim himself the judo champion of the world. Seattle judoka Ito Tokugoro gained the attention of European-American fans after notching victories over several prominent wrestlers, including Eddie Robinson and Ted Thye. Santel and Ito met twice in San Francisco in 1916; Santel won the first bout after Ito's head struck the floor, rendering him unable to continue (Burdick, 1999; Hewitt, 2005; Svinth, 2003). In the re-match, Santel "gave a couple of gurgles, turned black in the face and thumped the floor, signifying he'd had enough" of Ito's chokehold (LAT, February 1, 1917).

These mixed matches were tremendously popular, consistently earning higher billing and receiving greater media attention than wrestler vs. wrestler or judoka vs. judoka matches. In particular, these contests seemed to appeal to fans that rooted for competitors based on race. A Japanese-American judoka was cheered on by "a crowd of jabbering Japanese enthusiasts" (LAT, December 9, 1917), while in another contest "[t]he white element tried hard to make as much noise as the Japs, but the brown men howled continually" (LAT, May 31, 1909). In one match, "the white people" — including the unabashedly partisan sportswriter — "shouted for the white man and we did all that we could to make him win, but the Japs outnumbered us and they outdid us in the matter of enthusiasm" (OT, April 2, 1909). When a lone European-American woman, "a certain ordinary-looking person who was dressed as a lady" — the implication of course being that such a woman could not actually be a "lady" — lent her support to a Japanese-American judoka, "it called forth the cat calls and hisses of the house and the things that were said about this certain young person would not look well in print." Not only did most fans choose their loyalties based upon race, but those that failed to do so could find themselves subject to harassment by spectators and even insults by journalists.

III. What Was the Appeal of These Matches?

European-Americans were interested in judoka/wrestler matches for a number of reasons. One was a simple interest in Japanese culture. After all, Japan had until only recently been closed to westerners, so the exposure to judo gave a glimpse into the society that produced it. But European-Americans also enjoyed the way in which these matches reinforced stereotypes about Japanese-Americans. For example, a judoka's ability to defeat a larger opponent emphasized the supposed smaller physical stature of Japanese people. Thus, even when praising the skill of a judoka, European-American journalists would dismissively refer to him as a "hardy little Jap" (SFC, March 27,1904) or "little brown gentleman" (LAT, February 18, 1918). In addition, some journalists seem to delight in quoting, often at length, the broken English of immigrant judoka in order to present them as less intelligent than native speakers (see, e.g., LAT, April 3, 1919). Judoka were also portrayed as excessively polite, in contrast to the rough-and-tumble western wrestlers, which presented contrasting notions of masculinity. One is described as an "inoffensive fellow" while another "smiled and maintained his good humor" throughout a rough match (Edgren, 1905). Respectful judo competitors are depicted "formally kowtowing to each other," while when "American boys wrestle, they do it in an impromptu and rather reckless fashion which would shock the convention-bound Jap" (ST, March 10, 1907). In another account, a judogi (judo uniform) was referred to as "a jaunty Japanese nightie" and the judoka as "a saucy little bantam" up against a "husky white man" (LAT, December 9, 1917). Regardless of the outcome of the bout, the reader was left with no doubt who the "real man" in the contest was (see also Sabo, 1985).

As the modern nation-state is a relatively recent phenomenon, so to is nationalism, which can be defined "as a condition of mind, feeling, or sentiment of a group of people living in a well-defined geographical area, speaking a common language, possessing a literature in which the aspirations of the nation have been expressed, and, in some cases, having a common religion" (Snyder, 1990). The regrettable flipside to the communal good feelings towards other members of the state takes the form of racism and xenophobia towards those living outside the state; if nationalism instills in us a belief that our culture is superior, other cultures must therefore by inferior. In the wake of the Civil War, American nationalism was on the rise. This nationalism often took the form of what Billig (1995) terms "banal nationalism," which includes routine expressions of nationalist sentiment, such as children's recitation of the Pledge of Allegiance before school or the use of patriotic symbols on postage stamps and currency. Banal nationalism found routine expression in sporting contests of the day "as the nation was 'represented' in competition short of war" (McCrone, 1998). Athletes in international competition embody the state and their successes and failures are shared by their fellow citizens (Betts, 1974; Copeci and Wilkerson, 1983; Germs, 2006; Guttmann, 1988; Guttman, 1994; Hobsbawn, 1990; Loy and Elvogue, 1970; Kiku, 2004; Mandell, 1984; Mogull, 1981; Mrozek, 1983; Pope, 1997; Rainville et al., 1978; Schneider and Eitzen, 1979).

Much of the European-American interest in these matches arose out of anxiety over the larger socio-political context. Westerners felt threatened by Japanese immigration, which was effectively shut off by a 1907 "gentleman's agreement" between President Roosevelt and the Japanese government. Japanese-Americans, even those of the second generation, were denied citizenship under the Naturalization Act of 1790, which only applied to "free white persons." More locally, the California Alien Land Law of 1913 barred Asian-Americans from owning real property. Despite these restrictions against Japanese-Americans, western laborers still feared an influx of low-paid, foreign workers. Similarly,

Japan's 1905 military victory over Russia, the first victory by an Asian power over a European country, gave rise to fears of Japanese imperialism (Burdick, 1999; Germs, 2006; Wilson, 2000). In fact, many in the West attributed Japan's victory to the study of judo; one writer went so far as to recommend the study of jujutsu "for Anglo-Saxon readers" so that "peace congresses will soon be a thing of the past" (SFC, October 16, 1904).

In order to understand how these socio-political anxieties influenced sports fans during this period, it is useful to look at studies of modern professional wrestling, which, it should be noted, is far more theatrical than the early twentieth century judoka/wrestler matches (many of which were legitimate athletic contests). Modern professional wrestling fans "are low income workers, welfare recipients, or immigrants who are finding little success in what is supposed to be the land of opportunity" and enjoy the vicarious thrills of "sports entertainment" (Campbell, 1996). These groups are particularly interested in storylines in which a "foreign menace" reflecting a current military or economic threat to the United States is defeated by an American hero, who is almost always of European descent. Ethnicity is often used to distinguish "good guys" from "bad guys." European-American wrestling fans of the pre-World War I era would likely have felt similar motivations, particularly due to the tense political and economic climate in which they lived. Moreover, the fact that the athletic contests they watched had at least the perception of legitimacy, they may have invested more emotionally in their support of a favorite athlete as opposed to modern fans who know they are watching "muscular theater" (Archer and Svinth, 2005; Mondak, 1989; Deeter-Schmeltz and Sojka, 2004).

Conclusion

The contests between wrestling and judo in the first two decades of the twentieth century show an American West that is both intrigued by and in fear of Japanese-Americans and the burgeoning power of their native land. Much of these sentiments were expressed in an ugly nationalism, which is fortunately absent—at least in such obvious terms—from modern political dialogue. But nationalism and even racism remain driving forces in modern sports, where many of our more cosmopolitan instincts are drowned out in the heat of battle. By better understanding the origins of these forces, we may achieve the Olympian goal of truly casting aside cultural differences in the name of athletic competition.

BIBLIOGRAPHY

Archer, J. and Svinth, J. (2005). Professional wrestling: Where sport and theater collide. *InYo: Journal of Alternative Perspectives.* Available: http://web.archive.org/web/20070818163456/ejmas.com/jalt/jaltframe.htm.

Betts, J. (1971). Home front, battlefield and sport during the Civil War. *Research Quarterly* 42:113-32.

Betts, J. (1974). *America's sporting heritage: 1850–1950.* Reading, MA: Addison-Wesley Publishing Co.

Billig, M. (1995). *Banal nationalism.* London: Sage Publications.

Burdick, D. (1999). The American way of fighting: Unarmed defense in the United States, 1845–1945. Doctoral dissertation, Indiana University, Bloomington.

Campbell, J. (1996). Professional wrestling: Why the bad guy wins. *Journal of American Culture* 19(2):127–132.

Carr, K. (1993). Making way: War, philosophy and sport in Japanese judo. *Journal of Sport History* 20(2):167–188.

Copeci, D. and Wilkerson, M. (1983). Multifarious hero. *Journal of Sport History* 10(3), 5–25.

Deeter-Schmelz, D. and Sojka, J. (2004). Wrestling with American values: An exploratory investigation of World Wrestling Entertainment as a product-based subculture. *Journal of Consumer Behaviour* 4(2):132–143.

Edgren, R. (1905). The fearful art of jiu jitsu. Outing, 322–28. Reprinted in Svinth, J. (ed.) (2000). *Journal of Combative Sport*. Available: http://ejmas.com/jcs/jcsart_edgren1_0300.htm.

Fielding, L. (1975). Reflections from the sport mirror: selected treatments of Civil War sport. *Journal of Sport History* 2:132–144.

Fielding, L. (1977). War and trifles: sport in the shadow of Civil War Army life. *Journal of Sport History* 4:151–168.

FILA (2004). History of wrestling. International Wrestling Hall of Fame. Available: http://www.filahalloffame.com/historyofwrestling.html.

Germs, G. (2006). *The athletic crusade: Sport and American cultural imperialism*. Lincoln, NE: University of Nebraska Press.

Gorn, E. (1985). "Gouge and bite, pull hair and scratch": The social significance of fighting in the southern backcountry. *American Historical Review* 90(1):18–43.

Guttmann, A. (1988). *A whole new ball game: an interpretation of American sports*. Chapel Hill: University of North Carolina Press.

Guttmann, A. (1994). *Games and empires: Modern sports and cultural imperialism*. New York: Columbia University Press.

Guttmann, A. and Thompson, L. (2001). *Japanese sports: A history*. Honolulu: University of Hawai'i Press.

Hewitt, M. (2005). *Catch wrestling: A wild and wooly look at the early days of pro wrestling in America*. Boulder, CO: Paladin Press

Hobsbawn, E. (1990). *Nations and nationalism since 1780*. Cambridge: Cambridge University Press.

Kiku, K. (2004). The development of sport in Japan: Martial arts and baseball. In Dunning, E., et al. (eds.), *Sports histories: figurational studies of the development of modern sports* (pp. 153–171). New York: Routledge.

Loy, J. and Elvogue, J. (1970). Racial segregation in American sport. *International Review of Sport Sociology* 5, 5–23.

Mandell, R. (1984). *Sport: A cultural history*. New York: Columbia University Press.

Mogull, R. (1981). Racial discrimination in professional sports. *Arena Review* 5(2): 12–15.

Mondak, J. (1989). The politics of professional wrestling. *Journal of Popular Culture* 23(2): 139–149.

Morton, G. and O'Brien, G. (1985). *Wrestling to rasslin': Ancient sport to American spectacle*. Bowling Green, OH: Bowling Green State University Popular Press.

Mrozek, D. (1983). *Sport and American mentality, 1880–1910*. Knoxville: University of Tennessee Press.

Pope, S. (1997). *Patriotic games: Sporting traditions in the American imagination, 1876–1926*. Oxford, UK: Oxford University Press.

Rainville, R. et al. (1978). Recognition of covert racial prejudice. *Journalism Quarterly* 55(2): 256–259.

Rickard, J. (1999). "The spectacle of excess": The emergence of modern professional wrestling in the United States and Australia. *Journal of Popular Culture* 33(1):129–137.

Rosenblum, M. (1981). Martial arts poetics. *Journal of American Culture* 4(3):148–153.
Sabo, D. (1985). Sport, patriarchy, and male identity. *Arena Review* 9(2):1–30.
Savenga, D. (1995). The problem of wrestling 'styles' in the modern Olympic Games: A failure of Olympic philosophy. *Citius, Altius, Fortius* (now *Journal of Olympic Sport History*) 3(3):19–29.
Schneider, J. and Eitzen, D. (1979). Racial discrimination in American sports. *Journal of Sport Behavior* 2(3):136–142.
Shun, I. (1998). The invention of the martial arts: Kano Jigoro and Kodokan judo. In S. Vlastos (ed.), *Mirror of modernity: Invented traditions of modern Japan* (pp. 163–173). Berkeley, CA: University of California Press.
Snyder, L. (1990). *Encyclopedia of nationalism*. New York: Paragon House.
Svinth, J. (2000a). Sizing 'em up: Statistical relationships between various combative sports in the Japanese American communities of the Pacific Northwest, circa 1910 to circa 1942. *In Yo: Journal of Alternate Perspectives*. Available: http://ejmas.com/jalt/jaltart_svinth1_0300.htm.
Svinth, J. (2000b). Women who would not be sheep. *In Yo: Journal of Alternate Perspectives*. Available: http://ejmas.com/jalt/jaltart_svinth4_1199.htm.
Svinth, J. (2001). The evolution of women's judo, 1900–1945. *In Yo: Journal of Alternate Perspectives*. Available: http://ejmas.com/jalt/jaltart_svinth_0201.htm.
Svinth, J. (2003). *Getting a grip: Judo in the Nikkei communities of the Pacific Northwest, 1900–1950*. Guelph, Ontario: Electronic Journals of Martial Arts and Science.
Terry, T. (1902). Jiu-jutsu, Japanese self-defense without weapons. *Outing* 41, 12–18.
Wilson, G. (Ed.)(2000). The history of Japanese immigration. *Brown Quarterly* 3(4). Available: http://brownvboard.org/brwnqurt/03-4/03-4a.htm.

Newspapers:	Referred to as:
Chicago Record-Herald	CRH
Harper's Weekly	HW
Los Angeles Times	LAT
Mind and Body	MAB
New York Times	NY
Oakland Tribune	OT
Salt Lake Herald	SLH
San Francisco Call	SFC
Seattle Times	ST

chapter 21

The Way of Kata in Kodokan Judo
by Llyr C. Jones, Ph.D., and Michael J. Hanon, Ph.D.

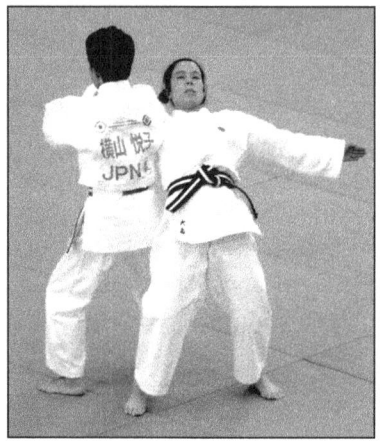

Illustrations courtesy of Carl DeCrée,
except where noted.

Introduction

In an article De Crée and Jones (2009) explain how Kodokan[1] Judo, developed by Kano Jigoro (1860–1938), is an all-around cooperative education, teaching system (pedagogy), and philosophy—based, among other things, on neo-Confucianist values, traditional school Japanese martial arts, and modern Western educational principles. In particular, judo emphasizes the holistic educational value of training in attack and defense, so that it can be a "path," or way of life, that all people can participate in and draw benefit from. In this way, and contrary to popular debate judo is neither a "martial art" nor a "combat sport."

> [J]udo in the larger sense aims to transcend the sporting context and . . . include aspects related to education, health and both physical and emotional self-defense.   – Gutiérrez Garcia, Pérez Gutiérrez and Svinth (2010:127)

The most complete definition of judo available in the literature is that due to Oda Join[2] (1929). Therein, he uses and builds on an original quote by Kano Jigoro that featured in the Kodokan periodical *Judo* (Kano, 1915). Oda writes: "Judo is the most effective way to use the power of the mind and body. Its training cultivates the body and spirit through the practice of attack and defense; the essence of this principled moral code (or "path") is learning through self-awareness. Therefore, judo was innovated so that the ultimate objective is to perfect oneself and benefit from life. In summary, judo is the most effective way of using the mind and body for the benefit of oneself and others" (Oda, 1929:8).

Kano Jigoro expressed judo's core concepts via the sayings "good use of mind and body" and "mutual welfare and benefit." A spirit of generosity and mutual assistance is therefore integral to judo. Kano envisaged that through the application of judo principles to everyday life a judoist achieves balance and self-mastery, thereby becoming better enabled to deal with routine stresses and to interact with other human beings in positive and mutually beneficial ways.

On the Techniques of Judo

The physical aspects of judo's techniques are based primarily on the Tenjin Shin'yo-ryu, Kito-ryu, and Yoshin-ryu styles of traditional school jujutsu. However, as already explained, the most significant aspect of judo is its blend of physical and mental education to help its practitioners develop well-balanced bodies and minds that will, through a spirit of generosity and mutual assistance, act to improve society as a whole. As such, the techniques of judo are only vehicles to greater goals. They themselves are not the goal. The techniques in judo are actually only of use as a tool to enable a judo practitioner to realize these greater ambitions.

The Elements of Judo Instruction

Writing in the journal *Kokushi* during the early years of the Kodokan's inception, Kano (1899) explains how judo instruction had four components:

- **Free Practice (*randori*):** Practice sparring sessions in which both participants practice attacking and defending, using freely applied throwing and/or pinning techniques (Kawamura and Daigo, 2000:109–110).
- **Forms (*katas*):** Formal movement pattern exercises containing idealized model movements illustrating specific combative principles (Ibid:86).
- **Lectures (*kogi*):** Lectures on judo principles were viewed as an essential part of judo education. Kano believed that training for matches or combat was enhanced greatly by teaching theory via lectures.
- **Dialogue (*mondo*):** "Question / answer" sessions between students and teachers were also considered important to reinforce the practical and formal learning.

Murata Naoki, the present curator of the Kodokan museum and library, adds contest (*shiai*) to this list, stating that contest is an important supplementary component of the judo learning process (Murata, 2007).

It is also important to recognize that the way of teaching judo outlined above was actually never implemented beyond Japan. A notable exception, though, was Trevor Leggett's (1914–2000) two-hour, invitation-only Sunday class at the Budokwai, London. Hoare (2000) writes how those sessions "were always packed," with the class itself "being a mixture of grinding hard work, contest and instruction on every aspect of judo." Similarly, Hicks (1996) recalls that for Leggett "judo was an ethical and educational training which opened doors of understanding far beyond the dojo," and how even "his most dedicated pupils were sometimes alarmed when required to write essays."

Why was no tradition of formal judo education through lectures and dialogue ever established and embedded on a wide-scale basis outside of Japan? In judo's formative years it was Kano himself and other senior teachers who directed the lectures and dialogue. Despite Kano and the other seniors undertaking considerable international travel, they were primarily resident in Japan. With only very limited exceptions, teachers of comparable knowledge who could lead formal learning simply did not exist elsewhere. For this reason, no such instructional practice was established.

Furthermore, with the continued internationalization of judo and the International Judo Federation's (IJF) ever-increasing emphasis on sports competition, even the practice of kata became marginalized and viewed as a historical oddity. This left behind a pared-down and distorted judo consisting of only free practice and contest, which is today what most judo practitioners think of as being the totality of judo.

Kata Practice in Current Times

In the article "Competition, Kata and the Art of Judo" (Jones, 2005) it was explained how the practice of the kata in judo had become deemphasized. In his article Jones outlined how the IJF's and national governing bodies' (NGB) emphasis on the sports-competitive aspects of judo and winning medals had produced generations of fighters and coaches who believed that kata practice was outdated and had no relevance or value.

Jones's views were later echoed by Alessio Oltremari in an online article: "Competition and fighting has enchanted generations of judo practitioners and, through applying principles from several sports to judo, they have forgotten its origins and meaning. The important thing is to win—never mind if the technique used is dirty, vulgar and dangerous .... Although technique is absent it does not matter when brute force is enough to achieve the win. Better to be weight training rather than wasting time on deepening technique" (Oltremari, n.d.).

In recent years however, there has been a resurgence in the popularity of kata—one driven not by an appreciation of the self-improvement that accrues from regular kata practice, but by the medal-winning opportunities provided by the rapidly expanding phenomenon of "kata championships." Indeed, such is the growing popularity of kata as a competitive pursuit that the development of training strategies for achieving success in kata championships is starting to feature as a research topic, for example, see Sheedy (2010).

THE KATAS OF KODOKAN JUDO

Kata as a Living Textbook

Kata practice is an important training method in most modern and traditional Japanese martial arts. Finn (1991:211) is particularly insightful, writing that katas are "prearranged forms[3] in Japanese martial arts that are like a living text book. They contain all the fundamental information in animate form, with which to perfect technique and understanding of the particular skill."

The Listed Katas

There exist ten "listed"[4] Kodokan katas (De Crée and Jones, 2009). This is despite several popular sources incorrectly claiming that there would be only seven, eight, or nine official Kodokan katas. The ten katas are detailed in Table 1, which itself is structured based on how the katas are commonly categorized according to purpose (Kotani, Osawa, and Hirose, 1968:1; Otaki and Draeger, 1983:32–33).

In his opening lecture to the 2008 Kodokan Summer Kata Course, Daigo Toshiro[5] gave a brief overview with some history of each currently practiced and recognized kata, listing nine distinct katas overall (Kano, n.d., in Daigo, 2008; Kotani and Otaki, n.d., in Daigo, 2008-2009). Daigo's lecture subsequently formed the basis of his broad multi-part article on kata which was serialized in seven parts in the Kodokan's periodical, *Judo* (Daigo, 2008-2009).

In counting nine Kodokan katas, Daigo inexplicably omits the female self-defense kata, Joshi Goshin Ho, which is an officially approved but uncommon Kodokan kata. Additionally, such counting of Kodokan kata ignores both the "Forms of Decision" (*Kime Shiki*) and the "Forms of Gentleness" (*Ju Shiki*), two katas which were considered separately in the past, but today are regarded as being part of the Sei-ryoku-zen'yo Kokumin-Taiiku. There also exist several non-Kodokan approved katas of both Japanese and non-Japanese origin. This chapter will not consider any of these unapproved katas.

Table 1: The Katas of Kodokan Judo

FORMS OF FREE PRACTICE	**RANDORI-NO-KATA**
- Forms of Throwing	- Nage-no-kata
- Forms of Grappling or Holding	- Katame-no-kata
FORMS OF SELF-DEFENSE	**SHOBU-NO-KATA**
- Forms of Decisiveness	- Kime-no-kata
- Kodokan Forms of Self-Defense	- Kodokan Goshin Jutsu
- Methods of Self-Defense for Women	- Joshi Goshin Ho
FORMS OF PHYSICAL EDUCATION	**RENTAI-NO-KATA**
- Forms of Gentleness & Flexibility	- Ju-no-kata
- Forms of (proper use of) Force	- Go-no-kata
- National Physical Education according to (the principle of) best use of energy	- Sei-ryoku-zen'yo Kokumin-Taiiku
FORMS OF THEORY	**RI-NO-KATA**
- The Five Forms	- Itsutsu-no-kata
- The Antique Forms	- Koshiki-no-kata

It is beyond the scope of this chapter to present the technical ("how to") details of the ten Kodokan katas. Full technical details on eight of the ten katas (the two omissions being the Joshi Goshin Ho and the Go-no-kata) are provided in the book *Kodokan Judo*[6] (Kano, 1986:145-251). For the technical details of the Joshi Goshin Ho, the reader is directed to the text *Kata of Kodokan Judo* (Kotani et al, 1968:124-153). Similarly, for the technical details of the Go-no-kata, the reader is directed to a recent booklet by Mori (2008).

The Purpose of Kata Practice in Judo

In the early days of the Kodokan, Kano Jigoro's teaching method was to start the students off on free practice and allow them to assimilate katas naturally. However, this approach quickly became unsustainable.

Writing in the Kodokan periodical *Sakko* ("Awakening") in 1927, Kano Jigoro explained how katas were created as a teaching framework in response to the fact that the Kodokan was expanding rapidly, and that he (Kano) could not deliver his syllabus just by himself and there were no trained instructors. Kano wrote: "The main reason why the kata[s] were created was because of the ever increasing number of students at the Kodokan. It became impossible to teach students individually as had been the case in the early days, and a system to teach . . . any students simultaneously was required" (Kano, 1927).

It is a wrong, but widely held, belief that the objective of kata practice in judo is the development of technical refinement and the perfection of technique.[7] This is only a minor component of kata practice, since technique can be perfected in other ways. Proper kata study contributes to improving one's understanding[8] of judo and, as part of this learning, one needs to equate the "perfection of technique" with "perfection of oneself" (Otaki and Draeger, 1983:35–46, 58–61).

All of the Kodokan katas reflect an ideal goal of judo—"good use of mind and body"—through transmitting the concepts of proper action/reaction, exploiting a moment of opportunity (*debana*), balance breaking (*kuzushi*), and "remaining mind" (*zanshin*). Additionally, each Kodokan kata makes a specific contribution to teaching different inherent judo principles and aspects of control—for example, control of breathing, control of posture and balance, control of speed, control of body movement (*tai-sabaki*), timing, and ultimately emotional control. Even the Koshiki-no-kata and the Itsutsu-no-kata, katas that seem in first instance to be very remote from everyday judo, are valuable. The understanding that can be derived from their proper practice importantly contributes to the development of "inner feeling" (*kimochi*), a "sense of balance breaking, and a "sense of positioning and set-up" (*tsukuri*).

In the book *Judo* marking the centenary of Kano Jigoro's birth, Kodokan officials stated: "Each . . . kata, while demonstrating a number of classical movements, possesses a deep significance. The more kata is practiced the stronger is the feeling that they are a cultural asset embodying the essence of Judo" (Kodokan, 1961:65).

Looking Deeper into the Kodokan Katas

Each Kodokan kata has its own subliminal thread or theme running through it. However, when one first starts to learn any particular kata, it is usually just its superficial mechanical movements that are learned. Indeed, it is only after much practice and self-exploration that the kata's pervading principles and themes as they apply to judo practice as a whole become revealed. The following pages will look deeper into each of the Kodokan katas to facilitate the development of their more detailed understanding.

Forms of Free Practice

Together, the Nage-no-kata and the Katame-no-kata are known as the Randori-no-kata (forms of free practice). They provide a framework that facilitates the development of free practice skills, and it is essential that they are practiced with the attitude that one would bring to free practice, i.e., gusto and commitment and certainly no "theatrical pretence."

It will now be explained how the learning extractable from the Nage-no-kata transcends that of merely developing skills in throwing techniques. For this purpose the first set of the kata, namely "hand techniques," will be considered. The sequence of techniques is "floating drop," followed by "back-carry throw," followed by "shoulder wheel" (*uki-otoshi* → *seoi-nage* → *kata-guruma*).

For the benefit of further explanation, it is now appropriate to introduce two terms common to judo: *tori* and *uke*. During controlled practice, tori is the person who applies a throw or another technique. Uke is the person who receives the technique.

- **Floating drop (*uki-otoshi*):** When uke attacks tori he does so with all his might regardless of his situation and is thrown with a floating drop. Uke never again attacks tori in such an unchecked manner and learns from each failed attack. Moreover, tori adapts to each new attack.
- **Back-carry throw (*seoi-nage*):** Next, uke attacks tori with an explosive, down-ward forceful blow to the top of the head. Tori repositions his body and directs that force away from his head and down to the ground, using a back-carry throw. As such tori allows uke to throw himself over tori's body, using his (uke's) own force and strength. There is no block; tori merely turns then throws. The purpose of this technique is to demonstrate a key principle in judo (that of nonresistance) with uke being undone by the force of his own attack. Tori does not throw in the conventional sense of the word, but merely utilizes uke's own action to defeat him. "Maximum efficiency with minimum effort."
- **Shoulder wheel (*kata-guruma*):** Uke attacks again, but this time keeps his body rigid and stiff to avoid the throwing responses he has already received. Once again, though, uke is overcome by the understanding of tori who throws him with a shoulder wheel.

This pattern repeats itself across the entire kata. In the complete Nage-no-kata, uke will attack tori fifteen times, and each time tori will neutralize that attack and use the force or action of uke's own attack to prevail. Therefore, as tori progresses with the study of Nage-no-kata, he develops insight into basic and complex biomechanics, in particular how to apply himself to overcome the actions of an attacking uke. Tori also learns good technique and in doing so becomes able to cross-reference this learning with that from free practice. Finally, tori learns how his own body and mind react under physical and psychological stress, and also how to adapt to a given situation utilizing both his body and his mind in an effective and productive manner.

The Katame-no-kata is concerned with learning control, in particular, how tori can best use his body in an efficient manner to control uke on the ground. Tori must work on his versatility and show excellent body movement while grappling, and uke must strive to escape and exploit any weaknesses in tori's techniques. Moreover, each and every time the Katame-no-kata is practiced, uke should continue to test tori by looking for his weak points and then attacking them. Similarly, tori should find new ways of nullifying uke's new escape attempts. Both tori and uke should assimilate this learning from the Katame-no-kata and leverage it for the benefit of their free practice and contest efforts.

Forms of Self-Defense

The Kime-no-kata, the Kodokan Goshin-jutsu, and the Joshi Goshin Ho are classified as Shobu-no-kata (forms of self-defense). These katas reflect what is crucial when involved in a "real" fight to the death (*shinken shobu*), where the central objective is to defeat an adversary and survive. They teach effective body movement, speed, coordination, and control of posture while controlling another person, irrespective of the particular technique or kata being studied.

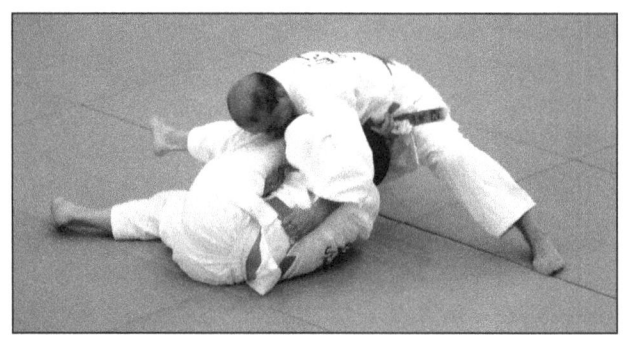
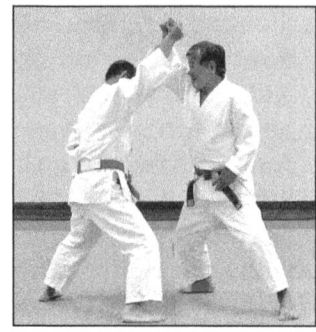

Forms of Physical Education

The Ju-no-kata, the Go-no-kata and the Sei-ryoku-Zen'yo Kokumin-Taiiku are grouped together as Rentai-no-kata (forms of physical education), where the foremost objective is to educate the body to remain healthy. In particular, the Ju-no-kata teaches the principles of resistance and non-resistance, flexibility, and suppleness; the Go-no-kata teaches the principle of the appropriate use of controlled force and develops physical conditioning; and the Sei-ryoku-Zen'yo Kokumin-Taiiku builds up physical development and coordination, as well as laying a foundation for the development of basic judo skills.

The Ju-no-kata does not teach "fighting techniques" in any conventional sense or with the idea of literally using those techniques in combat. Rather, the Ju-no-kata includes a number of attacks and defenses to demonstrate the efficient redirection of force and movement. In addition, as neither tori nor uke is thrown or held down during the course of the kata, it can be practiced anywhere by anyone, even those who are old or nervous. The Ju-no-kata conveys the principle of not countering force with force; it teaches how to respond to action with a reaction that instead of force (*go*) is yielding (*ju*). Uke attacks tori and tori neutralizes that attack, using the attack itself to prevail. For this reason, those who practice the Ju-no-kata merely as fifteen physical movements are missing the purpose of the kata. While the physical element of the kata provides vital lessons in the application of yielding, the Ju-no-kata is actually a set of exercises in tori controlling his mind and emotions to find inner harmony and then blending that harmony with uke. The Ju-no-kata is aptly named and is regarded by many as the finest of all the Kodokan katas.

The Go-no-kata provides a framework for the correct learning of the basics of judo without throwing. It teaches tori to use force effectively, without ever relying on force as the primary means to overcome uke. Additionally, the Go-no-kata teaches the precision use of one's body, especially how to use both focused strength and yielding at critical timings during judo techniques. The Go-no-kata also assists in the development of physical strength itself and contributes to increased willpower and "spiritual energy" in the sense of "a healthy spirit in a healthy body" (De Crée and Jones, 2009).

Both the Ju-no-kata and the Go-no-kata convey the meaning of *ju-no-ri*, i.e., the core principle of jujutsu whereby one avoids opposing an opponent's force and power directly in favor of using it to one's advantage. They also accord with a core principle of judo, which can be expressed in a number of ways: "softness overcomes hardness," "flexibility overcomes stiffness," "gentleness controls strength," or "win by yielding" (Ibid).

The Sei-ryoku-Zen'yo Kokumin-Taiiku is not a strict kata, but rather a physical education exercise[9] that may be practiced in a very informal manner with considerable degrees of freedom. (Note also that the word "kata" does not even feature in the name, reflecting that it is even freer in nature than a series labeled *ho* or "method.") It is divided into two main types of exercise: solo practice (*tandoku renshu*) and partnered practice (*sotai renshu*).

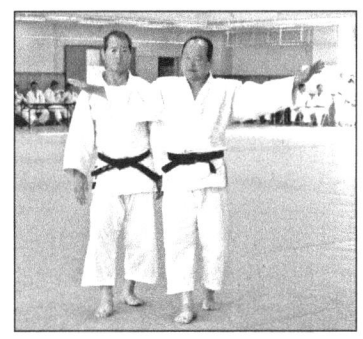

The solo exercises have strikes and kicks, as well as a number of other exercises designed to build muscle tone and harmoniously develop a balanced physique. Most typically, every movement is repeated five times, left and right, before moving on to the next. However, freedom exists to increase the number of repetitions, should it be desired.

The partnered exercises are divided into two main groups: *Kime Shiki* (forms of decision) and *Ju Shiki* (forms of gentleness). The Kime Shiki techniques contain simple versions of several techniques found in the Kime-no-kata including grabs, blows, and attacks with weapons. The Ju Shiki section has two groups of five techniques each, taken directly from the Ju-no-kata.

Forms of Theory

The Itsutsu-no-kata and the Koshiki-no-kata are grouped together as Ri-no-kata (forms of theory). Both of these katas are rooted in traditional school jujutsu and convey principles from their historical schools of origin. It should, though, be noted that these principles are totally unknown to most people;[10] however, some concepts, such as an "immovable mind" (*fudoshin*), are somewhat known.

The Itsutsu-no-kata expresses the principles of attack and defense in movements evocative of natural phenomena and can be regarded as a physical manifestation of the "philosophical mind" of judo. Discussing the Itsutsu-no-kata in the publication *Judo* (1961), Kodokan officials stated: "It is an artistic and meaningful kata calling for natural movements (the movement of water, the movement of heavenly bodies etc.) to be skillfully expressed by the human body" (Kodokan, 1961:67).

In this sense, the Itsutsu-no-kata can be considered the kata of "motional principles," a sort of "judo-physics." While the Itsutsu-no-kata is officially attributed to Kano Jigoro (Kano, 1986), recent research by De Crée (2010) indicates that it was not created by Kano, and that it clearly existed in Tenjin Shin'yo-ryu jujutsu under the name "Five Step Oral Teachings" (*Kuden Gohon*).

The Koshiki-no-kata was placed in the Kodokan repertoire as a reminder of judo's heritage being partially in Kito-ryu jujutsu, in particular its Takenaka-ha style (Ibid). Accordingly, the Koshiki-no-kata is also known as the Kito Kata and can be thought of as the kata of "judo tradition" or "judo history."

According to the Kodokan (1961) the first movement of the Koshiki-no-kata, the "ready posture" (*tai*), is the basis of the entire kata: "Tai is the basis of the Kito Kata. It teaches that it is important to adopt a calm posture; to quiet the spirit; to clear the mind and, by these means, to discern the opponent's strength and weaknesses. So the original object of the Koshiki-no-kata was to teach not so much technique as methods of training the mind" (Kodokan, 1961:69).

The core purpose of the Ri-no-kata is to develop a higher understanding of the fundamental and deeper "essence" and perhaps even "esoteric" principles of judo (De Crée and Jones, 2009). The Ri-no-kata involve the mental state of the attacker, and the principles of physics, anticipation, and reaction. They require developing an understanding of the mental state of the attacker at the point of attack ("What is he trying to accomplish?" and "How does one anticipate the attack?"), and what laws of physics and principles of yielding should one apply to that situation. These are very complex ideas, and it is the synthesis and compression of all those concepts into individual katas that make the Itsutsu-no-kata and the Koshiki-no-kata so difficult and beyond the comprehension of most judo practitioners at any given point in their judo career.

The Ri-no-kata are therefore the logical final stage of the kata-learning process. They cannot be properly studied until the Randori-no-kata, the Shobu-no-kata, and the Rentai-no-kata have all been mastered.

Inner Feeling

It has already been explained how kata in judo involves the synthesis of a whole group of physical and mental concepts and disciplines in the performance of extremely challenging routines and exercises, and how this makes the kata study a complete education in itself. "The concept of kata is often misunderstood. Although various techniques are executed, kata should not be considered a catalog of designated responses to specific dangerous situations. Rather, kata is a method of transmitting core principles and concepts" (Cunningham, 2008:10).

Katas, therefore, are about inner feeling (*kimochi*) and are as much about training the mind as the body. If katas are performed as "mere movements" then these educational aspects are missed.

Kata, Intrinsic Energy, and No-Mindness

Guy Pelletier, the world's highest Kodokan ranked judo practitioner of non-Japanese descent (Kodokan eighth-degree rank), considers the relationship of kata, intrinsic energy (*ki*), and "no-mindness" (*mushin*), writing:

> A good kata is more than just a number of physically correct actions. It is the mental attitude of the two partners who realize the *kiai*, or concentration of spirit. Therein lies the essence of kata. The flow of mental energy is very noticeable when attending a quality demonstration.
>
> Uke, like tori, must show their "ki" or mental energy. Their external attitude is one of calm, quiet vigilance and self-confidence. You and your partner's ki unite and rely on kiai, which in turn induces a mental state called Muga-mushin. This however is not attained until after much experience. *Muga-mushin* means "no self, no mind." It is a state of indifference that frees the consciousness of the actions undertaken. In this state, the spirit solves problems automatically, so to speak, hence its importance in self-defence and judo.
>
> Kata is the best way for a [judo practitioner] to do judo in a state of ignorance of the specific actions he is doing. A [judo practitioner] is an expert when he reaches this stage. Kata refines the spirit, enabling him to carry out actions faster than through itself, in this way the art becomes an "art without art."
> – Pelletier, n.d.

Protect, Break, Separate

Shu-ha-ri is an educational concept rooted in the martial arts and other classical Japanese disciplines, such as flower arranging, puppetry, theater, poetry, painting, sculpture, and weaving. According to Takamura (1986), it has been instrumental in the survival of many of these older knowledge traditions. Shu-ha-ri describes the learning curve to mastery through the stages of "protect" (imitation/absorbing,) "break" (understanding /detaching/digressing), and "separating" (consolidation/transcending the physical).

Using a lecture note by Ukichi, Daigo (2008) explained how one progresses from the basic form through to a deep understanding of kata using this concept:

Shu First stage (protect): The stage of *shu* consists in studying a teacher's lesson correctly. The teaching of a particular school must be studied faithfully without any change. This is the stage of imitation. In short, it is the way to preserve and protect the integrity and the dignity of a school. This is the stage of *shu*.

Ha Second stage (break): After progressing more after repetitive kata practice, a student begins to question and discover by himself. He separates from his master and inquires beyond the superficial instruction of kata movements. After, self-individuality is harnessed. The width of the style is expanded. The meaning of kata is investigated deeply. This is a stage of *ha*.

Ri Third stage (separate): Furthermore, kata practice is treated freely and spontaneously. It is in the realm of the new creation which is made by oneself. This is a stage of *ri*.

– Ukichi, n.d., in Daigo, 2008

Further insight into the application of shu-ha-ri to kata study in the martial arts is provided by Takamura (1986) and Klens-Bigman (n.d.). The material presented therein is as relevant to judo as it is to the specific arts considered in the articles themselves.

Harmony, Concentration, Immersion, and Purity

In a personal communication with the authors, the noted judo practitioner Paul Nogaki (sixth-degree rank) recalled the teachings that he received from Daigo in 1980 regarding the thought process that one should strive to achieve when practicing kata. He stated that "kata in judo is about learning mental and physical discipline, and connecting the two together in attempting extremely difficult routines and exercises. Even the words to describe the ultimate goals to be attained in kata—*in'yo-wago, senshin, seiboku*, and *genshitsu*—are really almost impossible to translate correctly into another language [other than Japanese]" (Nogaki, 2009).

Both Nogaki (2009) and De Crée (2009) kindly provided translations of the concepts introduced by Daigo to explain the ultimate goal of "kata Nirvana."

- **In'yo-wago:** In'yo-wago means a harmony or balance between yin and yang energies[11] (and what they mean in the martial arts) leading to strength. This concept no doubt originates from Kito-ryu and not from judo. Obtaining this yin/yang balance is a lengthy process, and not one that judo consciously discusses or tackles. Arguably, it is something that is the goal of the Ri-no-kata, although practicing other katas could also help.
- **Senshin:** *Senshin* literally means "committed," "undivided attention" or "concentration"—important components in the development of spiritual power. However, in judo, the concept of ki is not cultivated in that sense, though Kano Jigoro used and talked about *sei-ryoku* or "optimization," which is the equivalent. (This was a conscious choice, in order to demystify ki). For Kano, sei-ryoku existed in two components: a physical component (*chikara*), and a spiritual component (without such being some mystical superior power). Using the two in harmony (as per *in'yo-wago*) resulted in "optimization," often known in judo as "efficient (or best) use of energy."
- **Genshitsu:** Genshitsu literally means "commitment." This can be extrapolated to mean "total immersion."

- **Seiboku**: Seiboku means "to be gentle and pure" and thus different from powerful, abrupt judo. The purity refers to proper technique and use of balance breaking, timing, and setup. If so, then no force is necessary, much like Mifune Kyuzo's "empty jacket" judo.[12]

The above is a key original contribution of this chapter, as the authors are unaware of any other written sources that present this insight. Additionally, they are unaware of any sources where the concepts discussed are related to kata practice.

THE KATA CHAMPIONSHIPS AND THE SPORTIFICATION OF KATA

Under this heading, a critical evaluation of the impact that the "sportification" of kata is having upon this important element of judo is presented. In doing so, the questions posed by Oltremari (n.d.) will be indirectly answered: "Can the exercise of kata in judo be considered a sport? Can the performance of an exercise in judo forms be likened to an exercise in gymnastics" (Oltremari, n.d.)?

History

Kata championships are not new. The British Judo Association (BJA) held its first National Kata Championship (together with the first British Veterans Championship) at Woolwich College in London in 1981. Recent years, however, have seen a marked increase in the number and level of kata championships, and events now regularly take place at regional, national, continental, and world levels.

At the continental level, for example, the first European Kata Championships were hosted by the BJA and held in Burgess Hill, Sussex, in 2005. (A European Masters [veterans] Championship was also held at the same time.) The proceedings were attended by Daigo from the Kodokan and dominated by kata pairs from Italy. Subsequent European Kata Championships have been held under the auspices of the European Judo Union (EJU) in Italy (2006), Germany (2007), Malta (2008), and Romania (2009). Other Continental associations have also organized their own kata championships.

At the world level, championships have been organized since 1999 by the World Masters Judo Association (WMJA). The WMJA is an entity founded in Ottawa, Canada, in 1998 with the purpose of encouraging participation in competition judo and kata for judo practitioners aged thirty years plus, in a fun, friendly, and family-orientated manner. The first such event was held in Welland, Canada. Subsequent WMJA kata (and contest) championships have been held in Canada (2000), the United States (2001), UK (2002), Japan (2004), Canada (2005), France (2006), Brazil (2007), Belgium (2008), and the United States (2009).

The IJF itself was somewhat slow off the mark in organizing kata championships, with the first IJF event, known as the Kata World Cup, taking place in Paris, France, in November 2008, the event essentially being a rehearsal for the first official IJF Kata World Championships that were held in October 2009 in Valetta, Malta. The second such IJF event was held in Budapest, Hungary, in May 2010.

In parallel to organizing its own masters' event, the IJF discharged additional actions that could be interpreted as a conscious effort to marginalize and smother the efforts of the WMJA.[13] In 2009, the WMJA finally gave in to the inevitable and agreed to disband itself in 2010. The final WMJA event was held in Montreal, Canada, in August 2010, after which sole organizational control of world-level masters judo passed to the IJF. It is only the passage of time that will reveal whether the IJF will be able to preserve the spirit of masters judo as originally intended and established by the WMJA.

The first Kodokan Judo Kata International Tournament championships, organized under the joint auspices of the Kodokan Judo Institute and the All Japan Judo Federation, took place in October 2007 at the Kodokan Judo Institute in Tokyo. This significant event is described by Gatling (2008).

Kata Championships: The Positive

It is clear that the introduction of a competitive element has provided the competitive judo player with a source of motivation for studying katas, i.e., the tangible goal of a medal. It should also be stated that some of the kata performances achieved in kata competition are outstanding in all respects, particularly those by judo practitioners from Italy, Japan, and Spain. Such spirited performances though are often the exception to the rule.

It is also clear that as a direct consequence of kata championships, there are currently more judo practitioners aware of and practicing katas than at any time in the recent past. Without this competition-led revival, there is a high probability that kata practice would have silently and progressively vanished from judo, leaving behind only the undignified and increasingly commercialized "jacketed wrestling sport" that the IJF has made judo into.

Given the above, it is often remarked, "Without kata championships, kata would be dead." This chapter will now argue that due to the values and constraints imposed by kata championships, kata as the learning aid envisaged by Kano Jigoro is already "near death." Oltremari (n.d.) writes: "The same barbarism that has pervaded *shiai* [contest] and turned it into an inferno conducted in a pit in an arena is about to break forth on kata. A new gymnasium for the triumph of the ego is about to rise, while a scheme [kata] created for completely different purposes slowly disappears. The introduction of the principles of modern sport in this discipline [kata] will distort its essence and meaning, first condemning it to its cultural contextualization and then to its very ending" (Oltremari, n.d.).

Kata Championships: The Negative

It will now be explained how kata championships are eroding the underlying benefits and fundamental principles of kata training and why their very concept (i.e., the sportification of an educational tool) should be regarded as being fundamentally flawed.

Kata championships do not accommodate individuality, have no room for interpretation, and rigidly limit any creative endeavor in the performance of any particular kata. They consider only how well the "kata performance"[14] has complied with a given marking scheme, regardless of the impact that this has on the development of the performers as judo practitioners. The impact of this is that in order to achieve success at kata competition, kata practitioners are compelled to train not for enhanced insight or personal growth or to improve their own kata practice, but rather to present "carbon copy" duplicates of the physical movements of the kata as shown in the relevant teaching film. The sole purpose of this charade is to enable kata judges to conduct "like-for-like" evaluations, with the victors being the performers who can demonstrate the best-looking "kata copy" or "kata clone," irrespective of the spirit and realism. By dint of this approach, kata championships focus entirely on the *shu* ("protect") aspect of kata study and pay no respect at all to the *ha* ("separate") or *ri* ("leave") elements.

If the focus of kata practice becomes success at a kata championship rather than self-improvement, then the entire training will become imbalanced due to overemphasizing minor technical aspects and conventions[15] that should not be a source of concern in regular training. By slavishly copying the ritualized movements captured in a teaching film, both the original educational intent of kata practice and the associated holistic learning that results from proper kata practice are being lost. The resulting kata renditions often end up empty and fake, as they are devoid of any meaningful action/reaction component. In reality, katas can never be copied, and all kata performances are, of course, nonrepeatable. This is because no two performing pairs are the same (in terms of physique and psychology), and no two circumstances are ever encountered again, even between the same pair.

Even if one is prepared to accept the principle that kata can be evaluated, the concept of summing the scores of individual techniques in a complete kata to see how one set of performers compares against others and then to award medals (à la figure skating or gymnastics) based on this ranking, is unsound. Every kata is a complete representation from its beginning to its end, and any evaluation of a kata must therefore be for the kata as a whole and not the sum of its individual parts.

The absurdity of the "sum of the individual parts" approach to evaluating kata performance can be illustrated by the example of Daigo, who was demonstrating Nage-no-kata at a Kodokan "New Year's rice-cake cutting ceremony" (Otaki and Draeger, 1983:432). Daigo was the victim of an error of his uke, who attacked with a technique out of sequence and began the third ("rear sacrifice techniques," *ma-sutemi-waza*) set of the kata with a blow, instead of engaging and taking a grip as prescribed for the correct throw in the sequence, the "circle throw" (*tomoe-nage*). Daigo reacted seamlessly and effectively: unable to take the prescribed grip, he simply stepped in and executed the correct, logical response to the attack, the "rear throw" (*ura-nage*). He then performed this throw to the left. Thereafter, he executed *tomoe-nage* (as the second set of techniques) and then proceeded to perform the correct third set of techniques. Such was the intensity of Daigo's actions and so well coordinated were his reflexes and reaction that many spectators were totally unaware of what had happened.

Daigo's response was the best one possible in the circumstances and much better than hesitating, pausing completely, or starting again. However, in the context of the Nage-no-kata the overall performance still contained an "error." The question then becomes the consequence of an "error" in kata. In a kata competition, an error such as that made by Daigo's uke would be viewed as being "very poor" and would have resulted (as a minimum) in a zero score (IJF, 2010; 2010a) for that particular technique. In a kata competition this would have meant that they would have had no chance of medaling.

However, when what happened is evaluated in the broader context of judo, the error can be regarded as trivial, it only being an error in the logical progression of the Nage-no-kata. Daigo should have been praised for his flexible mind and for executing an appropriate response against the particular attack. Great judo is not how one performs under benign conditions, but how one performs, acts, and responds under hazardous or unanticipated conditions.

It is particularly disheartening to those wishing to promote the serious study of judo and its katas that as a direct consequence of the current emphasis on competition the true purpose and place of judo kata practice as a learning tool is being lost. Additionally, ignorant and incorrect information on kata is being promulgated, a particularly heinous example being the worthless description of kata proffered by the director of communications and media relations for USA Judo (the NGB for judo in the United States), Nicole Jomantas: "Kata is a forms-based judo discipline in which two athletes perform a set routine of judo techniques which are then scored by a panel of judges" (Jomantas: 2009).

Jomantas' definition reflects the wretched attitude toward kata that permeates contemporary judo, i.e., the obsession of NGBs with the competitive, as opposed to educational, aspects of judo. It is also clear that Jomantas has thought nothing about the logic of her definition, since cursory consideration of the question "If a kata is performed without judges, is it not still a kata?" should have revealed just how flawed it was.

judo
柔道

"the felxible way"

Illustration courtesy
of www.iStockphoto.com

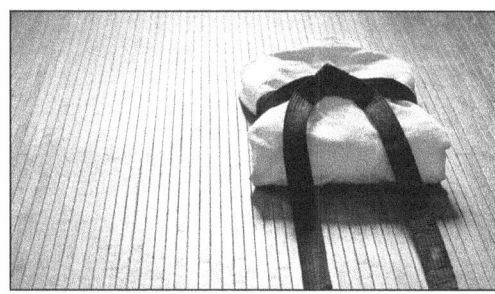

Questioning the Purpose of Kata Practice

Katas were not created to be "judged" or to be studied as an exercise in "how to perform a ceremonial kata demonstration"; rather, they were developed as a living and breathing tool to support the correct learning and practice of judo principles.

Envisaged by Kano, katas were primarily intended as a type of practice. However, when one sees katas today, it is always as a demonstration, and virtually never as a true practice of technique or self-defense, or even simple pre- or post- training exercises. In Kano's time, kata practice need not have been a complete ceremonial performance, but simply an activity to improve one's understanding of judo, or to warm up, or to strengthen one's muscles, or to enhance one's reflexes, flexibility, coordination, and focus, or to really learn how to defend oneself against a certain attack.

When katas are first studied, it is easy to become overinvolved with their ceremony, ritual, and mechanics. Notwithstanding the genuine importance of those aspects, they should not be allowed to detract from the greater lessons of the kata, and to understand those lessons it is necessary for judo practitioners to question and ask "what is a kata?" more deeply and with greater understanding and appreciation. While training for a kata competition will support the learning of the specific technical moves in a kata, it will not, however, lead to an under- standing of why one studies katas, the benefits, the intentions of the creators of katas, or the tradition and psychology of kata practice.

Katas should always be studied for their educational content and never just to "look good." Katas belong to every judo practitioner as an individual and cannot be a clone of any other person's. In this way, all kata renditions should be different, and at a fundamental level, for a kata rendition to be "correct," it is only the order of the techniques, the protocol of the kata in question, and the appropriate spirit that are essential to preserve.

Set against the original purpose and intent of kata, it is clear that the only justifiable rationale for kata championships is the opportunity they provide to be critiqued by one's peers and seniors. However, peer and senior feedback should be readily obtainable with any form of competition with others. Indeed, the concept of competing against others in kata performance should be anathema to anyone with even the most rudimentary under- standing of Kodokan judo. "How can one possibly compete in an exercise that is about personal development?" "How can one judge one human being against another?" And since judo is the education of the physical and emotional being that one is, "How can such judgments be reached (since one's kata practice is a manifestation of one's judo and thus of oneself)?"

Katas performed well and with understanding can be a thrilling and interesting spectacle for an observer, as well as enjoyable and rewarding for the participants.

Mechanistically cloned kata demonstrations are worthless for both participant and observer. As explained earlier, the spirit and mental attitude in a person doing a kata dictate its feel and flow, and this can be about as individual as anything can be in judo. As Damblat writes: "Learning a kata is relatively easy, but knowing a kata is only the first step. The ultimate goal is to discover, to understand or grasp its raison d'etre and the message it conveys. One must first assimilate, then feel, and it [the kata] must be alive.... The execution of a kata should never be done mechanically and without soul. It need not be demonstrative, but simply living and logical while demonstrating the governing principles of judo so that the practice is beneficial and contributes to some evolution and understanding of judo. The aesthetics of a kata must reflect the sincerity of control, specific techniques and a perfect communion of mind of both partners" (Damblat, n.d.:3).

At this point, the authors will register their disappointment that the Kodokan has condoned and embraced the concept of kata championships. Although Kano Jigoro recognized the value of contest, kata used as a surrogate competition was never part of his thinking. The authors do acknowledge, though, that the Kodokan's motives for doing so were sincere and well intentioned (Kano, 2007):[16]

> We can see today increasing interests in learning kata, not only in Japan but also throughout all the countries of the world. As a result, the 1st Kodokan Judo Kata International Tournament 2007 is being held ... I sincerely hope that all judokas will contribute to the development of judo through learning kata.
>
> Most of the competitors and judges participating in this event are totally involved in judo as instructors. I have high expectations that all the participants will take this opportunity to recognize the essence of Kodokan judo anew through kata and promote authentic judo.

Despite its genuine motivation for supporting kata tournaments, it is the Kodokan that is the guardian of Kano Jigoro's legacy, and it should discharge this function in part through the setting and maintenance of appropriate standards. The promotion of kata that is fake, empty, and without action/reaction is not judo, and the concept of competing against others in kata performance is totally contrary to the philosophy and intent of the founder.

In closing this section it is worth noting that perhaps "some light exists at the end of the tunnel," as some serious study is now underway at the Kodokan, which could be interpreted as part of an ongoing effort to address the issue of kata evaluation and perhaps address the recent deteriorations (Murata and Todo, 2007; 2009).

The main purposes of Murata and Todo's work are to research how to develop a simple and clear method of evaluating kata performances, and to make recommendations as to how to modify the present systems. In so doing, they examined the European and Japanese kata evaluation methods with the following findings (Murata and Todo, 2007):

- The European "reduction only" system is not good because it does not recognize positive aspects of performance, only the negative;
- The Japanese system does not allow for differentiation between good and better, or poor and worse kata performances;
- Neither system clarifies the principles to be judged;
- The absence of an official kata championships referee system.

Murata and Todo's formal conclusions were as follows: "Kata techniques exist on rational mechanism of *tsukuri* and *kake*, and this mechanism should be called Waza no Ri (principle of techniques). Neither students nor teachers could learn and teach any kata without knowing the Waza no Ri. No judges could evaluate any Kata performance without knowing this Waza no Ri" (Ibid). Tsukuri is body positioning in preparation for executing a throw. Kake is the finishing or execution of the throw.

Murata and Todo (2009) recently extended their work with a specific focus on the Koshiki-no-kata and this study remains to be evaluated by the authors.

Conclusions

We live in very different times compared to the days and era of Kano Jigoro and, as we become removed further and further from them, our understanding of many of judo's essential aspects becomes less and less. Katas are vital learning tools and to complete one's judo, one needs to learn, practice, and understand them. Moreover, one should also exploit the lessons that kata imparts in both free practice and contest.

An argument could be advanced that the proper teaching and evaluation of kata demand a considerable intellectual level. In today's judo (where belt ranks are largely awarded on the basis of current or past competitive prowess, rather than deep judo knowledge and skill), a nonintellectual high-degree holder has large hierarchical supremacy over a highly intellectual lower grade. This creates problems when it comes to the accurate teaching of katas.

In the main, the judo kata landscape is a wilderness populated with well-intended, but often uninformed, teachers. Accordingly, most kata instruction focuses on the mechanical aspects of kata (movements, timing, and distance), and says nothing about feeling or techniques on how to understand and improve spirit. Frequently this is not strictly the fault of the teachers, as they are often unaware of any deeper purpose behind what they teach, and thus have no knowledge to pass on to their students beyond the superficial physical movements.

What Fraguas (2001) wrote about karate-do is equally true for judo: "Unfortunately, 95 percent of the people don't understand kata, only the outside movements which are irrelevant without understanding" (Fraguas, 2001:283).

Moreover, as discussed in this chapter, the introduction of kata competitions has only reinforced the emphasis on the mechanics of kata to the virtual exclusion of all their other aspects. Accordingly, a paradoxical situation now exists whereby kata practice is becoming more popular with rank-and-file judo practitioners, but the true purpose and spirit of kata usage is becoming increasingly lost.

If one returns to premodern, i.e., pre-kata competition, ways of doing kata, one does not acquire the form of movement that most judo practitioners seem to think that kata practice entails. Instead, one acquires an exercise that encapsulates judo principles, which, once understood and felt, can be experimented with to any degree of "aliveness" that one wants within the confines of one's training—for example, working with real live blades in the Kime-no-kata and the Kodokan Go-shin-jutsu, or wearing traditional armor (*yoroi*) for the Koshiki-no-kata. Such practice and experimentation would produce katas that are very different from the robotic, sequenced forms seen in most contemporary kata competitions.

Studying katas the way they were originally developed is not about learning judo's history; rather, it is about doing judo correctly in the first place. While good teachers produce good judo practitioners, great teachers can help their pupils achieve greatness in life. "Real" kata is one of the tools a "real teacher" uses.

Glossary

Debana	出端	Koryu	古流
Fudoshin	不動心	Kuzushi	崩し
Gendai budo	現代武道	Mushin	無心の心
Genshitsu	言質	Sakk	作興
In'yo-wago	陰陽和合	Seiboku	清穆
Joshi Goshin Ho	女子護身法	Senshin	専心
Kagami Biraki	鏡開き	Shu-ha-ri	守破離
Kata	形	Mushin no shin	無心の心
Ki	気	Tai-sabaki	体捌
Kimochi	気持ち	Tenjin Shin'yo-ryu	天神真楊流
Kito-ryu	起倒流	Tsukuri	作り
Kodokan	講道館	Yoshin-ryu	楊心流
Kokushi	國士	Zanshin	残心

ACKNOWLEDGMENT

The authors would like to thank Professor Carl De Crée and Paul Nogaki for sharing their wisdom and knowledge. The quality of this chapter has been significantly enriched by their many insights and contributions.

Editor's Note: The use of "katas" in this paper to denote the pluralization of "kata" is to conform with the editorial style used in the *Journal of Asian Martial Arts*.

NOTES

[1] Kodokan, the headquarters of judo, was originally founded in 1882 by Kano Jigoro, the creator of judo.

[2] Many publications wrongly write Oda's first name as Tsunetane, as opposed to Join.

[3] One of the issues when translating words from one language to another is that subtle meanings and nuances of the original words are often lost. This is very much the case with the word kata. Although the accepted translation of kata in judo is "form," other words, such as "template," "pattern," or "style," might be better suited. The word kata is also often used in Japanese culture to describe standard of posture. This is also appropriate.

[4] The term "listed kata" is due to John Cornish (7th-degree judo, 8th-degree aikido) (Cornish, 2004). It refers to formally written sets of choreographed exercises and techniques grouped to illustrate specific principles as opposed to ad hoc prearranged sequences of judo techniques.

[5] Daigo Toshiro (b. 1926) was for many years the chief instructor at the Kodokan Judo Institute. He was promoted to 10th-degree rank in 2006 and is arguably the world's greatest kata expert. See Sidney (2003:144–153) for a detailed profile of Daigo.

6. Although Kano Jigoro is presented as the author of this book, it is in fact a compilation by the Kodokan Institute that dates after the founder's death.
7. The practice of any kata, no doubt importantly contributes to developing technical refinement, since to do kata one must be able to "sense" (or "feel") one's partner. It is possible, though, to prevail in free practice and contest without "feeling," by using mainly the elements of surprise, speed, and force. These elements are effective and even important aspects of judo, but they do not represent judo in its entirety. Moreover, they will ultimately fail, as one can always encounter an opponent who is faster and stronger.
8. Here, understanding does not simply mean intellectual understanding, but principle and bodily understanding.
9. Despite Kano's enormous efforts in promoting the Sei-ryoku-Zen'yo Koku-min-Taiiku as a kata of physical exercise, it was not appreciated as much as he wished, partly because of the timing of his death and partly because of the disruption caused by the Second World War.
10. With the exception of some very senior Kodokan teachers, virtually no one, either Japanese or Westerner, is able to completely explain the essence and applicability of the Itsutsu-no-kata and the Koshiki-no-kata and how they integrate with the broader judo syllabus.
11. In Chinese theory, yin and yang: the fundamental principle of two mutually interdependent and constantly interacting polar energies that sustain all living organisms.
12. Mifune Kyuzo (10th-degree rank) was known for the softness of his techniques. He was able to defeat students twice his size while barely seeming to expend any effort. People who trained with him later said, "It was like fighting with an empty jacket."
13. In 2009 the IJF and the EJF refused permission for referees and kata judges to officiate at any WMJA event. Additionally, Budapest, the original planned venue for the WMJA 2009 event, withdrew its candidacy at short notice—allegedly in the face of pressure applied by the IJF.
14. With respect to kata, the oft-used word "performance" is also troublesome to the authors. Performance implies an activity done to entertain or please others. As already explained, kata is done for the benefit and education of the two judo practitioners doing the kata. Any judge who really understands kata should easily be able to differentiate between a pair of judo practitioners genuinely "doing" the kata and a pair who are only "performing" the kata.
15. The IJF has produced a "competition formula" (IJF, 2010; 2010a) that detail how many points to deduct for various categories of "technical errors" in a competitive kata performance. Consequently, when practicing, judo players place much emphasis on avoiding these mistakes at the expense of the overall spirit or realism of the kata.
16. Kano Yukimitsu (b. 1932) is the grandson of Kano Jigoro and was the fourth president of the Kodokan. He stepped down from his post in 2009.

BIBLIOGRAPHY

Cunningham, D. (2008). *Samurai weapons: Tools of the warrior.* Tokyo: Tuttle Publishing.

Cornish, J. (Spring 2004). What is kata? *The Bulletin,* 10:1–2. Available online and from The Kano Society. URL: http://www.kanosociety.org/bulletins/bulletinx10.htm (Retrieved, July 2010).

Daigo, T. (2008). Jigoro Kano, Kodokan Judo-no-kata 1964. Lecture notes from the Kodokan Summer Kata Course. 29 July 2008. Tokyo: Kodokan Judo Institute.

Daigo, T. (2008–2009). *Kodokan Judo Kata ni Tsuite* (1–7) (About the Kata of Kodokan Judo, Parts 1–7). *Judo,* 79(10): 52–57; 79(11): 7–12; 79(12): 18–23; 80(1): 16–22; 80(2):

43–50; 80(3): 12–16 and 80(4): 3–9. In Japanese.

Damblant, R. (n.d.). Judo – Les katas ou formes: Leur histoire, leure raison d'Être et leurs valeurs (Judo – Kata or forms: Their history, their rationale and their values). Article online and available from Judo Quebec's Website, URL: www.judo-quebec.qc.ca/img/pdf/les_kata_ou_formes.pdf. In French. Retrieved, July 2010.

De Crée, C. (2009). Personal correspondence with Professor Carl De Crée on matters of Japanese-English translation pertaining to the ideals of kata.

De Crée, C. (2010). *Ryu-setsu. Judo no musha shugyo – As snow on a willow. A pilgrimage in judo.* Cambridge: Cambridge University Press (In preparation).

De Crée, C. and Jones, L. (2009). Kodokan judo's elusive tenth kata: The Go-no-kata— "Forms of proper use of force," Parts 1–3, *Archives of Budo*. 5, 55–73; 75–82 and 83–95. Articles online and available from the Archives of Budo website, URL: http://www.archbudo.com/fulltxt.php?ICID=878157 (Part 1) http://www.archbudo.com/fulltxt.php?ICID=878158 (Part 2) http://www.archbudo.com/fulltxt.php?ICID=878159 (Part 3)

Finn, M. (1991). *Martial arts: A complete illustrated history.* Leicester: Blitz Editions.

Fraguas, J. (2001). *Karate masters.* Burbank, CA: Unique Publications.

Gatling, L. (2008). The First Kodokan Judo Kata International Competition and its katas. *Journal of Asian Martial Arts, 17*(1), 68–77.

Gutiérrez Garcia, C., Pérez Gutiérrez, M. and Svinth, J. authors (2010). Judo. In Green, T. and Svinth, J. editors. (2010). *Martial arts of the world: An encyclopedia of history and innovation,* 1. Santa Barbra: ABC-CLIO.

Hicks, J. (1996). Interviewed Trevor Leggett. Article online and available from *The World of Judo* magazine's archives, URL: http://www.twoj.org/archives/2000/autumn/aut00_news5.html (Retrieved July 2010.) (Originally in: *The world of judo* (1996). Edition No. 6.)

Hoare, S. (2000). Trevor Pryce Leggett 1914–2000. Article online and available from *The World of Judo* magazine's archives, URL: http://www.twoj.org/archives/2000/autumn/aut00_news5.html (Retrieved July 2010.) (Originally in: *The World of Judo* (2000). Edition No. 24.)

International Judo Federation (2010). *World Kata Championships 2010 Budapest, Hungary, Competition Rules.* Budapest: International Judo Federation.

International Judo Federation Data Commission (2010a). *Kata competition 2010.* International Judo Federation.

Jomantas, N. (2009). Team USA to compete at first ever Kata World Championships this weekend (13 October 2009). Article online and available from USA Judo's website, URL: http://judo.teamusa.org/news/article/28266 (Retrieved, July 2010).

Jones, L. (2005). Competition, kata and the art of judo. *Journal of Asian Martial Arts, 14*(3), 72-85.

Kano, J. (n.d.). In Daigo, T. editor. (1964 and 2008). *Kodokan Judo no kata* (The kata of Kodokan judo). Tokyo: Kodokan Publications. Reprinted for the 2008 Kodokan Summer Kata Course. Tokyo: Kodokan Judo Institute.

Kano, J. (1899). Kodokan Judo kogi (Kodokan judo lectures). *Kokushi, 1*(4). (In Japanese.)

Kano, J. (1915). Kodokan Judo gaisetsu (Outline of Kodokan Judo). *Judo.* 2. (In Japanese).

Kano, J. (1927). *Kano Jigoro judoka,* 12 (Kano Jigoro the judoka, Part 12). *Sakko.* 5(12). (In Japanese).

Kano, J. (1986). *Kodokan judo.* Tokyo: Kodansha International.

Kano, Y. (2007). Welcome Address. Souvenir Program of the 1st Kodokan Judo Kata International Tournament 2007. pp. 26–27.

Kawamura, T. and Daigo, T. (Eds.) (2000). *Kodokan new Japanese-English dictionary of judo.*

Tokyo: Kodokan Institute.

Klens-Bigman, D. (n.d.). Creativity, bound flow and the concept of shu-ha-ri in kata. Article online and available from FightingArts.com's website, URL: http://fightingarts.com/reading/article.php?id=173 (Retrieved, July 2010).

Kodokan (1957–1999). Qualification for dan promotion. Information online and available from the Kodokan's website, URL: http://www.kodokan.org/e_basic/shoudan.html (Retrieved, June 2010).

Kodokan (1961). *Judo*. Osaka: Nunoi Shobo Co.

Kotani, S., Osawa, Y. and Hirose, Y. (1968). *Kata of Kodokan judo*. Kobe: Koyano Bussan Kaisha Ltd.

Kotani, S. and Otaki, T. (1971). In Daigo, T. editor. (2008). *Kodokan Goshin-jutsu* by [Saishin judo no kata]. Reprinted for the 2008 Kodokan Kata Kaki Koshukai (Kodokan Summer Kata Course). Tokyo: Kodokan Judo Institute.

Mori, O. (2008). *An introduction to Go no kata*. Tokyo: Private publication based on Kuhara, Y. (1976). *Judo Mizu Nagare*. Tokyo: Shudokan Kuhara Dojo. (in Japanese).

Murata, N. (2007). What is kata? The congratulatory address to the 1st Kodokan Judo Kata International Tournament. Souvenir Program of the 1st Kodokan Judo Kata International Tournament 2007, 26–27.

Murata, N. and Todo, Y. (2007). A study on evaluation of judo kata performance. *Bulletin of the Association for the Scientific Studies on Judo*, Kodokan. Report XI. (In Japanese, abstract in English.)

Murata, N. and Todo, Y. (2009). A study on evaluation of judo kata performance II Koshiki no Kata. *Bulletin of the Association for the Scientific Studies on Judo*, Kodokan. Report XII. (In Japanese, abstract in English).

Nogaki, P. (2009). Personal correspondence with Paul Nogaki on the ideals of kata.

Oda, J. (1929). *Judo taikan*. Tokyo: Shoshikan. (In Japanese).

Oltremari, A. (n.d.). Kata, sport e gare (Kata, sports and competition). Article online and available from freeBudo's website, URL:http://www.freebudo.com/articoli/judo%20tradizionale/articoli%20judo/1%20kata%20sport%20e%20gare/1%20kata%20sport%20e%20gare.htm (In Italian) (Retrieved, July 2010).

Otaki, T. and Draeger, D. (1983). *Judo formal techniques*. Tokyo: Charles E. Tuttle Company.

Pelletier, G. (n.d.). Kata. Article online and available from Guy Pelletier and André Andermatt's website, URL: http://pagesperso-orange.fr/pelletier.andermatt/5kata0.html (In French) (Retrieved, July 2010).

Sheedy, J. (2010). Judo kata competitions: A review of practice strategies for the Goshin Jitsu [sic]. Article online and available from the Judo Information website, URL: http://judoinfo.com/new/techniques/formsof-judo-kata/671-practice-strategies-for-goshin-jitsu (Retrieved, July 2010).

Sidney, J. (2003). *The warrior's path: Wisdom from contemporary martial arts masters*. Boston: Shambhala Publications.

Takamura, Y. (1986). Teaching and shu-ha-ri. Article online and available from the Takamura-ha Shindo Yoshin Kai website, URL: http://www.shinyokai.com/essays_teachingShuhari.htm (Retrieved, July 2010).

Ukichi, S. (n.d.) Matsumoto, T. and Davidson, P. translators. (n.d.) in Daigo, T. editor (2008). *Eternal kendo*. Reprinted for the 2008 Kodokan Kata Kaki Koshukai (Kodokan Summer Kata Course). Tokyo: Kodokan Judo Institute.

chapter 22

A Taxonomy of Principles Used in Judo Throwing Techniques
by Linda Yiannakis, M.S.

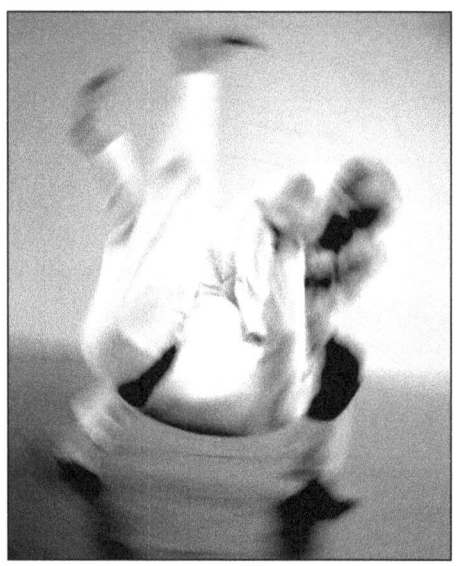

All photographs courtesy of David J. Higgins.

Techniques and Variants

Judo offers many throwing techniques. Some are considered standard throws, while others are seen as variants of those throws. How can we identify exactly which throw we have seen, or even which throw we are practicing? While there are no hard and fast rules about defining variants, an examination of a technique's properties can help in the following ways:

1) to identify it
2) to address the critical properties for practicing it
3) to foster innovations
4) to help in teaching the technique to others

All of the techniques presented in the central throwing syllabus of judo, *Five Sets of Techniques* (Gokyo no waza, 1920) represent models of throwing. For a visual overview, points can be placed on a grid to represent techniques that form a systematic plan for teaching a complete repertoire of movements. Each throw is defined by what happens when it is executed: the general movement pattern or path, level of complexity, and associated actions such as reap, hook, sweep, etc.

Techniques, Principles, and Operative Ranges

Generally speaking, techniques are not principles. A principle is a law or property that operates consistently where it is applied. Techniques are identifiable sets of actions that are driven by principles. Principles have an optimal range of operation and are less effective or ineffective once outside that range. For example, to make best use of the principle of leverage in hip techniques, the thrower (*tori*) typically must drop his center of gravity below that of his partner or receiver of the action (*uke*). If he tries to apply leverage outside of this range of optimal operation he will have difficulty. Similarly, a successful foot sweep depends upon tori's sweeping action occurring at the moment uke transfers his weight onto or off of his foot. If uke's weight is fully on the target leg, the intended sweep is more likely to function as a kick. In other techniques, tori's and uke's relative positions will either help or hinder the best application of the principles for that particular technique, depending on the operative range of the principles involved.

CONSTRUCTION OF TECHNIQUE

We can better understand both the standard throwing forms and their variants by examining how the techniques are constructed. Each technique has a set of structural elements as well as internal operational principles or processes. We build techniques from combinations of structural elements and operational principles in a variety of configurations and directions of throwing. We can look at the structural and operational properties as discrete elements, but in actual application they overlap and integrate when techniques are executed.

Structural Elements:
1) the stance of both tori and uke
2) the physical orientation of tori to uke
3) the direction of the breaking of balance
4) the configuration of the fitting in and positioning portion of the throw (*tsukuri*)
5) the placement of limbs for various actions

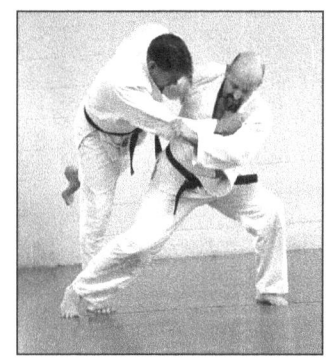

We can call these features of placement, intended direction, and shape or contour of construction. As the actions of the throw progress, some of these elements of structure may shift. For example, the position or orientation of the arms in the pulling hand and the lifting hand may change as tori moves through the throw. We can see this in a technique such as the one-arm back-carry throw, where tori's lifting hand begins at the lapel but shifts across uke's body to a new position under his arm as tori moves into position. In the lifting-pulling hip throw, tori's stance and the relative positions of uke and tori shift as tori moves from a higher to lower position in front of uke. Looked at this way, structural elements are snapshots of critical features of tori's technique at particular moments during his performance of the throw.

Examples of Structural Elements

These photos illustrate various elements of structure, such as hand placement, leg placement, orientation of tori and uke, and higher or lower stance, at a particular point in the throw.

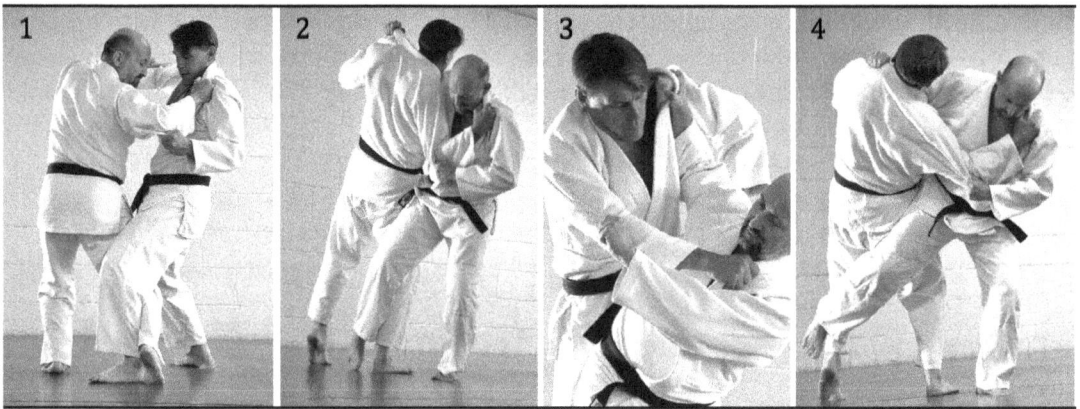

1) Major inner reaping throw.
2) Lift-pull hip throw.
3) Major outer reaping throw.
4) Major outer wheel.

Operational Principles

1) centered action in body management and power generation
2) turning with conversion of energy
3) generating momentum (*hazumi*)
4) the actions of the pulling hand and the lifting hand
5) the active staging of the breaking of balance, positioning, and technique execution (*kuzushi*, *tsukuri*, and *kake*).

This category also includes:
6) the use of leverage,
7) sweeping, reaping, hooking, or other leg actions,
8) the sacrificing of the standing position,
9) winding or wrapping actions
10) "slipping by" actions,
11) other actions from tori's center.

The structural elements of tori's orientation to uke and the placement of tori's hands, arms, or legs as he moves through a technique allow him to achieve the operations necessary for a particular throw. As an example, tori must achieve a certain orientation to uke and must place one leg outside of uke's leg in order to accomplish the reaping action in the major outer reaping throw. If he adopts a different orientation, i.e., turns his back to uke or places his leg between uke's legs, he will not be able to execute the major outer reaping throw. But he will be in position to move into a technique that has the structural and operational features for that orientation or leg placement, such as the inner thigh throw. The operational processes of the fitting-in stage of the throw are also often accompanied by changes in tori's arm placement, orientation to uke, or other structural characteristics.

Examples Using Operational Principles

1a–c: These illustrate tori's body control and turning in the big wheel throw.
2a–c: These show the use of momentum in the side wheel throw.
3a–c: These illustrate the principle of abandoning the standing position and using tori's dropping center to destabilize and throw uke.

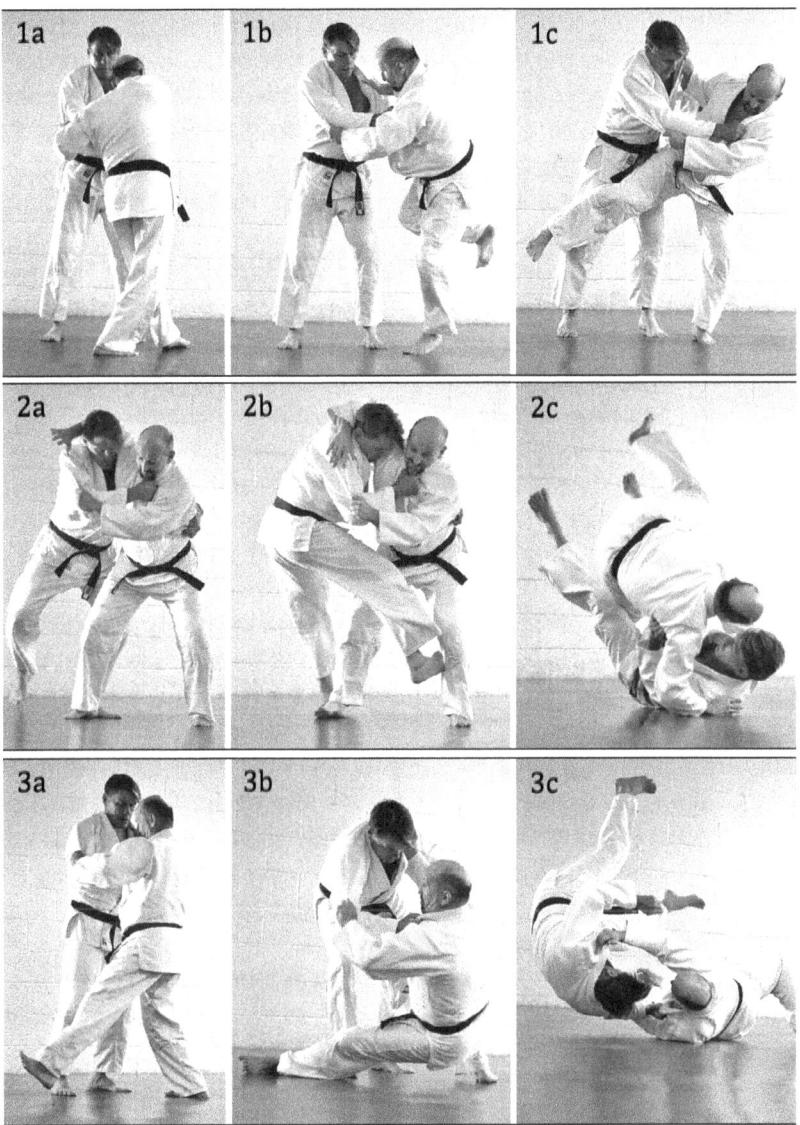

Contextual Principles

Structural and operational principles may be supplemented by contextual principles. Contextual principles apply in situations or contexts of technique execution. This category includes principles:

        1) initiative strategies (*sen*)
        2) control of distance (*maai*)
        3) creating momentum (*hazumi*)
        4) yielding and redirecting (*ju*)
        5) continuousness (*renzoku*)

Contextual principles operate in the interaction or synergy of movement between uke and tori. They may be applied as highly technical skills or as powerful, athletic movements. Some principles, such as the use of momentum, may operate both as a dynamic process internal to the throw (operational principle) and/or independently as a contextual principle. Judo players often work to create momentum when moving around with uke as a means of helping to establish the breaking of balance and allowing more efficient entry into techniques. Momentum can also be seen as an operational application within techniques such as the side wheel, the knee wheel, or the side drop, where internal momentum occurs as a result of tori's actions as he fits into the throw. Other contextual principles, such as continuousness (*renzoku*), aren't thought of as internal processes, but as operations that take place in the technique's environment. In the case of continuousness, two or more discrete techniques become seamlessly linked, but the principle itself is not part of the structural or operational features of the individual techniques that it brings together.

What tori does in the moments immediately before moving into a throw will directly affect how the operational principles of the technique come into play. Judo practitioners sometimes ask, "Which comes first, breaking balance or fitting into position?" While we summarize throwing principles as breaking balance, then fitting in, and finally execution, this is not a compartmentalized sequence of events that is engraved in stone. These three principles overlap and interact as a throw progresses. In either case, breaking balance and fitting in are complementary processes that culminate in the completion of the throw. Without a doubt, execution is the final phase, but what about breaking balance and fitting in? Breaking balance may precede or follow the fitting-in stage, but in either case, it must be continuous after it has begun. Tori's actions in the context that gives rise to the technique determine which operational principles come into play next. If these contextual actions are dominated by a high degree of reliance on athleticism, power, speed, or superb timing, then the resulting processes of positioning may take precedence over the breaking of balance as an initiating element. That is to say, breaking balance may be a result of a dynamic fitting-in movement. As one example, tori may deal with uke by using strong gripping strategies both as a defensive maneuver and to prepare his own posture for a sudden drop under uke into a very low shoulder throw. Tori may drop into the throwing position with perfect timing and speed without necessarily destabilizing uke first. The breaking of balance occurs as tori moves rapidly through fitting in under uke and continues into the execution phase of the technique.

On the other hand, if elements such as the use of initiative strategies, control of distance, yielding and redirecting, action-reaction, or the seamless continuation of one technique into a second one are used to break the opponent's stance or to create an opening, then the breaking of balance may more likely precede positioning. Tori may attempt a knee wheel throw against uke's right knee, which uke evades by pulling or stepping back with his right foot. Tori, using the principle of continuousness, blends his movement with uke's retreating leg action and moves smoothly into a major outer reaping throw. Tori uses the energy and direction of uke's retreating action to stage the overbalancing of uke as tori continues into position for the major outer reaping throw.

Examples Using Contextual Principles

Using uke's energy or movement in combination techniques (*renzoku*) to unbalance the opponent (*kuzushi*) for a follow-up throw. These photographs (1a–d) show tori attempting a kneel wheel and uke retreating by pulling his attacked leg back. Tori blends his forward movement with uke's retreating movement and steps forward with his left foot into the major outer reaping throw.

These photographs (1a–d) show tori beginning a foot sweep on uke's left foot. As uke withdraws his left foot, tori continues sweeping his own right foot across to position it in front of uke's right foot. Tori continues to turn, and uses his rotation outward to unbalance uke and enters for a one-arm back carry throw.

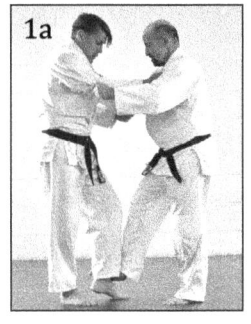
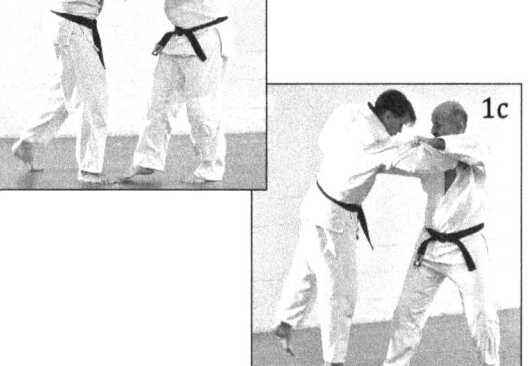
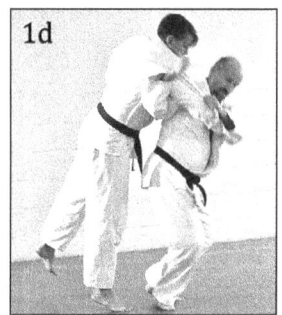

The Standard Syllabus of Judo Throws and Katas

In judo the Kodokan's standard syllabus of throws is a primary resource for studying the structural and operational principles of techniques, and for understanding the relationships among the techniques. Prearranged forms such as Nage-no-kata (forms of throwing) fill out the study of techniques with examples of situations that require the application of a variety of contextual principles. For example, the first technique in Nage-no-kata is the floating drop. This technique provides lessons in responding to uke's advancing action with a synchronous retreating action. It also teaches tori to use control of distance as a means of staging overbalance. Tori's deliberately extended third step back increases the distance between himself and uke and breaks uke's posture forward for the throw's successful execution. The kata provides practice in executing techniques in dynamic interactions with uke that require the understanding of structural, operational, and contextual principles.

Moving out from the original central models in the Gokyo, we can also learn variations in techniques. These may involve changes in hand or leg placement or action, fitting-in actions, throwing direction, etc. Yet the throw may be still identified as the one of the same name in the Gokyo, or as a close relation. The variations may change some aspects of the outward appearance of the throw, but retain enough of its structural and operational features for a useful reference to the original. At times a throw that is essentially a variant of another has come to be regarded as a separate technique, rather than simply a variant. The one-arm back-carry throw was once considered a variant of the two-hand back-carry throw (Kano, 1986:67). It is now placed as a separate technique in the newly accepted techniques of judo. Similarly, the minor outer hook was once regarded as a variant of the minor outer reap, but due to operational principles that differ, it stands on its own (Kano, 1986:76).

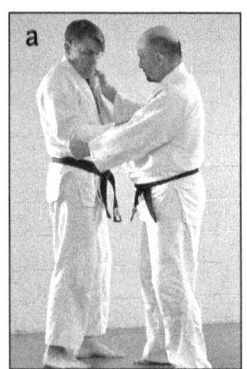
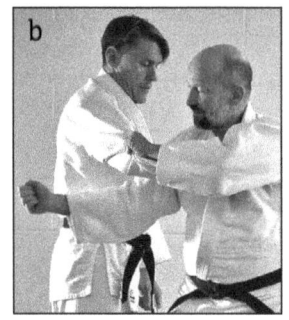
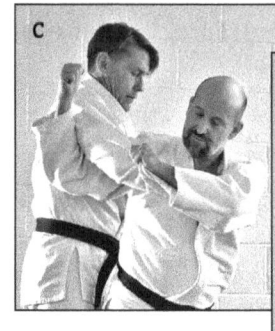
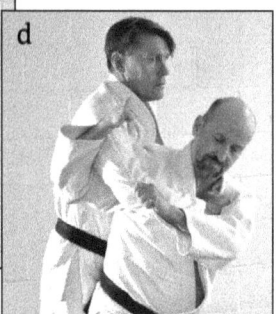

One-arm back-carry throw (a–d).

Homogenization of Technique

At other times changes take place that result in a homogenization of technique so throws that are actually distinct become variants of each other. Although main elements may remain, some of the internal operational principles may get dropped out or changed. When this happens, the lines between techniques begin to blur. Throws that were placed in the Gokyo as separate techniques with distinct operations now coalesce into variants of each other. This happens largely in techniques with similar outward appearances.

As an example, we sometimes see the leg wheel and big wheel presented in modern judo as essentially the same throw. What differentiates them from each other in this way of thinking is primarily the leg placement: very high for the big wheel, and lower on the thigh for the leg wheel. In a case like this, the structural and operational principles that distinguish them from each other have been lost.

However, as actual distinguishing principles in the leg wheel, the leg acts to hold uke as tori turns out away from him, rotating uke over his out-stretched leg. There is no sweeping or cutting action by the leg, and the leg placement can vary somewhat. In the big wheel, the situation is very different. The outstretched leg is quite active in the big wheel, uke must be extended farther forward by tori than in the leg wheel, and tori's leg makes a definite rotating action back toward uke.

In the leg wheel, uke is essentially rotated over a stationary barrier, while in the big wheel, the top part of his body is brought forward while the bottom half is pressed and actively rolled over through the action of tori's leg. These differing properties between the techniques require that more differences in action must take place beyond simply changing the position of the leg. When tori understands each technique's operational principles, he can address adopting any additional skills required for such differentiated techniques. This increased proficiency results in an expanded repertoire of movement skills. This type of understanding also provides instructors with additional resources for guiding and helping students to grasp the properties of techniques and to be better equipped to self-correct during their practice.

Similarly, we sometimes see the lifting hip throw taught as a version of the major hip throw with a belt hold. But *tsuri* refers to a particular action of lifting that doesn't occur in *ogoshi*. In order to achieve the tsuri action in the lifting hip throw, tori uses a type of hip action somewhat similar to that found in the floating hip throw, but with a fuller hip insertion somewhat closer to the major hip throw, as well as different corresponding upper-body actions.

As another example, the major outer wheel operates differently than the major outer reaping throw, and so is more than the major outer reaping throw done on both of uke's legs. The relative positions of uke and tori differ somewhat in the two techniques, as does the desired weight distribution on uke's legs and the actions needed by tori to achieve this for each technique. These differing structural and operational elements result in differing leg actions by tori against uke's leg(s) in the execution of the throw.

A variety of approaches to capturing different techniques occurs when uke and tori engage in free play or contest. The interplay of the many variables in movement between uke and tori provides opportunities for applying the contextual principles.

Kano organized the *Gokyo* as a guide to systematically teach the application of principles. He provided a curriculum of specific movement types and operations across increasing levels of complexity. When separate techniques become melded into variants without clear understanding of what has happened, some of that educational benefit is lost.

Showing Differences Between Techniques That Look Very Similar
Leg wheel (*ashi guruma*) ↔ big wheel (*oguruma*)

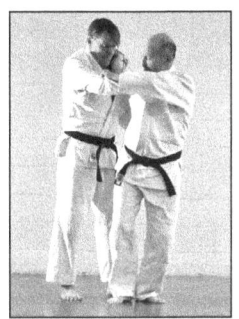 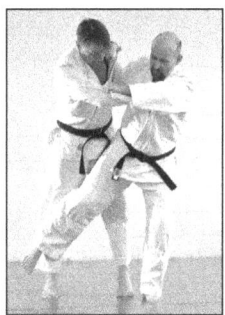

Leg wheel throw. Tori's blocking leg is stationary and uke is rotated over it by tori's continued turning action.

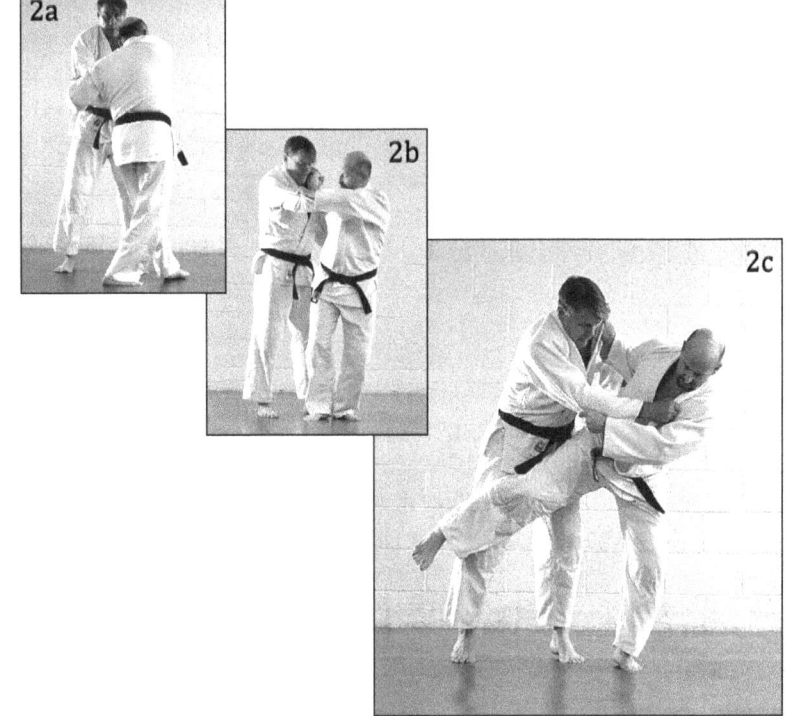

Big wheel throw. Tori's outstretched leg actively rotates back into uke in this throw (2a–c).

Major outer reaping throw (*osoto gari*) ↔ major outer wheel (*osoto-guruma*)

Major outer reaping throw (l.)
Tori drives uke back onto his right heel or outside of his right foot and then uses a reaping action to throw uke.

Major outer wheel (r.)
Tori drives uke back on both legs and rotates him over his outstretched leg.

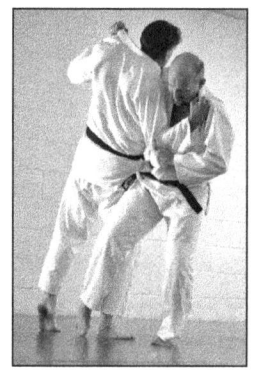
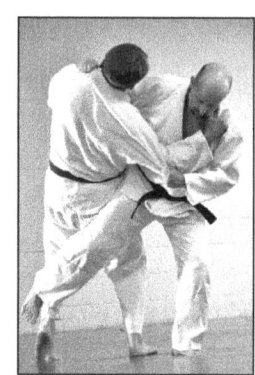

Applicability to Contest
 Someone who is interested in judo only as a competitive sport may not want as broad a curriculum as provided in the *Gokyo*. But it is still advantageous to understand the critical properties of the throws in individual competitive arsenals in order to make the techniques as powerful and as adaptable as possible in the high-speed, rapidly shifting demands of contest situations. An understanding of the original techniques' properties also allows for preservation of underlying processes and elements. These are important both in themselves and as a basis from which to consider innovation or to pass on to others.

Preservation and Change
 Systems change over time in response to perceived needs or pressure from outside influences. One method of preservation and change in Japanese martial art is known as *shu ha ri* (Shimabukuro, 2008:59–60). In this method, the preservation of the principles that define a system is built into whatever changes are made over the years. Any changes must conform to the defining principles of the system; otherwise, the very nature of the system becomes compromised. In the protective or imitative learning stage *shu* (守), the student strives to copy the teacher's actions as closely as possible, and to acquire a critical mass of the fundamentals on which the system is built. This stage lasts several years. In the change or divergence stage (*ha* 破), the student (now well into the black-belt level of the art) begins to move outside the boundaries of the carefully prescribed program of the ha stage. Nevertheless, his experimentation at this stage is still driven by close adherence to the principles that govern the system. He applies the fundamentals learned in the shu stage to more variations, or applies more individualistic interpretations of those fundamentals. In the final separation stage (*ri* 離), the student—now a high-ranking practitioner—has achieved a high level of understanding and skill within the system. In this stage, he moves out more freely into areas of innovation and transcends technical boundaries. He now has the knowledge to make changes to the system without corrupting its essential nature. In this way the art is both preserved and moved forward.
 Judo has become subject to many changes over the years by high-ranking teachers at the Kodokan and elsewhere, as well as from the innovations that have arisen from competitors. However, coming from such diverse sources, modification in judo has not been entirely systematic, or necessarily in accord with the original principles of the system. This makes cataloging innovation much more difficult than if a process such as shu ha ri were in place today. For this reason, the framework of principles suggested in this chapter may be helpful in allowing creative innovators to better articulate and share their contributions, as well as allowing them to see how their innovations fit into or change judo.

Summary

The essential principles underlying judo throwing techniques may be organized into structural, operational, and contextual categories. The elements and processes within these categories interact, overlap, and combine during the moving application of techniques.

The structural principles of technique may be thought of as those that answer questions that begin with "where" or "what," while the answer is a noun or an adverb: "What is my stance relative to uke?" "Where do I place my leg?" "Which is the optimal direction to off-balance an opponent?" Structural principles may be examined statically at any moment in time.

Operational principles of technique are those that mainly answer the question "How?" The answer involves a dynamic process or action. "How do I destabilize uke?" "How do I fit into position?" "How do I drop to the floor without pulling uke on top of me?"

Contextual principles answer the questions "when," "where," and "how," and are applied in the situation preceding or continuing into actual execution of the technique.

"When do I start my approach?" "Where do I enter for this technique?" "How do I make uke step so that I can apply the technique?" "How do I follow the first technique with the second?" These principles cannot occur in static isolation, but only during dynamic interactions.

We can practice techniques with structural and operational principles alone to highlight and clarify their operative processes. For example, all of judo's throwing techniques may be addressed individually in practice, if desired, with little or no resistance from uke. However, when studied in attack situations, free play, competitive "set-ups," contest, and routine practice (kata), they are supplemented with the contextual principles that allow them to be executed in an endless number of dynamic situations with a partner or opponent.

The framework presented here is offered as a tool and aid in clarifying the many overlapping, complex, and sometimes challenging actions that come together through best use of energy to result in the beautiful throws of Kano Jigoro's judo.

REFERENCES

Daigo, T. (2005). *Kodokan judo throwing techniques*. Tokyo: Kodansha.
Kano, J. (1986). *Kodokan judo*. Tokyo: Kodansha International Ltd.
Shimabukuro, M., and Pellman, L. (2008). *Flashing steel: Mastering Eishin-Ryu swordsmanship*, second edition. Berkeley, CA: Blue Snake Books.

ACKNOWLEDGMENTS

Many thanks to David J. Higgins for the photography and to Mark Fraser and Andrew Frye, who gave generously of their time and energy to serve as tori and uke in the illustrations for this chapter.

Judo Terminology

ashi guruma	足車	leg wheel
Gokyo no waza	五教之技	five sets of techniques
hiza guruma	膝車	knee wheel
ippon seoinage	一本背負投	one-arm back-carry throw
kosoto gake	小外掛	minor outer hook
kosoto gari	小外刈	minor outer reap
kuzushi	崩し	breaking of balance
makikomi	巻込	winding or wrapping actions
morote seoinage	双手背負投	two-hand back-carry throw
Nage-no-kata	投の形	forms of throwing
nage-waza	投げ技	throwing techniques
ogoshi	大腰	major hip throw
oguruma	大車	big wheel
osoto gari	大外刈	major outer reaping throw
osoto guruma	大外車	major outer wheel
seiryoku zenyo	精力 善用	best use of energy
sukashi	透	"slipping by" actions
sutemi	捨身	sacrificing body position
tai sabaki	体捌き	body management
tenkan	転換	turning with conversion of energy
tsuri goshi	釣腰	lifting (belt) hip throw
tsuri komi goshi	釣込腰	lifting-pulling hip throw
uchi mata	内股	inner thigh throw
uki goshi	浮腰	floating hip throw
uki otoshi	浮落	floating drop
yoko guruma	横車	side wheel
yoko otoshi	横落	side drop

chapter 23

Rhythm, Patterns, and Timing in Martial Arts as Exemplified Through Judo
by Linda Yiannakis, M.S.

Introduction

We live in a world of patterns and rhythms. The tides roll, the seasons change, and our own internal rhythms ebb and flow. There are also patterns and rhythms that we create in our daily or weekly activities that we overlay on our lives and world.

Musashi, the great swordsman of seventeenth-century Japan, wrote about the importance to the martial artist of understanding timing and rhythm (*hyoshi*) in the *Earth Scroll* (Chi no Maki) from his book *Go Rin No Sho* (The Book of Five Rings):

> Rhythm is something that exists in everything, but the rhythms of martial arts in particular are difficult to master without practice. Rhythm is manifested in the world in such things as dance and music, pipes and strings. These are all harmonious rhythms. In the field of martial arts, there are rhythms and harmonies in archery, gunnery, and even horsemanship. In all arts and sciences, rhythm is not to be ignored. There is even rhythm in being empty.
> – Cleary, 1994:30

How conscious are you of varying rhythms in your technique applications? Trying to barrel through every technique at exactly the same pace can result in frustration or failure. An awareness of rhythm in martial arts can help us fine-tune what we are trying to accomplish. The art of judo offers us a great many examples.

Judo practitioners should know that everything we do does not happen at the same speed or rhythm. Rhythm is not the same as speed. The Merriam-Webster dictionary defines speed as "swiftness or rate of performance or action: velocity." The definition of rhythm in reference to movement is given as "movement, fluctuation, or variation marked by the regular recurrence or natural flow of related elements." A movement's rhythm may therefore contain segments or cadences of varying speeds, and may be perceived as a pattern. While speed or lack of speed of application is something we can see easily in judo, rhythms can be subtler and less apparent unless we are looking for them.

Contextual Processes

One way to think about achieving an entry to a throw is to add a consideration of rhythms to the "when" and "how" of our approach to the receiver of the action (*uke*). What are the elements of rhythm that bring the thrower (*tori*) right to uke's doorstep, so to speak? These involve the movements that allow tori to be in position to move into the

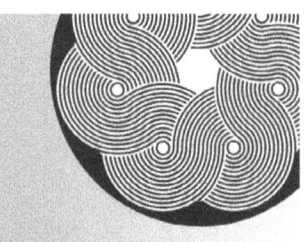

Sidebar: Uke and Tori

Uke and tori are designations for roles taken by two judo players in interactions with each other. Uke receives the action tori makes. Tori may be executing a throw, or just fitting in for one—or he may be applying a choke, armbar, pin, or other action against uke. Uke may be cooperative and compliant, or he may resist tori's actions in a variety of ways, but the relationship is the same. Although the dynamics of the interaction change in different situations, uke is ultimately the receiver of an action that tori completes.

fitting-in phase (*tsukuri*) of the technique. These actions occur in the context immediately preceding tori's initiation of his entry, and contribute to his being in the right place at the right time. At this point in tori's impending attack we can see patterns emerge in the use of a variety of strategies and principles, such as gripping strategies, stepping patterns, body management (*tai-sabaki*), the creation of momentum, and others.

Stepping Pattern

When you use a normal walk (*ayumi ashi*), a following step (*tsugi ashi*), or another type of movement, you can establish directional patterns. The basic, common patterns are (1) advancing straight forward, (2) retreating straight backward, (3) moving laterally to the left or the right, (4) moving forward to the left or right corner, (5) moving backward to the left or right corner, and (6) circling. Each of these patterns may be performed at a variety of speeds or combined with another. Of course, these directions are only selected, representative points from 360 degrees of possibility of movement, but they allow you to structure your practice in the major directions.

Speed

Every encounter is characterized by a particular speed or tempo, which may vary throughout the interaction. One partner may seek to control the tempo while the other partner either follows or attempts to impose his own pace. Tempo can vary from nonstop, rapid motion to slow, almost static, cautious stepping.

Stride Length

The length of your stride, or the space between one step and the next, varies from judoka to judoka, from technique to technique, and sometimes between defensive and offensive movement.

Rhythms in Pattern Matching

How do we actually use the understanding of rhythms to improve our positioning for an entry in free play or contest? It is easy to become familiar with various rhythms in gross movements by starting with exercises that center on matching patterns with your partner using the characteristics identified above.

Mirroring

A simple exercise is to work with a cooperative partner and have one person follow the other's movements by mirroring them. The two take grips, and the leader begins the exercise by moving in a relaxed manner, in natural posture (*shizentai*), in any direction he chooses. The follower's job is to mirror his partner's relaxed posture and movements. Without resistance, this exercise allows both participants to concentrate on fluid, centered action, and to be aware of their partner's movements and changes in direction.

The mirroring exercise can be modified in many ways. One way to change it is to require the follower to mirror the leader, but to follow reluctantly. The follower gives some resistance, but still mirrors the leader's pattern. The leader then has to focus on maintaining fluid movement and making his follower move by use of the leader's own centered action, and not by muscling or yanking to make his partner follow.

Resistance by the follower can be ramped up in stages to full-fledged resistance in the defensive posture called *jigotai*, if desired. The leader's objective remains the same: to move his partner using centered action, and not with a reliance on upper-body strength. By changing the follower's role, both participants can experience discerning the other's movement patterns under varying conditions of cooperation and resistance.

Stepping Pattern in Mirroring

When using the mirroring exercise, the leader can focus on particular patterns of movement at any level of resistance by the follower. The six basic directional patterns are discussed above. The leader can choose one, two, or all six patterns to move through as he leads his partner, who must perceive each movement and follow seamlessly. These exercises can also be expanded by requiring the leader to change directions and to make entries into throws with adequate overbalancing in all of the directions of movement. As the agreed-upon resistance by the follower increases, the leader will need to continue to use centered action to achieve the overbalance. If he finds that he is beginning to rely on too much muscle power to break his partner's posture, he should drop back to a step with less resistance by the follower and work more at that level.

Speed in Mirroring

The leader chooses movement directions and the level of resistance from the follower. He also chooses the speed at which he will move through his patterns or into his entries. The follower must match the speed. The leader may vary the tempo throughout the movement exercise, and his partner must match this and the changes in direction of movement, as well as maintain the desired level of cooperation or resistance.

Stride Length in Mirroring

Finally, the leader also establishes a particular stride length as he leads his partner through the mirroring exercise. As with the first two elements described above, the leader may change this feature at will during the exercise. The follower must match stride length as well as direction and speed of movement throughout the exercise.

Varying the Elements of Rhythm and Pattern

By varying the main factors of direction or stepping pattern, speed, and stride length, the leader gains experience in moving efficiently in a variety of ways. He also must achieve overbalance of his partner and be able to move into position for a throw under a variety of conditions. In addition, he becomes more aware of commonly occurring patterns involving all of these elements. As the leader establishes patterns or rhythms and then continually changes them throughout the interaction, the follower's awareness of these patterns, rhythms, and changes to them by his partner is also enhanced through this structured exercise.

The exercise may be further expanded by the following:
1) requiring work on both left- and right-side techniques,
2) specifying different grips,

3) continually shifting posture from natural to defensive and back,
4) requiring partners to work in same stance or opposite stance (*kenka yotsu*),
5) limiting the types of throws the leader may attempt
   (i.e., just hip techniques; just sweeps, etc.),
6) focusing on awareness of the follower's weight transfers
   onto and off of his feet as he moves,
7) requiring the follower to block, evade, or counter
   each time the leader makes an entry, or
8) requiring the leader to focus on continuous
   combination attacks (*renzoku waza*), and
9) any other feature you want to build into the exercise.

Disruption of Rhythm

When engaged in free play (*randori*) or in contest, we don't want to get caught in the predictability of an established pattern or rhythm. Further, if we match our partner's pattern for more than a step or two at a time, it can be difficult to achieve overbalance or begin an entry for a throw because he will see the pattern match and be ready to block or counter. But establishing, however briefly, any of the movement patterns mentioned above in order to disrupt them provides the thrower (*tori*) with an opportunity to move into his throw.

Yagyu Munenori, head of the Yagyu Shinkage-ryu in the seventeenth century, wrote, "Deliver the kind of strokes that do not harmonize with the opponent's strokes" (Tabata, 2003:6). Although he was referring to swordwork, the same principle applies to other types of movement.

Tori may set up a particular stepping pattern that uke follows or responds to, even if only for a couple of steps. For example, tori may initiate a series of small, advancing steps (or even one advancing step). Uke may then retreat in response. As soon as tori perceives that uke has fallen into the pattern, he disrupts the rhythm by stepping sideways or diagonally, or by changing his speed or stride length. This sudden change, controlled by tori, gives him a small opportunity to attack outside of the brief rhythm of the pattern, where uke is not expecting him to move.

Setting and Disrupting a Stepping Pattern

Mark and Andrew begin in the left natural posture (*hidari shizentai*) (A1). Mark steps forward with his right foot. Andrew mirrors this by stepping back with his left foot (A2). Mark then disrupts this brief pattern by stepping out to the side with his left foot, drawing Andrew off balance as he does so (A3). *Uke: Andrew Frye; Tori: Mark Fraser.*

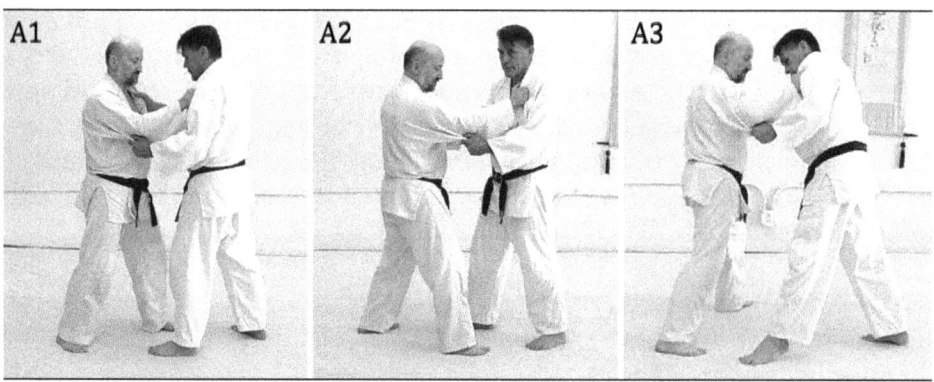

As an example, tori initiates the advancing pattern with his right foot in preparation for moving into a major outer reaping throw (*osoto-gari*) to uke's rear. If uke retreats with his left leg, tori can continue to move forward with uke's backward movement. As tori then begins to advance with his left foot, uke retreats with his right. But here tori allows his left leg to lag behind for just a brief moment. This allows uke time to complete his withdrawing movement with his right leg and to transfer his weight to it, which is what tori wants for this throw. At the moment uke commits his weight to his right leg, tori changes his speed and stride length to bring his left foot forward and then achieve placement of his reaping (right) leg against uke's now-weighted right leg. Tori has implemented a rhythm of slowing down and then suddenly speeding up. This control of tempo in the approach to the throw provides tori an opportunity to attack uke's leg before he has a chance to move it farther back and out of reach. It gives tori the opportunity for a more efficient attack by reducing the problem of having to catch up to uke's retreating leg before uke transfers the weight off of it as he continues moving backward.

Timing the Entry for the Major Outer Reaping Throw (*Osoto-gari*)

Mark steps forward with his right foot, and Andrew responds by stepping back with his left foot (B1). Mark then presses forward and begins to move his left foot forward, but allows it to lag slightly behind (B2). Andrew, expecting Mark to take a full step forward with his left as he had with his right, steps back with his right (B3). As soon as Andrew's weight is committed to his right leg, Mark moves in quickly for a major outer reaping throw (B4). *Uke: Andrew Frye; Tori: Mark Fraser.*

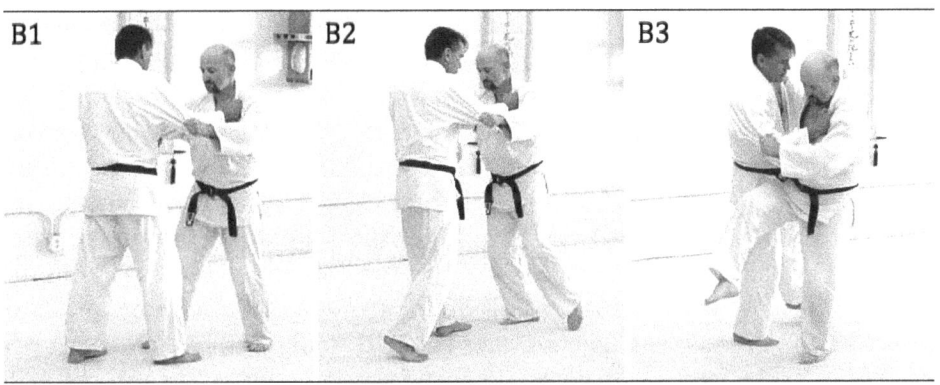

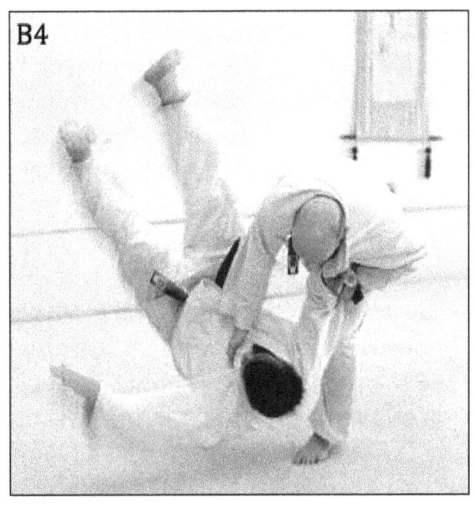

Uke's Rhythm

Just as important as the rhythms you initiate and control as tori are the rhythms that uke puts in place. Uke will also establish various stepping patterns, speeds, and stride lengths. You need to be aware of exactly what uke is doing. By honing your awareness and perception of his actions, you can use the same methods of disruption that you use when you establish the pattern, by altering any of the elements of direction, speed, or stride length (or a combination of these).

For example, let's say uke has begun to retreat. He can be using any type of stepping movement, taking small, cautious steps or longer, more definitive steps backward. As tori, you can follow him in this pattern and try to achieve a throw to uke's rear. Or, you can suddenly disrupt the pattern and timing with a rapid "jumping in" entry to the front, where you allow his legs to continue to retreat but keep his upper body drawn forward as you enter for a sweeping loin throw (*harai goshi*), a back carry throw (*seoi-nage*), or other forward throw. Similarly, you can disrupt his pattern by stepping sideways or to the corner, or by imposing your own rhythm by speeding up or slowing down.

Once the entry has been achieved, there are further rhythms to consider: those that occur as part of completing the positioning and execution of the throw. At that point we are considering the operational principles, or the dynamic processes, of the technique itself.

Operational Processes and Internal Rhythms

It is clear to most judoka that different techniques have different "feels" to them. Those differences arise partly from the various actions that tori makes with his torso, arms, and legs as he fits in and disturbs uke's balance, but also from the differences in timing that result from these varied actions. Thus different techniques can be seen to have their own unique rhythms. For example, the thrower's timing for the side separation throw (*yoko wakare*) can seem abrupt when compared to the rhythm of coming around his partner to enter for the side wheel throw (*yoko guruma*). By the same token, the timing for the advanced foot sweep (*de ashi barai*) is very different from the timing for a larger technique, such as the major hip throw (*ogoshi*) or the large wheel throw (*oguruma*).

My sensei's sensei, Taizo Sone, used to tell him, "Waza wa hito nari." The sense of this phrase is that the technique takes on a life of its own. You need time for all of these movements and forces to come together and play out in their unique rhythmic patterns. You must consider the interaction of tori, uke, and the dynamics of the technique itself.

The time we are speaking of is fractions of a second. This is easy to see in foot sweeps, where sweeping slightly too soon or too late will result in a failed technique. A mistimed, early sweep in the following or double foot sweep (*okuri ashi barai*) or in the lifting-drawing foot sweep (*harai tsurikomi ashi*) provides lessons in the understanding of the need for a little patience in the execution of certain techniques.

As another example, it is useful to compare the control of rhythm in the major outer reaping throw (*osoto-gari*) with the minor outer hooking throw (*ko soto gake*). Both of these techniques throw uke to the rear. In the major outer reaping throw, tori's inside leg is used to create a large reaping motion against uke's near leg. In the minor outer hooking throw, tori's outside leg comes across to uke's near leg in a hooking motion.

For the minor outer hook, tori advances with his right foot and uke retreats with his left foot, as in the example of the major outer reaping throw described previously. Now tori has set up the suggestion of a pattern of movement. Tori next inclines his upper body slightly and begins to bring his left leg forward as if to advance with his left. Instead, as uke withdraws his right leg, tori lets his left foot lag behind while he allows his left hand to follow uke's movement backward. As uke steps down onto his withdrawn right foot, tori changes rhythm by very quickly moving his left foot ahead so it is outside of uke's right. Just as quickly, he skips his right foot forward to take the place of his left, which then presses against the outside/back of uke's right foot and clips it out from under him in a hooking movement as tori continues to drive forward with his center through the technique.

While this "lagging" method utilizes rhythm in the same manner as in the major outer reaping throw, the rhythms in each of the two techniques feel quite different due to the dynamics of leg movement and placement for tori's inside leg or his outside leg, as well as differences in the upper-body movements for each throw.

Changing the Rhythm for the Minor Outer Hook (*Ko Soto Gake*)

Andrew steps forward with his right foot and Mark retreats with his left foot in response (C1). Andrew then begins to bring his left leg forward as if to advance with his left but lets his left foot lag behind while Mark steps back with his right foot (C2). Andrew allows his left hand to follow Mark's movement backward (C3). As Mark steps down onto his withdrawn right foot, Andrew changes rhythm by quickly moving his left foot forward outside of Mark's right (C4). Just as quickly, he skips his right foot forward to replace his left, and then presses his left foot against the outside/back of Mark's right foot and clips it out from under him in a hooking movement as he drives through the technique (C5). *Uke: Mark Fraser; Tori: Andrew Frye.*

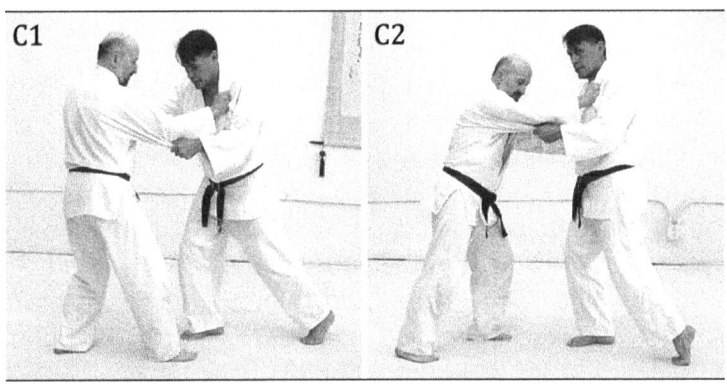

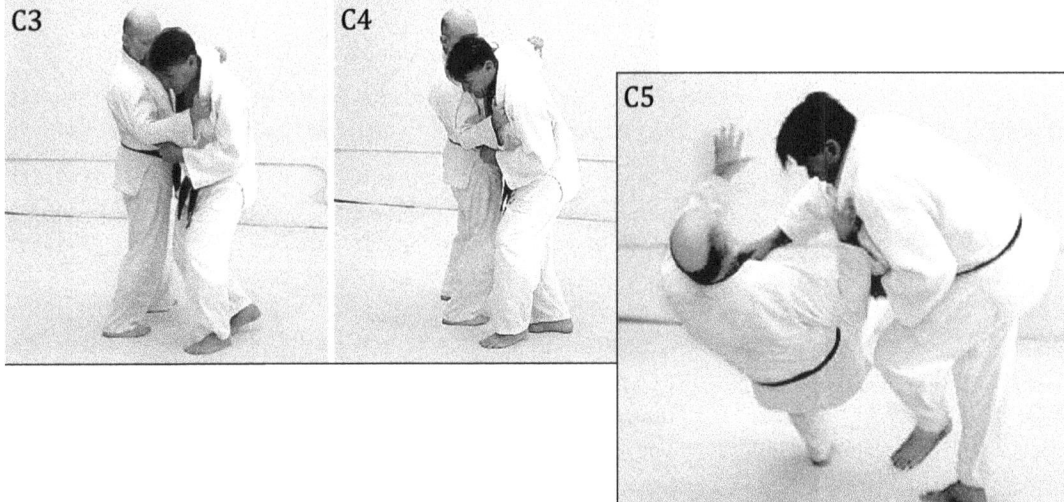

Perceiving the Pattern Change in Combination Attacks

Judoka often use techniques in combinations. Combinations may be done as discrete, sequential techniques, often in an action-reaction dynamic. This type of combination is known as *renraku waza*, in which the techniques are connected in sequence. Combinations may also be done as renzoku waza, in which the second technique flows continuously from the action of the first technique. Both types of combinations require that tori initiate an approach or entry to a throw. In effect, a throw is a pattern of specific movement involving breaking of posture (*kuzushi*), fitting in (*tsukuri*), and, if successful, execution (*kake*). However, if uke detects the initiation of the pattern in time, he will move to disrupt it by evading, blocking, or countering with a technique of his own. When tori initiates a technique, he must be aware of any shifts in movement that uke makes so that tori can follow uke's shift with a second technique—a combination—based on what uke has done to disrupt tori's original pattern or throw. Essentially, the thrower begins a pattern, uke disrupts it, and the thrower follows uke's disruption with a second technique. Successful combination throwing depends upon tori's ability to perceive pattern changes made by uke and to respond to them with appropriate follow-up movements.

Other Applications of Rhythm: Repetitive Practice

A common exercise in judo is repetitive fitting practice, or *uchi-komi*. There are many ways to perform this exercise, but we will use a basic, common method as the example here. In this method of repeated practice, uke stands in whatever posture the thrower, tori, designates—usually basic natural posture, or right or left natural posture, but it can also be defensive posture. The thrower selects one technique at a time for his repetitive practice exercise. He enters for the throw, bringing uke into an overbalanced position, but does not complete the throw beyond that point of overbalance. The thrower then reverses his movement and returns to his starting position. Typically, an uchi-komi exercise like this will be repeated a set number of times in rapid succession. It is sometimes extended to include an actual throw at the end of the repetitions, when tori will complete the technique and execute the throw on the final entry. For example, tori may perform nine rapid entries with overbalance for the sweeping hip throw, and on the tenth trial complete the technique, taking uke over and to the ground. Then tori will begin another round of repeated practice with the same throw or with a different one.

For uchi-komi to be beneficial, each of tori's entries must contain all of the necessary elements for a successful completion of the throw. This means that if tori is doing rounds of ten—nine entries plus one throw—each entry must look and feel and operate like the final one when tori actually throws uke. If the entries preceding the final throw in each set are different from the final product, the exercise has not contributed to tori's practice of actually throwing. The final throw should be a smooth continuation of the entry and off balancing that tori has achieved in each of his first nine entries in that set of repeated practice.

One of the benefits of this type of practice is the use of rhythm as an organizing device in the construction of throws. As tori moves smoothly in and out through his ten entries and into his final throw, he establishes an overall rhythm that helps him bring together the various elements of off balancing, fitting in, and correct body and limb orientation to uke for optimal efficiency in each particular throw. When tori switches to a different throw, or type of throw (e.g., from a hip throw to a foot sweep), he finds that the overall rhythm changes because the internal elements and operational processes of the two throws are different from each other. The rhythmic pattern that tori creates for each technique in repeated practice exercises helps him to coordinate all of the necessary forces at the right time for smooth and efficient throwing and to develop a feel for each type of technique.

The organizing concept of rhythm in uchi-komi is also found in repetitive throwing practice, or *nagekomi*. Nagekomi also involves awareness of appropriate rhythms as tori performs repeated throws, whether standing still or moving. When moving, tori must find the best moment of opportunity to begin his throw, and must wrap this together with all of the critical elements that come into play as part of the throw itself.

Repetitive Practice

Here Mark sets up a rhythm that organizes his movements during repetitive practice (*uchi-komi*). *Uke: Andrew Frye; Tori: Mark Fraser.*

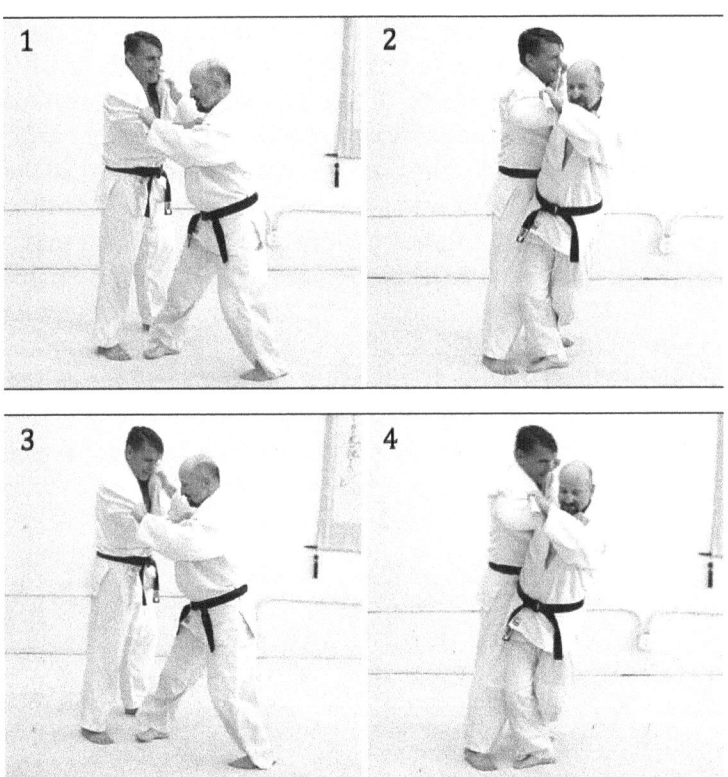

Falling or Receiving (*Ukemi*)

Another area where we can see the use of rhythm is in the practice of falling ways. Ukemi practice can be structured to make use of rhythm as an organizing force in various exercises. The standard method for practicing falling as part of or after a warm-up involves performing back, side, and front falls and rolls from varied distances from the floor. Key points include attention to breathing, controlling the head and body in space, and managing the impact properly. But in addition to these important elements, falling practice can facilitate body control through attention to the rhythm of the movements.

Self-Defense Techniques (*Goshin Waza*)

Striking techniques in judo (*atemi waza*) are jujutsu strikes and were developed to be used as an end in themselves and as a means of breaking posture (*kuzushi*) to allow entry into throwing, joint locking, or strangling techniques. Overall rhythms in an exchange with an opponent will vary according to type of offense or defense involved, directionality, and intensity of the opponent's movement, as well as environmental factors such as terrain, obstacles, walls, additional attackers, involvement of weapons, and tori's ultimate intentions for the outcome of the encounter (to escape, to immobilize the assailant, or to cause injury to the assailant). The timing and rhythm of judo atemi waza and other self-defense techniques fit into this larger whole of closing distance while moving into the opponent to finish the encounter.

Other Examples of Larger Rhythms: Types of Initiatives

Each of the major types of combat initiatives—direct (*sen*), following or countering (*gonosen*), or leading (*sen sen no sen*)—involves its own timing. The rhythm of gonosen, for example, involves a period of waiting—a very short period—that does not occur in the same way in a direct initiative attack. The "go" in gonosen refers to something "behind" or "after"—your attack must follow behind or after another attack. The rhythm of initiation in gonosen is governed by tori's perceiving uke's attack and allowing it to proceed to a certain point. At that time tori collects the energy that uke has given him and counters with his own technique, utilizing the motion and energy provided by uke. The difference may at times be subtle between a lightning-fast counter and a rapid direct attack, but ignoring these subtle differences between sen and gonosen may result in tori's rushing the counter. A counter that is attempted too early in uke's attack may end with uke's blocking or evading the counter, and tori's failure. Each of the three main initiative types is characterized by timing appropriate to its approach and implementation of technique.

Countering the Inner Thigh Throw (*uchi-mata*) with a Hip Throw

Mark attempts a right-side inner thigh throw (uchi-mata) (E1). Andrew waits for the appropriate moment (E2), evades Mark's leg (E3), takes Mark's energy (E4), and moves into a left-side hip throw to counter (use of gonosen) (E5). *Uke: Mark Fraser; Tori: Andrew Frye.*

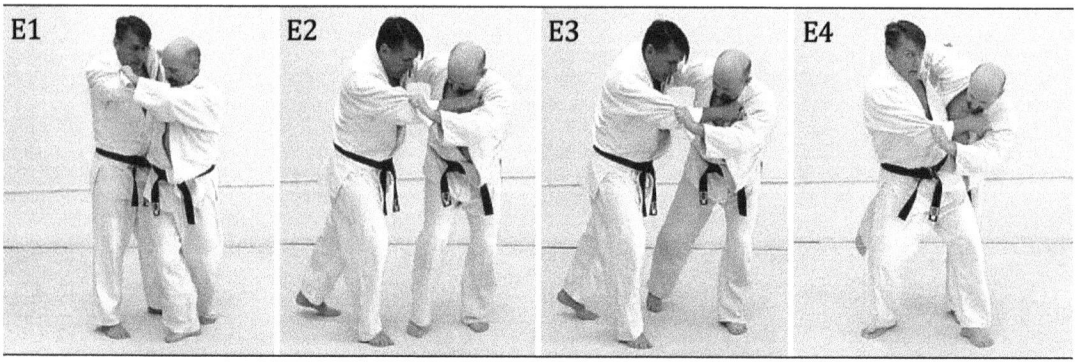

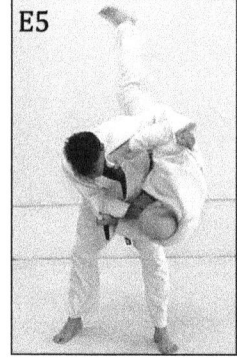

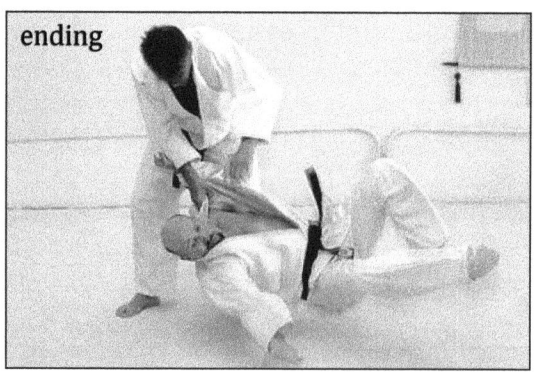

Countering the Major Outer Reaping Throw (*osoto-gari*) with the Floating Drop (*uki-otoshi*)

Andrew approaches Mark for a major outer reaping throw (osoto-gari) (F1). As Andrew commits himself to reaping his leg through (F2), Mark evades the reap by stepping back and dropping (F3), countering Andrew's major outer reaping throw with a floating drop (uki-otoshi) (F4-5). *Uke: Andrew Frye; Tori: Mark Fraser.*

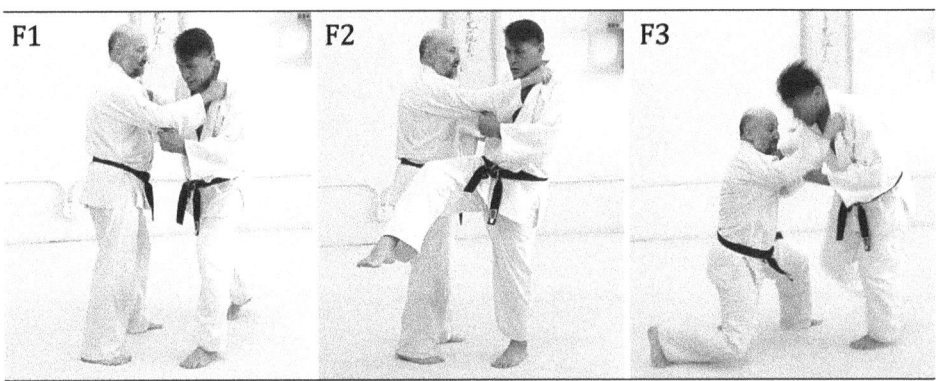

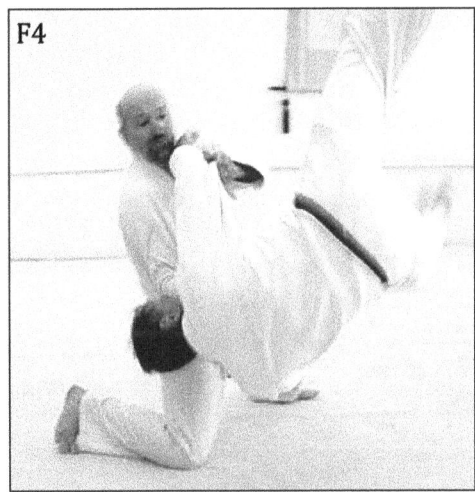

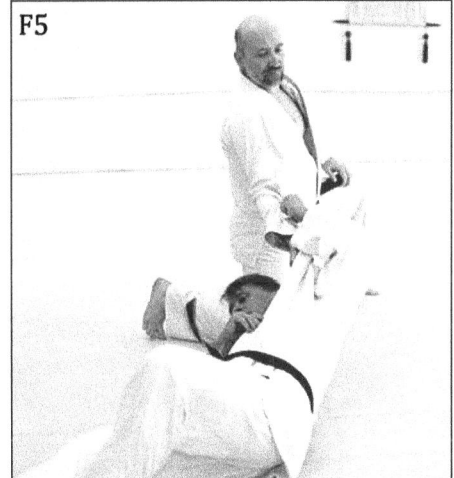

Kata

The various forms (*kata*) of judo provide opportunities to observe, study, and work within prescribed rhythms for the specific purposes of each kata. Draeger (1983:133) calls attention to the differences in the overall rhythms of the Forms of Throwing (*Nage-no-kata*) and the Forms of Grappling (*Katame-no-kata*):

> Unlike Nage no Kata, this kata [Katame-no-kata] is a mixture of paces or tempos, easy to recognize, but quite difficult to achieve except for the most experienced judoists. The burden of keeping the proper rhythm rests with Tori, who frequently must move in and out on both the lateral and longitudinal axes as well as between them to apply his techniques.... Hesitations and mistakes in positioning by either partner make for bad timing and easily shatter the rhythm of this kata. As an alternation of slow, smoothly executed preliminary movements and faster, more actively executed techniques, this kata lacks the metronomic rhythm of the Nage no Kata.

Within Nage no Kata itself, a use of similar rhythm was noted by Leggett in both the opening and closing techniques as they were done in earlier days:

> Ukiotoshi is the simplest of throws in principle—rhythm is imposed on uke, and then the very long step breaks the rhythm and uke cannot recover psychologically in time to adapt. In Ukiwaza at the end, tori reverts to the same principle, including the long step. – Leggett, 1982:69

Similarly, practice of the Forms of Gentleness (Ju-no-kata) involves a study of moments of opportunity for evading and countering continuing attacks. A harmonious rhythm is built from perceiving and reacting to actions, countering actions, and countering the countering actions. "One must manage timing by blending with the partner, demonstrating the principle of Ju in reciprocal tai-sabaki. The pair must make an effort to move accurately and smoothly by the practice of correct timing" (Fukuda, 2004:6).

Other katas of Kodokan judo also include studies of rhythm and timing related to the principles expressed in those forms.

Summary

Timing, patterns, and rhythm in martial arts play an important role, one that is too often overlooked. Understanding, perceiving, and directing the many rhythms involved before and during an exchange can give you an added edge in an encounter. Although each is brief in nature, the successive rise and fall of rhythms during a confrontation can constitute significant elements of the interaction. Learning to perceive and act on these rhythms is an important part of training.

As Musashi advises:

> The rhythms of the martial arts are varied. First know the right rhythms and understand the wrong rhythms, and discern the appropriate rhythms from among great and small and slow and fast rhythms. Know the rhythms of spatial relations, and know the rhythms of reversal. These matters are specialties of martial science. Unless you understand these rhythms of reversal, your martial artistry will not be reliable.
>
> The way to win in a battle according to military science is to know the rhythms of the specific opponents, and use rhythms that your opponents do not expect, producing formless rhythms from rhythms of wisdom. In individual martial arts it also happens that an adversary will get out of rhythm in combat and start to fall apart. If you let such a chance get by you, the adversary will recover and thwart you. It is essential to follow up firmly on any loss of poise on the part of an opponent, to prevent him from recovering.
> – Cleary, 1994:31; 91–92

BIBLIOGRAPHY

Aida H. and Harrison, E.J., trans. (1956). *Kodokan judo.* London: W. Foulsham.
Cleary, T., trans. (1994). *The book of five rings.* Boston: Shambhala.
Fukuda, K. (2004). *Ju-no-kata: A Kodokan textbook.* Berkeley: North Atlantic.
Koizumi, G. (1960). *My study of judo.* New York: Cornerstone Library.
Ishikawa,T., and Draeger, D. (1999). *Judo training methods.* Boston: Tuttle.
Leggett, T.P., and Kano, J. (1982). *Kata judo.* London: W. Foulsham and Co.
Leggett, T.P. and Watanabe, K. (1994). *Championship judo.* London: Ippon Books.
Otaki, T. and Draeger, D. (1983). *Judo formal techniques.* Vermont: Tuttle.
Tabata, K. (2003). *Secret tactics: Lessons from the great masters of martial arts.* Boston: Tuttle Publishing.
Tokitsu, K. (2005). *Miyamoto Musashi: His life and writings.* Boston: Weatherhill.
Wilson, W.S., trans. (2002). *The book of five rings: Miyamoto Musashi.* Tokyo: Kodansha International Ltd.

chapter 24

Kodokan Judo's Self-Defense System: Kodokan Goshin-jutsu
by Llyr C. Jones, Ph.D, Martin P. Savage, B.Ed., and W. Lance Gatling, M.A., M.P.S.

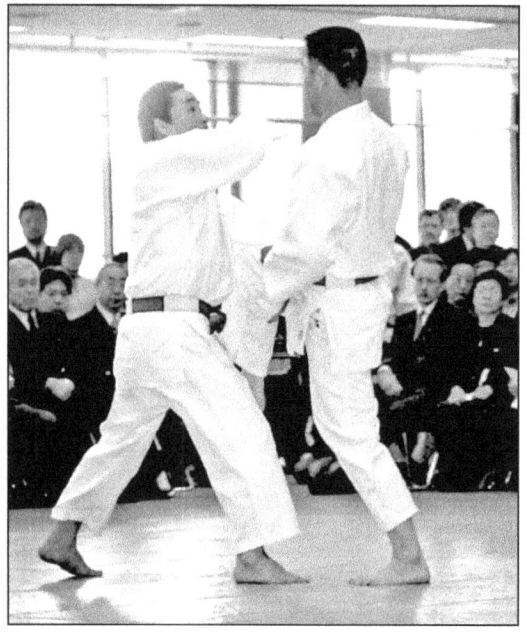

Introduction

Kodokan[1] Judo (*judo*) [the flexible way] developed by Jigoro Kano *shihan* [head teacher[2]] (1860–1938) is an all-round cooperative education, teaching system (pedagogy) and philosophy—based inter alia on conservative Confucianism values, *koryu*[3] [traditional (or old) school] *jujutsu* [flexible art, "the old samurai art of fighting without weapons" (Lindsay and Kano, 1889)] and European liberal educational philosophy (Stevens, 2013: 43). In particular, judo emphasizes the holistic educational value of training in attack and defense, so that it can be a "path", or way of life, that all people can participate in and benefit from.

Judo's *Kodokan Goshin-jutsu* [literally Kodokan Self-Defense Techniques] is an exercise developed in the early 1950s by that era's greatest Kodokan teachers, including Hideichi Nagaoka, Kyuzo Mifune, Kaichiro Samura, Shozo Nakano, Tamio Kurihara, Sumiyuki Kotani, Tadao Otaki, Kenji Tomiki, and others. Today, Kodokan Goshin-jutsu is included in the list of *kata* [forms] officially recognized by the Kodokan.

Purpose, Scope and Structure of this Chapter

Finding information about the technical contents and mechanics of Kodokan Goshin-jutsu is not difficult. Having existed for just sixty years, it is the youngest of all the Kodokan kata, and is well documented by some of the main people involved in its development. Moreover, since Kodokan Goshin-jutsu dates from after Kano's death, there are no original writings by the Shihan, nor any rare historic books on the exercise to be found. However, the texts that go beyond describing Kodokan Goshin-jutsu's mechanical movements (be they in Japanese, English or another Western language) are either out of print or rare, and this makes accessing detailed information on its historical background, theoretical foundations and fundamental principles more challenging.

To address this challenge the present chapter, published to coincide with the sixty-year anniversary of the establishment of Kodokan Goshin-jutsu, provides an accessible and detailed English language study into the exercise. In doing so it contributes to furthering judo knowledge. However, presenting full details on how to perform the complete Kodokan Goshin-jutsu is out of scope, and for this, the reader is directed to the various learning resources referenced herein. In terms of organization, this chapter follows a structure analogous to that found in other work on kata by De Crée and Jones (2009; 2011) and De Crée (2015).

THE POSITION OF KODOKAN GOSHIN-JUTSU IN THE KODOKAN KATA

Kata in Judo

Kata are "formal movement pattern exercises containing idealized model movements illustrating specific combative principles" (Kawamura and Daigo, 2000:86)—which together with *randori* [free practice], *kogi* [lectures] and *mondo* [dialogue] comprise the four critical pillars of Kodokan judo education (De Crée and Jones, 2009; 2011; De Crée, 2015).

Writing (in Japanese) in the early Kodokan journal, *Sakko* [Awakening], Kano explained how judo's kata were formulated in response to the fact that the number of students at the Kodokan was growing, and that he himself could not directly teach each one individually:

> In those [early] days I taught kata personally, to each student, but gradually their numbers increased. To give all students individual instruction became a very time-consuming process... It was shortly thereafter that I realised that new judo kata were needed.
> – Kano, n.d. cited in Watson, 2008

In this context, kata are merely short, predetermined attack and defense sequences that are both a teaching tool, and a training drill. However, in judo, what are most often thought of as kata are the formally recorded sets of choreographed techniques synthesized to illustrate specific principles. Cornish (2004) calls these exercises the "listed kata".

The Listed Kata

In his opening lecture to the 2008 Kodokan Summer Kata Course, Toshiro Daigo[4] gave a brief overview, with some history, of nine "official" listed kata currently recognized by the Kodokan—see Table 1.

Table 1 *Kata*	Intellectual &/or Moral	Physical Conditioning	Attack & Defense	Aesthetic
Nage-no-kata [Forms of Throwing]	O	△	O	△
Katame-no-kata [Forms of Grappling / Holding]	O	△	O	△
Kime-no-kata [Forms of Decisive Techniques]	△		O	
Ju-no-kata [Forms of Gentleness & Flexibility]		O	△	△
Kodokan Goshin-Jutsu [Kodokan Self-Defense]	O		O	
Itsutsu-no-kata [Five Forms]	O			O
Koshiki-no-kata [Ancient Forms]	O		△	O
Go-no-kata [Forms of (proper use of) Force]		O		
Sei-ryoku-zen'yo Kokumin-Taiiku [Forms of Maximum Efficiency National Physical Education]		O	△	
Key. O Significant △ Less Significant				

Daigo's lecture notes (Daigo, 2008) included, inter alia, translated extracts from Kotani and Otaki's 1971 book *Saishin Judo-no-Kata Zen* [The Latest Judo Kata Complete] (Kotani and Otaki, 1971) and also from *Kodokan Judo-no-kata* [The Kata of Kodokan Judo] published by the Kodokan in 1964 (Showa 39). Moreover, the lecture subsequently formed the basis of Daigo's comprehensive, multi-part article on kata—"Kodokan Judo Kata ni Tsuite" ["About the Kata of Kodokan Judo"], which was serialized in seven parts in the Kodokan's periodical *Judo* from October 2008 to April 2009 (Daigo, 2008–2009).

The nine kata each contain various spheres of principles that help teach the *judoka* [a person who practices judo] the overall meaning of *ju-no-ri* [principle of flexibility]—where one avoids directly opposing an opponent's force and power, in favor of using it to one's own advantage (Kawamura and Daigo, 2000:83).

While not a means of formally grouping[5] the various kata per se, Table 1 shows how these principles come to the fore in each kata (Osamu Mouri, personal communication, 13 September 2015).

In counting nine Kodokan kata, Daigo omits the female self-defense kata, Joshi Go-shin-ho, which is an officially sanctioned, but uncommon Kodokan kata[6] (De Crée and Jones, 2011). Additionally, such counting ignores both *Kime Shiki* [forms of decision] and *Ju Shiki* [forms of gentleness]—two kata that were considered as distinct in the past, but today are regarded as being part of Sei-ryoku-zen'yo Kokumin-Taiiku.

Underlying Principles

Towards the end of his life Jigoro Kano (at the age of 75) wrote an important short article on general principles in judo—"The True Significance of Judo and the Purpose of Training" (Kano, 1934 in Imperial Japan Oratory Society, 1934). In the article Kano explained that all applications in judo were created from the fundamental principle of *seiryoku zen'yo* [best use of energy]. Originally in Japanese:

> I taught the principles [of judo], not the application of the principles... If something goes wrong with the application [technique], be it technical or mental, then return to the basic principles and test how closely they are reflected in the application.... if any of the techniques do not conform to the principles, then they are not my teachings, and a mistake has been made in the application of the principle ...
> – Ibid.

This approach goes directly to the very heart of judo, and indicates, inter alia, that kata is not an application, or mere mechanical movements, but rather, is a direct expression of judo's *riai*[7] [underlying principles]. For example, the 15 techniques in Nage-no-kata were deemed sufficient to learn the principles of the entire Gokyo-no-waza [five sets of techniques]—the standard syllabus of judo throwing techniques for randori (O. Mouri, personal communication, 25 January 2007).

Moreover, the principles are timeless and unbounded, and so, for example, Nage-no-kata is equally relevant for learning the Gokyo's subsequent evolutions and additions, such as the Shinmeisho-no-waza [newly accepted techniques]. Principles are also subliminal, and in regular practice today, almost every judoka is actually applying principles that can be found, for example, in Koshiki-no-kata, whether or not they have any knowledge of that particular form, or awareness that they are doing so (Ibid.).

Is Kodokan Goshin-jutsu a kata or not, and why?

Kodokan Goshin-jutsu is not called Kodokan Goshin-jutsu-no-kata [forms of Kodokan self-defense], though this inaccurate name quite often features in some of the less informed material on the exercise. Given the intentional omission of "-no-kata" from the name, it is valid to pose the question "Is Kodokan Goshin-jutsu a kata or not, and why?" To address this issue, this study will use reliable and pertinent material from both primary and secondary sources.

From one standpoint, the compact, but comprehensive, *Kodokan New Japanese-English Dictionary of Judo* by Kawamura and Daigo (2000) indicates that Kodokan Goshin-jutsu is a kata. This perspective of course is consistent with its present-day treatment by the Kodokan:

> *Kodokan Goshinjutsu* (Kodokan Self-Defense Forms): A set of Kodokan Judo formal exercises (*kata*) designed to teach ways and means of self-defense using throwing, grappling and striking techniques, formally devised in 1956 to meet modern needs. – Ibid.:92

However, the literature also contains alternative standpoints, also from serious sources. For example, Steven Cunningham[8] presently USJA[9] 6th dan in an interview with Linda Yiannakis, discusses the content and development of several judo kata, including Kodokan Goshin-jutsu. The interview was serialized as a two-part article in *American Judo*—the journal of the USJA. Therein, Yiannakis (2002:19–21; 2003, 20–24) reports Cunningham's observations:

> Also in the Kodokan syllabus is the Kodokan Goshin-jutsu. Notice that it isn't called Goshin-jutsu no Kata. This is because the Goshin-jutsu is thought to be a plan of study of self-defense techniques (*goshin waza*), as opposed to being formally a kata, although it's often demonstrated that way. – Yiannakis, 2002:20

Cunningham is therefore explaining that it was not intended for Kodokan Goshin-jutsu to be a kata, in the proper sense of "kata", but rather a collection of techniques grouped together to represent defenses against several kinds of attack.

Arguably, the most authoritative answer to the original question comes from Daigo. In a personal exchange, first formally reported in De Crée and Jones (2011), Daigo expressed a revised position to the one he had implied earlier (Kawamura and Daigo, 2000; Daigo, 2008–09):

There are no kata after the death of Kano Jigoro. Sei-ryoku zenyo kokumin taiiku was never meant to be a kata (solely) for judoka but for general physical education (for the general public). Joshi goshinho is more an application than a set of principles, thus consequently intended to be more practical, which is understandable, particularly if we consider the social environment in which it was made by Nango.[10] For the same reason, Kodokan Goshin-jutsu is not given a suffix of '-kata'. – De Crée and Jones, 2011

Daigo's statement is unambiguous—Kodokan Goshin-jutsu is not a kata in the strictest of formal senses, even though today the Kodokan formally treats it as if it were one. Daigo indicates that Kodokan Goshin-jutsu, and the other two[11] exercises without "-no-kata" in their names, are actually *ho* [methods]— that is, sequential groups of related techniques in a framework of principles, whose "performance" as formal demonstration was never intended. Strictly interpreting Daigo's statement yields an "official list" of seven Kodokan kata—namely Nage-no-kata, Katame-no-kata, Ju-no-kata, Go-no-kata, Kime-no-kata, Itsutu-no-kata and Koshiki-no-kata.

Earlier, the senior British judoka Syd Hoare[12] presently BJA13 8th dan had presented an identical viewpoint to Daigo—similarly arguing that there could be no new kata after the death of Kano, and intimating that any such creations would lack legitimacy and authority in the absence of his personal endorsement:

From a Japanese point of view judo froze in time in 1938 when Kano died. He created Kodokan Judo which ipso facto made him the master (or *shihan*) of the school. What he created could of course be changed by him while he was still alive but not after his death... attempts to create new kata in judo have always foundered on this point. – Hoare, 2010

THE CREATION OF KODOKAN GOSHIN-JUTSU

A New Kodokan Self-defense System

Kodokan Goshin-jutsu was formally established on 8 January 1956. Yiannakis (2002) presents Cunningham's observations on its historical origin and nature:

The Goshin-jutsu is a construction of the 1950s, when 21 masters came together to construct a modernized form of self-defense to be taught in the Kodokan. The most influential and probably the best known to us in the West of those members was Tomiki. Kenji Tomiki had been a student of Kano and had also, by arrangement of Kano, studied under Ueshiba, of the Aikido school. Tomiki was also sent around to other of the traditional ryu, by Kano, to people that Kano knew and had made arrangements with, like Aoyagi at Sosuishi-ryu (also pronounced Sosu-ishitsu-ryu) and others. All of that old knowledge was brought to bear in the construction of the modern Goshin-jutsu. There were earlier Goshin-jutsu which are no longer practiced. They were discarded, hidden away for various reasons, and there was a feeling that there was a need for a Goshin-jutsu but the Kodokan wanted a modernized version. And so that was why they called together these instructors and asked them to construct this art. So this is designed to teach the goshin waza, whereas the Nage and Katame-no-kata teach the randori waza. – Yiannakis, 2002:20

These remarks however are incorrect. Around 1930, Kano in fact sent two judoka—Jiro Takeda and Minoru Mochizuki[14] to study under Morihei Ueshiba (1883–1969), the eventual founder of what is now known as *aikido* [the way of unifying spirit, or, the way of spiritual harmony]. Tomiki himself had already been studying *aiki-jujutsu*[15] [the martial art of unifying spirit] directly under Ueshiba since 1926 (Shishida, 2011).

Unfortunately, Cunningham provides no specific references for his view that other Goshin-jutsu methods already existed before the war, but were subsequently concealed. One example of such an earlier method would be *Mifune Soen Goshin-jutsu* [Mifune's Personal Self-defense Techniques]—an exercise, as its name suggests, developed by Kyuzo Mifune. However, at no point was it hidden away. Mifune Soen Goshin-jutsu will be described and referenced later in this chapter when more relevant for the further content.

Relationship to Kime-no-kata

To fully understand the motivation for Kodokan Goshin-jutsu's creation, it is necessary to explore the history, position in judo, and principles of Kime-no-kata.

Kime-no-kata was intended as a kata for real combat, which was reflected in its original name—Shinken-Shobu-no-kata [forms of real fighting][16]. The number of techniques in the kata was initially ten, and this number was then increased to 13 or 15. The kata was later expanded again to give today's 20-technique form, and at the same time was renamed Kime-no-kata. The kata drew upon techniques from unattributed koryu jujutsu schools, as well as on Kano's own ideas.

Standardization, codification and unification of Kime-no-kata proved to be challenging, and due to a failure to agree, it was not ratified at the 24 July 1906's famous conclave of leading koryu jujutsu and judo masters held at the Kyoto Butokuden [Hall of Martial Virtues] of the Dai Nippon Butokukai (DNBK) [Greater Japan Martial Virtue Society]. Nevertheless, the Kodokan continued to use it, and eventually it was formally adopted as a Kodokan kata (Kano Sensei Biographic Editorial Committee, 2009:63–65; Hoare, 2009:62, 114–115; Kano (n.d.) cited in Watson, 2008;79–80). However, it was never formally adopted by the DNBK.

Kime-no-kata supports the study of the theoretical basis of attack and defense. Its 20 techniques are divided into two sections—eight *idori* [kneeling] used while in *seiza* [formal seated position], and 12 *tachiai* [standing] used whilst standing. Each of these two sections contains practical and realistic defenses against empty-handed and armed attacks, and involves the safe practice of counter-attacking and control techniques prohibited from daily judo randori and shiai.

The main underlying principles for the defenses in Kime-no-kata are *tai-sabaki* [body movement],[17] *shisei* [good posture], leverage and the use of *katame waza* [controlling techniques] (Kotani et al, 1968:92–123). By understanding and developing a mastery of Kime-no-kata, one acquires the decisiveness, focus, strength of character and skills relevant to a variety of critical situations.

Kime-no-kata was formalized during the Meji period[18] but its heritage is in Edo-period[19] Japan. It therefore features defenses against typical real-world attacks from that time—including those from assailants armed with a *daisho* [literally, big-little sword set] comprising a *katana* [long, single-edged Japanese sword] and a *wakizashi* [short sword], and also those armed with a *tanto* [knife]. The idori section of the kata reflects the scenario of a samurai visiting a *daimyo* [feudal lord] and leaving his katana at the entrance[20], but retaining his wakizashi and tanto (Carl De Crée, personal communication, 30 January 2006).

In everyday Kime-no-kata practice, a *bokken* [wooden sword] represents the katana, while a wooden[21] tanto doubles as the tanto and also the wakizashi (Ibid.). The tanto is used multiple times, in both the idori and tachiai sections, and also twice in a manner representing a wakizashi in the *kirikomi* [downward slash] attacks, both standing and seated. At some unknown time, it was deemed unnecessary to actually use two different short weapons in the kata since at the upper extreme of the tanto and the lower extreme of the wakizashi, the weapons are fairly similar in length, though the attacks with them are distinctly different. Also, the use of a tanto to represent a wakizashi simplifies the weapons handling protocol in the kata and removes the awkwardness of carrying three weapons on the tatami. When the wooden knife is being used as a tanto it is secured inside the jacket of the *judogi* [traditional uniform for judo], and when it represents a wakizashi it is secured in the belt outside the jacket.

Example techniques from Kime-no-kata are shown in the vintage photographs of Figures 1 and 2. The photographs date from the early 20th century, and are from the personal collection of one of the authors (WLG). Figure 1 shows *Ude-hishigi-hara-gatame* [arm crushing stomach armlock] from *yoko-tsuki* [side thrust] in the idori section, and Figure 2 shows *kataha-jime* [single-wing choke] from *nuki-gake* [sword unsheathing] in the tachiai section. Yoko-tsuki and nuki-gake are the eighth and eleventh techniques of the idori and tachiai sections respectively.

Figure 1 (left):
Ude-hishigi-hara-gatame [arm crushing stomach armlock] from *yoko-tsuki* [side thrust] in the *idori* [kneeling] section of *Kime-no-kata* [forms of decisive techniques].

Figure 2 (right):
Kataha-jime [single-wing choke] from *nukigake* [sword unsheathing] in the *tachiai* [standing] section of *Kime-no-kata* [forms of decisive techniques]. Hideichi Nagaoka is *tori* [the one demonstrating the technique] and Yoshitsugu Yamashita is *uke* [the one attacking].

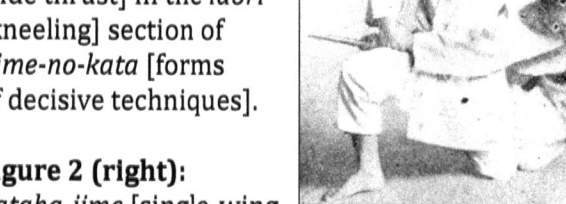
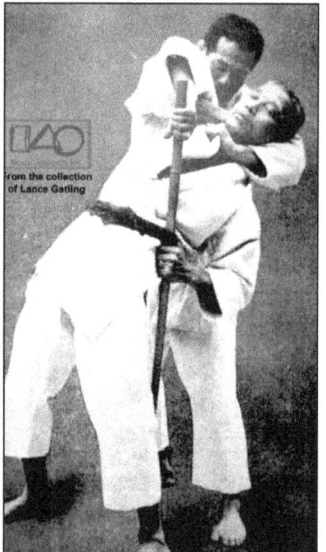

The identity of the two judoka in Figure 1 is not known to the authors, but the two in Figure 2 are among the Kodokan's most distinguished judoka ever, with tori and uke[22] being respectively Hideichi Nagaoka (1876–1952) and Yoshitsugu[23] Yamashita (1865–1935). At the time both held the rank of Kodokan 7th dan, and both subsequently went on to hold the exceptional rank of Kodokan 10th dan. Most notably, Yamashita was the Kodokan's first[24] ever 10th dan holder.

Through a series of government edicts in the late nineteenth century, the open carry of swords became all but outlawed in Japan. Additionally, sitting in seiza became much less common. With these changes in lifestyle, Kime-no-kata gradually became considered outmoded for practical self-defense, and it was therefore necessary to devise a new exercise better suited to more modern circumstances. Recognizing this need, in 1952, the Kodokan established a dedicated research team (or committee) for this purpose[25].

The new exercise was to include defenses against a broader range of unarmed attacks than Kime-no-kata, and also against attacks involving more contemporary weapons—specifically, a tanto, a *jo* [staff] and a *kenju* [pistol]. Attacks with the sword and short sword were discarded.

The Research Team

The Kodokan research committee charged with creating the new self-defense exercise began work in September 1952. There were no less than 25 members of the team, all holding rank of 7th dan or higher, though the composition of the team did vary, both in personnel and numbers, over the time that it took to complete the task.

The names of the 25 main committee members and their historical rank (that is, at the time Kodokan Goshin-jutsu was created) are presented in Table 2 (O. Mouri, personal communication, 10 March 2014).

Table 2: The Kodokan Goshin-jutsu Research Team

Rank	Research Team Members
10th dan	Hideichi Nagaoka[26], Kyuzo Mifune, Kaichiro Samura
9th dan	Join Oda, Tamio Kurihara, Shozo Nakano
8th dan	Gensui Arai, Koki Ito, Goichi Ebii, Chu Kawakami, Yoji Kikuchi, Kazuzo Kudo, Masao Koyasu, Sumiyuki Kotani, Itsuyo Sawa, Kiyoshi Suzuki, Kisaburo Takahashi, Hamakichi Takahashi, Isao Nagahata, Masaru Hayakawa, Tadao Otaki
7th dan	Fusataro Sakamoto, Chugo Sato, Kenji Tomiki, Yoshizo Matsumoto

From Table 2 it can be seen that the theoretical and practical contribution for the development of Kodokan Goshin-jutsu came from the preeminent Kodokan teachers of the time, with three of the team, Hideichi Nagaoka,[27] Kyuzo Mifune (1883–1965), and Kaichiro Samura (1880–1964), holding the rank of Kodokan 10th dan. Two of these 10th dan holders had koryu experience—specifically Nagaoka in Kito-ryu [school of the rise and fall] jujutsu, Noda-ha [Noda clan lineage], and Samura in Takeuchi Santo-ryu jujutsu [a now extinct koryu jujutsu style centered on the city of Kumamoto] (De Crée and Jones, 2011; C. De Crée, personal communication, 30 March 2012).

The third 10th dan holder, Mifune, had no known koryu experience, but had experimented extensively with judo's connections to both jujutsu and *torite*[28] [literally, "grasping hands"]. Despite being ideologically very different to Kano, Mifune had one of the most original and technically brilliant minds in judo. He had already contributed significantly to judo self-defense through a strong involvement in developing Joshi Goshin Ho, and also through the creation of Mifune Soen Goshin-jutsu (De Crée and Jones, 2011; De Crée, 2015).

Created sometime between 1937 and 1942, or perhaps earlier, Mifune Soen Goshin-jutsu mainly incorporates koryu and torite techniques. The exercise can be seen on a 2005-produced DVD of the famous 1955 film project—*Judo no Shinzui* [The Essence of Judo], with Mifune himself (as tori) demonstrating the techniques, and his dedicated *deshi* [student]—Sei'ichi Shirai (as uke) attacking and being defeated (Mifune, 2005). At the time of filming Mifune was 72 years old, yet still very vigorous.

Two of the team's three 9th dan holders were posthumously promoted to 10th dan—specifically Shozo Nakano (1888–1977) promoted to 10th dan in 1977, and Tamio Kurihara (1896–1979) promoted to 10th dan in 1979. One of the team's 8th dan holders was also to later achieve the rank of 10th dan—specifically Sumiyuki Kotani (1903–1991) who was promoted to that rank, during his lifetime, in 1984. Also prominent among the committee's 8th dan holders were Kazuzo Kudo[29] (1898–1970) and Tadao Otaki[30] (1908–1992)—both later promoted to 9th dan.

From the team, it is Kotani (Figure 3) and Tomiki (Figure 4) who arguably became the greatest and best-known experts of Kodokan Goshin-jutsu. Kotani's personal performance of the exercise was known to be very impressive—particularly his *tekubi-waza* [wrist techniques]. A rare color recording of him performing Kodokan Goshin-jutsu does exist—though, to date, it has not been made available on modern media.

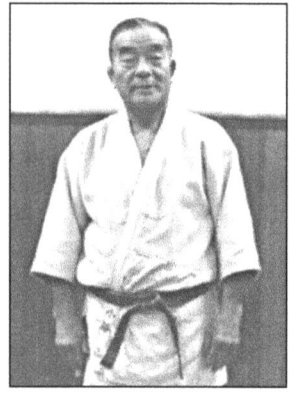
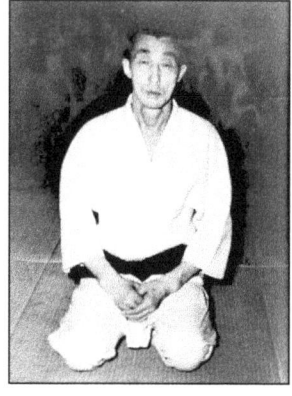

Figure 3
Sumiyuki Kotani
(1903–1991).

Figure 4
Kenji Tomiki
(1900–1979).

As well as having a very high level of personal proficiency, Tomiki's contribution to the development of Kodokan Goshin-jutsu was particularly significant, and will be detailed now.

Role and Contribution of Kenji Tomiki

The name from the research team that is most closely associated with the formulation of Kodokan Goshin-jutsu is undoubtedly Kenji Tomiki (1900- 1979). He wrote the first and most important textbook on the exercise—*Kodokan Goshin-jutsu* (Tomiki, 1958), Figure 5, and also the slightly earlier and highly original book, *Judo, Appendix: Aikido* later renamed *Judo and Aikido* (Tomiki, 1956; 1967). *Judo, Appendix: Aikido*, Figure 6, explains how judo and aikido complement each other, with the book's aikido appendix being among the earliest English language text on that system.

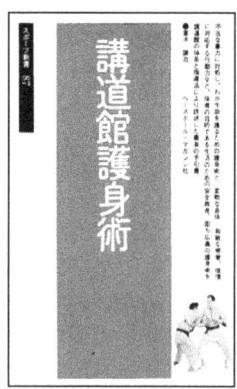
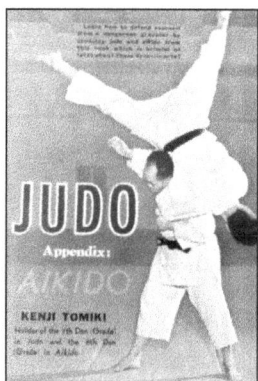

Figure 5
Kodokan Goshin-jutsu by Kenji Tomiki was published in 1958 and was the first textbook on the exercise.

Figure 6
Judo, Appendix: Aikido by Kenji Tomiki was published in 1956 and takes a highly original approach to both styles.

Tomiki was born on 15 March 1900 in Kakunodate, Akita Prefecture. He was one of the earliest students of Morihei Ueshiba, and also a direct student of Kano-shihan. A graduate of the Political Economic Department of Waseda University[31], Tomiki later became Professor of Calligraphy, and also head of the Physical Education Department, at his alma marter. Additionally, he was a member of the Kodokan's Special Direction Committee and an official of the All Japan Judo Federation. Tomiki was also central to continuing and executing some of the theoretical work to reinforce the martial aspects of judo that Kano started to reconsider near the end of his life.[32] Shishida (2010; 2011; 2012; 2013) describes a number of these plans.

In a formative article in the development of Kodokan Goshin-jutsu, Tomiki (1953) explored the relationships between judo as a martial art, as self-defense, and as a restricted subset of koryu jujutsu. Some of the key themes in this chapter will now be presented as they provide important background context to Tomiki's contribution to Kodokan Goshin-jutsu.

Originally, koryu jujutsu schools taught a broad range of techniques, including many of those in the *bugei juhappan* [the "traditional" eighteen martial arts] that every samurai should know[33]. These arts include *so-jutsu* [art of spear], *naginata-jutsu* [art of halberd], *kyu-jutsu* [archery], *ken-jutsu* [art of sword], *bo-jutsu* [art of staff], *jo-jutsu* [art of short staff], even *ba-jutsu* [martial horse-riding] and *sui-jutsu* [combative swimming].

Examples of schools, still extant, that would teach such a large number of armed and unarmed techniques today include Takeuchi-ryu [one of the oldest koryu schools founded by Hisamori Takenouchi who instituted the school during the late Muromachi period], Araki-ryu [believed to have been founded by Araki Muninsai, and originally taught in the area near modern Nagoya] and Sosuishitsu-ryu [School of Grasping the Two Waters]. These are known as *sogo bujutsu* [integrated or comprehensive martial arts] as opposed to a single purpose school like archery or swordsmanship.

Koryu jujutsu's techniques include those for situations such as when gripping one's opponent [*kumu*]—throwing, pinning, choking, and crushing; those for when separated and not gripping one's opponent—striking, thrusting, and kicking; those for when unarmed and facing an armed opponent—defending against strikes with sword, spear, staff, and finally those for when armed—using weapons such as sword, spear and staff. In his judo, Kano restricted koryu's multiple complex techniques in favor of throwing and grappling techniques, with striking techniques being restricted to kata.

In his seminal article, Tomiki highlighted that there are two methods of ensuring that an attacker's violence cannot be directed against oneself—simply to injure, or not to injure, the adversary. Tomiki also emphasized that there are two types of joint techniques—the first type being direct attacks to vulnerable areas for inflicting, or threatening to inflict damage to the adversary's joints, and the second type being indirect attacks against mechanically vulnerable areas to destroy the assailant's balance. Furthermore, Tomiki highlighted that there are two ways of considering atemi-waza. First, as techniques used against the opponent's physiological weak points [*kyusho*] to injure or kill them, and secondly as techniques used against his biomechanical weak points to take his balance [*kuzushi*] and throw him.

Tomiki's innovative concept was to use judo for close range, and aikido from at a distance, and while there is no direct mention of Kodokan Goshin-jutsu in the text of *Judo, Appendix: Aikido*, there is content very closely associated with it. Unsurprisingly, this material is found in the aikido appendix, alongside some of the ideas presented in the 1953 article (Tomiki, 1956; 1967:101–180). For example, Figure 7 shows Tomiki executing defenses against an attacker armed with a pistol (Ibid.:166–167). These have clearly been incorporated, albeit in a slightly modified form, into Kodokan Goshin-jutsu (Ibid.:170–171).

Tomiki's role in developing Kodokan Goshin-jutsu is often overstated, particularly by Western authors, with many incorrectly suggesting that either he would have personally created, or compiled, the exercise, or else would have been the Chairman of the committee that did so. In 1956 when Kodokan Goshin-jutsu was established, Tomiki held the judo rank of Kodokan 7th dan, and the *aiki-budo*[34] [the martial way of unifying spirit] rank of 8th dan[35]. Tomiki was not the committee Chairman, since at the time, six of its members were 9th or 10th dan holders, with 15 others holding 8th dan, and all therefore senior to him. Given the strong hierarchical structure of Japanese society, protocol and respect for seniority would have made Nagaoka, Mifune and Samura the leaders.

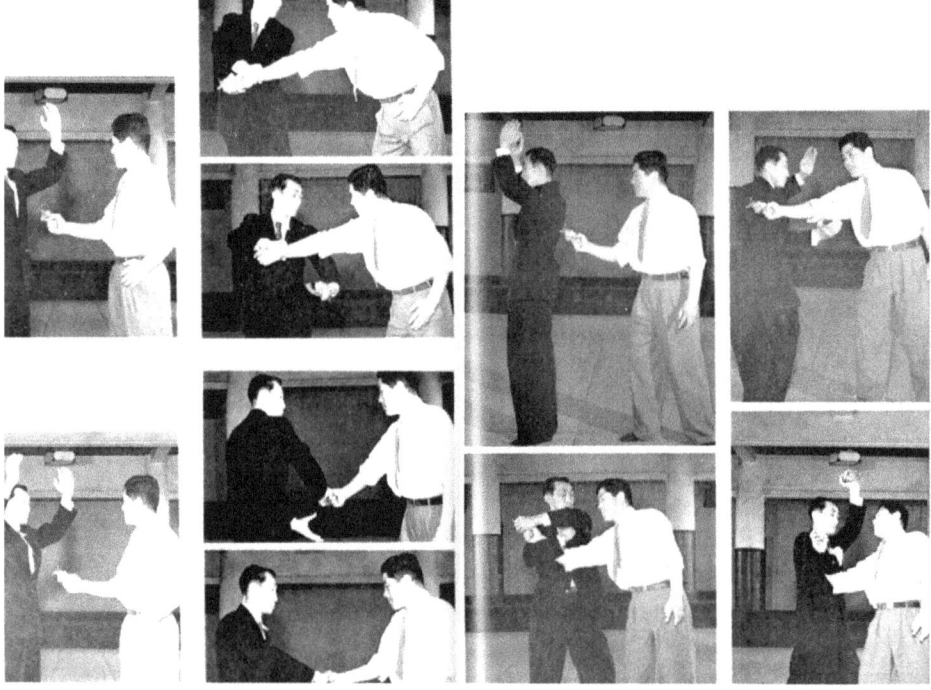

Figure 7: Kenji Tomiki showing a number of aikido defenses against an attacker armed with a pistol. From his own book, *Judo Appendix Aikido*.

Notwithstanding, Tomiki was a major technical contributor to the development of Kodokan Goshin-jutsu—providing, in particular, a very strong aiki-jujutsu input. Risei Kano (1900–1986), the (third) Kodokan Kancho from 1946 to 1980 (and the Shihan's son) specifically highlighted Tomiki's contribution in his preface to the original 1958 Kodokan Goshin-jutsu textbook. Originally in Japanese:

> Kano-shihan made every effort possible to complete judo as a modern physical education, but could not yet systematize the self-defense aspect of judo which is contained in classical jujutsu, even though he did study it deeply. That he was very much concerned about the self-defense aspect of judo is clearly seen from the fact that he sent some of his students to Ueshiba-sensei to study aiki-jujutsu, and also invited an expert on jo-jutsu to the Kodokan for a seminar. Some of the self-defense techniques are incorporated into Kime-no-kata which

is well known to all. After WWII, quite a few judoka abroad showed interest in the self-defense aspect of judo, and the Kodokan organized a panel to create and publish the Kodokan Goshin-jutsu. As stated earlier, since the Kodokan had already started its study, it was fairly easy to reach consensus. The writer of this book, Professor Kenji Tomiki has deep understanding of judo as a Professor at Waseda University and also as an authority on research of aiki-jutsu in the light of judo principles. In formulating Goshin-jutsu, he played a leading role in the panel. I am firmly convinced, therefore, that this book will become the best guidebook for all practitioners of judo self-defense.

Risei Kano, December 1958   – Tomiki, 1958:3–4

Additionally, Tomiki was tori in the first public demonstration of Kodokan Goshin-jutsu during the Kagami Biraki ceremony held at the Tokyo Budokan in January 1956. His fellow committee-member, Otaki, was uke. In this demonstration, Kodokan Goshin-jutsu was shown as an unceremonial and practical self-defense method based on judo principles, rather than a formal kata[36]. Highlights from this demonstration can be seen on the DVD *Classic Judo Kata* edited by Hal Sharp[37] (2013), and also on the most recent DVD release of the Kodokan-produced Kodokan Goshin-jutsu instructional film (Kodokan, 2009)—see later.

Tomiki was promoted to the judo rank of Kodokan 8th dan in 1971, and died on 25 December 1979. He was 79 years old.

STRUCTURE AND TECHNICAL CONTENTS OF KODOKAN GOSHIN-JUTSU

The Name Kodokan Goshin-jutsu

Goshin-jutsu means "self-defense", and is merely a set of applications that can be used in conflict situations. The inclusion of the term "-jutsu" does not imply that Kodokan Goshin-jutsu is part of *bujutsu*[38] [martial art/science]—it is of course part of judo, a martial way [budo[39]], where there is greater emphasis on principles and educational aspects, than on the use of techniques in actual combat.

Tomiki explains, in a matter-of-fact way, why "Kodokan" was affixed to the title of the new exercise. Over the first 38 pages of the original Kodokan Goshin-jutsu textbook (Tomiki, 1958), he emphasizes that judo self-defense must be a practical application of judo techniques that are derived from judo principles. In so doing, Tomiki is placing Kodokan Goshin-jutsu firmly within the context of judo, and is primarily for this reason that today the exercise is regarded as a member of the Kodokan kata family.

Including the word "Kodokan" as a prefix was natural, as it clearly differentiated the new exercise from the archaic Kime-no-kata. Whereas in Kime-no-kata one could maim, or kill, an attacker, Kodokan Goshin-jutsu was a more modern adjunct for self-defense purposes only. Kodokan Goshin-jutsu was also designed to be consistent with a core principle of judo, namely seiryoku zen'yo, with its aim being not to damage or punish an attacker, but to immobilize or incapacitate them, so that no further attack was possible (Cornish, 1984:7).

Past Names for Kodokan Goshin-jutsu

Kodokan Goshin-jutsu has, in the past, been infrequently referred to by two other names—Ippan-yo Goshin-no-kata [Regular Use Self Defense Forms] and Shin-Kime-no-kata [New Kime-no-kata].

Ippan-yo Goshin-no-kata

The opening paragraph of Chapter X, "General Description of the Prearranged Forms of Judo" in the text *Illustrated Kodokan Judo* mentions for the first time a self-defense kata called Ippan-yo Goshin-no-kata [Regular Use Self-Defense Forms]:

> There are nine kinds of kata or forms generally taught today at Kodokan. They are ... (3) Kime-no-kata (Forms of Decision) or Shinken-shobu-no-kata (Forms of Actual Fighting) ... (8) Fujoshi-yo-Goshin-no-kata (Forms of Self-Defence for Girls and Women); and (9) Ippan-yo-Goshin-no-kata (Forms of Self-Defence for Men).
> – Kodokan, 1955:161

Ippan-yo-Goshin-no-kata was the unofficial temporary designation ("working title") for Kodokan Goshin-jutsu during its development phase, which by when Illustrated Kodokan Judo was first published in 1955, was almost at an end. It is not known why Ippan-yo Goshin-no-kata was wrongly translated in the book as "Forms of Self-Defence for Men", though it can be speculated that the erroneous inclusion of the phrase "for Men" could have been an attempt to distinguish it from the self-defense exercises for women, which, through Joshi Goshin Ho[40] had been available since 1943. The inclusion of the phrase "Regular Use" in the proper translation suggests that the exercise was intended for the general public, and not just for professionals like security operatives, law enforcement officers and other individuals working in high-risk environments.

Mikinosuke Kawaishi (1899–1970) DNBK / Kodokan 7th dan, FFJDA[41] 10th dan[42] mentions similar self-defense kata in his significant book[43] *The Complete 7 Katas of Judo*:

> At the Kodokan they still study the Seiryoku-zenyo-kokumin-taiku-no-kata, or Kata of Physical Training, and also two derived from the Kime-no-kata, a Kata of Defence for Women and another a little different for Men.
> – Kawaishi, 1957:11

While the Japanese names of these two other self-defense kata is omitted, the clear parallels between Kawaishi's text and that previously cited, would suggest that they are Joshi Goshin Ho and Ippan-yo-Goshin-no-kata respectively.

Inexplicably, Ippan-yo Goshin-no-kata continues to be mentioned in the later and expanded (299 pages cf. 285), reprint of *Illustrated Kodokan Judo*. This is despite Kodokan Goshin-jutsu having by then been established for 20 years, summarized in Chapter X[44] (Kodokan, 1976:163), and described in detail in Chapter XIV (Ibid.:209–216).

> There are nine kinds of kata or forms generally taught today at Kodokan. They are.... (3) Kime-no-kata (Forms of Decision) or Shinken-shobu-no-kata (Forms of Actual Fighting); (4) Kodokan-Goshin-jutsu (Forms of Self-Defence) ... (9) Fujoshi-yo-Goshin-no-kata (Forms of Self-Defence for Girls and Women); and (10) Ippan-yo-Goshin-no-kata (Forms of Self-Defence for Men).
> – Ibid.:161

The statement "There are nine kinds of kata ..." with the subsequent listing of ten exercises indicates editorial quality control shortcomings with the reprint. Beyond this error, by separately numbering Ippan-yo-Goshin-no-kata and Kodokan Goshin-jutsu, the reprint is implying that they are different exercises, which, as already explained, is incorrect. Additionally, inserting Kodokan Goshin-jutsu into fourth position in the list, instead of being appended at the end, is an error and source of confusion, as it causes the other, and earlier, Kodokan kata to be wrongly ordered.

Note that the 1986 revised and update version of *Illustrated Kodokan Judo*, published by Kodansha under the simple title of *Kodokan Judo* (Kano[45], 1986), makes no mention of Ippan-yo-Goshin-no-kata. This reliably establishes the obsolescence of this 1950s interim designation and the discontinuation of its use.

The final named mention of Ippan-yo-Goshin-no-kata in the literature is in Cunningham's wide-ranging interview with Yiannakis. Therein, Yiannakis remarks:

> There are other kata which are not currently recognized by the Kodokan, such as Go no Kata, Ippon Yo Goshin-jutsu no Kata [sic], Gonosen no Kata, and others. What are the origins and nature of these so-called "lost kata" and why do you think they are no longer widely known?   – Yiannakis, 2003:20

Cunningham responds:

> As for the other kata, for example, there were earlier Goshin Jutsu. There was Ippon Yo Goshin Jutsu no Kata [sic] and Fujoshi Goshin-jutsu no Kata. Ippon Yo Goshin-jutsu no Kata—*ippon yo* means "general; it's the general self-defense art that was taught to everybody. There had to be some place to learn all the goshin waza, which was the other half of judo. You have randori waza and goshin waza, and if you're going to teach the full syllabus, you have to teach both.
>
> There was also Fujoshi Goshin-jutsu no Kata, which was the women's version. What it really meant was that it was the techniques which are special to women's attacks. It focused on those specifically. These two kata, like the Go no Kata, were sort of lost before WWII, quite deliberately I think, and the loss of them gave rise to the Joshi Goshinho and Kime Shiki that appeared in the Women's Division during WWII, and the new Goshin Jutsu which appeared in the 1950s as a result of the research group that I mentioned earlier.
> – Ibid.:20

Cunningham does not provide any references for his view that Ippon Yo Goshin Jutsu no Kata [sic] was an early self-defense form, and that it, together with some other kata such as Go-no-kata, were lost pre-war. Moreover, there are several material errors in his answer to Yiannakis. First, Kime Shiki pre-dates Joshi Goshin Ho by a decade or more. Next, while it is correct that Go-no-kata is seldom taught or practiced today, it is not "lost" having been preserved mainly by the efforts of the late Yoshiyuki Kuhara (1906–1985) Kodokan 9th dan and his nephew Toshiyasu Ochiai, presently Kodokan 8th dan (De Crée and Jones, 2009; Ochiai, 2012). Finally, as already explained, Ippan-yo Goshin-no-kata was merely Kodokan Goshin-jutsu's working title, and so clearly post-war. Given the litany of errors in this answer, Cunningham's observations on Ippan-yo Goshin-no-kata should be discarded.

Shin-Kime-no-kata

The kata books written by Sumiyuki Kotani, in combination with various other authors, have long been a reference text for serious judoka. One of the most detailed treatments of Kodokan Goshin-jutsu is contained in the book *Kata of Kodokan Judo*, and its reprint, the *Kata of Kodokan Judo Revised* (Kotani et al, 1968:54–91):

Kodokan Goshinjitsu [sic.] is the new form formulated by Kodokan Judo Institute in January 1956 and is composed of, as its name manifests, 21 techniques suitable for defending ourselves from unexpected attacks of others.... It may be called as Shin-Kime-no-kata (New Forms of Self-defense).   – Ibid.:54

Similarly, John Cornish[46], in his detailed booklet on Kodokan Goshin-jutsu writes:

The Go-shin-jutsu is sometimes called the *Shin* (new) Kime-no-kata, and as it contains different defence moves from those in Kime-no-kata, even where the attack is the same, it can be thought of as an addition to Kime-no-kata.
– Cornish, 1984:3

Additionally, Daigo's previously mentioned lecture note presents a brief overview of Kodokan Goshin-jutsu, together with some of its history. This material is a translated excerpt from Kotani and Otaki (1971):

This kata was made at Showa 31 (January 1956). It is almost the same as Kime no kata. It should be called Shin kime no kata (New Kime no kata).
– Kotani and Otaki, 1971 cited in Daigo, 2008)

Notwithstanding these references from senior judoka, the name Shin-Kime-no-kata, although sometimes heard, was never officially in use, and so should be discarded.

Etiquette in Kodokan Goshin-jutsu

The *reiho*[47] [etiquette] in Kodokan Goshin-jutsu, has tori standing with *joseki* [seat of seniority] to his right. This is a reversal of the positions in the more basic, Randori-no-kata, but identical to those in Ju-no-kata. After the initial standing bow, uke turns through 90° to face joseki, walks forwards, kneels in seiza and then places the weapons on the *tatami* [mat]—see Figure 8. Uke then returns to his original position and stands facing tori. Both tori and uke then step forward into *shizen-hontai* [basic natural posture] ready to begin.

Note that the reiho within Kodokan Goshin-jutsu has changed over time. Originally, a seated bowing ceremony was featured, and then for an interim period, either a sitting or a standing bow[48] was accepted. Finally, normalization of Kodokan Goshin-jutsu standards resulted in the standing bowing ceremony that is always seen today.

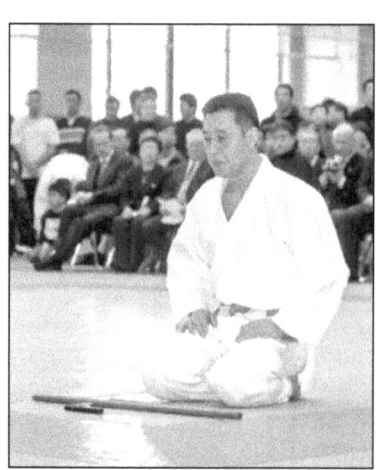

Figure 8
Etiquette in Kodokan Goshin-jutsu shown by Masaru Sato.

Technical Contents of Kodokan Goshin-jutsu

A schematic overview of the structure and contents of Kodokan Goshin-jutsu is presented in Table 3 where it can be seen that the exercise is divided into two main sections—each containing defenses against distinct and differentiated attack types—*toshi-no-bu* [unarmed attacks] and *buki-no-bu* [armed attacks].

Structural and Functional Overview of Kodokan Goshin-jutsu

Table 3	*Kodokan Goshin-jutsu* [Kodokan Self-defense]	
TOSHU-NO-BU [UNARMED ATTACKS]		
Kumitsu-kareta-baai [When held]	*Hanareta-baai* [When attacked from a distance]	
1. *Ryote-dori* [Two-hand hold] 2. *Hidari-eri-dori* [Left-lapel hold] 3. *Migi-eri-dori* [Right-lapel hold] 4. *Kataude-dori* [Single-hand hold] 5. *Ushiro-eri-dori* [Collar hold from behind] 6. *Ushiro-jime* [Choke from behind] 7. *Kakae-dori* [Seize and hold from behind]	1. *Naname-uchi* [Slanting strike] 2. *Ago-tsuki* [Uppercut] 3. *Gammen-tsuki* [Thrust-punch to face] 4. *Mae-geri* [Front kick] 5. *Yoko-geri* [Side kick]	
BUKI-NO-BU [ARMED ATTACKS]		
Tanto-no-baai [Knife attacks]	*Tsue-no-baai* [Staff attacks]	*Kenju-no-baai* [Pistol attacks]
1. *Tsukkake* [Thrust] 2. *Choku-tsuki* [Straight thrust] 3. *Naname-tsuki* [Slanting stab]	1. *Furiage* [Upswing] 2. *Furi-oroshi* [Downswing] 3. *Morote-tsuki* [Two-hand thrust]	1. *Shomen-zuke* [At the front] 2. *Koshi-gamae* [Held on hip] 3. *Haimen-zuke* [At the back]
VOCALS		
By *Uke*	By *Tori*	
Kiai for all *atemi-waza* "*Te wo ageru*" for all *Kenshu-no-bai*	Kiai for all *atemi-waza*	

The names of the individual attacks themselves follow an established and highly efficient naming convention, as described by Cornish:

> The Japanese names used for the techniques in the kata only describe parts of the attack. To use a comprehensive description of all the attack and the defence would make the name too long-winded and, for the non-Japanese, difficult to remember whereas these short names should prove no difficulty at all. The English... is not meant to be a transcription of the Japanese names, like them it is meant only as a memory aid. – Ibid.:3

The Toshu-no-bu section contains 12 attacks, split into two subsections. The first one, called Kumitsukareta-baai, consists of seven attacks from an assailant that one is already in contact with, or who is close by. The second, called Hanareta-baai, contains five attacks at a distance, with the attacker suddenly coming in from afar. Example techniques from Toshu-no-bu are shown in Figures 9a and 9b. Specifically, Figure 9a shows *Kote-hineri* [wrist twist] from *Ryote-dori* [two hand-hold] and Figure 9b shows *osoto-otoshi* [major outer drop twist] from *naname-uchi* [slanting strike]. Recall from Table 3 that Ryote-dori and naname-uchi are the first attacks in the Kumitsu-kareta-baai and Hanareta-baai subsections respectively.

The Buki-no-bu section contains nine named attacks, split into three subsections, of three attacks each. The first subsection, named Tanto-no-baai comprises three knife attacks. The second, named Tsue-no-baai comprises three staff attacks. The third, named Kenju-no-baai comprises three pistol attacks. Example techniques from Buki-no-bu are shown in Figures 10a, 10b and 10c. Figure 10a shows tori taking away uke's knife from *naname-tsuki* [slanting stab], Figure 10b shows tori throwing uke down from *furi-oroshi* [downswing], and Figure 10c shows tori throwing uke from *haimen-zuke* [pistol at the back]. Again, recall from Table 3 that naname-tsuki is the third attack in the Tanto-no-baai subsection, furi-oroshi is the second attack in the Tsue-no-baai subsection and Haimen-zuke is the third attack in the Kenju-no-baai subsection.

Figure 9a (left): *Kote-hineri* [wrist twist] from *ryote-dori* [two hand-hold] in the *toshi-no-bu* [unarmed attacks] section.

Figure 9b (right): *Osoto-otoshi* [major outer drop twist] from *naname-uchi* [slanting strike] in the *toshi-no-bu* [unarmed attacks] section.

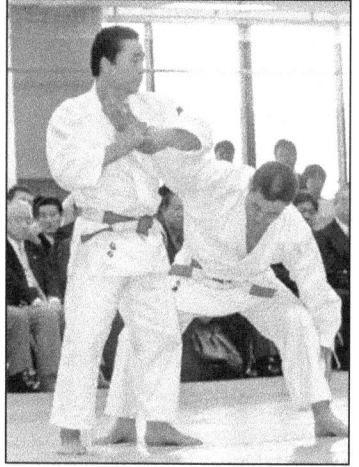
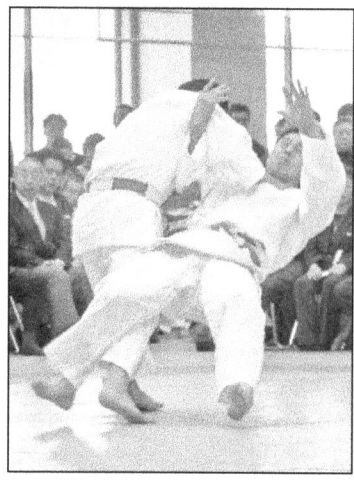

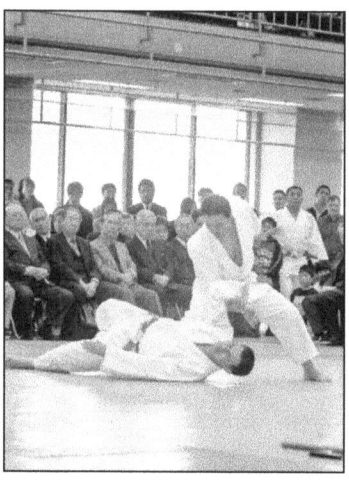
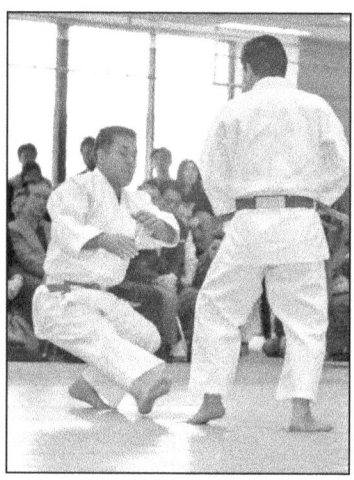
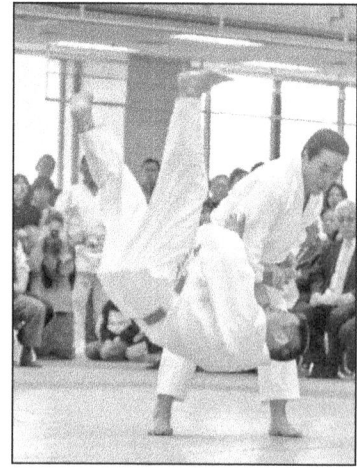

Figure 10a (left): Taking away the knife from *naname-tsuki* [slanting stab] in the *Buki-no-bu* [armed attacks] section. **Figure 10b** (center): Throwing uke down from *furi-oroshi* [downswing] in the *Buki-no-bu* [armed attacks] section. **Figure 10c** (right): Throwing uke down from *haimen-zuke* [pistol at the back] in the *Buki-no-bu* [armed attacks] section.

The photographs of Figures 9a to 10c are from the Kodokan Goshin-jutsu performance at the 2002 Kodokan Kagami Biraki. Tsueno Sengoku presently Kodokan 8th dan is tori [the one demonstrating the technique] and Masaru Sato presently Kodokan 8th dan is uke [the one attacking].

To date, the Kodokan has reviewed the Kodokan Goshin-jutsu three times since its inception—in July 1987, in December 1992 and in July 2004. The July 1987 review by the Kodokan's Kodokan Goshin-jutsu Research Committee, chaired by Kotani, was the most extensive and significant and was aimed at unifying and standardizing the exercise. This included clarifying many of its key technical points, the protocol for handling the weapons and the positioning of tori and uke. Following the review, a new Kodokan teaching booklet was published (Kodokan, 1987).

Foundations of Kodokan Goshin-jutsu

The composition and structure of Kodokan Goshin-jutsu was influenced by that of the other Kodokan kata, which, in their finalized form, contain either 15 techniques—Nage-no-kata, Katame-no-kata and Ju-no-kata, or 20–21 techniques—Kime-no-kata and Koshiki-no-kata. Note that although Go-no-kata and Itsutsu-no-kata only contain ten and five techniques, respectively, both these kata were unfinished by Kano, and most likely would have been later revised and expanded to include more techniques.

The division of Kodokan Goshin-jutsu into unarmed and armed sections was logical, and the number of attacks in each section was of course initially arbitrary. However, some underlying structural logic was necessary, and the armed section eventually followed a similar pattern to Kime-no-kata, with equal number of attacks per weapons type. Under this approach, having two attacks per weapon-type produced a total of six defense sequences, and having three, produced nine. This would leave either 12 or 15 attacks available for the unarmed section. The structuring of this into subsections for "when held" and "at a distance" would, due to Tomiki's influence, come later.

As well as introducing new attack types into judo, Kodokan Goshin-jutsu also preserved, and built upon, a number of attack forms already contained in Kime-no-kata[49] and, to a much lesser degree, in Ju-no-kata.[50] As part of updating Kime-no-kata, the attacks in Kodokan Goshin-jutsu were however usually executed in a modified way, or on a different side. Kodokan Goshin-jutsu also introduced alternative defenses. Table 4 lists the similar attacks found in Kime-no-kata and Kodokan Goshin-jutsu.

Table 4	Similar Attacks in *Kime-no-kata* and *Kodokan Goshin-jutsu*	
ATTACK	KIME-NO-KATA (TACHIAI SECTION)	KODOKAN GOSHIN-JUTSU
Two-hand hold	Ryote-dori	Ryote-dori
Single-hand (sleeve) hold	Sode-dori	Kataude-dori
Hold from behind	Ushiro-dori	Kakae-dori
Single-fist thrust punch	Tsukkake	Ganmen-tsuki
Uppercut	Tsuki-age	Ago-tsuki
Front kick	Ke-age	Mae-geri

As an example, consider Ryote-dori. In Kime-no-kata this attack concludes with tori applying a *katame waza* [controlling technique]—specifically the *kansetsu-waza* [joint-locking technique] *ude-hishigi-waki-gatame* [arm crushing armpit armlock] against uke's left arm. Kodokan Goshin-jutsu provides tori with an additional method for freeing his right wrist, and concludes with him applying a different kansetsu-waza—this time *Kote-hineri* [wrist twist] against uke's right arm.

Another example is the attack comprising a single-fist thrust punch to the face. This attack is known as *tsukkake* in the tachiai section of Kime-no-kata, and Ganmen-tsuki in Kodokan Goshin-jutsu. In both exercises the attack concludes with tori applying a katame waza—specifically the same *shime-waza* [strangulation technique] *hadaka-jime* [naked choke] in both cases.

PRINCIPLES WITHIN KODOKAN GOSHIN-JUTSU

The central objective in Kodokan Goshin-jutsu is to use judo self-defense principles to defeat an adversary and survive. Every defense in the exercise has fundamental principles for its effective execution, and in learning the exercise, it is these principles that have to be understood and mastered. However, in English-language texts on Kodokan Goshin-jutsu, it is only Kotani et al, (1968:54–91) and Cornish (1984) that pay proper attention to the principles as being the exercise's most vital aspect. Hopefully, one of the contributions of the current chapter will be to further an understanding of these principles, by assisting in making them more accessible to the interested judoka.

Self-Confidence and Focus

What matters most in any self-defense situation is the individual, and their personal ability to handle real life conflict, both physically and emotionally. For this reason, it is largely irrelevant what bujutsu, budo, or even combat sport one has studied. Remaining composed, under stress, is more important for self-defense than being technically skilled, or physically in good condition. This is because if an individual cannot control their own mind, their potential for being able to control another person is similarly limited.

Kotani et al highlight the role of Kodokan Goshin-jutsu in fostering self-confidence:

> ... practice of Goshinjitsu [sic.] aims to acquire the techniques and the self-confidence which can be applied effectively and timely for defending ourselves from unexpected attacks of others ...   – Kotani et al, 1968:57

Through practicing Kodokan Goshin-jutsu, tori develops decisiveness and the confidence to use tai-sabaki to quickly get into the correct position to parry attacks and execute defenses—depending on the *maai*[51] [interval or spacing] and *debana* [opportunity]. Practice also helps foster mental capabilities through furthering *mushin*[52] [no-mindedness] and *zanshin*[53] [awareness (in case of further attacks)]. Both aspects improve as tori becomes more proficient in executing Kodokan Goshin-jutsu's various defenses, and begins using them against a variety of random attacks such as those shown in Cornish (1984:30–32).

Kuzushi

The most critical technical principle in Kodokan Goshin-jutsu is *kuzushi* [balance breaking], with the aim being to create a safe opportunity for tori to counter-attack, and ultimately control uke. Without kuzushi, tori cannot easily achieve the necessary control, and in such circumstances, the defenses become unrealistic and even dangerous for tori to attempt. This is because a uke that is not unbalanced can simultaneously counter-attack tori.

The original informal Kodokan Goshin-jutsu was a great training in kuzushi, due mainly to Tomiki's contribution, however, over the years that focus has been largely lost. Proper practice of Kodokan Goshin-jutsu helps teach tori kuzushi skills for use in non-sports competitive judo situations—including against an armed attacker, where it is impossible, or very difficult, to grip uke and perform basic *Happo-no-Kuzushi* [eight directions of unbalancing] (Cornish, 1984:7).

Kodokan Goshin-jutsu teaches tori how to use both indirect, and direct action to generate kuzushi. Tori's indirect actions mainly involve correct tai-sabaki, with him moving and repositioning his whole body. Tori's direct actions often involve *atemi-waza* [striking techniques][54] to provide kuzushi—prior to applying a decisive technique such as a *nage-waza* [throwing technique] or katame waza. Direct action using atemi-waza is also used to create mental kuzushi—where it is uke's concentration, more than his body that is disturbed. This distraction produces an instantaneous opportunity for tori to counter-attack.

Execution of Technique in a Dynamic Situation

Kodokan Goshin-jutsu introduces the concept of dynamic displacement into judo self-defense, with its attacks and defenses being executed from moving situations. This contrasts with the predominantly static situations in Kime-no-kata. Against uke's attacks, tori must quickly use tai-sabaki to prepare his movements and get into the correct position to control or throw uke. In so doing, it is vital that tori maintains control of his own balance and posture, while moving himself, and controlling uke.

Controlling Distance

Kodokan Goshin-jutsu exposes judoka to the combat principles that result from working with an increased maai compared to that normally found in everyday judo including the other Kodokan kata. In particular, the maai in the Toshu-no-bu section is significantly greater than that in ordinary judo randori, and the use of weapons in the Buki-no-bu section increases the maai even further.

The Kumitsu-kareta-baai and Hanareta-baai subsections of the Toshu-no-bu in Kodokan Goshin-jutsu teach very different principles from Kime-no-kata. Whereas in Kime-no-kata, tori and uke are in a fixed, close-in, positions, and there are no real attacks from distance[55], the Hanareta-baai subsection of Kodokan Goshin-jutsu specifically teaches tori how to cope with attacks from an assailant suddenly coming in from afar.

Note that it is the scenarios where there is some distance between tori and uke, that Tomiki made his greatest contribution—not just to Kodokan Goshin-jutsu, but to judo as a whole (Tomiki, 1956; Shishida, 2010; 2011).

Proper Use of Leverage

The effective use of leverage is an essential element of most of the defenses in Kodokan Goshin-jutsu. Through practice, tori learns how leverage can be effectively applied to different components of uke's body, depending upon the actual defense being executed, and both his own and uke's movements.

Defense Against a Pistol

Kodokan Goshin-jutsu introduces, for the first time, the concept of defenses against guns into formal Kodokan training, and hence judo. In the Kenshu-no-baai scenarios, uke threatens tori with a pistol to gain compliance and take his wallet. Uke has no real set intention of shooting tori, but the scenario is that he might do so if compliance is not forthcoming.

A critical point in the gun attack scenarios is that uke looks down as he reaches for tori's wallet. This break in focus provides tori with the opportunity to take the initiative, move out of the line of fire, and counter-attack. Uke's brain must first register that tori has moved, and subsequently must process a decision whether, or not, to pull the trigger. Action beats reaction, and providing his hands are held up at shoulder height, and not above his head, tori should have sufficient time to control the gun and disarm uke.

The Kenshu-no-bai subsection therefore introduces new principles into judo that are not found elsewhere. Most important is the principle that tori only starts to counter-attack, when uke's attention is not on him. Tai-sabaki is critical, and tori must have turned to always have his own body out of the gun's line of fire. Also, tori must always attack the hand holding the gun, or the gun itself, seizing the barrel, warding it off, and using it as a lever to disarm or throw uke.

The principles which are sine quo non for the Kenshu-no-baai are very well illustrated in the third gun attack—haimen-zuke. This is not only the last attack of the Kenshu-no-baai, but also the final attack of the entire Kodokan Goshin-jutsu.

In haimen-zuke, uke is standing behind tori, and as tori walks forwards, uke follows. Drawing the pistol with his right hand uke commands "*Te wo ageru*" ["hands up"]. Tori stops and slowly complies. Uke then steps forward with his right foot, places the pistol muzzle against the middle of tori's back, and reaches for tori's wallet. During this time tori has already glanced out of the corner of his eye to see which of uke's arms has the gun.

As uke reaches down to tori's pocket for the wallet, tori uses tai-sabaki by slightly lowering his hips and turning to his right, dropping his right hand under uke's gun hand as he does so. Tori then raises his hand up and over, catching his right forearm in the crook of uke's arm in the process. Tori then pulls forward and uses pressure to trap uke's right (gun) arm. Subsequently, tori disarms uke by capturing the gun with his other (left) hand.

In Tomiki's original text (1958) haimen-zuke concludes here, with tori being poised to strike uke in the head with the gun. This ending is consistent with the two preceding pistol defenses that finish in a similar manner. The photographic sequence of Figure 11 shows this original form, with Tomiki as tori and Mr. Sakamoto of Waseda University as uke (Tomiki, 1958).

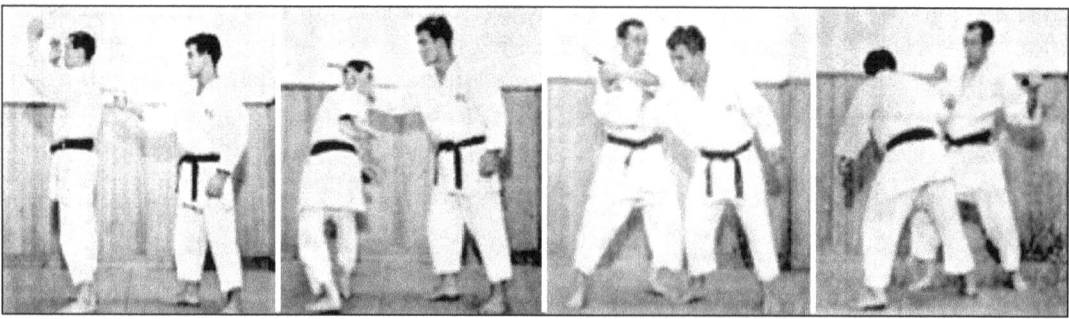

Figure 11: The original form of *haimen-zuke* [pistol at the back] the final technique of Kodokan-Goshin-jutsu concluding with tori simply disarming uke. Kenji Tomiki is *tori* [the one demonstrating the technique] and Mr. Sakamoto is *uke* [the one attacking].

However, in quite short order, a modified ending to haimen-zuke started to feature, with tori throwing uke to the ground using a *kote-gaeshi* [wrist reversal] type technique.

The first documented example of this (known to the authors) actually has Tomiki himself as tori, and features in the book *Judo* (Kodokan, 1961) which was published in 1961 to mark the centenary of Jigoro Kano's birth. Most interestingly, while the photographs in the book clearly show tori throwing uke, the supporting text makes no mention of the throw and only refers to tori disarming uke. Similarly, in the book *Saishin Judo-no-Kata Zen* [The Latest Judo Kata—Complete] (Kotani and Otaki, 1971) a throw is shown in the photographs without any supporting text. This is not unusual as in Japanese-authored books the text always takes precedence over any photographs. The photographic sequence of Figure 12 shows this modified form of haimen-zuke, with Tomiki as tori, and his close friend and colleague Hideo Oba (1910–1986) Kodokan 6th dan, aikido 9th dan, as uke (Kodokan, 1961).

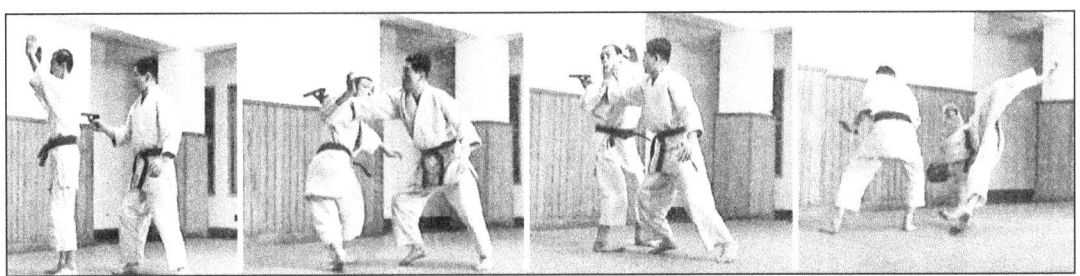

Figure 12: The modified form of *haimen-zuke* [pistol at the back] the final technique of Kodokan Goshin-jutsu concluding with tori throwing uke with a *kote-gaeshi* [wrist reversal] style technique. Kenji Tomiki is *tori* [the one demonstrating the technique] and Hideo Oba is *uke* [the one attacking].

Note that where most texts consider only one of the endings to haimen-zuke, the 2007 book *Judo Kata—Les Formes Classiques du Kodokan* by Inogai[56] and Habersetzer[57], considers both. While the illustrations only show the throw, the narrative (originally in French) states:

> Tori may seek not to throw [uke]: he can simply seize the gun with his left hand and then strike the back of uke's head with the butt, remaining standing and simply leaning forward slightly.
> The same as in the previous two techniques.
> – Inogai and Habersetzer, 2007:208

Whilst it might be assumed that making a significant modification to Kodokan Goshin-jutsu, such as introducing a throw into haimen-zuke, would have been the subject of extensive debate amongst Kodokan seniors, it seems that this change became assimilated through informal practice, and only officially sanctioned once it was established as the norm.

The possibility of having two different concluding techniques for haimen-zuke is of course entirely consistent with the philosophy for Kodokan Goshin-jutsu, and indeed all of judo. Core principles have to be followed throughout, but the application of those principles is permitted to vary. Accordingly, the absence, or presence, of the concluding throw in haimen-zuke is of limited relevance, since from a self-defense perspective, both endings are valid, and there is no compelling reason why uke has to be thrown in the way he is today.

It was only in the mid-1980s that the Kodokan's "Kodokan Goshin-jutsu Research Committee" formally decided that uke should be thrown after tori had snatched the pistol. Naturally, it was only after the taking of this decision that authoritative Kodokan Goshin-jutsu teaching material began including both photographs showing, and text describing, haimen-zuke culminating with a throw.

Sequential Self-defense

The greatest insight into Kodokan Goshin-jutsu is obtained by considering it as containing 21 self-defense "sequences" as opposed 21 distinct "techniques". These sequences are significantly more complex than those found in everyday randori and sports competition judo, and involve, inter alia, atemi-waza, tai-sabaki, kuzushi, nage-waza and katame waza, for which a limitless number of permutations and combinations exist.

This complexity of the sequences in Kodokan Goshin-jutsu is now illustrated by considering the first defense, Ryote-dori. As soon as uke reaches the proper maai, he steps forwards, grasps both of tori's wrists and attacks tori's groin [kokan] with an atemi-waza—*hiza-ate* [knee strike] using his right knee. Tori cannot block or deflect, this incoming knee, so he responds logically with tai-sabaki—evading the attack, by stepping back with his left foot, turning slightly to the left and taking uke's balance—kuzushi.

Simultaneously, tori breaks free from uke's left-hand grip by using leverage and stretching uke's elbow. He accomplishes this by extending the fingers of both his hands and bending his right arm inwards. Tori then applies an atemi-waza to uke's right temple [*kasumi*]—striking it with his right *te-gatana* [hand blade] thereby psychologically unbalancing uke, and destroying his concentration—mental kuzushi.

Tori then controls uke by locking his right wrist with *kote-hineri*—clamping uke's right arm under his own left arm as he does so. Tori then uses tai-sabaki—stepping back with his right foot and turning his body to his right, thus further off-balancing uke. Tori finally controls uke with Ude-hishigi-waki-gatame.

Acquiring the Principles

To build a thorough understanding of the riai in Kodokan Goshin-jutsu, its defenses and counterattacks should be practiced deliberately and properly. Greater speed can be progressively introduced as tori improves his avoidance, escape and counter attack skills (Cornish, 1984:6–7).

For example, recall Ryote-dori. As previously described, tori's reactions to uke grabbing his wrists are multiple—stretch the fingers, withdraw the left leg diagonally to the left, and bend the right arm towards the inside. These actions must occur simultaneously and automatically. Mouri (personal communication, 13 September 2015) recollects being regularly directed by an elderly Kodokan sensei to continually practice the sequence until he could execute it instinctively. Like for all judo, *uchi-komi* [repetition training], where a particular technique is practiced repeatedly to learn the specific kuzushi, tai-sabaki and other technical aspects, has an important role in learning Kodokan Goshin-jutsu. Specifically, uchi-komi helps tori imbed the defenses of Kodokan Goshin-jutsu so that they can be readily applied in a physical emergency.

The role of uke in supporting tori to develop an understanding of the principles is also crucial (Ibid.:5–6). Cornish explains:

> Uke of course plays an intrinsic part in kata. Some maintain the most important part and we must add his attempted techniques to the knowledge we gain by doing kata. Even though uke's attempts never succeed his techniques must be

perfectly feasible and truly attempted. Otherwise both uke's and tori's training will be impaired. – Ibid.:6

Further guidance on acquiring the principles within Kodokan Goshin-jutsu is provided later where its teaching and learning challenges are explicitly considered.

Kodokan Goshin-jutsu as a "Point of Departure"

Real combat always requires the adaptation of previous learning to the genuine attack being experienced. Since the particulars of the actual conflict will never be identical to those in the exercise, it is essential that Kodokan Goshin-jutsu should not be considered in isolation as a prescribed and rigidly fixed success formula, for specific self-defense situations only. Rather, Kodokan Goshin-jutsu should be regarded as a judo exercise that encapsulates a series of self-defense examples that teaches principles that are part of a greater whole, and which through practice helps tori develop and embed self-defense responses that are most likely to result in favorable outcomes. In the engagement, it is uke's actions and tori's own experiences and capabilities that determine which tools to use.

In this way, Kodokan Goshin-jutsu in its standard form was meant to be a "point of departure", with the sequences and techniques therein merely a range of options that could be experimented with during training. Specifically, once the principles of sequential self-defense in the basic form have been mastered, then modifications and variations, consistent with these concepts, can be added and practiced.

Cornish (1984:30–32) presents examples of many such "alternatives" in his booklet, where he provides solution options to the challenges arising were uke to respond differently than expected. He achieves this by drawing on his extensive personal experience in aikido, and also by substituting other techniques from elsewhere in Kodokan Goshin-jutsu to cope.

The principle in operation here is that one can use judo to survive in shinken shobu, with tori having complete freedom of action to respond how he wants, and Kodokan Goshin-jutsu having helped prepare him mentally and physically for the challenge. In this way Kodokan Goshin-jutsu is a valuable part of a broader judo curriculum, and a reminder of, and bridge to, the self-defense aspects of judo that are typically ignored nowadays[58].

TEACHING AND LEARNING KODOKAN GOSHIN-JUTSU

Some of the issues associated with teaching and learning, Kodokan Goshin-jutsu will now be reflected upon. Included in this will be a review of a selection of Kodokan Goshin-jutsu learning resources that are available to support both teachers, and students.

Teaching and Learning Challenges

Like many other aspects of judo, Kodokan Goshin-jutsu only makes sense when one personally has a high degree of judo understanding, technical sophistication and competence. This is usually predicated on one having been expertly taught[59], and for this purpose the annual Kodokan Summer Kata Course is popular with judoka looking to improve their competencies through direct instruction from senior Kodokan teachers. Figure 13 shows judoka practicing the staff attacks from Kodokan Goshin-jutsu's Buki-no-bu during the 2015 Kodokan Summer Kata Course.

As a teaching approach, it is recommended that Kodokan Goshin-jutsu be first placed in its proper context. This should include an explanation of the purpose of the exercise, including the historical background to its development and the intentions of its creators.

Kodokan Goshin-jutsu's defenses against the standard attacks can be taught and learnt next. As a learning approach, grouping the sequences into holistic sets of related actions, rather than considering each one individually, is helpful (Cornish, 1984:5) as it enables the principles to be introduced. When considering the physical mechanics of the defenses, prominence should also be given to ensuring realism and strong spirit.

Once progress is made in learning Kodokan Goshin-jutsu's mechanics ("the how"), then greater understanding of the *riai* or reasons and principles behind each and every movement ("the why") should be developed. Acquiring this understanding is best achieved through a twin-track process that simultaneously addresses both the fundamental and the specific principles. For example, kuzushi and tai-sabaki skills are fundamental principles to all of judo, whereas self-confidence, situational awareness, escape methods, atemi-waza and their linkages to nage-waza or katame waza in a conflict situation are principles more specific to Kodokan Goshin-jutsu.

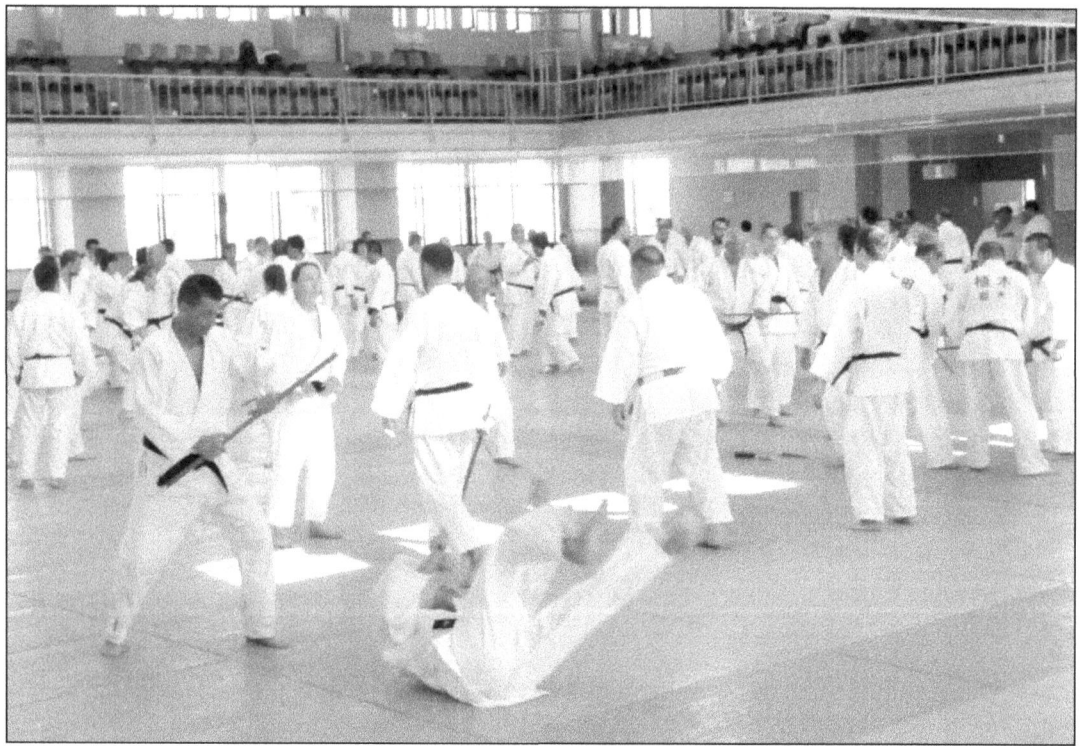

Figure 13: The *Tsue-no-baai* [staff attacks] from the Buki-no-bu section of Kodokan Goshin-jutsu being practiced during the 2015 Kodokan Summer Kata Course.

RESOURCES FOR LEARNING KODOKAN GOSHIN-JUTSU

A range of the written and filmed material for teaching and learning Kodokan Goshin-jutsu is now be reviewed. Note that texts by Tomiki (1958), Kotani (1962), Kotani et al (1968), Kodokan (1976), Cornish (1984), and Hamot et al (1985) all show the original conclusion to haimen-zuke where uke is merely disarmed and not thrown.

1958, Kenji Tomiki: *Kodokan Goshin-jutsu*

Tomiki's 1958 book *Kodokan Goshin-jutsu* (shown earlier in Figure 5) is the first and most important book on the exercise. The 144-page text provides an illustrated explanation of the complete Kodokan Goshin-jutsu—including step-by-step black and white photographs of the attacks and defenses, line drawings of the footwork patterns, and advice on how to execute the wristlocks and various atemi-waza. However, consistent with the informal intent for Kodokan Goshin-jutsu, no emphasis is given to any reiho aspects. Recall in this original text, the final technique, haimen-zuke concludes with tori simply disarming uke by capturing the gun.

The demonstrators are Tomiki himself as tori, and Mr. Sakamoto, a former captain of the Waseda University Judo Club as uke. Regrettably as with many Japanese judo books of that vintage, the paper is delicate and the printed photographs are of poor quality. The text is only available on the used book market, and given its historical significance, the asking price is often high. For these reasons its major usefulness is for reference and research purposes, rather than a practical text for studying Kodokan Goshin-jutsu.

1955 and later 1976 reprint, Kodokan, editors: *Illustrated Kodokan Judo*

The original 1955 edition of this classic text from the Kodokan does not contain Kodokan Goshin-jutsu, as it was still in development. However, the later 1976 reprint does. Chapter XIV (Kodokan, 1976: 209-216) presents a well-illustrated explanation of the exercise's mechanical movements and a succinct summary of its purpose and content:

> The Kodokan Goshinjutsu (methods of self-defence) includes, together with the Kime-no-kata (forms of self-defence), devices for actual fighting. In this category are included the best and most typical devices against conceivable grappling, choking, striking, thrusting or kicking attacks from the opponent, as well as tricks against various forms of violence— the dagger, the staff and the pistol. When these methods were finally established by the Kodokan in 1956, much consideration was necessitated to make them suitable and up-to-date, and yet distinct from those techniques of the Kime-no-kata (forms of self-defence). In these methods, all the tricks of the punching technique, the throwing technique and the seizing technique culminate . . .
>
> – Ibid.:209

Despite being small, the black and white photographs serve well as a memory aid, and for an experienced judoka are sufficient for starting to learn the exercise. In the photographs, tori is the late Masao Koyasu, Kodokan 9th dan and uke is thought to be the late Kiyoji Suzuki, Kodokan 9th dan (Kodokan, personal communication, 20 November 2015).

1961, Kodokan: *Judo*

The book *Judo*, which was published in 1961 to mark the centenary of Jigoro Kano's birth, devotes six pages to *Kodokan Goshin-jutsu* (Kodokan, 1961:74–79). A summary descriptive paragraph on the exercise is included, and a series of large black and white photographs, used to show five representative techniques from across the entire exercise. The photographs show two sequences drawn from the Oshu-no-bu section and three from the Buki-no-bu section. In the photographs, Tomiki is tori and Oba is uke.

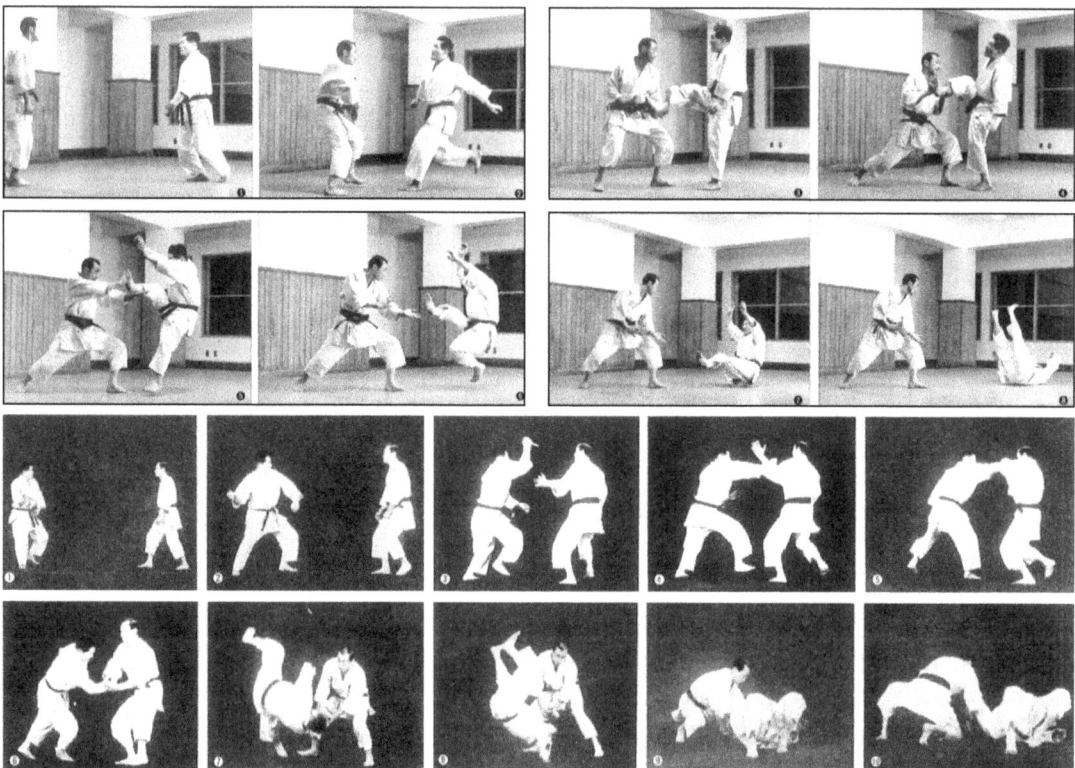

Figure 14: Outtake from the Kodokan Goshin-jutsu pages from the 1961 book *Judo* which was published to mark the centenary of Jigoro Kano's birth. The techniques shown are *maegeri* [front kick] and *nanametsuki* [slanting stab]. Kenji Tomiki is *tori* [the one demonstrating the technique] and Hideo Oba is *uke* [the one attacking].

The two Toshu-no-bu sequences are Ushiro-jime from the Kumitsu-kareta-baai, and maegeri from the Hanareta-baai. The three Buki-no-bu sequences are Naname-tsuki from the Tanto-no-baai, Morote-tsuki from the Tsue-no-baai, and haimen-zuke from the Kenshu-no-baai. Very limited de- scriptive text on the sequences is provided—see Figure 14 for the mae-geri and Naname-tsuki examples. Recall also that haimen-zuke in this book ends with tori throwing uke with kote-gaeshi, and that this is the first example of this conclusion known to the authors (Ibid.:78).

The book is not really a learning resource for Kodokan Goshin-jutsu, but is highly desirable for its historical content. It would be a valuable addition to the library of anyone interested in the history of judo.

1968, Sumiyuki Kotani, Yoshimi Osawa and Yuichi Hirose: *Kata of Kodokan Judo* & *Kata of Kodokan Judo Revised*

The technical kata books written by Kotani and others in the late 1960s and early 1970s remain the primary reference texts for the serious study of kata. With respect to *Kodokan Goshin-jutsu*, Kotani et al's, translated, *Kata of Kodokan Judo*, Figure 15, and its near-identical reprint *Kata of Kodokan Judo Revised* were, prior to Cornish (1984), the most technically detailed study texts available in the English language (Kotani et al, 1968: 54–91). It is worthy to note that as well as Kotani, another of these books' co-authors went on to receive the illustrious grade of Kodokan 10th dan, with Yoshimi Osawa (born 1926), Figure 16, being promoted to that level in 2006.

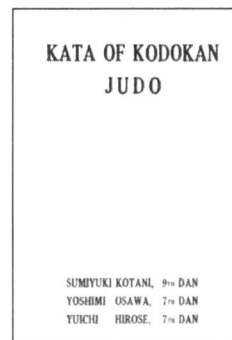 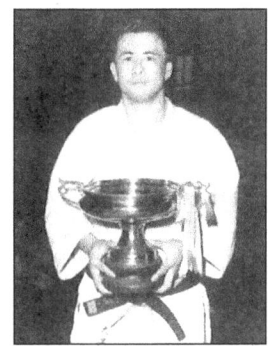

Figure 15: *Kata of Kodokan Judo* by Kotani et al. was published in 1968 and is a detailed text for studying the various Kodokan kata.
Figure 16: Yoshimi Osawa (born 1926)—pictured here in 1958.

Beyond explaining Kodokan Goshin-jutsu's mechanics, the books also describe its important principles, and provide helpful guidelines for practice. They also contain relatively small black and white photographs of the exercise's mechanical movements, as well as footwork patterns for each sequence (Ibid.). In the photographs, Kotani is tori and Yuichi Hirose is uke.

Note that the placement of the weapons shown in these books is the opposite of what is standard today, with the gun, rather than the knife, being closest to uke (Ibid.: 56). This however is most likely a simple mistake, rather than a different historical convention, and in no way detracts from their overall merit.

1971, Sumiyuki Kotani and Tadao Otaki: *Saishin Judo-no-Kata Zen*

The previously mentioned Japanese language book *Saishin Judo-no-Kata Zen* by Kotani and Otaki (1971) is a 324-page text containing seven Kodokan kata. To this day it remains the kata textbook of choice for dedicated Japanese judoka. The book, Figure 17, contains a relatively detailed description of Kodokan Goshin-jutsu, though again only relatively small, black and white photographs (Ibid.:119–169). Katsuyoshi Takata, a noted Kodokan sensei in his own right, see later, was the photographer.

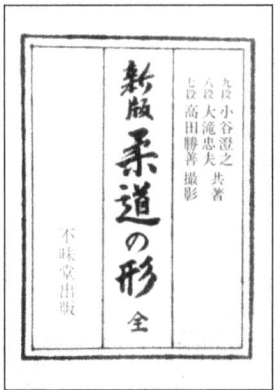 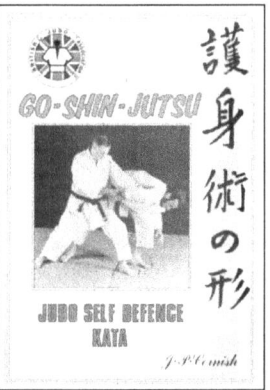

Figure 17 (left): *Saishin Judo-no-Kata Zen* by Kotani and Otaki was published in 1971 and remains the kata textbook of choice for keen Japanese judoka.
Figure 18 (right): *Kodokan Goshin Jutsu* by John Cornish was published in 1984 and is an in-depth English language resource for learning the exercise.

1984, John Cornish: *Go-Shin-Jutsu – Judo Self Defence Kata*

John P. Cornish (born 1929) is a senior British judoka (presently BJA 7th dan) and aikidoka (presently 8th dan). He studied judo from 1952 at the London Budokwai[60] under the celebrated British judoka, author, broadcaster and scholar Trevor (T.P.) Leggett (1914–2000) Kodokan 6th dan. From 1958 to 1964 he practiced both systems in Japan—specifically, judo at the Kodokan as a member of the Kenshusei [research student] class, and aikido and the Hombu [Headquarters] dojo. In particular, he studied Kodokan Goshin-jutsu as a direct student of Kenji Tomiki. After his return to the UK, he taught both judo and aikido at the Budokwai until his retirement in 2010.

In the early 1980s Cornish published a booklet entitled *Go-Shin-Jutsu— Judo Self Defence Kata* (Cornish, 1984), Figure 18. Together with Kotani et al's 1968 translated texts, it is the most technically detailed written resource on Kodokan Goshin-jutsu available in the English language. As well as benefiting from large and clear black and white photographs of the exercise's mechanical movements, it presents a complete dissection of each attack and defense sequence—including a valuable explanation of the underlying principles at work, as well as guidelines for "further study".

While clearly effective, the *Kodokan Goshin-jutsu* shown by Cornish is of its time, and differs in several places from today's accepted standard. As a direct student of Tomiki, it is unsurprising that what Cornish presents is comparable to that in Tomiki's original text (Tomiki, 1958). None of these differences detract from the merit of Cornish's booklet, and it is highly recommended as essential reading for anyone seriously interested in the exercise.

1985, George Parulski: *Black Belt Judo*

In the book *Black Belt Judo* published under the auspices of the now defunct American Society of Classical Judoka, George Parulski Jr. presents a summary description of Kodokan Goshin-jutsu:

> KODOKAN GOSHIN-JUTSU: Translated as the 'Kodokan's method of self-defense', this kata was invented in the '50s by a staff of masters at the Kodokan. Their intention was to update the techniques of the Kime-no-kata for modern times. This kata contains methods of throwing, holding, evading kicking, striking and choking. There are defenses against bare hands, staffs, knives and guns.
> – Parulski, 1985:74

Parulski provides no further specific content on Kodokan Goshin-jutsu. He does however provide detailed instructions on various self-defense techniques—including various atemi-waza (Ibid.:157–173), and also some self-defense sequences (Ibid.:174–181). These are interesting in their own right.

1985, Claude Hamot, Guy Pelletier and Claude Urvoy:
Katame no Kata Kodokan Goshin Jutsu

Hamot, Pelletier and Urvoy's 1985 French-language book *Katame no Kata Kodokan Goshin Jutsu* presents clear black and white photographs with limited accompanying narrative that deals only with the mechanics of Kodokan Goshin-jutsu. The attacks and defense movements shown are like those in Tomiki (1958), Kotani and Otaki (1971) and Cornish (1984). As mentioned earlier, the etiquette involves sitting bowing arrangements.

Note that one of the authors, Guy Pelletier (1921–2011) Kodokan 8th dan, FFJDA 9th dan, was until his death, the world's highest ranking Kodokan-graded judoka of non-Japanese descent. For this reason alone, the book is of historical interest.

1986, Jigoro Kano: *Illustrated Kodokan Judo*

This book, published by Kodansha, and presenting Jigoro Kano as its author, was actually compiled by a Kodokan editorial committee long after the Shihan's death. It is a more recent update of the original 1955 *Kodokan Judo*, and contains descriptions of all formally recognized techniques, and eight judo kata—including Kodokan Goshin-jutsu.

Like in the 1976 expanded reprint of the 1955 standard, the instructional text on Kodokan Goshin-jutsu is concise and focuses on mechanical movements only. Similarly, the black and white photographs, this time with the late Kazuhiko Kawabe, Kodokan 8th dan as tori and Tsuyoshi Sato, Kodokan 8th dan as uke, are small. The book however is a good resource for starting to learn Kodokan Goshin-jutsu, and given its availability in Japanese, English, French and German, probably represents the most popular introductory text.

1987 and 1992, Kodokan: *Kodokan Goshin-jutsu* (K. Takata and T. Sengoku)
Following the conclusion of the review by the Kodokan's Kodokan Goshin-jutsu Research Committee, a new teaching booklet was published (Kodokan, 1987). This booklet aimed to present a unified and standardized Kodokan Goshin-jutsu, and clarified some of the exercise's key points—including the protocol for weapons handling, and the positioning of tori and uke. The booklet was available in both Japanese and English, with the English version being a full, Kodokan-produced, high quality translation of the Japanese original (Kodokan, personal communication, 11 December 2015). In the photographs, Katsuyoshi Takata is tori and Tsueno Sengoku is uke—at the time holders of Kodokan 8th dan and 7th dan respectively. Additionally, and most notably, the conclusion of haimen-zuke in the booklet had tori throwing uke with a kote-gaeshi, type technique and the photographs for this technique were accompanied, for the first time, by a suitably detailed instructional narrative (Ibid.:45–46).

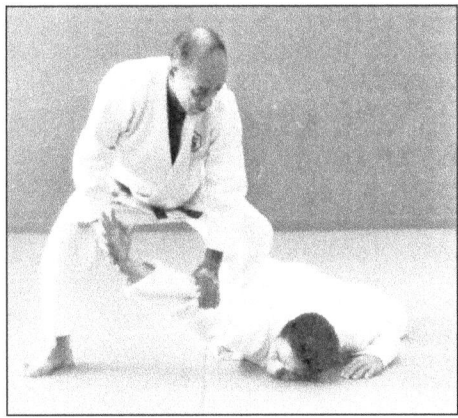

Figure 19: *Ude-hishigi-te-gatame* [arm crushing hand armlock] from *hidari-eri-dori* [left-lapel hold] in the *toshi-no-bu* [unarmed attacks] section of Kodokan Goshin-jutsu as shown in the 1987 Kodokan-produced instructional booklet. Katsuyoshi Takata is tori and Tsueno Sengoku is uke.

Both Takata and Sengoku have been important Kodokan teachers of Kodokan Goshin-jutsu, and for this reason, further information on these two senior judoka is now provided.

Katsuyoshi Takata (1921–2000), Figure 20, was a dynamic and inspirational Kodokan teacher and a prominent kata expert in the period following the retirement[61] of Kotani. Takata, like his mentor Kotani, was known to focus extensively on Kodokan Goshin-jutsu's principles—emphasizing in particular its aiki-jujutsu heritage in his search for maximum effectiveness.

Takata was also nicknamed "Mr. Hanegoshi" due to his well-known mastery of the technique[62] [*hanegoshi* = spring hip throw], and authored a bilingual (Spanish and English) book describing thirteen different methods of executing the throw (Takata, 1961). Takata achieved the rank of Kodokan 8th dan during his lifetime, and on his death in 2000 was posthumously promoted to Kodokan 9th dan (Oltremari, n.d.).

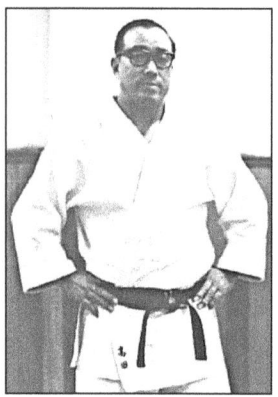 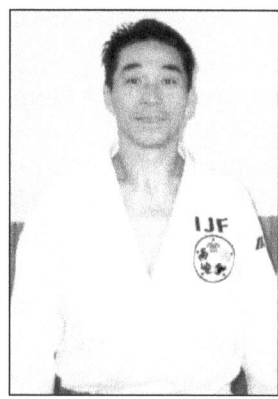

Figure 20 (left): Katsuyoshi Takata (1921–2000).
Figure 21 (right): Tsueno Sengoku (born 1945).

Tsueno Sengoku (born 1945) presently Kodokan 8th dan, Figure 21, has been a Kodokan teacher and member of its core kata staff. Additionally, he has been a senior judo instructor at the Keishicho [Tokyo Metropolitan Police Department] and is also highly experienced in *taiho-jutsu* [arresting art]—a well-established system for law enforcement professionals, synthesized from koryu, *gendai budo* [modern martial ways][63] and Western boxing. As well as being a dedicated uke to Takata, Sengoku is probably best known, along with Tadashi Sato presently Kodokan 8th dan, as a demonstrator in Daigo's definitive book on nage-waza—*Kodokan Judo: Throwing Techniques* (Daigo, 2005). Currently Sengoku resides in Indonesia where a large modern judo center, the Sengoku International Judo Hall, has been built in Bali, and named after him.

1998, Pedro Dabauza:
Kata Judo-Jujitsu: Formas Antiguas y Modernas de Defensa Personal

Pedro Rodríguez Dabauza (born 1949) is a Spanish budoka who holds high-dan rank in both judo—presently DNBK 8th dan, RFEJYDA[64] 8th dan, and non-koryu jujutsu. He is a multi-published author, a producer of several budo instructional films and a regular teacher and participant at international budo seminars.

Kata Judo-Jujitsu: Formas Antiguas y Modernas de Defensa Personal [Judo-Jujitsu Kata: Old and Modern Forms of Self Defence] is a Spanish-language text that, as its title suggests, covers both the old, Kime-no-kata, and modern, Kodokan Goshin-jutsu, self-defense forms. Also included is a concise overview on Kano's contribution to judo as well, as several souvenir photographs of the author with many noted Kodokan teachers (Dabauza, 1998: 129–155).

The Kodokan Goshin-jutsu section (Ibid.,17–69) contains true, still black and white photographs of the exercise, with Dabauza himself, then a 6th dan, as tori, and Jorge Cuevas, then a 5th dan, as uke. Succinct instructive text for all of the sequences is provided, as well as a summary of their main principles.

2003, Kisaburo Watanabe: *Essential Judo Katas*

Kisaburo Watanabe (born 1936) Kodokan 8th dan is a past Asian Games judo champion, and was resident coach at the London Budokwai from 1962 to 1966. To coincide with the 1993 kata championships, organized by the now-defunct World Masters Judo Association[65] (WMJA), he produced a 214-page book with instructions for five Kodokan kata. Kodokan Goshin-jutsu is the fifth one described therein (Watanabe, 2003:165–213).

The book was printed in limited numbers and was not openly for sale. The book contains black line drawings and simple, limited instructions. For these reasons it represents a helpful quick-reference guide for use on the tatami, rather than a resource for serious learning.

2004 and 2015, *Kodokan: Kodokan Goshin-jutsu* (with K. Onozawa and K. Komata)

Between 2004 and 2008 the Kodokan published a series of kata instructional booklets for use in conjunction with the appropriate Kodokan teaching film. Six booklets were produced, covering seven Kodokan kata, with Itsutsu-no-kata and Koshiki-no-kata featuring in the same booklet. Originally available in Japanese only, the booklets contained a limited narrative but were well illustrated with black and white photographs. These however, were non-crisp snapshots taken from the video title.

The *Kodokan Goshin-jutsu* booklet, Figure 22, was published in 2004 and replaced the earlier volume featuring Takata and Sengoku. Being derived from the film, the new booklet (Kodokan, 2004) also had Onozawa as tori and Komata as uke. Presently, both Onozawa and Komata hold the rank of Kodokan 8th dan.

In 2015 the Kodokan released five of the kata booklets in the English language—including *Kodokan Goshin-jutsu* (Kodokan, 2015), Figure 23. These were based on an official translation of the 2004–2008 booklets, with significantly expanded contents provided by the translator, Lance Gatling, working with a number of senior Kodokan instructors. Additional, purpose-shot, black and white photographs were introduced throughout, as well as more details of the various kata's mechanical movements.

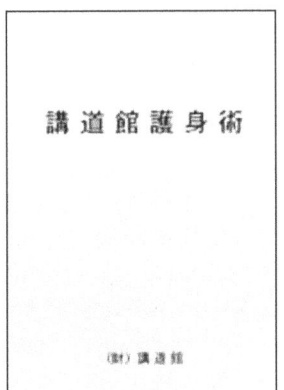 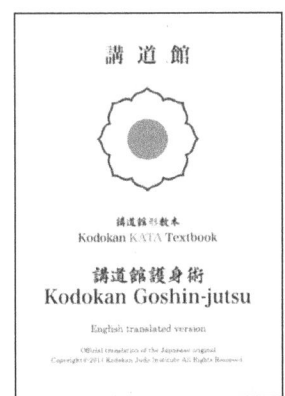

Figure 22: The Kodokan's study booklet for Kodokan Goshin-jutsu—produced in 2004, originally in Japanese only. **Figure 23:** The Kodokan's expanded English language study booklet for Kodokan Goshin-jutsu released in 2015.

2005, Masao Takahashi (and Family): *Mastering Judo*

The book *Mastering Judo* presents a broad based overview of judo's philosophy, history, techniques, tactics, and training methods. The authors—Masao Takahashi and family—(wife, June and children Allyn, Phil, Ray, and Tina) all hold high dan rank in judo, and between them have over 200 years of judo experience. The principal author and family patriarch, Masao Takahashi presently holds the rank of Judo Canada 8th dan.

The book presents a tabulated description of the mechanics of Kodokan Goshin-jutsu, with separate summary descriptions of the roles of uke and tori for each attack and defense sequence (Takahashi, 2005:55–56). Takahashi provides no illustrations of Kodokan Goshin-jutsu itself, however later, detailed well illustrated instructional material on various judo self-defense techniques (Ibid.:169–194) is provided.

2007, Tadao Inogai and Roland Habersetzer:
Judo Kata—Les Formes Classiques du Kodokan

Tadao Inogai (1908–1978) Kodokan 8th dan in conjunction with the French budoka Roland Habersetzer (born 1942), has several French language judo books to his name. The text, *Judo Kata–Les Formes Classiques du Kodokan* [Judo Kata–Kodokan Classic Forms] which has become an essential source for serious French judoka, presents eight Kodokan kata through clear, two-color, line drawings and reasonably detailed instructions. Despite the erroneous use of the name Goshin-jutsu-no-kata throughout (Inogai and Habersetzer, 2007:161–210), the book does represent a very helpful, quick-reference, guide that enables the exercise's mechanical movements to be readily learnt.

2009, Shu Taira: *La Essencia del Judo*

La Essencia del Judo [The Essence of Judo], Figure 24, is an ambitious and meticulously prepared study of judo from a technical, historical and philosophical perspective, due to Shu Taira (born 1942), presently RFEJYDA 9th dan. Shu Taira has resided in Spain since 1967, and is the son of Tsuson Taira (1901–1988), himself a Kodokan 8th dan.

La Essencia del Judo was first published, in two (sold together) volumes, in 2009, and reprinted in 2015. The first volume is about the history of judo, nage-waza and katame waza, while the second focuses on kata and also contains the appendices. The section on Kodokan Goshin-jutsu (Taira, 2009:253–314) contains a good explanation of the exercise's history, principles and mechanics, and is lavishly illustrated with high quality photographs, with Taira himself as tori, and an unknown uke. The book is very desirable, relatively expensive and available in Spanish only. Nevertheless, it is highly recommended to all serious judoka.

Post 2009, FFJDA: *Kodokan Goshinjitsu*

The "Guide du judoka" series of booklets and accompanying DVDs created by the FFJDA are training resources designed for both judo teachers and students to discover, or rediscover, the technical subtleties of kata practice. Produced in the French language, the materials are approved by the FFJDA's National Technical Directorate and the High Grades Commission. The third booklet and DVD in the series feature Kodokan Goshin-jutsu and are undated—however, they are known to have been produced sometime after 2009, as the preceding booklet and DVD on Katame-no-kata, the second in the series, is dated for then.

The booklet and DVD themselves are entitled *Kodokan Goshinjitsu*, Figure 25, which is a common error made by those unfamiliar with the nuances of transliteration from Japanese writing systems to the Roman alphabet.

Involved in the preparation of the material were FFJDA high grades Michel Algisi, Michel Casse, Michèle Lionnet, Patrice Berthoux and André Boutin along with French international kata competitors Frédéric Guillaume and Sevestre Esteve.

As would be expected from the FFJDA, the booklet itself is well produced. Each attack and defense series is illustrated with three photographs which are stills from the DVD. The narrative for each sequence is structured into three sections—general principles, how to perform the series and overall advice.

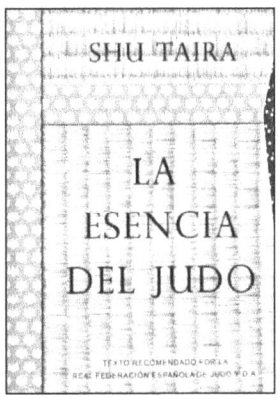 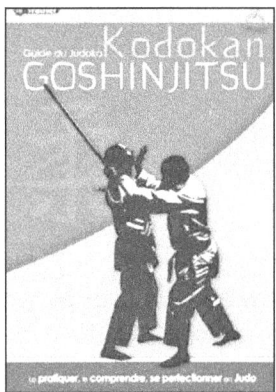 

Figure 24 (left): *La Esencia del Judo* by Shu Taira was published in 2009 and is a Spanish-language in-depth study of judo from a technical, historical and philosophical perspective. **Figure 25 (center):** *Kodokan Goshinjitsu* (sic.) produced by the FFJDA is a well produced French-language guide for learning the exercise. **Figure 26 (right):** *Kodokan Goshin Jutsu* by Blonk et al. was published in 2010 and is a good Dutch-language guide for learning the exercise.

2010, Mas Blonk, Richard de Bijl and Ferry van Dijk: *Kodokan Goshin Jutsu*

In *Kodokan Goshin-jutsu*, Figure 26, the fifth book of their series on the Kodokan kata, Mas Blonk (born 1944) and Richard de Bijl (born 1952), supported by Ferry van Dijk (born 1933), address the issue that the exercise is barely described in the Dutch judo literature. The authors are kodansha of the JBN[66], with Blonk and de Bijl presently holding the rank of JBN 8th dan and van Dijk, JBN 7th dan.

It is correctly acknowledged in the book that Kodokan Goshin-jutsu is not formally a kata, and that although the order of the sequences is defined, tori has considerable freedom in how he performs the defenses. In this way the authors are faithfully describing the spirit originally intended for Kodokan Goshin-jutsu, though they do suggest a normalized set of attacks and defenses. The book contains clear descriptions of the sequences and is well illustrated with insightful photographs. In this way it is an important guide for the proper practice of Kodokan Goshin-jutsu.

**FILMED INSTRUCTIONAL MATERIALS
FOR KODOKAN GOSHIN-JUTSU**

A selection of recommended filmed materials on Kodokan Goshin-jutsu are now reviewed.

1998 & 2009, *Kodokan: Kodokan Judo Kata Series–Kodokan Goshin-jutsu*

In January 1998 the Kodokan produced on VHS tape a 45-minute long Kodokan Goshin-jutsu instructional film (Kodokan, 1998). Recall that this film, with Onozawa and Komata, forms the basis of the subsequent Kodokan teaching booklets (Kodokan, 2004; 2015). As well as presenting a demonstration of the complete exercise, the film provided commentary on the correct forms of each technique including a precise explanation of the correct mechanical movements.

The film was re-edited in September 2009 and released on DVD (Kodokan, 2009). A welcome addition was the inclusion of some excerpts from Tomiki and Otaki's original 1956 demonstration.

2006, Kano Society: *Kodokan Goshin-jutsu*

The Kano Society was founded in 2000 by a group of senior British judoka concerned that judo was no longer being taught or practiced according to the principles espoused by Kano. Their goal was to promote the style of judo that was once prevalent.

In support of this purpose the Society has been compiling a number of DVDs—including a two-part Kodokan Goshin-jutsu teaching film, featuring John Cornish teaching (in October 2005) at the now closed "Sleeping Storm Aikido" dojo in Epsom, UK. The discs are separately sold with "Part 1—*Toshu* (against an unarmed attack)", and "Part 2—*Buki* (against an armed attack)" (Kano Society, 2006). The Kodokan Goshin-jutsu shown on the DVDs is identical to that presented in Cornish's booklet (Cornish, 1984). The earlier comments on that work also apply here.

As already highlighted, Cornish's teaching is rooted in his own judo background and he regards all kata as a training resource. The DVDs do not present a complete ceremonial performance of Kodokan Goshin-jutsu and are caveated:

> This series of instructional videos are intended as an aid to
> study of the Kata (and not as a formal 'demonstration').
> – Ibid.

Cornish's commitment to Kodokan Goshin-jutsu is clear from the film, and even at an advanced age his enthusiasm for the exercise is undiminished. While the vital kuzushi is not emphasized in all the demonstrations, the wrist techniques are clearly strong and effective.[67] The teaching style throughout the films is relaxed and genial, and as Cornish retired from all teaching in 2010 these films represent the best opportunity to benefit from the experience of someone who learnt Kodokan Goshin-jutsu at source—that is directly from its creators in its formative years.

INTERNET SOURCES

Nowadays, Kodokan Goshin-jutsu demonstrations and teaching materials are freely viewable on videosharing websites such as YouTube and Vimeo. These include film recordings made at the Kodokan Summer Kata Course and also at various kata championships—see later. Some archive film footage of great teachers such as Tomiki, Kotani and Takata is also available. Such material is easily found using any search engine and will not be specifically referenced here. Finally, while most of the web-based material really only helps with Kodokan Goshin-jutsu's mechanics, and is not of benchmark standard, it can still be helpful and inspiring.

PERFORMING AND COMPETING IN KODOKAN GOSHIN-JUTSU

Performance Aspects

As explained earlier, kata were designed as a learning resource and the original intent for kata practice was that judoka would select a few sequences from a listed kata, say and simply study them as a core part of training. Therefore, it was never intended that ceremonial performances of complete kata would be the most common form of practice, and despite formal renditions of whole kata being today's norm, such presentations were initially only intended to be part of a judo *enbu* [ceremonial demonstration] to an audience.

In a personal communication, Cornish reinforces this point, and explains how complete performances with high degrees of finesse are unnecessary.

> In my years as a British National Coach for kata I have, and still do, try to explain that the demonstration of kata is not important, it is the training, and what [principles] you learn from the training, that counts. For so much of judo, kata is the only way that training in safety can be carried out.
> – J.P. Cornish, personal communication, 3 June 2000

The above point is particularly true for Kodokan Goshin-jutsu, which is the application of a pedagogical system (judo) to self-defense. As has been explained, the primary goal, and mindset, for practice should not be one of "perfecting" the mechanical movements of the complete performance sequence, but rather one of developing an understanding of the principles of judo self-defense.

Kotani et al also counsel:

> ... judo players ... are apt to practice only the forms of Goshinjitsu [sic.] and forget acquiring the essentials of Goshinjitsu [sic.] ..." – Kotani et al, 1968:57

The Impact of Kata Competitions

No contemporary article on kata in judo would be complete without considering the impact being made by kata competitions, which have markedly grown in popularity in recent years (Jones and Hanon, 2010).

One consequence of the Kodokan formally treating Kodokan Goshin-jutsu as a proper kata is that it now features in most organized kata competitions. Interestingly however, there was no Kodokan Goshin-jutsu category in the first, and so far only, Kodokan Judo Kata International Tournament. This event was organized jointly by the Kodokan and the All Japan Judo Federation, and held in Tokyo in October 2007 (Gatling, 2008).

The Positives and Negatives

It is evident that the introduction of kata-specific tournaments has broadened the appeal of kata by providing judoka with new sources of motivation for its study. These include the prospect of winning a medal, or of becoming an international-level competitor via the alternative pathway that "competitive kata" provides.

As a direct consequence of kata championships, there are presently more judoka aware of, and practicing kata, than at any time in the recent past. However, in the long-term, the drift of kata into the "realm of sport", especially under the rules of the IJF with a scoring system[68] that focuses on mistakes and points deductions (for deviations from a supposed reference standard) could do more harm than good. Of particular concern is the idea that there exists an ideal standard kata, as such thinking contradicts the principle of *shu-ha-ri* [protect-break-separate][69]—the traditional route of progressing from basic knowledge to mastery in Japan[70]. Specifically, the current approach to judging kata is overly weighted on the shu component, with minimal scope in the scoring system to accommodate the ha or the ri elements (Jones and Hanon, 2010).

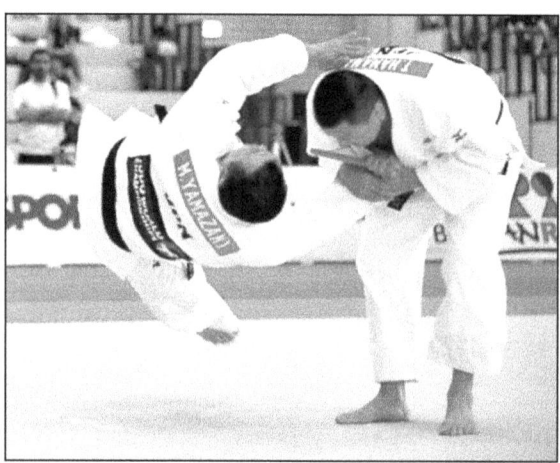

Figure 27: Tomoo Hamana as tori and Masayoshi Yamazaki as uke, winning the Kodokan Goshin-jutsu category at the 2011 International Judo Federation (IJF) World Judo Kata Championships held in Frankfurt, Germany. The technique shown in the photograph is *kote-gaeshi* [wrist reversal] from *naname-tsuki* [slanting stab].

In the case of Kodokan Goshin-jutsu, the emphasis on the principles within has diminished[71], and that on mechanical movements increased. For this reason, the Kodokan Goshin-jutsu performances seen in contemporary kata tournaments are sometimes over-stylized self-parodies with unrealistic techniques, and markedly different from Tomiki and Otaki's first demonstration (Kodokan, 2009; Sharp, 2013) which was full of realism, spirit and effective technique.

Authors' Comments

Kata were not created to be "judged" or to be studied as an exercise in "how to perform a complete ceremonial kata demonstration"—rather they were developed as a living and breathing educational tool to support the correct learning and practice of judo principles (Jones and Hanon, 2010). However, for better or worse, competitive kata is here to stay, and with this the risk of future generations of judoka believing this significant misrepresentation of kata is the norm. This is exemplified by the particularly uninformed definition of kata from USA Judo[72]:

> Kata is a forms-based judo discipline in which two athletes perform a set routine of judo techniques which are then scored by a panel of judges.
> – Jomantas: 2009

Given the original intent for kata, participation in competitive kata should ideally be viewed as an opportunity to validate one's training, improve one's judo under highly stressful circumstances and obtain feedback for future improvement. However, this requires that the judges doing the critiquing have themselves an in-depth knowledge of kata that goes beyond the capability to notice IJF-specified mistakes.

CREDIBILITY OF KODOKAN GOSHIN-JUTSU FOR SELF-DEFENSE

Much in the way that many think Nage-no-kata and Katame-no-kata are irrelevant to modern sports competitive judo, there are those who believe that Kodokan Goshin-jutsu is neither a complete, nor an effective system of self-defense (Michael J. Hanon, personal communication, 24 November 2013). Often, but not always, this unjust criticism comes from those persons whose learning has been limited to Kodokan Goshin-jutsu's performance aspects[73] and who have not studied and explored its core principles, or how they translate to self-defense (C. De Crée, personal communication, 25 November 2013). Since Kodokan Goshin-jutsu is nowadays treated as a kata, the remark of Fraguas (2001) is particularly relevant:

> Unfortunately, 95 percent of the people don't understand kata—only the outside movements which are irrelevant without understanding.
> – Fraguas, 2001:283

The principal points of criticism for Kodokan Goshin-jutsu are whether or not it provides one with the tools for effectively dealing with knife and pistol attacks. To a degree this is understandable, but again has at its source an over-emphasis on mechanical movements, and an under-appreciation of principles. To address this issue, further explanation of the defenses against knife and pistol attacks will now be presented. This will draw on Cornish (1984:22–24; 27–33) and Wolfgang Dax-Romswinkel (personal communication, 27 November 2013).

Knife Attacks

The knife attacks in Kodokan Goshin-jutsu include a sudden draw and thrust, a lunge, and a slanting slash from above. They encompass what would be the most common types of knife attack, and therefore represent a sufficiently complete set of generic situations for developing self-defense concepts and principles.

Defenses against a determined attacker armed with a knife are difficult and dangerous to execute, so tori has to study the Tanto-no-baai sequences very deeply. The essential principles in the defenses are tai-sabaki, to evade the attack and remain in a relatively safe position, and kuzushi to distract and disturb uke's equilibrium. These two aspects cannot be over-emphasized for knife defenses, and failure to perform them perfectly in a "real situation" could well result in tori's death. Above all else, the emphasis in their practice has to be on realism and effectiveness.

Consider, for example, the first knife-defense—Tsukkake, which arguably is the most difficult defense in all of Kodokan Goshin-jutsu. In this defense, tori foils uke's attack in the preparatory stage[74], with the intended attack being first countered with tai-sabaki in such a way as to shatter it. It is the errors in uke's own actions that provide an opportunity for tori to counter-attack and prevail.

Uke turns to his right to draw the knife from the (virtual) sheath inside his judo jacket, and as a result his left shoulder turns forward and inward. Uke's knife-holding (right) arm is (back) out of tori's reach, and so tori has no option but to attack the other (forward, left) arm. Tori steps forward to take up a position to uke's left rear, so as to be reasonably safe should his counter-attack fail. Tori instantly uses atemi-waza by applying a blinding strike [metsubushi] to uke's eyes with the outstretched fingers of his left hand. Tori then immediately grasps uke's left wrist and twists it up, while controlling uke's left elbow, pushing it towards his ear, and off balancing him—kuzushi. Then, as uke reacts and attempts to regain his balance, tori's right hand applies pressure onto the raised elbow and pulls uke diagonally forwards and down to the ground, to uke's left, with *hiki-otoshi* [drawing drop].

Even though the knife in uke's right hand remains free, uke does not have the opportunity to use it due to the blinding *metsubushi*, and the movement and distance that tori maintains from him. Tori then controls uke on the ground through with *ude-hishigi-te-gatame* [arm crushing hand armlock].

Gun Attacks

In his original book on Kodokan Goshin-jutsu, Tomiki seems to regard the Kenshu-no-baai gun defenses as something of an "adventure". This is in the sense that most judoka learning the exercise may not appreciate that the gun defenses are mainly built on the effective use of mental functions, more so than the mechanical movements. Tomiki writes:

> Needless to say, it is totally absurd to compare, or compete, the speed of bodily action against that of a bullet. But there can be various mental states in the mind of a gunman until he actually pulls the trigger. In the process of an attack, one should be able to take advantage of the slightest lack in an attacker's concentration. On the whole, there is no difference in the attitude of a person facing a weapon, be it a gun or something else, but in case of a gun, a scientific weapon, special caution is in order. Further on, Professor Kudo 9th dan at the Police Academy suggested three points of great importance in dealing with a similar situation:
>
> 1. Never make any move until a gunman comes within reach of your hands. While watching carefully his moves, stay alert, but very calm, so as not to cause any agitation.
> 2. Any defense action should start by first pushing the gun away, use your hands and hips but not your legs.
> 3. Once such action is initiated, it has to be decisive as you do it at the risk of your life.
>
> – Tomiki, 1958

Additionally, one of the high-ranking judoka at the Keishicho [Tokyo Metropolitan Police Department] supervised an empirical study that tested the practicality of executing the three Kenshu-no-bai defenses. In the experiments, the participants were wearing appropriate safety clothing and were using pistols that fired plastic bullets. The study concluded that some 80% of the time, tori was shot while attempting the techniques, and the concluding words regarding the practical application of the defenses was "Very difficult" (O. Mouri, personal communication, 6 April 2015).

It is beyond the scope of this chapter to second-guess such research, but the authors assume it very difficult to duplicate the gun attack situations envisioned in Kodokan Goshin-jutsu for training purposes—an untrained, unsuspecting, naive gunman[75] that has his attention diverted. In any instance, the conclusion reported above should be fully recognized, and the pistol defenses viewed for use only *in extremis*. Indeed, most military and law enforcement professionals with combatives[76] and defensive tactics experience, would not claim to have seen a sufficiently reliable technique for disarming a gunman, that they would recommend for use, unless they observed indicators that lead them to believe they were about to be shot.

Authors' Comments

Kodokan Goshin-jutsu makes a valuable contribution to judo, and none of the issues discussed in this section render it worthless. Indeed, the major criticism of its limited efficacy against guns would apply to all other elements in the entire judo syllabus.

Whether a technique works in "real life" depends on the skill level of the people involved—both attacker and defender. However, in self-defense situations, skill is not the only factor, and recall from earlier, that the ability to physically and emotionally cope with real life conflict and stress, is paramount.

The authors' recommendations to those who believe that an exercise developed by the greatest Kodokan sensei of the time, is fundamentally flawed and futile, is to revisit its learning under a knowledgeable and experienced teacher, focus on principles not mechanics, and then after many years of serious study, reexamine their views.

Concluding Remarks

In the context of judo principles for self-defense, establishing Kodokan Goshin-jutsu was entirely appropriate, since at that time, the only formal exercise for both men and women to study how to attack and defend was the archaic, but still valuable Kime-no-kata.

Knives, staffs and pistols still regularly feature in violent crime today, as do other cutting instruments and firearms. However, nowadays assailants also use new weapons originally developed for law-enforcement, or self-defense purposes, such as electroshock devices or Tasers, CS gas, mace, and pepper sprays. While Kodokan Goshin-jutsu is often referred to as being a "modern self-defense kata", the period for it actually being "modern" was over half a century ago. As Savage (2010; 2013; 2016) points out, critics might argue that Kodokan Goshin-jutsu is as obsolete today as Kime-no-kata was thought to be in the 1950s.

While judo is limited to what it can achieve in terms of defense against any of the aforementioned weapons, this is not a valid reason for discarding Kodokan Goshin-jutsu. The authors firmly believe that Kodokan Goshin-jutsu is fully deserving of its place in contemporary judo—not as a ceremonial performance exercise, or even a method of self-defense, but as a living textbook (Finn, 1991) to practice self-defense principles, and a framework to build and derive additional defenses.

ACKNOWLEDGEMENTS

The authors would like to register their gratitude to Shinro Fujita, Rie Kurashina and Keiko Otsuki of the International Department of the Kodokan Judo Institute for providing assistance and valuable information whenever requested. Additionally, Figures 11-14, 16 and 19 are reproduced with the permission of the Kodokan Judo Institute, a public interest incorporated foundation. Recall that Figures 1 and 2 are from the personal collection of one of the authors (WLG), whereas Figure 4 was kindly provided by Fumiaki Shishida, Professor of the Intellectual History of the Japanese Martial Arts at Waseda University, and a direct student of Kenji Tomiki. Figures 9a to 10c and that above the Abstract were made available by professional photographer and judoka, Bob Willingham, and professional photographer and judoka David Finch kindly provided Figure 27. The authors are also indebted to Osamu Mouri for sharing his knowledge of and personal insights into Kodokan Goshin-jutsu—a contribution that significantly enriched the quality of this chapter. Finally, one of the authors (LCJ) would like to dedicate this work to his own Kodokan Goshin-jutsu teacher—Robert (Bob) Thomas, IJF 8th dan— who inspired in him a deep and abiding interest in the exercise. Any and all errors are our own.

AUTHORS' NOTE

Japanese names in this chapter are presented given name first and family name second—instead of traditional Japanese usage that places the family name first.

FOOTNOTES

[1] The Kodokan (in full, the Kodokan Judo Institute) is the headquarters of the worldwide judo community. Literally, *ko* means "to lecture" or "to spread information," *do* means "the way," and *kan* is "a public building or hall," together translating roughly as "a place for the study or promotion of the way." The original Kodokan was founded in 1882 at the Eishoji Temple in the Higashi Ueno area of Taito-ku, Tokyo. Today, the Kodokan Judo Institute it is located in a modern eight-story building in Bunkyo-ku, Tokyo.

[2] Since in judo the term "*shihan*" is used exclusively for Kano, it could be translated as "master".

[3] *Koryu* is a general term for Japanese schools of martial arts that were primarily created by, and for, the warrior class of Japan's feudal period.

[4] Toshiro Daigo (born 1926) was for many years the Chief Instructor at the Kodokan. He was promoted to the rare rank of Kodokan 10th dan in 2006, and is arguably the world's foremost kata expert.

[5] The only formal grouping of kata used by the Kodokan is the collective consideration of Nage-no-kata and Katame-no-kata as Randori-no-kata [Forms of Free Exercise]. However, other authors have produced additional groupings for illustrative purposes—notably Kotani, Osawa and Hirose, (1968:1) and Otaki and Draeger (1983:32–33). These groupings are Combat, Physical Education, and Theory. Jones and Hanon (2010) provide Japanese terms for these groupings—respectively, Shobu-no-kata, Rentai-no-kata and Ri-no-kata.

[6] Joshi Goshin-ho was developed during the last days of the Second World War (WWII) (1939–1945), when inter alia there was great concern that Japanese women could be physically attacked by invaders. Its creation was ordered by retired Imperial Japanese Navy Admiral Jiro Nango (1876–1951), a nephew of Kano-shihan, and the second Kodokan Kancho [Head] from 1939 to 1946 (De Crée and Jones, 2011). Careful study of

Joshi Goshin-ho reveals that it is tailored towards women in the days when they were mostly clad in kimono, and while judo principles are intermittently applied, the exercise is more founded on a number of specific tricks.

7 In the context of kata, the term *riai* refers to executing the kata in proper accordance with its principles and theory (Dax-Romswinkel, 2015:44).

8 Dr. Steven Cunningham is a mathematician, economist and former Technical Director of the USJA.

9 USJA = United States Judo Association—one national association for judo in the United States of America.

10 Nango did not personally devise Joshi Goshin-ho—he merely ordered its creation (De Crée and Jones, 2011).

11 Recall that these two exercises are Sei-ryoku Zen'yo Kokumin Taiiku and Joshi Goshin-ho.

12 Sydney (Syd) R. Hoare (born 1939) is a former Chief Instructor of the London Budokwai [sic.] and the London Judo Society, a 1964 Tokyo Olympian and a former Chairman of the BJA. Hoare spent four years training in Japan, is fluent in Japanese, and inter alia is a multi-published author.

13 BJA = British Judo Association (BJA)—the National Governing Body (NGB) for judo in the United Kingdom (UK).

14 Minoru Mochizuki (1907–2003) Kodokan 8th dan was a direct student of both Jigoro Kano and Morihei Ueshiba. He founded the composite system Yoseikan Budo [Yoseikan = "Place where the Truth is Taught" or "Place for Practicing what is Right"] and first taught it at his dojo [place of the way = formal training place] in Shizuoka in 1931. Mochizuki held *kodansha* [high dan] rank in many different budo styles.

15 *Aiki-jujutsu* was the first (short) term used to describe the jujutsu style more formally known as Daito-ryu Aiki-jujutsu [The Great Eastern School of the Martial Art of Unifying Spirit] (Shishida, 2011).

16 *Shinken shobu* denotes a real fight to the death, or to a true submission.

17 *Tai-sabaki* is a general term for movements to shift the position of one's body and change direction in the process of reacting to an opponent's technique and setting up and applying techniques of one's own (Kawamura and Daigo, 2000).

18 The Meiji period extended from 8 September 1868 to 30 July 1912. During this period major socio-political change took place in Japan—with society moving from being isolated and feudal to its modern form.

19 The Edo (or Tokugawa) period is a Japanese era between 1603 and 1868, when society was under the rule of the Tokugawa bakufu [shogunate] and 300 regional Daimyo [feudal lords]. The period was characterized by economic growth, strict social order, isolationist foreign policies, and popular enjoyment of arts and culture.

20 Samurai were forbidden from entering a daimyo's house, or to be in the presence of the Shogun or the Emperor, while carrying a katana.

21 Note that some who have trained to a very high level in Kime-no-kata are known to practice with live blades. This introduces absolute realism into training, and advances the learning and understanding of the kata.

22 During controlled practice, *tori* and *uke* are the individuals that apply, and receive, a technique, respectively. In Kime-no-kata and Kodokan Goshin-jutsu, uke makes the initial attack, and tori demonstrates the defensive technique.

23 Also known as Yoshiaki Yamashita.

24 Yamashita was posthumously promoted to 10th dan by Kano on 26 October 1935. However, Kano dated his promotion certificate for two days earlier—thereby making it

appear as a substantive promotion.
25. The idea to "modernize" Kime-no-kata had existed since the 1920s, when Jigoro Kano and Kodokan members started to practice *bo-jutsu* [staff technique] at the Kodokan (Shishida, 2011).
26. Three variations of Nagaoka's given name are often seen—Hidekazu Nagaoka, Shuichi Nagaoka and Hideichi Nagaoka. The correct given name was finally identified via the US National Archives and Records Administration, and the US Immigration Passenger Arrival Records, since when Nagaoka visited Seattle in 1934 he personally signed his entry in romaji as "Nagaoka Hideichi".
27. The influence of Nagaoka might be questioned as being minimal, since he died in November 1952. However, with his koryu background and periods teaching at the Dai Nippon Butokukai and the Busen (its martial arts specialist school) he was an influential figure in Kime-no-kata. By dint of this, it could be considered that he had an impact on the practical combat training of many committee members.
28. *Torite* is a type of self-defense containing technique for restraining, or escaping from, an attacker.
29. Kudo wrote separate master-volumes on the throwing and grappling techniques of judo under the collective title "Dynamic Judo" (Kudo, 1967; 1967a).
30. Otaki, along with the notable US budoka Donn Draeger (1922-1982) wrote "Judo Formal Techniques" (Otaki and Draeger, 1983) which is to this day the most comprehensive manual on Randori-no-kata.
31. Waseda University is a private university mainly located in Shinjuku, Tokyo.
32. Towards the end of his life, Kano became increasingly aware of certain failings of judo—not necessarily because of its own flaws, but because the way it was being practiced was increasingly deviating from his original ideas, and also the technical challenges of dealing with assailants using Western boxing techniques attacking from beyond reach. He tried to remedy this by conceding that judo might benefit from an infusion of techniques from koryu jujutsu and even Western boxing. However, this effort apparently never formalized and waned after his death—due to the dislocation caused by WWII, the leadership of Nango, and the subsequent outlawing of martial arts training in public facilities under the Allied occupation of Japan. It was emphasizing judo as a sport that facilitated its eventual return to public facilities.
33. There is no authoritative single list, but a number of different lists with significant overlap.
34. The term aiki-budo [the martial way of unifying spirit] began to be used by Ueshiba's pupils (instead of aiki-jujutsu) around 1933. In 1942 aiki-budo was renamed aikido—the name still used today (Shishida, 2011).
35. Tomiki was awarded the first 8th dan of aiki-budo by Ueshiba in 1940.
36. For example, there are instances of uke attacking, and tori either failing to grasp him at the first attempt, or else uke breaking free, and tori having to grasp him again.
37. Harold (Hal) E. Sharp (born 1927) is a senior American judoka, and presently a USJA 9th dan. He is Japanese-trained, the author of several popular judo books and also the editor of several judo films of historical interest.
38. *Bujutsu* may be defined as "... combative systems designed by and for warriors to promote self-protection and group solidarity..." (Draeger, 1973:19).
39. *Budo* may be defined as "... spiritual systems, not necessarily designed by warriors, or for warriors, for the self-protection of the individual..." (Ibid.:19).
40. Fujoshi-yo-Goshin-no-kata was at one time a suggested name for Joshi Goshin-ho (De Crée and Jones, 2011).

[41] FFJDA = Fédération Française de Judo, (Jujitsu, Kendo, Aikido) et Disciplines Associées = French Federation of Judo, (Jujitsu, Kendo, Aikido) and Associated Disciplines—the NGB for judo in France.

[42] Kawaishi was posthumously promoted to 10th dan by the FFJDA—the first promotion to this rank by a Western judo NGB (De Crée, 2015).

[43] The English language book is a translation by the British journalist, author and judoka Ernest (E.J.) Harrison of the original 1955 French-language text "Les Katas Complets de Judo" by Kawaishi and Jean Gailhat.

[44] The summary of Chapter X wrongly states that Kodokan Goshin-jutsu was established in 1958. Recall that 1958 was the year of publication of Tomiki's original book on Kodokan Goshin-jutsu, and that the exercise itself was established two years earlier in 1956.

[45] Although Jigoro Kano is presented as the author of this book—it is in fact a compilation by the Kodokan Judo Institute that dates from long after the founder's death.

[46] John P. Cornish is a senior British judoka, BJA 7th dan, and *aikidoka* [a person who practices aikido], 8th dan. He is Japanese-trained and was a direct student of Kenji Tomiki—see later.

[47] For clarity, *reigi* is the concept of etiquette and *reiho* is its physical manifestation.

[48] During this interim period a few countries, such as France, continued mainly with sitting bowing arrangements—see Hamot, Pelletier and Urvoy (1985).

[49] This is excepting of all of the idori section and all of the katana attacks.

[50] Ju-no-kata includes a number of attacks and defenses that show the efficient redirection of force and movement. They are not "fighting techniques" in the conventional sense, and there is no notion of literally using them in combat.

[51] *Maai* is a complex concept that goes beyond the mere physical distance between the combatants. It is an integration of that distance, with timing, speed, distance, angles, coordination and rhythm of attack.

[52] *Mushin* is a mental state into which very highly trained budoka are said to enter during combat. The term is shortened from mushin no shin, a Zen expression meaning "mind of no mind", i.e. a mind not fixed or occupied by thought or emotion, and thus open to everything.

[53] *Zanshin* is a state of awareness that continues even after throwing your opponent, maintained to allow further action and response should he continue with a counterattack.

[54] In judo, atemi-waza are most often used for the purposes of kuzushi. This contrasts with their use in karate-do [empty hand way] where they are an objective in their own right.

[55] This is with the exception of one fist attack—Tsukkake and one sword attack—*kiri-oroshi* [downward cut], both in the tachiai section.

[56] Tadao Inogai (1908–1978) Kodokan 8th dan has, along with co-author Roland Habersetzer, several judo books, published in the French language, to his name.

[57] Roland Habersetzer (born 1942) is a senior French practitioner of Japanese and Chinese martial arts and is the author of several reference books on multiple styles.

[58] Similarly, Kime-no-kata still remains of great value, as it too teaches several core principles that remain directly relevant to judo and self-defense.

[59] Any lack of appreciation of the powerful ideas in Kodokan Goshin-jutsu is often due to shortcomings in teaching.

[60] The Budokwai [Society of the Martial Way], or to use its full official name The Budokwai (The Way of Knighthood Society), was founded in London in 1918 by Gunji Koizumi (1885–1965) Kodokan 8th dan, and initially offered tuition in jujutsu (later transitioning to judo) and kendo [way of the sword]. It is one of the oldest such societies (or clubs)

[61] in Europe. The name Budokwai, as opposed to Budokai, arises from the conversion of Japanese to the Roman alphabet using an earlier system of transliteration that the one commonly used today. To this day, the continued use of Budokwai remains the club's preference.

[61] Kotani retired from the Kodokan in 1988 and returned to his home prefecture of Hyogo, in the Kansai region of Japan.

[62] Takata himself could throw in any (360°) direction with hane-goshi.

[63] Gendai budo are modern Japanese martial ways which were established after the Meiji Restoration of 1868.

[64] RFEJYDA = Real Federación Española de Judo y Deportes Asociados = Royal Spanish Federation of Judo and Associated Sports—the NGB for judo in Spain.

[65] The World Masters Judo Association (WMJA) was an entity founded in Ottawa, Canada in 1998 with the purpose of encouraging participation in competition judo and kata for "masters" judoka—that is, those aged 30 years plus, in a fun, friendly and family orientated manner. It "voluntarily disbanded" in 2010, ceding organisational control of masters' judo events to the IJF.

[66] JBN = Judo Bond Nederland = Dutch Judo Federation—the NGB for judo in the Netherlands.

[67] Two of the authors (LCJ and MPS) have personal experience, as uke, of the effectiveness of Cornish's *Kodokan Goshin-jutsu*, and are fully appreciative of the power of his technique.

[68] The IJF have produced "competition formula" (IJF, 2015) that detail how many points to deduct for various categories of "mistakes" in a competitive kata performance. Consequently, when practising, judoka place great emphasis on avoiding these mistakes over and above any other aspects.

[69] *Shu* is focused on the mechanical movements of a kata, and copying what a teacher shows. *Ha* involves developing a deeper understanding, by reflecting on the kata's principles after the mechanics have been learnt. *Ri* involves going beyond the original teachings, and developing personal variations based on the principles.

[70] Ukichi (n.d.) cited in Daigo's (2008) lecture notes from the 2008 Kodokan Summer Kata Course, emphasises the shu-ha-ri approach to kata study.

[71] Dax-Romswinkel (2015:44) comments on a similar trend for Ju-no-kata, where its aesthetic component has faded due to the influence of kata competition.

[72] USA Judo is the NGB for judo in the US.

[73] The performance aspects of Kodokan Goshin-jutsu encompass its mechanical movements—including the timing and distance of individual techniques.

[74] Note that the defense against the first staff attack—*furiage* [upswing against staff] is also launched before uke's strike. In this way the defenses against the attacks with the knife and the staff have some similarities.

[75] A trained, suspicious and experienced gunman will not get within arms' reach of any opponent.

[76] Combatives is a term for hand-to-hand combat training and techniques.

REFERENCES

Blonk, M., DeBijl, R. and Van Dijk, F. (2010). *Kodokan Goshin Jutsu*. Den Haag: Paagman. (In Dutch).

Cornish, J.P. (1984). *Go-Shin-jutsu—Judo self defence kata*. United Kingdom: FJR Publishing for the British Judo Association.

Cornish, J.P. (1985). Koshiki-no-Kata. *British Judo Magazine, 8*(4), 6.

Cornish, J.P. (2004). What is Kata? *Kano Society—The Bulletin*, 10, 1–2.

Dabauza, P.R. (1988). *Kata Judo-Jujitsu.* Barcelona: Editorial Alas. (In Spanish).

Daigo, T. (2005). *Kodokan Judo—Throwing techniques.* Trans. F. White. Tokyo: Kodansha International.

Daigo, T. (2008). Jigoro Kano—Kodokan Judo-no-Kata—Kodokan Published Showa 39 (1964). Lecture notes from the Kodokan Summer Kata Course, 29 July 2008. Tokyo: Kodokan Judo Institute.

Daigo,T. (2008-2009). Kodokan Judo Kata ni Tsuite (1)-(7) [About the Kata of Kodokan Judo—Parts 1-7]. *Judo.* 79(10), 52–57; 79(11), 7–12; 79(12), 18–23; 80(1), 16–22; 80(2), 43–50; 80(3), 12–16 and 80(4), 3–9. (In Japanese).

Dax-Romswinkel, W. (2015). Ju No Kata: The application of riai and its physical benefits. *Judoka Quarterly*, 1, 42–48

De Crée, C. and Jones, L. (2009). Kodokan Judo's Elusive Tenth Kata: The Go-no-kata— "Forms of Proper Use of Force" Parts 1-3, *Archives of Budo*, 5, 55–73; 75–82 and 83–95.

De Crée, C. and Jones L.C. (2011). Kodokan Judo's Inauspicious Ninth Kata: The Joshi go-shiho—"Self-Defense Methods for Women" Parts 1-3. *Archives of Budo*, 7(3), 105–123; 125–137; 139–158.

De Crée, C. (2016). Kodokan Judo's Three Orphaned Forms of Counter Tech- niques–Part 1: The Gonosen-no-kata—Forms of Post-Attack Initiative Counter Throws; Part 2: The Nage-waza ura-no-kata—Forms of Reversing Throwing Techniques; Part 3: The Katame-waza ura-no-kata—Forms of Reversing Controlling Techniques. *Archives of Budo*, 11, 93–123; 125–154; 155–171.

Draeger, D.F. (1973). *Classical bujutsu: The martial arts and ways of Japan volume 1.* New York: Weatherhill.

FFJDA. (n.d.) Kodokan Goshinjitsu. Collection guide de judoka (3). Talence: Trainer. (In French).

Finn, M. (1991). *Martial arts: A complete illustrated history.* Leicester: Blitz Editions.

Fraguas, J.M. (2001). *Karate masters.* California: Unique Publications.

Gatling, W.L. (2008). The First Kodokan Judo Kata International Competition and its katas. *Journal of Asian Martial Arts, 17*(1), 68–77.

Hamot, C., Pelletier, G. and Urvoy, C. (1985). *Katame no Kata Kodokan Goshin Jutsu.* Bolo-gne-Billancourt: SEDIREP. (In French).

Hoare, S.R. (2009). *A history of judo.* London: Yamagi Books.

Hoare, S.R. (2010). Go No Kata (The kata of resistance). Available online from URL: http://www.sydhoare.com/GO%20NO%20KATA.pdf

IJF (International Judo Federation—Kata Commission.) (2015). *Kata Competition—Criteria for the Evaluation.* International Judo Federation.

Inogai, T., author, and Habersetzer, R., compiler. (2007). *Judo kata—Les formes classiques du Kodokan.* Paris: Amphora. (In French).

Jomantas, N. (2009). Team USA to Compete at First Ever Kata World Championships This Weekend (13 October 2009). Available online from URL: http://judo.teamusa.org/news/article/28266 (Accessed: July 2010.)

Jones, L.C. and Hanon, M.J. (2010). The way of kata in Kodokan Judo. *Journal of Asian Martial Arts, 19*(4), 8–37.

Kano, J. (1934). The significance of judo and its objectives. Imperial Japan Oratory Society, editors.

Budo Hokan [Martial Arts Treasures]. Tokyo: Imperial Japan Oratory Society Discussion Group. 290–294.

Kano, J. (1986). *Kodokan Judo*. Tokyo: Kodansha International.

Kano Sensei Biograpic Editorial Committee. (2009). Bennett, A. editor and translator. *Jigoro Kano and the Kodokan—An Innovative Response To Modernisation*. Tokyo: Kano Risei, Kodokan Judo Institute. English publication Tokyo: Bunkasha International Corporation.

Kano Society. (2006). Cornish, J.P. teacher. Go-Shin-Jutsu—Part 1: Toshu (against an unarmed attack); Part 2: Buki (against an armed attack). 2-part DVD set. London: Dial Media.

Kawamura, T. and Daigo, T. editors. (2000). *Kodokan new Japanese-English dictionary of Judo*. Tokyo: Kodokan Institute.

Kawaishi, M. (1956). Gailhat, J., editor. *Les katas complets de judo*. Paris: Impr. de J. Cario. (In French).

Kawaishi, M. (1957). Harrison, E.J., translator. *The complete 7 katas of judo*. London: W. Foulsham and Co. Ltd.

Kodokan. (1961). *Judo*. Osaka: Nunoi Shobo Co. Ltd.

Kodokan. (1976). *Illustrated Kodokan Judo*. Tokyo: Kodansha.

Kodokan. (1987 and 1992). *Kodokan Goshin-jutsu*. Tokyo: Kodokan. (In Japanese and English).

Kodokan. (1998). Kodokan Judo kata series: Kodokan Goshin-jutsu. VHS Edition. Tokyo: Kodokan, Kodokan. (2004). Kodokan Goshin-jutsu. Tokyo: Kodokan. (In Japanese). https://www.hint.jp/cgi-bin/kshop/kshop.pl/page=bo021.html/SID =1440791991.47807

Kodokan. (2009). Kodokan Judo kata series: Kodokan Goshin-jutsu. DVD Edition. Tokyo: Kodokan, https://www.hint.jp/cgi-bin/kshop/kshop.pl/page=dvk06.html/SID= 1440 891385.48090 http://kodokanjudoinstitute.org/en/waza/forms/textbook/

Kodokan. (2015). Kodokan Goshin-jutsu. Tokyo: Kodokan. Available online from URL: http://kodokanjudoinstitute.org/en/docs/goshin_jutsu.pdf (Accessed: March 2015)

Kotani, S., Osawa, Y. and Hirose, Y. (1968). *Kata of Kodokan Judo / Kata of Kodokan Judo revised*. Kobe: Koyano Bussan Kaisha Ltd.

Kotani, S. and Otaki, T. (1971). *Saishin judo no kata zen* [The latest judo kata— Complete]. Tokyo: Fumaido Shuppan. (In Japanese).

Kotani, S. and Otaki, T. authors. (1971). In Daigo, T. editor. (2008). *Kodokan Goshinjutsu* [from Saishin Judo no Kata Zen]. Reprinted for the 2008 Kodokan Kata Kaki Koshukai (Kodokan Summer Kata Course). Tokyo: Kodokan Judo Institute.

Kudo, K. (1967). *Dynamic judo: Throwing techniques*. Tokyo: Japan Publications Trading Company.

Kudo, K. (1967a). *Dynamic judo: Grappling techniques*. Tokyo: Japan Publications Trading Company.

Lindsay, T. and Kano, J. (1889). Jiujutsu: The old samurai art of fighting without weapons. *Transactions of the Asiatic Society of Japan*, XVI(II). Yokohama. 1915 reprint. 202–217.

Mifune, K. (1955). *Mifune soen goshin-jutsu* [Mifune's personal self-defense].

On: (2005). Shingi Mifune Judan (Kanzenhan): Judo no Shinzui [The divine Mifune 10th dan (complete edition): The Essence of Judo]. [DVD]

Nihon Eiga Shinsha. Tokyo: Quest Co., Ltd. DVD SPD-3514, ca.: 06'21" (In Japanese).

Ochiai, T. (2012). Jones, L.C. and Mouri, O. translators. *Go-no-Kata*. Tokyo: Fuji Tosha-Do/ Fuji Printing.

Oltremri, A. (n.d.). Takata Katsuyoshi 9°Dan: Hane Goshi. freeBudo. Available online from URL: http://www.freebudo.com/articoli/judo%20tradizionale/tecnica%20judo/23.takata%20hane%20goshi/Takata%20hane%20gohi.htm (Accessed: March 2008). (In Italian).

Otaki, T. and Draeger, D.F. (1983). *Judo formal techniques*. Tokyo: Charles E. Tuttle Company Incorporated.

Parulski, G.R. (1985). *Black belt judo*. Chicago: Contemporary Books, Inc.

Savage, M.P. (2010). *A brief history and appraisal of Kodokan Goshin Jutsu*. British Judo Association 2010 Technical Congress, Leicester.

Savage, M.P. (2013). Kodokan Goshin-Jutsu. Judoka—Official Online Magazine of the British Judo Council, 121. Available online from URL: http://www.judoka.britishjudocouncil.org/issue/18/april-2013-issue-121/335/kodokan-goshin-jutsu.html (Accessed: April 2015).

Savage, M.P. (2016). Jones, L.C. editor. A brief history and appraisal of Kodokan Goshinjutsu [Kodokan self-defence]. *Kano Society—The Bulletin*. Issue 28, 1-4.

Sharp, H. (2013). *Classic judo kata*. Los Angeles: Rising Sun Productions.

Shishida, F. (2010). Judo's techniques performed from a distance: The origin of Jigoro Kano's concept and its actualization by Kenji Tomiki, *Archives of Budo*, 6(4), 165-171.

Shishida, F. (2011). Jigoro Kano's pursuit of ideal judo and its succession: Judo's techniques performed from a distance. Ido Movement for Culture. *Journal of Martial Arts Anthropology*, 11(1-4), 42-48.

Shishida, F. (2012). A judo that incorporates kendo: Jigoro Kano's ideas and their theoretical development. *Archives of Budo*, 8(4), 225-233.

Shishida, F. (2013). How does the philosophy of martial arts manifest itself? Insights from Japanese martial arts. Ido Movement for Culture. *Journal of Martial Arts Anthropology*, 13(3), 29-36.

Stevens, J. (2013). *The way of judo—A portrait of Jigoro Kano and his students*. Boston: Shambhala Publications Inc.

Taira, S. (2009). *La essencia del judo: Volume 2—Kata, apéndices*. Satori Ediciones: Gijón. (In Spanish).

Takahashi, M. (and Family). (1995). *Mastering judo*. Tokyo: Champaign: Human Kinetics.

Takata, K. (1961). *Estudio del hanehoshi*. Argentina: La Imprenta López. (In Spanish and English).

Tomiki, K. (1953). Goshin to shite judo ni tsuite [Concerning judo as self- defense]. *Judo*. May 1953. 45-49. (In Japanese).

Tomiki, K. (1956). *Judo, appendix: Aikido*. Tokyo: Japan Travel Bureau.

Tomiki, K. (1958). *Kodokan Goshin-jutsu*. Tokyo: Kodokan / Baseball Magazine. (In Japanese).

Ukichi, S. author (n.d.) Matsumoto, T. and Davidson, P. translators (n.d.) in Daigo, T. editor. (2008), *Eternal kendo*. Reprinted for the 2008 Kodokan Kata Kaki Koshukai (Kodokan Summer Kata Course). Tokyo: Kodokan Judo Institute.

Watanabe, K. (2003). *Essential judo katas*. Richmond Hill, Ontario: World Master Judo Association.

Watson, B.N. (2008). *Judo memoirs of Jigoro Kano*. Victoria: Trafford Publishing.

Yiannakis, L. with Cunningham, S. (2002). The kata of judo—Part I of a series. *American Judo—A Journal of the United States Judo Association*, Fall 2002: 19-21.

Yiannakis, L. with Cunningham, S.R. (2003). The kata of judo—Part II of a series. *American Judo—A Journal of the United States Judo Association*, Fall 2003: 20-24.

chapter 25

The Logic of Kodokan Judo Kata
by Llyr C. Jones, Ph.D.

This chapter is on Kodokan judo's Nage-no-kata ("forms of throwing") and Katame-no-kata ("forms of control"). Together, these katas form the Randori-no-kata ("forms of free practice"), and their study helps facilitate the development of free practice (*randori*) skills.

During my formative years in judo, the emphasis in the United Kingdom was only on sports competitive judo, and kata practice had essentially been eliminated. There were no teachers with kata experience local to me, and so my early study of kata was self-directed through books. After developing competence in the mechanical movements of the Randori-no-kata, I sought instruction from those judoka who had kept the kata flame alive in the UK, and over the years refined my skills under the guidance of some of the country's foremost kata experts, including Dai (David) Ball, the late Graham Wright, and Bob (Robert) Thomas. I would like to record my gratitude to those teachers now.

As an experienced judo player, I was privileged to develop further insight into katas through a memorable period of judo study in Japan. During my time spent at the Kodokan International Judo Institute in Tokyo and at various dojos in Kanagawa prefecture, I came to understand how the learning extractable from katas transcends that of merely developing physical skills and perfecting technique. While in Japan I cemented my belief that the link connecting judo's past, present, and future lies in the accurate teaching and practice of kata and it is this philosophy shapes my own kata practice, research, and teaching to this day.

Kata study is a challenging activity and achieving any degree of mastery will require many hours of patient and diligent study under the guidance of a knowledgeable teacher. However, as tips for their physical practice, the following elements should be considered essential. (In the following explanations, *tori* is the person who applies the technique, and *uke* is the person who receives the technique.)

- **Understanding:** An understanding of the fundamentals of the kata being demonstrated.
- **Logic:** Every movement in the kata must have a sensible purpose and be done in a sensible way. As such, one should always keep in mind the fundamental principles being demonstrated and the reason for the application of any particular technique.
- **Active Thought:** Katas should not be robotic, so one should actively think about one's role (as either tori or uke) and whether one is initiating or responding, attacking or defending, escaping or adjusting, etc.
- **Composure:** Proper concentration, decorum, and attitude.
- **Commitment:** Real attacks and real defenses.

- **Tempo:** Each kata has its own speed and tempo. Within some (e.g., the Nage-no-kata) the tempo also varies from move to move, while others have one tempo.
- **Fluidity:** The kata must "flow" since any performance will break down if there is hesitation during application.
- **Posture:** Balance and body control.
- **Coordination:** Between tori and uke in the techniques themselves, but also in the movements and transition between techniques.
- **Positioning:** Awareness of one's location on the mat with proper engagement distance, direction, and spacing.
- **Reigei:** Correct etiquette.

Kata practice should go beyond merely performing physical movements, and during practice one should always think about how kata can improve one's judo in the broader sense. The following are tips on assimilating and leveraging the lessons of Randori-no-kata into everyday judo.

- **NAGE-NO-KATA:** Consisting of five sets of three throws, each performed to the left and right sides, this kata helps develop an understanding of the theoretical basis of judo and the processes involved in kuzushi, tsukuri, and kake—i.e., how to assume the correct position for applying a throwing technique once uke's balance has been broken, and how to apply and complete a technique. This kata has uke attacking tori fifteen times—each time learning and adjusting his attack based on tori's previous response. Tori neutralizes uke's attack each time by applying himself and using the force or action of the attack itself to prevail. Tori also learns how his own body and mind react under physical and psychological stress, and also how to adapt effectively to changing circumstances utilizing both his body and mind.
- **KATAME-NO-KATA:** Consisting of three sets of five grappling techniques, this kata helps develop an understanding of the theoretical basis for learning control through executing and evading each technique. Tori learns how to best use his body in an efficient manner to control uke on the ground through working on his versatility and body movement while grappling. Similarly, uke, through striving to escape, learns how to exploit any weaknesses in tori's technique. Each and every time the Katame-no-kata is practiced, uke should continue to test tori by looking for his weak points and then attacking them, while tori should find new ways of nullifying uke's new escape attempts.

Sequence 1
1a) Shoulder wheel (*kata-guruma*) from the first set—hand techniques (*te-waza*).
1b) Lift-pull hip throw (*tsurikomi-goshi*) from the second set—hip techniques (*koshiwaza*).

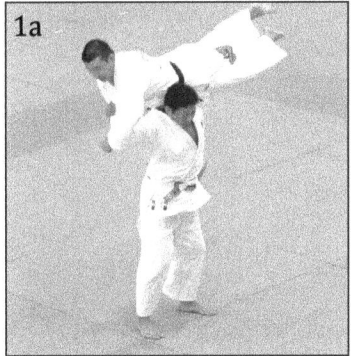
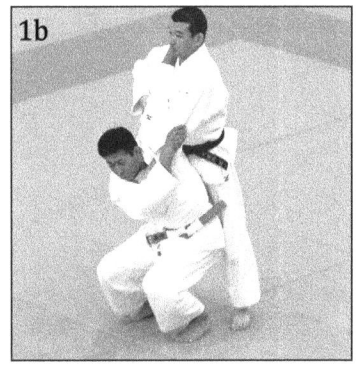

1c) Inner-thigh throw (*uchi-mata*) from the third set—leg techniques (*ashi waza*). 1d) Rear throw (*ura nage*) from the fourth set—supine sacrifice techniques (*ma-sutemi-waza*). 1e) Side hook (*yoko-gake*) from the fifth set—side sacrifice techniques (*yoko-sutemi-waza*).

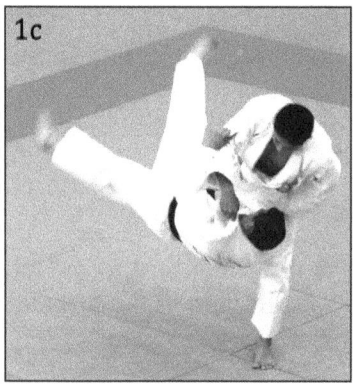
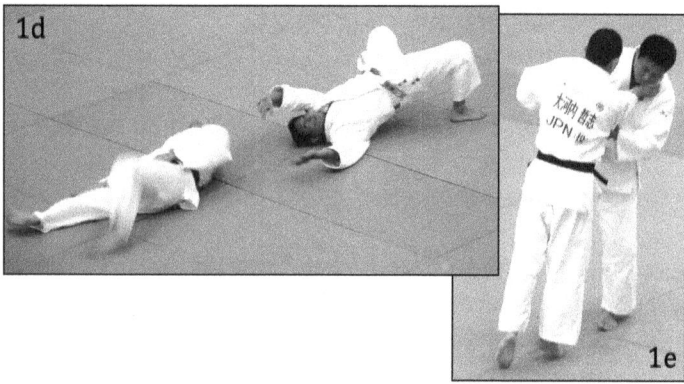

Sequence 1 is from a Nage-no-kata performance at the First Kodokan Judo Kata International Tournament, 2007. Tori: Katsuyuki Kondo, 6th dan. Uke: Tetsushi Okouchi, 5th dan.

Sequence 2

2a) Broken top four-corner hold (*kuzure kami shiho-gatame*) from the first set—holding techniques (*osaekomi-waza*). 2b) Naked lock (*hadaka-jime*) from the second set—strangling techniques (*shime-waza*). 2c) Arm crush (*ude gatame*) from the third set—joint techniques (*kansetsu-waza*).

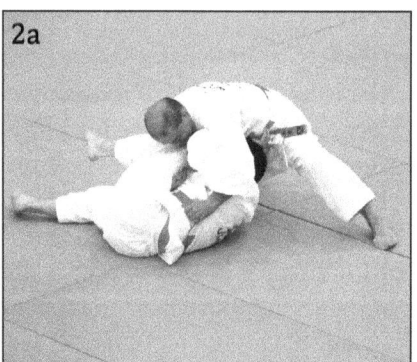
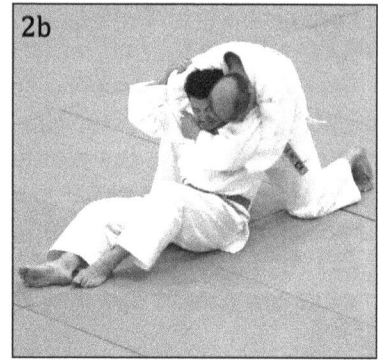

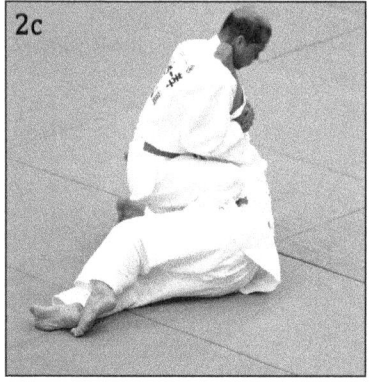

Sequence 2 is from a Katame-no-kata performance at the First Kodokan Judo Kata International Tournament, 2007. Tori: Kazutaka Yamamoto, 7th dan. Uke: Hirao Nasu, 6th dan.

All photographs copyright Carl De Crée (2007) and used with permission.

chapter 26

The Budokwai Centennial
by Brian N. Watson

Introduction

January 26, 2018 marked the 100th anniversary of the founding of the Budokwai, also known as GK House, by Gunji Koizumi in 1918. The following are thoughts on some of the notable events and the inspirational leaders who spearheaded the critical development of the Budokwai and judo throughout the UK and Europe over the past century.

Jigoro Kano

Jigoro Kano, born on 28th October 1860, started to study jujutsu in his teens and became a master of this art. He went on to create a new type of jujutsu and stressed its moral and spiritual value and named it 'Kodokan Judo'. After graduation from Tokyo Imperial University, he first became a lecturer, then at age 25, a professor of political science and economics. In the late 1880s, he and his leading students began the promotion of judo throughout Japan. From the early 1900s, however, Kodokan experts were increasingly sent abroad, most at the behest of Kano. Shortly thereafter his career began to span out: he was elected the first chairman of the Japan Amateur Sports Association; he later headed two important colleges, became a politician, and served on the International Olympic Committee for some twenty years.

The Early Dissemination of Judo Overseas

Jujutsu expert Yukio Tani (1881–1950), Figure 1, arrived in Britain in 1900 at the invitation of one of his students, Edward William Barton-Wright (1861–1951). Barton-Wright was an engineer, who had studied jujutsu in Japan from 1895 to 1898, while employed on the construction of a railway. Standing 5ft 2ins. and 50 kilos in weight, "Little Tani" as he was called soon became a household-name, especially throughout and following the boom period from 1902 to 1912. Jujutsu became a sensation. Most members of the general public were mesmerized when seeing such a small man defeat heavyweights, for it seemed to them like magic. Tani for years had huge success by trouncing his opponents of any weight in UK music hall prize-fights.

In 1902 Kano sent Yoshitsugu Yamashita (1865–1935), Figure 2, to the US where he instructed for some five years at Harvard University and at the US Naval Academy. President Theodore Roosevelt, Yamashita's most famous student, had a purpose-built dojo constructed at the White House where he took lessons. Mrs. Yamashita was also involved in teaching and gave judo tuition to American women.

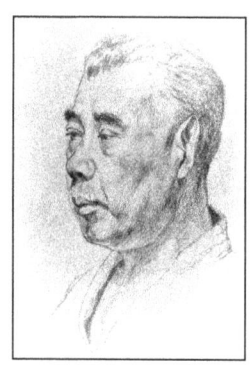 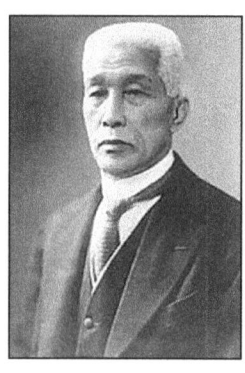 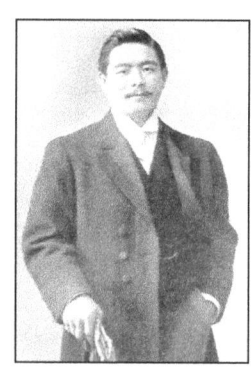

Figure 1, left: Yukio Tani (1881–1950), by Marcus Kaye.
Figure 2, middle: Yoshitsugu Yamashita (1865–1935).
Figure 3, right: Mitsuyo Maeda (1878–1941).

Among others heavily focused on the dissemination of judo overseas was the incredible Mitsuyo Maeda (1878–1941), Figure 3. He was born in Funasawa, Aomori prefecture, this area is now known as Hirosaki City. Maeda was given sumo lessons in boyhood by his father who was a keen amateur sumo man. He later went to Tokyo to attend the Tokyo Senmon School for his general education, and began the practice of Tenjin Shinyo-ryu jujutsu. Because he knew that Jigoro Kano was an expert in this particular style of jujutsu, Maeda decided to enrol at Kano's Kodokan. He soon grew adept at judo. Maeda was subsequently appointed judo team captain at Waseda University. He left Japan after graduating from Waseda and became active in the 1900s in North, Central, South America, and particularly so in Cuba and other countries.

Maeda finally settled in Brazil, where he trained among others Carlos Gracie (1902–1994). He became especially renowned in the Americas for his winning over 2,000 prize-fights during his long and well-paid career. Although Kano and his foremost instructors strove to make judo popular abroad, they were confronted with difficulties, one being that many foreigners were not so much interested in judo training as such, they merely wished to learn judo self-defense techniques. Furthermore, several of the early Japanese experts were more experienced in jujutsu than in judo, and by using their jujutsu skills in prize-fights, they gained lucrative income.

Although some Japanese were said to have given jujutsu lessons in the UK in 1900, the first dojo in the UK to be constructed as such was at Trinity College, Cambridge University. This amateur dojo was opened in 1906 by Mr. Evelyn Charles Donaldson Rawlins. He was born in 1884, and served for a time as president of this dojo. An expert linguist, Rawlins was said to have attained fluency in several foreign languages, a decided asset that no doubt served him well throughout his diplomatic career (1907–1940), which culminated in service as Minister to Bolivia (1937–1939). The dojo was private, however, and was used initially for the teaching of 25 members of Cambridge University. Since membership soon increased, Yukio Tani, Masutaro Otani (1896–1977), Figure 4, and Gunji Koizumi were each requested to travel periodically from London to Cambridge in order to give instruction.

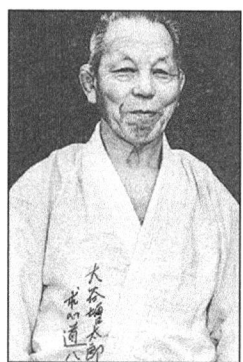 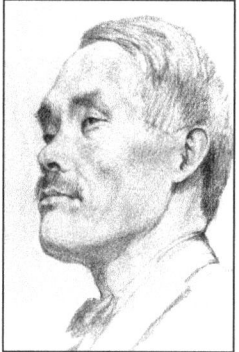

Figure 4, left: Masutaro Otani (1896–1977).
Figure 5, right: Gunji Koizumi (1885–1965), by Marcus Kaye.

Gunji Koizumi (1885–1965), Figure 5, often referred to as the "Father of British Judo," was a tenant farmer's son, born on July 8th 1885 in Komatsuka Oaza, a village north of Tokyo that is now part of Ibaraki Prefecture. His experience of budo was instigated with kendo lessons from the age of 12 to 15. Years later he said, 'At the time I did not fully realize it, but I owe much to this kendo master. The force of his personality and the kendo training had a strong influence in moulding my ego.' Koizumi also started to study English under the tutelage of a neighbor who had spent time in the United States. At 15 he left home and headed to Tokyo for training to become a telegraphist. At 16 he began to learn Tenjin Shinyo-ryu jujutsu. Shortly after qualifying as a telegraphist, he secured initial employment in Tokyo for a while before going to Korea where he worked for a railroad company. In 1904, Koizumi sailed to the US with the intention of studying electrical engineering. He worked his passage travelling via Shanghai, Hong Kong, Singapore and India.

Sometime later Koizumi left America for Britain and reportedly arrived penniless in May of 1906. He first stayed for one year in Liverpool where he gave instruction at the Kara Ashikaga School of Jujutsu. In 1907, he moved to London where he collaborated with famed prize-fighter Sadakazu Uyenishi (Raku) a teacher at a jujutsu school in Piccadilly Circus. Koizumi was engaged as a jujutsu trainer for a time at the London Polytechnic and at the Royal Naval Volunteer Reserve, following which he again went to the USA in 1907 where he found employment at the Newark Public Service Railroad Company. Unhappy with life in America, he returned to London in 1910 and attempted to set up an electrical appliance business. He met with little success, however, owing to insufficient capital. In 1912, he opened a lacquer ware studio at 83, Ebury Street, London, and fared somewhat better, for six years afterwards, at the age of 32, he founded the Budokwai which opened its doors on 26th January 1918. Shortly thereafter Koizumi engaged Yukio Tani as chief instructor. Tuition was initially offered in jujutsu, kendo and other kindred Japanese martial arts. Koizumi had long desired to operate a dojo for the study of martial arts and their related cultural aspects. This was based upon a twofold premise: to further interest in the martial arts, their philosophy and Japanese culture, and to repay his adopted country for its hospitality towards himself and his fellow compatriots. Unlike the privately-run Trinity College dojo, the Budokwai was reportedly the first judo club in the whole of Europe to accept members of the general public.

The original 36 students, however, were all Japanese. The 37th applicant was an Englishman who joined in March 1918. In the early days, famous judo instructors such as Hideichi Nagaoka (1876–1952), Sumiyuki Kotani (1903–1991), Ichiro Hata (1906–1983), and Kano's son-in-law who was the 1930 All Japan Judo Champion, Masami Takasaki, and others from Kano's Kodokan, all taught for a time at the Budokwai.

The relationship between Kano and Koizumi seems to have been a close and cordial one for Kano visited the Budokwai on six occasions, and was usually accompanied by high-grade instructors. For instance, Kano arrived in 1933 with two 6th dan grade holders, Sumiyuki Kotani and Masami Takasaki. Judging from Kano's comments and actions at that time it would appear that Kano wanted Kodokan branch dojos to be set up not only in Japan but also in principal cities around the world. On his 1933 August 26th visit, Professor Kano announced that he wished to merge the Budokwai with the Kodokan, thus in effect creating a London branch of the Kodokan. A general meeting was called and it was agreed without any dissent that the Budokwai would become a provisional branch of the Kodokan. Prior to Kano's departure, arrangements were made for Kotani to remain in London as judo master.

Unfortunately, Kotani was recalled by his employer, the Manchurian Railway Company, sooner than expected, nevertheless, he was able to instruct for three months during his leave of absence.

In the summer of 1934, Kano was again in London, this time accompanied by the illustrious 58-year-old Hideichi Nagaoka, 9th dan. Talks continued regarding the setting up of a Kodokan London branch. On July 24th 1934 Kano convened a meeting attended by Hideichi Nagaoka, Gunji Koizumi, Yukio Tani, Masutaro Otani, Marcus Kaye, Harold and Norman Hyde, Harold Tricker and Miss Woolhouse, with the intention of forming a Kodokan Yudanshakai (black belt association) of Great Britain. Following this gathering, Nagaoka remained to teach for some three or four weeks. However, this ambitious proposal by Kano for a Kodokan branch to take over the Budokwai, ultimately failed to materialize. This was mainly due to the deteriorating international situation that eventually led to worldwide hostilities.

Kano's demise on May 4th 1938 was followed by great international upheaval caused by the Second World War (1939–1945). As a result, there was precious little progress made in further promotion of judo until the mid 1940s. On July 26th 1948, at the Imperial College Union, Prince Consort Road, London, the European Judo Union was founded by a dedicated group of enthusiasts led by Gunji Koizumi. In attendance were Trevor Pryce Leggett, John Barnes, Dr. Feldenkrais, and F. Kauert representing Britain; P. Buchelli and F. Limfuhr on behalf of Austria; L. Thieme representing Holland; Signor Castella representing Italy and L. de Jarmy from France. During this meeting, Leggett was elected first chairman of the European Judo Union.

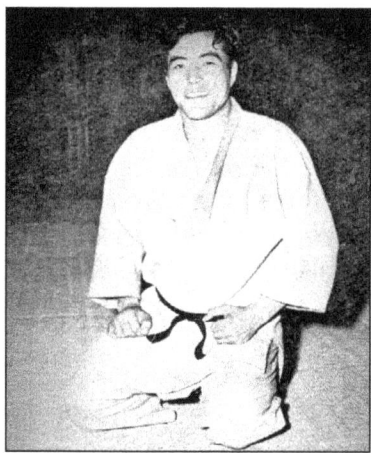

Figure 6. Teizo Kawamura (1922–2003).

Teizo Kawamura (1922–2003), Figure 6, a 6th dan, arrived in 1953, and was the first post-war Japanese instructor to be engaged at the Budokwai where he gave coaching until his return to Japan in 1955. To help popularize judo in response to the sporadic lacklustre recruitment periods, annual martial arts displays were instigated by the Budokwai membership from around 1930 until 1968. These well-attended demonstrations in later years attracted hundreds of curious spectators to such large London venues as Seymour Hall and the Royal Albert Hall.

Judo Included in the Olympic Games

Kano's endorsement of judo was life-long and resolute for he strove long and hard to scatter as much as possible the seeds of judo internationally. These seeds started to sprout 100 years after his birth when in 1960, in Rome, Italy; the International Olympic

Committee announced that judo was to be included in the 1964 Tokyo Olympic Games. This declaration initiated a sudden and globally determined rush by sports administrators to assemble, train and foster contestants for the initial upcoming weight category events at the 1964 Games. Also, the reputation of judo in the early 1960s was given a significant boost following international championship successes by non-Japanese judoka, in particular by Dutchman, Anton Geesink (1934-2010) who at the age of 27 stunned the global judo fraternity by his overwhelming of leading Japanese opponents when he captured the World Judo Championship in Paris in December 1961. He subsequently gained the Tokyo Olympic Open Weight gold medal in October 1964 and the +80kg category World Judo Championship in Rio de Janeiro, Brazil, in October 1965, following which he retired from contest judo at the age of 31.

After the hugely successful 1964 Tokyo Olympic Games, judo gained ever more rapid exposure from a powerful source. Judo techniques, often performed by an actress pitching a man in retaliation for harassment, were very much in vogue in movies and in TV drama scenes. Such throws were famously featured in the trendy 'James Bond' movies of the day. Thanks to this wide-reaching exposure, 1960 to 1970 was the decade that many women as well as men started to take a keen interest in the practice of judo. Likewise, succeeding decades saw other oriental fighting systems take the spotlight as they too achieved universal fame largely due to the movie exploits of stars such as Bruce Lee and Jackie Chan.

The Budokwai

In closing, I wish to highlight the significance of this venerable institution, for the Budokwai is much more than a dojo. It's a cultural asset, a symbol of the salient link that binds the budo tradition to British society and as such will, I'm sure, prove increasingly of benefit by the future promotion of this strong bilateral relationship, as long as the Budo-kwai remains at its current location, Figure 7, that is. Also, we must remember that the British judo fraternity owes a debt of gratitude to the memory of all those many staunch enthusiasts, both British and Japanese, who have gone before. They, through dint of hard work and dedication, have helped the Budokwai reach this important 100-year milestone. But above all, we should remember in particular, the four ardent members who built and maintained the solid foundations that enabled the Budokwai to survive during its critical years. These four adherents, who played crucial roles, were Yukio Tani (1881-1950), Gunji Koizumi (1885-1965), Dame Enid Russell-Smith, (1903-1989) and Trevor Pryce Leggett (1914-2000).

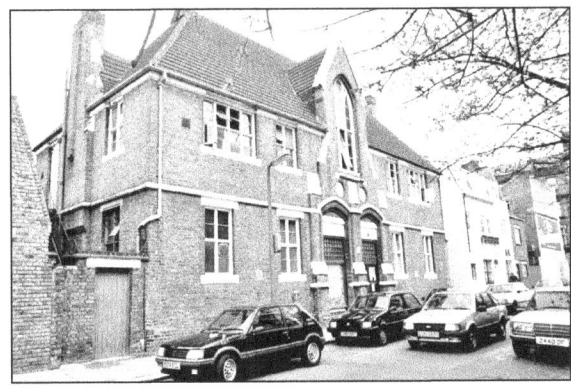

Figure 7: Exterior of the present Budokwai at 4 Gilston Road, Kensington, London.

Yukio Tani

Yukio Tani arrived in Britain, according to Richard Bowen's research, in September 1900 and soon achieved eminence as a jujutsu superstar. The diminutive Tani, toured the profitable music hall circuit issuing challenges for prize money to boxers and wrestlers of any weight. He was renowned in particular for his many surprising 'David versus Goliath' victories, against heavyweight opponents, and reportedly earned some 250,000 pounds in the process, a vast sum in those days.

Tani taught at the Budokwai from the early days. He suffered a stroke, however, in 1937 at the age of 57 putting an end to much of his active career. He did, nonetheless, continue to teach from the sidelines until a second stroke in 1950 led to his passing at the age of 69. He was married to Mary Alice Fearon. Their daughter, born in 1920, became Moya Ward upon marriage. Moya also trained in judo and taught British women at the Anglo-Japanese Judo Club in Strathmore Gardens, London, in the mid 1930s. This club was founded in 1901 by Tani's jujutsu collaborator Sadakazu Uyenishi who together with Tani successfully toured the music hall circuit as a prize-fighter for a time, before returning to Japan.

Dame Enid Russell-Smith, DBE

The first authoritative UK judo periodical to be issued regularly was the *Budokwai Quarterly Bulletin*, published throughout the 1940s and 1950s under the very capable editorship of Dame Enid Russell-Smith (1903–1989), Figure 8, who was, incidentally, one of the first British females to gain a judo 3rd dan. She carried out this important editorial task and other Budokwai clerical duties despite her heavy engagement in busy and essential work at the Ministry of Health from 1925 until retirement in 1963. Dame Enid was subsequently appointed Principal of St. Aidan's College at Durham University where she served until 1970. She died on 12 July 1989 aged 86.

In similar vein, mention should be made of the sterling efforts of G. A. Edwards and A. R. Menzies who for many years regularly issued the highly informative monthly magazine Judo. Without this valuable communicative organ, the dissemination of judo-related matters would have been severely handicapped.

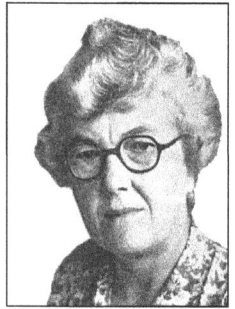

Figure 8
Dame Enid Russell-Smith
(1903–1989).

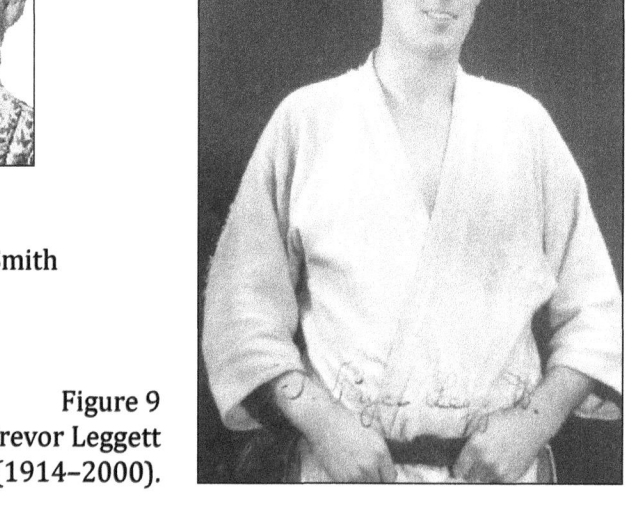

Figure 9
Trevor Leggett
(1914–2000).

Trevor Pryce (T.P.) Leggett

Trevor Pryce Leggett (1914–2000), Figure 9, was another of the Budokwai stalwarts. He started judo at the age of 16 under the guidance of Yukio Tani and Gunji Koizumi. He earned a degree in law from London University in 1934. A fanatically disciplined person, Leggett took to his training wholeheartedly and quickly gained promotion to 3rd dan before leaving in 1939 at the age of 25 for Tokyo where he was employed at the British embassy. He trained at Chuo University and the Kodokan. He was later awarded 5th dan in 1948, then 6th dan in 1955, reportedly the first non-Japanese to achieve this grade. Interned in Japan following the outbreak of the Pacific War in 1941, he was repatriated along with other embassy staff and left Japan in July 1942 aboard the Tatsuta Maru of the NYK Line. Once back in the UK, he entered the Ministry of Information and saw service in India as a British army major working in counter-intelligence where part of his duties was to interrogate Japanese POWs.

From 1946 Leggett worked at the BBC and in this same year at the age of 32 he suffered a stroke and was advised by his doctor to give up judo. Nevertheless, he continued judo practice. In later years, he was promoted head of the BBC Japanese Service. In 1959, at his own expense, Leggett founded the Renshuden Judo Academy, situated near Regents Park, London, where he led a number of young 5th dan experts; namely, Saburo Matsushita, Kisaburo Watanabe and British 4th dan holders John Newman and George Kerr in the training of the members, who were mostly British international contest men. The Renshuden, however, after more than a decade eventually closed its doors.

From the 1950s to the early 1960s Leggett trained many leading British judoka; especially those who were privileged to attend his much celebrated but physically demanding and exhaustive 'Sunday Class' at the Budokwai. Leggett retired from the BBC in 1969. He then turned more of his attention to writing and published some 30 full-length books covering subjects such as judo, Zen, yoga, Buddhism, and budo. In 1984 Leggett was awarded the Order of the Sacred Treasure by the government of Japan for his contributions in helping to introduce Japanese culture to Britain. He, like Kano, was a man devoted to learning and to self-improvement, and saw judo as a training for life. Leggett died of a stroke on 2nd August 2000, aged 86.

Gunji Koizumi

Gunji Koizumi was another remarkable man, who largely self-taught, managed to achieve some success in business and a high level of fluency in both spoken and written English. In April 1912, he married Ida Celine Winstanley. They had one child, a daughter, Hana, who later married judo instructor Percy Sekine. Koizumi was a man conscious of social ethics. As a result of the German aerial bombardment of London during the First World War, Koizumi and other Japanese formed a volunteer ambulance unit, and supplied all the necessary equipment themselves. Also, at this time, Koizumi served as General Secretary of the charitable Kyosai Kai (Mutual Aid Society) that was set up mainly by him in 1919 at an office in the Budokwai. The Japanese community wanted to be totally self-sufficient and had no wish for any distressed Japanese person to be a burden on the host British society. The Kyosai Kai, therefore, sought to provide medical, employment and housing assistance and also secured a communal burial area at Hendon Cemetery, London, for those among the thousand or so Japanese community residents in the UK who were at times in need. Britain became Koizumi's country of residence, for after his return from the US in 1910, he remained in the UK for the rest of his life. Koizumi taught judo as a method of character training in which he stressed both the moral and spiritual aspects. His judo career spanned some 64 years. During that time, he served in many capacities, including terms as president and as national coach to the British Judo Association. Koizumi wrote the following in the April 1945 issue of the *Budokwai Quarterly Bulletin*: "One day it (judo) will be recognized as the best form of mental and physical education and health-giving exercise."

Koizumi's days were mainly split between business interests as an art dealer and the Budokwai. Moreover, he wrote extensively not only on judo and related matters but also as a consultant on Chinese and Japanese lacquerware for the Victoria and Albert Museum. He penned *Lacquer Work: A Practical Exposition* published by Sir Isaac Pitman and Sons in 1923 and *My Study of Judo*, issued by Foulsham, in 1960. It was Koizumi who often paid the bills from his own pocket to prevent the Budokwai from sliding into bankruptcy, especially so prior to and during the Second World War (1939–1945) when funds dried up with so many members away on wartime service. At one stage the Budokwai owed Koizumi over 500 pounds, a considerable sum in those days. Years later he received an 8th dan grade from the Kodokan in recognition for his life-long efforts. On April 15th, 1965, he died by his own hand. He was 79. Mrs. Koizumi, his wife for some 34 years, had died earlier in 1947.

The following is the message that he left for the UK coroner:

> To the Coroner, and whom it may concern,
>
> This is my true testimony that the action I am about to take, to effect permanent rest to my physical life, is purely to accord to my philosophical conviction.
>
> In spiritual sense, the process of human life clearly indicates that the Divine Wisdom for creation was founded on the principle of progression and continuity, and each individual life is endowed with specific faculty to serve specific part in the Divine plan. Thus, the tenure of one's life depends on one's capacity for that service.
>
> Approaching to the 80th birthday, by the progressive and irretrievable state of mental and physical debilities, I have been persuaded to realize that the term of my service to the cause of life has now come to an end, and to linger on the futile existence is not only against my conviction but an evil burden to my friends and society. Hence this action.
>
> I am sorry to be a cause of wasteful nuisance to you all but I hope it will be taken as a lesser evil.
>
> Many thanks,
> G. Koizumi

Concluding Remarks

Finally, I hope that the great services that he rendered with such unremitting devotion to judo, to Japanese and British society and to his support of the Budokwai, will not be forgotten, for Gunji Koizumi was without doubt a credit to his race—The Human Race.

BIBLIOGRAPHY

Bowen, R. (2011). *100 years of judo in Great Britain, Vol. 2*, Indepenpress Publishing Ltd.

Bunasawa, N. and Murray, J. (2007). *The toughest man who ever lived: The story of Mitsuyo Maeda*. Costa Mesa, CA: Innovations Inc.

Cortazzi, H. (2002). *Britain and Japan biographical portraits, Vol. IV*. London: Routledge.

Itoh, K. (2001). *The Japanese community in pre-war Britain: From integration to disintigration*. London: Curzon Press.

Watson, B. (2014). *Judo memoirs of Jigoro Kano: Early history of judo*. Bloomington, IN: Trafford Publishing.

Wilson, B. (2012). *The father of judo: A biography of Jigoro Kano*. New York: Kodansha International.

Watson, B. (2012). *Memorias de Jigoro Kano: O inicio da historia do judo*. Sao Paolo: Editora Cultrix.

Watson, B. (2005). *Il padre del judo: Una biografia di Jigoro Kano*. Rome: Edizioni Mediterranee.

chapter 27

**Budokwai Kime-no-kata:
Budokwai Form of Decisive Techniques**
by Llyr C. Jones, Ph.D., H. John Bowen and David W. V. Finch

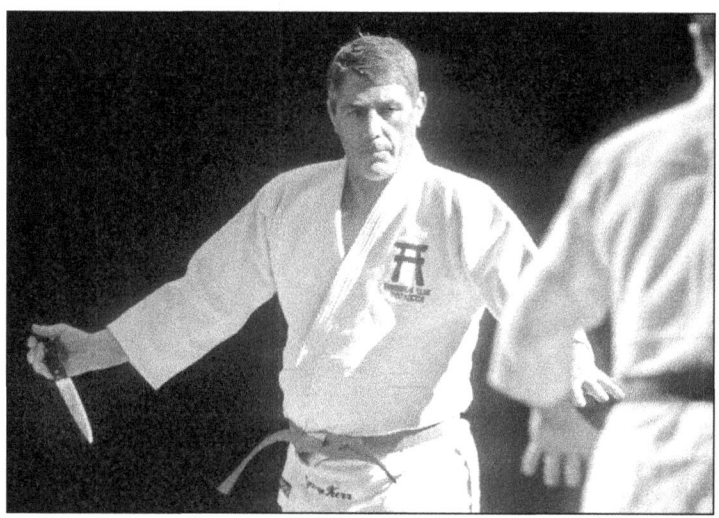

Introduction
Kodokan[1] Judo (judo, the flexible way) developed by Jigoro Kano *Shihan* (head teacher)[2] (1860–1938) is an all-round cooperative education, teaching system (pedagogy) and philosophy—based inter alia on conservative Confucianism values, *koryu* (traditional or old school) *jujutsu* (flexible art, "the old samurai art of fighting without weapons") (Lindsay and Kano, 1889) and European liberal educational philosophy (Stevens, 2013: 43). Judo emphasizes the holistic educational value of training in attack and defense, so that it can be a "path," or way of life, that all people can participate in and benefit from.

Katas in judo are "formal movement pattern exercises containing idealized model movements illustrating specific combative principles" (Kawamura and Daigo, 2000: 86)—which together with *randori* (free practice), *kogi* (lectures) and *mondo* (dialogue) comprise the four critical pillars of Kodokan judo education (De Crée and Jones, 2009; 2011; De Crée, 2015; Jones, Savage and Gatling, 2016).

The topic of this chapter is an innovative, unofficial judo self-defense kata, created around the 1930s/1940s at the Budokwai[3]—or in full, The Budokwai (The Way of Knighthood Society). Founded on 26 January 1918, The Budokwai is a prominent and highly influential institution for the Japanese martial ways situated in London, United Kingdom (UK), and one of the oldest such organizations in Europe (Callan, 2017; Budokwai, 2018).

The exercise, referred to throughout this chapter as Budokwai Kime-no-kata (literally Budokwai Forms of Decisive Techniques), consists of defenses (throws and locks) against the most common types of fist, stick, knife and pistol attacks, and quite often featured at *enbu* (martial arts displays) organized by The Budokwai.

Kime-no-kata

Kime, a Japanese word, is the noun form of the verb *kimeru*, meaning "to decide"[4] (Nakao, 1996:126). This chapter's use of the name Budokwai Kime-no-kata is to clearly distinguish the exercise from the official Kime-no-kata (forms of decisive techniques), which is "... a set of Kodokan Judo formal exercises (*kata*) designed to teach fundamental ways and means of defending against attacks using throwing, grappling, and striking techniques..." (Kawamura and Daigo, 2000:90).

The inclusion of the prefix "Budokwai" to distinguish the kata is natural, and fully reflects its heritage in the Society. Note though, that in the scant literature and audiovisual media that reference the exercise, it is sometimes called "Kime-no-kata," "Kime-no-kata of The Budokwai," or simply just "Budokwai Kata."

It is beyond the scope of this chapter to provide further detail on the official Kime-no-kata, other than to note that it is composed of twenty techniques divided into two sections—eight *idori* (kneeling) technique used while in *seiza* (formal seated position), and twelve *tachiai* (standing) techniques used while standing. Each of these two sections contains (similar) practical and realistic defenses against empty-handed and armed (with bladed weapons) attacks, and involves the safe practice of counter-attacking and control techniques prohibited from everyday judo *randori* (free practice) and *shiai* (contest). By understanding and developing a mastery of Kime-no-kata, the *judoka* (a person who practices judo) develops an understanding of the theoretical basis of attack and defense, and acquires the decisiveness, focus and skills relevant to a variety of critical situations. There does of course, exist an abundance of sources detailing the official Kime-no-kata, and, as a starting point, the interested reader is directed to the dedicated Kodokan Kime-no-kata textbook (Kodokan, 2015).

Purpose, Scope and Structure of this Chapter

Finding information about the history, technical contents and mechanics of Budokwai Kime-no-kata is difficult. It does not feature in any currently available judo text or teaching film, has not been performed in public for over twenty-five years, and is not presently taught at the Society, or elsewhere.

To rectify this deficiency, the present chapter, published to coincide with the centenary of the founding of The Budokwai, aims to provide an in-depth study into Budokwai Kime-no-kata. Inter alia it will consider under what circumstances, and by who the exercise was created, and also detail its technical contents and their theoretical foundation. In terms of organization, this chapter follows a structure like that found in other work on kata by De Crée and Jones (2009; 2011), De Crée (2015), and Jones et al. (2016).

UNOFFICIAL JUDO KATA

Unofficial judo katas are those formal exercises which were either (i) not created by Kano, (ii) did not receive a personal endorsement from the Shihan during his lifetime, or (iii) have not obtained the Kodokan's institutional endorsement after Kano's death. Practically, such katas include those created in Japan—but outside the formal structure of The Kodokan, and those created and/or popularized outside of Japan—by either expatriate Japanese judoka, or non-Japanese judoka.

Otaki and Draeger remark on such katas in their classic book *Judo Formal Techniques*:

> Different practices and uses for kata have been established by judoists outside of the Kodokan, though the majority of these versions hinge on the unchanged fundamental Principle of Kodokan Judo. These kata can be referred to as private variations patterns. Included here are those which have been developed by qualified Judo teachers; some of these teachers are Kodokan men. Because [some of] these kata have definite qualities and characteristics meaningful within the realm of Judo, they are most certainly worthy of preservation and use ...
> – Otaki and Draeger, 1983:33

Kata Created in Japan, but Outside the Formal Framework of the Kodokan

The best-known katas created in Japan, outside of The Kodokan, feature *kaeshi-waza* (also called *ura-waza*, counter or reverse techniques). The most complete, refined and coherent of these exercises had a strong contribution from the legendary Kyuzo Mifune[5] Kodokan 10th dan in their development. Specifically, these katas are *Nage-waza Ura-no-kata* (forms of reversing throwing techniques) (Mifune, 1956:229–240) and *Katame-waza Ura-no-kata* (forms of reversing controlling techniques) (Ito, 1970:1–111).

A lesser known unofficial kata worthy of mentioning is also due to Mifune. This is the self-defense exercise, Mifune Soen Goshin-Jutsu (Mifune's personal self-defense), which incorporates both koryu and *torite*[6] (literally, "grasping hands" techniques) (Mifune 1955, 2005; De Crée and Jones 2011; De Crée, 2015; and Jones et al. 2016). It is of course beyond the scope of this chapter to detail all the katas in this category, and for further information the interested reader is directed to De Crée (2015) and the references therein.

Katas Created and/or Promoted Outside Japan

These katas are either those created/promoted by Westerners outside of Japan, or else by a significant Japanese *sensei* (teacher) resident overseas. Examples of such exercises created by Westerners include *Hoho kata* (forms of methods) due to Wolfgang Hofmann, *Rensa-no-kata* (forms of chains) due to Gerhard Steidele and Renraku-no-kata (forms of combination techniques) due to Edward Szrejter. These aforementioned katas are usually not found in any of the serious judo literature, and do not teach judo's fundamental principles in a structured and integrated manner. Lacking in didactic theory, these exercises often just consist of a series of judo techniques bookended by some *reiho*[7] (etiquette).

The best-known unofficial kata promoted by a Japanese teacher based overseas is undoubtedly *Gonosen-no-kata* (forms of post-attack initiative counter throws). This exercise was popularized in Europe by Mikinosuke Kawaishi (1899–1969) DNBK[8] (Dai Nippon Butokukai) / Kodokan 7th dan, FFJDA[9] 10th dan,[10] and has often been linked with Waseda University[11] (Kawaishi 1956; 1957 and De Crée, 2015).

Consistent with the aims of this chapter, the origin, background and technical content of Budokwai Kime-no-kata will now be explored.

LITERATURE AND MEDIA FEATURING BUDOKWAI KIME-NO-KATA

A literature review to establish the current state of knowledge on Budokwai Kime-no-kata is the natural starting point for this chapter. This review will include consideration of the available audiovisual materials where the exercise can be viewed.

Following extensive research, the authors have concluded that there is very little information available on Budokwai Kime-no-kata, with only a paucity of primary sources existing. The exercise has never featured in any scholarly, or popular, judo book, nor does it feature in any currently commercially available film. The authors' research identified only three sources that contain a level of detail sufficient for an interested judoka to use them as a learning resources, and these will be reflected upon here. However, what could be the oldest source mentioning the exercise will be highlighted first.

First Appearance and Mention of Budokwai Kime-no-kata

The (most likely) earliest mention of Budokwai Kime-no-kata, known to the authors, occurs in the event program for an international judo meeting that took place on 29 November 1932. This meeting involved Oxford University Judo Club and a visiting German team.

The event program (Oxford University Judo Club, 1932) mentions a "Kime-no-kata display" featuring Yukio Tani (1881–1950) and Gunji Koizumi (1885–1965). Both men were from The Budokwai, and were originally *jujutsuka* (jujutsu practitioners) who had subsequently become judoka—see later. In the program, their so-called "Kime-no-kata" is described as: "Self-defence against attack with knife, pistol, stick . . ." (Ibid.)

Since pistol and stick attacks do not feature in the official Kime-no-kata, the exercise done by Tani and Koizumi was clearly an "alternative" Kime-no-kata, and most likely a personal creation. Given that what is also called Budokwai Kime-no-kata does indeed include attacks with such weapons, and that Tani and Koizumi both hailed from The Budokwai, it is not unreasonable to suggest that what they showed was most likely a very early version of that exercise.[12] It is also worthy to highlight that Tani and Koizumi's exercise certainly represented a very early introduction of defenses against guns into judo, as that concept was not officially incorporated into formal Kodokan training until 1956.[13]

Additionally, by using the name "Kime-no-kata," it can be reasonably assumed that Tani and Koizumi were indeed doing some sort of "kata"—that is, a previously established and preserved set of attack and defense sequences, that were always practiced and performed in the same sequential order.[14]

1948-1949 – Gunji Koizumi – Kime No Kata; Decisive Combat Forms

A nine-page article by Gunji Koizumi is the first, and only known to exist, technical work on Budokwai Kime-no-kata (Koizumi, 1948–49). The article was serialized in three consecutive issues (October 1948 to April 1949) of The Budokwai's in-house journal *Judo*, the *Quarterly Bulletin of The Budokwai*, which, for brevity, will henceforth be referred to by its popular name, *The Budokwai Bulletin*.[15]

Koizumi's seminal article contains concise instructions on how to execute Budokwai Kime-no-kata's mechanics, supplemented by rudimentary black line "stickman"[16] illustrations for the first eleven attack and defense sequences, and black and white photographs for the final two. The article also provides limited information on the more general aspects of "decisive combat forms," as well as helpful guidelines for practice. No emphasis is given to any etiquette, or *reiho* aspects. Given its uniqueness, and despite its age and brevity, Koizumi's article is, without question, the most vital reference for Budokwai Kime-no-kata.

1948 – The Budokwai – The 'Budokwai' Film
n.d. – Take Five Productions – The 'Budokwai' Film

In 1948, The Budokwai produced an instructional film, The 'Budokwai' Film, to mark its thirtieth anniversary (Budokwai, 1948). The film shows some basic judo throws and holds, as well as combinations, self-defense techniques, and five definite katas—including Budokwai Kime-no-kata.

The original black and white recording was shot in 16mm—a then popular and economical film gauge that was regularly used for non-theatrical film making. Many years later the film was rearranged, transferred to a VHS (Video Home System) format, Figure 1, and re-issued by Take Five Productions of Frinton-on-Sea, Essex, UK (Take Five Productions, n.d.). Contrary to what is often stated, the film was not shot in The Budokwai grounds, but rather at The Hurlingham Club[17] (R. Bowen, n.d.; 292).

The 'Budokwai' Film features most of the exceptional British players of that time, and the eminent judoka, judo teachers and broadcasters John Newman (1935–1993) British Judo Association (BJA)[18] 4th dan and Trevor Leggett (1914–2000) Kodokan 6th dan, later added some fine commentary. This commentary initially takes the form of an informal conversation between the two men, which later evolves into additional information on the techniques shown (Budokwai, n.d.).

Budokwai Kime-no-kata on the film is done by Gunji Koizumi and Edward (Ted) Mossom—see later. The exercise they demonstrate is identical to the one described by Koizumi in his technical article in *The Budokwai Bulletin* (Koizumi, 1948–49). Inexplicably though, the fifth technique—*ryote-dori* (both hands hold) is omitted.

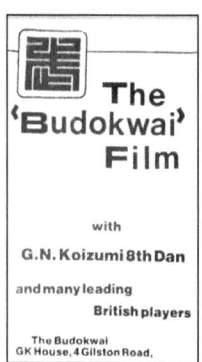

This film was originally made in 1949, but because of its contents, the BUDOKWAI have decided that all players interested in JUDO or JU JITSU should have the chance of seeing it, in full, as it shows KOIZUMI 8th Dan, showing his skills and proving what an outstanding teacher he was.

There are automatically faults with the filming, but this does not detract from the high standard of instruction shown, but should there be an Electronic 'Video' faults, then please return immediately to TAKE FIVE PRODUCTIONS, 15 Raglan road, FRINTON, ESSEX CO139HH. or direct to the BUDOKWAI.

This is a copyright film, and as it is being utalized to enhance the sport, any unlawful copying without permission from the BUDOKWAI will be dealt with accordingly.

Figure 1. *The 'Budokwai' Film* contains a black and white recording of Budokwai Kime-no-kata. Shown is an enhanced image of the front and copy of the text from the back cover of the case of the Take Five Productions VHS reissue.[19] Courtesy of Ian Whittlesea.

Even though the picture quality does not compare to modern high-definition digital DVD, the recording is highly recommended, as it is the only opportunity for the interested judoka to benefit from seeing Budokwai Kime-no-kata's physical mechanics demonstrated directly by its creator.

While no longer commercially available, The 'Budokwai' Film is freely viewable on the YouTube video-sharing website (Whittlesea, 2013a), where Take Five Productions' original error of crediting the film's year of creation as 1949 is innocently repeated.

1964 – Alan Menzies – Budokwai Show

On 31 October 1964, an enbu was held at the Royal Albert Hall.[20] Alan Menzies' account of that 1964 Budokwai Show describes the performance of an exercise that perhaps was Budokwai Kime-no-kata, though his report labels what was shown as "Go-shin-Jitsu-no-kata".

> The Goshin-Jitsu-no-kata, performed by Mr. M. Nishimura, 7th Dan and Mr. S. Yamada 6th Dan, was a celebrated first time event for this special kata devised by Mr. Gunji Koizumi, 8th Dan for the Budokwai many years ago. Mr. Koizumi

was, of course, there to watch, and no doubt approved of the rendering of his composition. Both of the performers are very experienced and their exposition of this highest form of Judo attainment was exceedingly exciting to watch.

– Menzies, 1964:30

Given that the exercise shown by Nishimura and Yamada is, in the report, called "Goshin-Jitsu-no-kata" [sic], and that the demonstration is described as a "first time event," it will now be considered whether what was shown was indeed Budokwai Kime-no-kata, or alternatively was, the 1956-created, *Kodokan Goshin-jutsu* (Kodokan self-defense).[21] It will be seen that this is a worthwhile evaluation, despite the text stating that Gunji Koizumi was the creator of the exercise demonstrated.

At the very highest level, Budokwai Kime-no-kata and Kodokan Goshin-jutsu have some similarities. Both are technically very different from the official Kodokan Kime-no-kata, and both contain defenses against armed and unarmed attacks. Note also that the contemporary weapons used in both Budokwai Kime-no-kata and Kodokan Goshin-jutsu are identical—namely a knife, a stick and a gun.

As to the claim that the 1964 Budokwai Show marked the (UK) premier of the "special kata," this chapter has already shown that Budokwai Kime-no-kata featured on *The 'Budokwai' Film* (Budokwai, 1948), and probably on earlier occasions too. While there is no reliable reference for the earliest UK demonstration of Kodokan Goshin-jutsu, it is known that the exercise's first ever public demonstration was at the January 1956 Kagami Biraki ceremony held at the Tokyo Budokan (Jones et al., 2016), with Kenji Tomiki[22] (1900–1979) then Kodokan 7th dan (later Kodokan 8th dan) as tori, and Tadao Otaki (1908–1992) then Kodokan 8th dan (later Kodokan 9th dan) as uke. The involvement of Tomiki will become relevant later.

With regard to the judoka involved in the 1964 Budokwai Show demonstration, M. Nishimura was Masami Nishimura (1917–1996) later Kodokan 8th dan who taught judo in South East Asia as well as in the UK, and S. Yamada was Senta Yamada (1924–2010) Kodokan 6th dan. Nishimura came to the UK around 1962 and was working for a Japanese company in London (Budokwai, 1962:25), whereas Yamada came to the UK in 1959 to teach judo and aikido at the (now defunct) London Judo Society (LJS).

In addition to his prowess in judo, Senta Yamada was a prominent *aikidoka* (a person who practices aikido) and had trained as an *uchideshi* (live in student) with Morihei Ueshiba (1883–1969), the eventual founder of what is now known as *aikido* (the way of unifying spirit, or, the way of spiritual harmony). Later, Yamada was to meet and study with Kenji Tomiki who impressed him with his vision of aikido that closely matched the principles and practice of judo. It was this vision of aikido that Yamada brought with him to the UK, where he remained until 1965.[23]

Given the above aspects, it cannot be determined with any real certainty what self-defense exercise was presented at the 1964 Budokwai Show. However, (i) the mention of the demonstration being a first-time performance, (ii) the involvement of Yamada (with his connections to Tomiki) and (iii) the inclusion of the label Goshin-Jitsu [sic] makes a strong case for the demonstrated exercise actually being Kodokan Goshin-jutsu. However, this conclusion cannot be asserted with complete certainty.

1968 – The Budokwai – The 50th Black-Belt Judo Display

On 30 November 1968, an enbu was again held at the Royal Albert Hall to mark the fiftieth anniversary of The Budokwai's founding—see Figure 2. The seventh item during the evening's display was Budokwai Kime-no-kata, done by George Kerr (then a BJA 5th dan) and Maurice Allan (then a BJA 2nd dan). See later.

The official commemorative booklet for the event (Budokwai, 1968), also in Figure 2, contains a succinct description of Budokwai Kime-no-kata. This description is entirely consistent with that provided by Koizumi in his technical article in *The Budokwai Bulletin* (Koizumi, 1948–49).

> Budokwai Kimenokata: The kata of decisive ends. The role of the attacker and attacked alternate.   – Budokwai, 1968

In correspondence with the authors, Allan stated that he learnt and practiced this exercise under the direction of Kerr in their native Edinburgh—adding that, for him, it was a highlight of their kata activity together (Maurice Allan, personal communication, 8 June 2017).

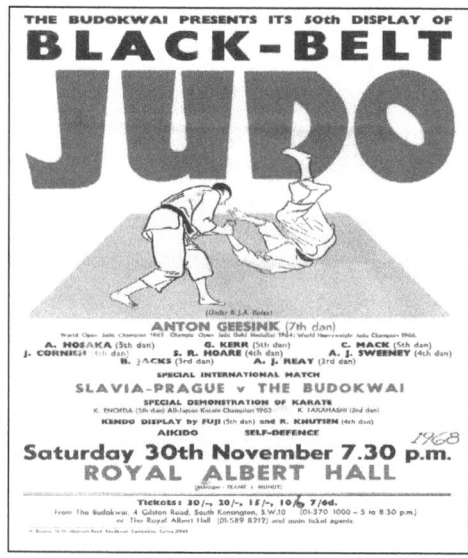

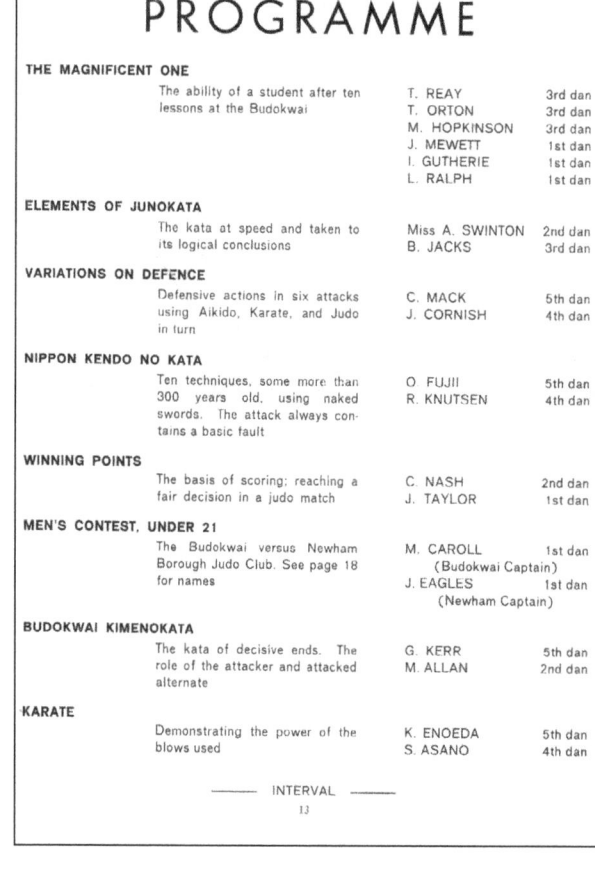

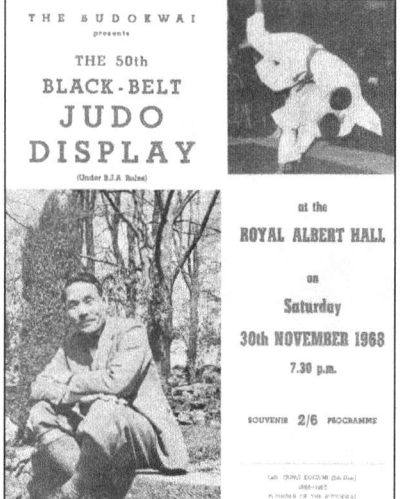

Figure 2. Poster and official commemorative booklet for The Budokwai's fiftieth anniversary show held at the Royal Albert Hall on 30 November 1968. Courtesy of Robert John Mewett.

1988 – The Budokwai – 70th Anniversary International Tournament
1988 – Fighting Films – The Albert Hall Show – The Budokwai International Judo & Karate Tournament

Twenty years later, on 27 November 1988, an enbu was yet again held at the Royal Albert Hall. The occasion this time, was to mark the seventieth anniversary of The Budokwai's founding.

Order of Programme

1. Judo display to music by children and Budokwai display squad.
2. Womens World Champions
3. Children's karate display
4. Judo International G.B. v W. Germany

   G.B.: Carl Finney, Mark Preston, Colin Savage, Paul Ajala, Raymond Stevens, Dennis Stewart, Elvis Gordon
   W.Germany: ....
   TEAM MANAGER: Neil Adams MBE
   TEAM MANAGER: ....

5. Mens karate display
6. George Kerr 7th Dan, "Budokwai Kata"

7. Royal Marines Unarmed Combat Display
8. Karate International G.B. v Spain

   G.B.: F. Brennan, J. Brennan, G. Harford, R. Christopher, R. Williams, M. Draper, G. Best
   SPAIN: ....
   TEAM MANAGER: A. Sherry
   TEAM MANAGER: ....

9. Neil Adams MBE 5th Dan demonstration – Judo
10. Judo demonstration by Brian Jacks and Angelo Parisi 6th Dan
11. Prof. K. Eneoda 8th Dan "Kata"
12. Angelo Parisi 6th Dan "One Against Ten"

INTERVAL

The Budokwai — Europe's Premier Martial Arts Club
Founded in 1918 by G. Koizumi, 8th dan
Founder Member of the British Judo Association
GK Houe, 4 Gilston Road, South Kensington, London SW10
Telephone: 01-370 1000/2088
OPEN 7 DAYS A WEEK
CLASSES AT ALL LEVELS IN JUDO – KARATE – AIKIDO
Beginners and visitors always welcome   For further details call or phone.

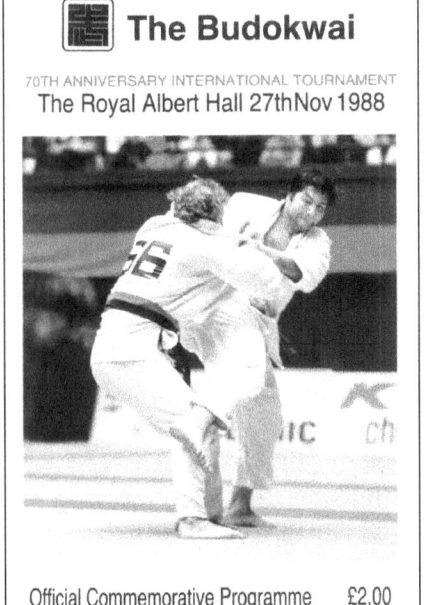

Official Commemorative Programme   £2.00

Figure 3. The Official Commemorative Booklet for The Budokwai's Seventieth Anniversary Tournament held at the Royal Albert Hall on 27 November 1988.

Inspection of the official commemorative booklet[24] for the event (Budokwai, 1988)—Figure 3, shows that the sixth item presented during the evening was an exercise called Budokwai Kata. This exercise—performed by George Kerr (by then a BJA 7th dan) and Rodger Bornowski (then a BJA 2nd dan) was, of course, Budokwai Kime-no-kata. Two authors of this chapter (Jones and Finch) were at the enbu and recall the dynamism of Kerr and Bornowski's demonstration (Figure 4 on following page), and how well-appreciated it was by the very judo-knowledgeable audience.

301

A high-quality VHS recording containing highlights from the entire enbu was produced by Fighting Films,[25] and made commercially available for purchase (Fighting Films, 1988)—see Figure 5. Produced by Simon Hicks (1955–2007) BJA 6th dan, this thirty-year old film contains the best quality, and only color, footage available of a Budo-kwai Kime-no-kata. The commentary on the exercise was provided by Simon Hicks' father, Gerald (Jerry) Hicks MBE, BJA 7th dan (1927–2014), who trained at The Budokwai under both Leggett and Koizumi. In the commentary, G. Hicks described Kerr and Bornowski's piece as a "historical item" and uses the exercise's full name—Budokwai Kime-no-kata".

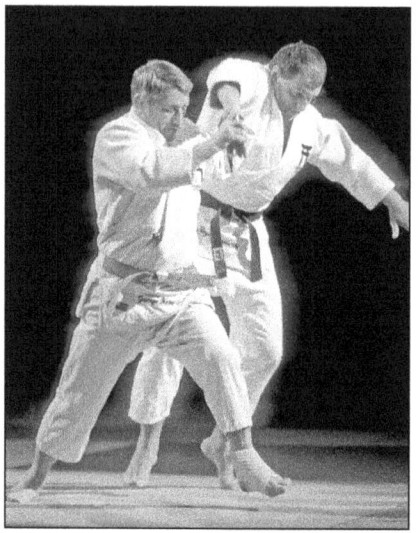

Figure 4:
George Kerr and Rodger Bornowski doing Budo-kwai Kime-no-kata at The Budokwai's Seventieth Anniversary Tournament.

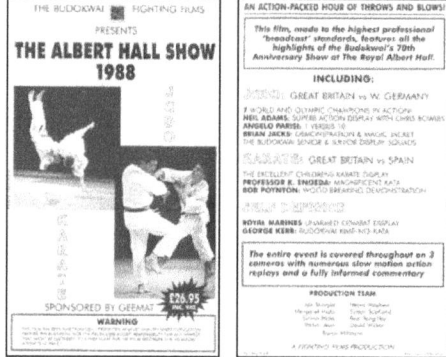

Figure 5, center and right: The Fighting Films video production of "The Albert Hall Show 1988—The Budokwai International Judo and Karate Tournament" contains a color recording of a version of Budokwai Kime-no-kata.

Regrettably, the recording of the Albert Hall event has not been made professionally available in any digital media format and is no longer available to buy from Fighting Films. However, it is freely viewable on the YouTube video-sharing website (Whittlesea, 2013b).[26]

Moreover, as will be explained later, Kerr and Bornowski's Budokwai Kime-no-kata contains significant technical differences, in terms of the attacks and defenses, to the exercise described in Koizumi's article (Koizumi, 1948-49), and hence the one found on The 'Budokwai' Film (Budokwai, 1948) with Koizumi and Mossom demonstrating. The Budo-kwai Kime-no-kata done at the 1988 enbu also contains a total of fifteen sequences, compared to the thirteen found in the original, as well as material differences in the reiho. These will be all be expanded upon later.

PROMINENT JUDOKA
ASSOCIATED WITH BUDOKWAI KIME-NO-KATA

Judoka featuring in the Literature and Media

Profiles of the judoka known to be associated with Budokwai Kime-no-kata are provided now. Their association comes from them featuring in the literature and/or appearing in audiovisual media. The judoka are Gunji Koizumi, Yukio Tani, Ted Mossom, George Kerr, Maurice Allan and Rodger Bornowski.

Gunji Koizumi

Gunji Koizumi "GK" (Figure 6) is a crucial figure in the development of judo in the UK. For his many contributions, he is the acknowledged "Father of British Judo." Koizumi's background is extensively described in his own book (Koizumi, 1960:17-18) and in work by others (Budokwai, 1965; R. Bowen, 2011a:273–296; R. Bowen, 2011b:i-xxx; Brousse, 2015:60–63; Callan, 2011; Fromm and Soames, 1982:6–17; Grant, 1965; Ito, 2001: 128–133; Watson, 2017). It is these references that form the basis of the biographical material that follows.

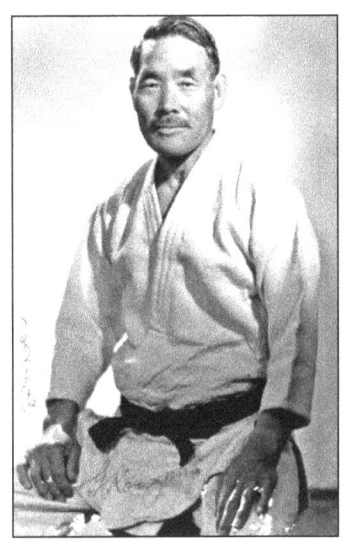

Figure 6. Gunji Koizumi (1885–1965).

Koizumi was born on 8 July 1885 in the village of Komatsuka (then some 30 miles north of Tokyo but now part of the Greater Tokyo Metropolis) in Ibaraki Prefecture. He was the younger son of a tenant farmer, Shukichi Koizumi, and his wife, Katsu, and had an elder brother, Chiyokichi, and a younger sister, Iku.

At age twelve Koizumi began training in *kenjutsu* (art of sword) under an inspirational school-teacher, Wataro Eizuka. Concurrently, he began to learn English from a neighbor who had been to the United States (US). Uninspired by the options available to him as the family's younger son[27] he left home around his fifteenth birthday to seek his fortune in Tokyo.

After trying a few different jobs, Koizumi enrolled as a trainee telegrapher under a government scheme. In 1901 he began practicing Tenjin Shin'yo-ryu[28] (divine true willow school) jujutsu at the dojo of Tago Nobushige, where the teaching was led by Nobushige's assistant, N. Takagaki. Once qualified as a telegrapher he worked for two years at the Tokyo Central Post Office, and at that time harbored ambitions to enter the Naval College. However, frustrated by the bureaucracy of working life at the Post Office, he rethought his plans and decided that he wanted to study electrical engineering. He also concluded that the most suitable place to do so was in the US. However, he did not have a clear strategy for realizing this ambition.

In 1903, Koizumi left Japan for Korea where he worked as a telegrapher for both the Pusan Post and the Korean Railway. In 1904, he trained at the jujutsu and kenjutsu dojo of Nobukatsu Yamada (a former samurai, member of the Japanese warrior class) where he learnt Shin Shin-ryu (true new school) jujutsu and *katsu* (resuscitation). In 1905, still with the aim of ultimately getting to the US, he left Korea and travelled through Shanghai, Hong Kong, Singapore, and India, working as he went. While in Singapore, in 1905, he practiced

Akishima-ryu (Akishima School) jujutsu under Tsunejiro Akishima and became an assistant teacher to Akishima Sensei.

Continuing his odyssey, Koizumi arrived in the UK on 4 May 1906—landing in Mostyn, North Wales aboard the S.S. Romford. He first travelled to Liverpool and worked there for three months as the instructor at the dubious "Kara Ashikaga School of Jujitsu [sic]" before relocating to London on 5 August 1906. In the capital, he taught at Sadakazu Uyenishi's jujutsu school in Golden Square, the Regent Street Polytechnic, the Royal Navy Volunteers, and probably elsewhere. Jujutsu was very popular in the UK at that time, with many jujutsuka touring the music halls—see later.

After several months in London, Koizumi departed for New York, where he arrived in May 1907 and secured work at the Newark Public Service Railway Company. However, after three years he was back in London where he struggled to start an electric lighting company in Vauxhall Road. In January 1912, Koizumi established a lacquerware studio in Ebury Street which thrived with a prestigious client base. On 6 April 1912 Koizumi married Ida Celine Winstanley (1876-1947) and in 1920 the couple had a daughter, Hana (Figure 7). Hana later married Percival (Percy) Yasushi Sekine (1920-2010) Kodokan 8th dan, BJA 9th dan (Figure 8) who was one of Koizumi's judo students, and who went on to become one of the UK's most senior judoka. From 1912 onwards, London became Koizumi's permanent home.

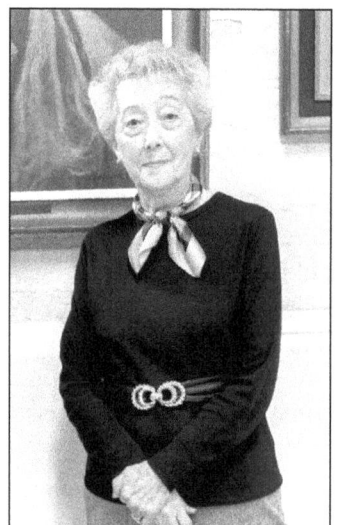 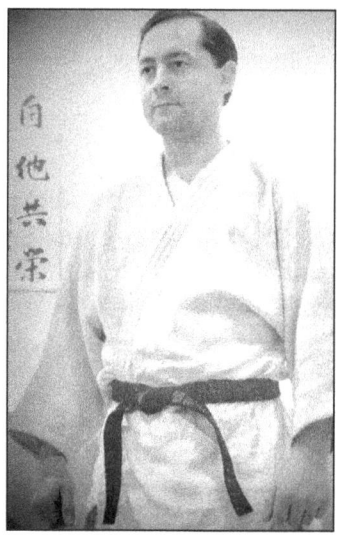

Figure 7, left. Hana Sekine, nee Koizumi, (born 1920).
Figure 8, right. Percy Sekine (1920-2010).

In 1918, Koizumi personally funded the founding of The Budokwai. The Society officially opened on 26 January 1918 at 15 Lower Grosvenor Place (Figure 9) near Buckingham Palace, and initially offered tuition in *jujutsu* (later transitioning to judo) and *kendo* (way of the sword). Yukio Tani, ultimately Kodokan 4th dan, was the Society's first lead instructor.

In 1919, Koizumi helped establish the *Zaiei Dobo Kyosai Kai* (Japanese Mutual Aid Society of Great Britain) to provide medical, employment, and housing assistance to Japanese people in the UK. The Society operated out of The Budokwai's premises, and Koizumi served as its General Secretary.

In July 1920, Kano Shihan visited The Budokwai while in transit to the Olympic

Games in Antwerp. Because of this visit, Koizumi and Tani agreed that The Budokwai should adopt the principles of Kodokan Judo, and Kano graded them both to 2nd dan in his judo. In 1922, Koizumi, was appointed as a consultant to the Victoria and Albert Museum—later cataloging the museum's entire lacquerware collection. His book *Lacquer Work: Full Description of the Process and the Preparations How to Identify the Age and the Quality of Lacquer* was published in 1925 (Figure 10; Koizumi, 1925) and contains a practical exposition of the art of lacquering, together with valuable notes for a collector. Around 1926/27 Koizumi made a significant contribution to the worldwide growth in popularity of judo through introducing a colored belt system for *mudansha* (those without dan) grades.[29]

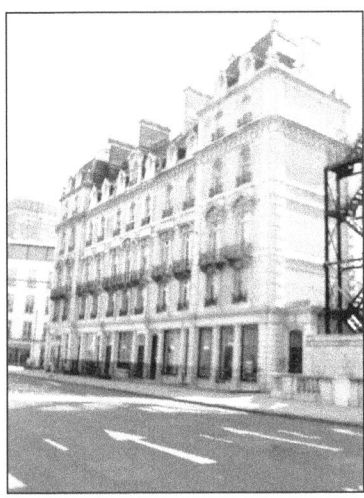

Figure 9.
The original location of
The Budokwai at 15 Lower
Grosvenor Place, London.

Figure 10.
*Lacquer Work: Full
Description of the Process
and the Preparations
How to Identify the Age
and the Quality of Lacquer*
by Gunji Koizumi was
published in 1925.

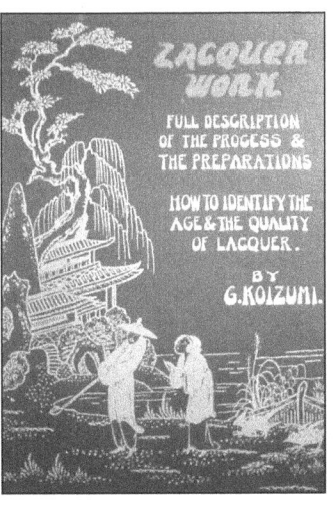

Throughout the Second World War (WWII) (1939–1945), judo practice continued at The Budokwai, but was heavily subsidized by Koizumi who was not personally restricted in any way over the conflict period. In 1948 and 1949 he was prominent in the activities that resulted in the formation of the British Judo Association (BJA) and subsequently the European Judo Union (EJU).[30] Three years later, in 1951, Koizumi was influential in the formation of the International Judo Federation (IJF). Around the same time, he stepped back from his business activities to focus full-time on judo.

On 19 September 1954, The Budokwai relocated to a new, larger, premises at 4 Gilston Road in South Kensington (Figure 11), where it remains to this day. Soon after, Koizumi visited Japan for the first time in half a century—discovering a very different country to the one he had left (Koizumi, 1955).

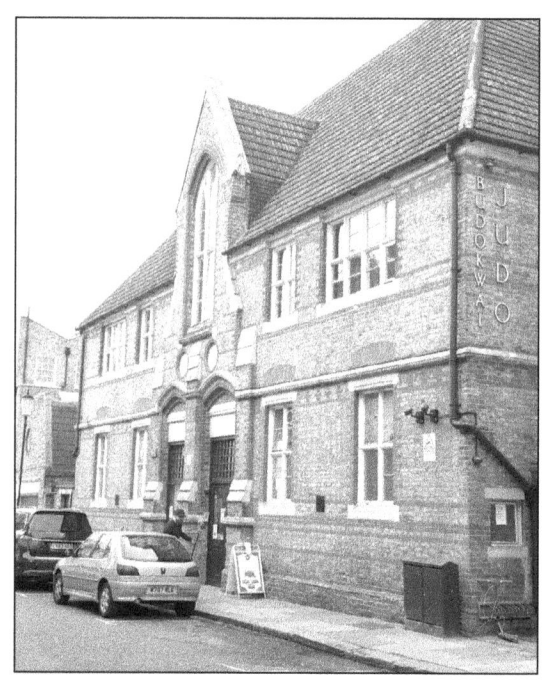

Figure 11. The present-day exterior of The Budokwai at 4 Gilston Road, South Kensington, London.

After his Japanese trip, Koizumi returned to the UK where he continued to teach judo throughout the early 1960s. Around this time, he also authored two judo instructional books—specifically *Judo: The Basic Technical Principles and Exercises* (Koizumi, 1958; Figure 12) and *My Study of Judo: The Principle and the Technical Fundamentals* (Koizumi, 1960; Figure 13).

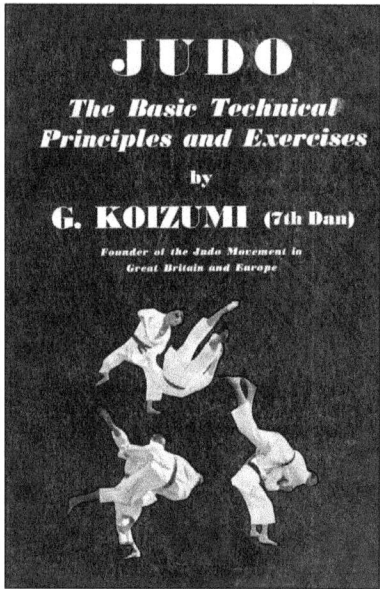
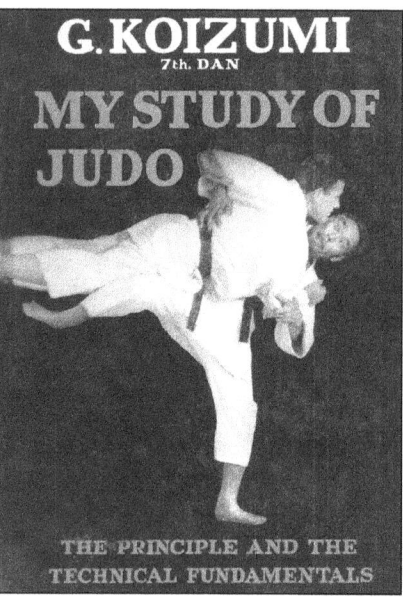

Figure 12. *Judo: The Basic Technical Principles and Exercises* by Gunji Koizumi was published in 1958. It introduces the student to the basic principles of judo along with its contest rules and grading syllabus.

Figure 13. *My Study of Judo: The Principle and the Technical Fundamentals* by Gunji Koizumi was published in 1960, and is a compact, well-illustrated, book containing some interesting original ideas and uncommon techniques.

Regarding his judo grades, Koizumi was promoted by The Kodokan to 4th dan in 1932, to 6th dan in 1948,[31] to 7th dan in 1951, and finally to 8th dan in 1962.[32]

Koizumi was known to have disliked the transformation of judo into a sport. He was of the view was that judo was an education. In January 1965, he was known to be working on an article entitled "Judo and the Basic Human Education" (Callan, 2011).

Gunji Koizumi took his own life on 15 April 1965 after feeling he had contributed as much as he could to humanity. Two days before he died he was asked what he would like to happen. He answered, "To see people think for themselves and not be led like sheep" (R. Bowen, 2011b, xxix).

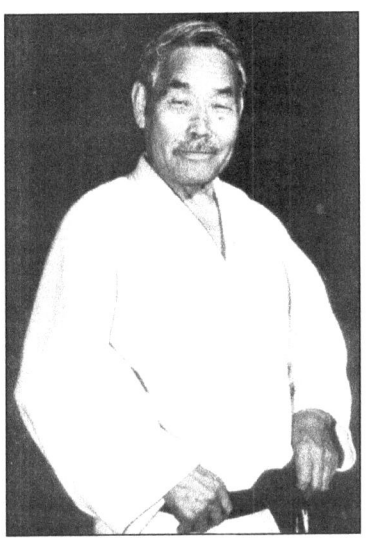 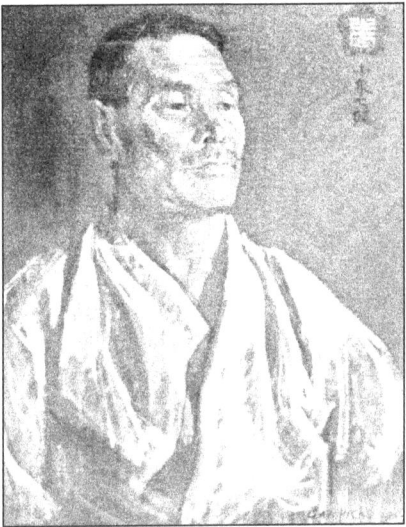

Figure 14. The last known photograph of Gunji Koizumi taken by Cliff Nash on 13 April 1965.

Figure 15. "G.K."— a portrait of Gunji Koizumi by Jerry Hicks MBE. This painting still hangs in the main dojo of The Budokwai.

Yukio Tani

Born in Japan in 1881, Yukio Tani ("The Pocket Hercules") (Figure 16) was a jujutsu and judo instructor, and professional challenge wrestler (Noble, 2000). The precise details of Tani's training in koryu in Japan are uncertain, but he is understood to have studied Fusen-ryu jujutsu under Mataemon Tanabe in Kobe, and Yataro Handa in Osaka (Diana Pho, writing as "Ay-leen the Peacemaker," 2011). Fromm and Soames (1982; 7) also state that Tani studied Shin-no-Shinto-ryu—one of the parent arts of Tenjin Shin'yo-ryu.

The physically small (1.60 m/5'3") Tani was 18 years old when, in 1900, he, along with two other[33] jujutsuka, was brought over to the UK by the British engineer and entrepreneur Edward William Barton-Wright[34] (1860–1951) (Noble, 1999). Barton-Wright, a self-defense and physical therapy enthusiast, had seen the jujutsuka fight in Japan and believed that the men, particularly Tani, had something special to offer. The pairing of Barton-Wright, as manager, with Tani, a skillful contest-man and natural showman, led them to visit music halls, where Tani would challenge anyone willing to wrestle him. Tani also taught jujutsu for some time at Barton-Wright's "Bartitsu School of Arms and Physical Culture" in London's Soho.

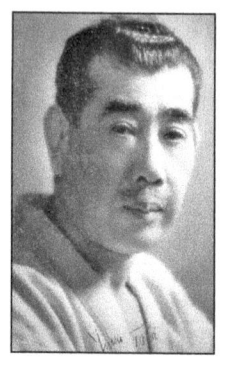 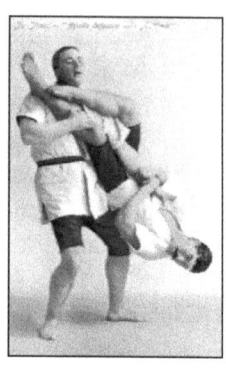

Figure 16. Yukio Tani (1881–1950).

Figure 17. Rare color promotional postcard, c. 1906, of Yukio Tani demonstrating a flying armlock on his then new manager, William "Apollo the Scottish Hercules" Bankier. Courtesy of Tony Wolf, Bartitsu Society.

After a disagreement, Tani split from Barton-Wright in 1903. He then teamed up with veteran promoter William Bankier (1870–1949), who had himself been a music hall performer under the name of "Apollo, the Scottish Hercules". Under Bankier's management, Tani continued to be active on the music hall circuit, where he was a formidable opponent for anyone. One of his favorite techniques was a "flying armlock" (Figure 17) which he would use to defeat much larger wrestlers. Over his eight- to nine-year music-hall challenge career, the only credible account of Tani being defeated was to another Japanese jujutsuka, Taro Miyake (1881–1935), who overcame him at the Tivoli theater, Strand, London, in December 1904. Notwithstanding this defeat, Tani went on to partner Miyake in several ventures. In 1904, they established the Japanese School of Jujutsu at 305 Oxford Street, London, and in 1906, they co-authored the book, The Game of Ju-jitsu (Miyake and Tani, 1906; Figure 18).

In 1918, Tani became the first professional teacher at The Budokwai where he initially taught jujutsu. Recall that in 1920 (after a visit by Kano Shihan) The Budokwai formally adopted the curriculum of Kodokan Judo, and at that juncture Tani was awarded the judo grade of 2nd dan. Regarding further judo grades, Tani was promoted to Kodokan 3rd dan in 1928, and to his final judo grade of Kodokan 4th dan on 10 January 1932 (Rie Kurashina, personal communications, 15 September 2016; 12 May 2017).

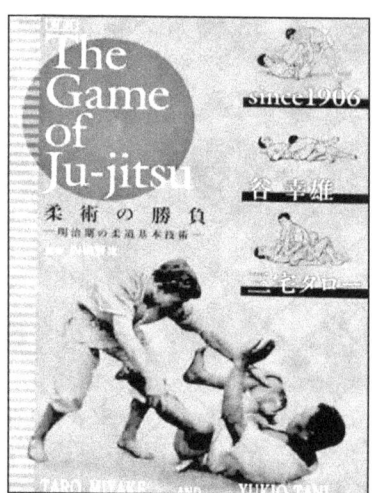 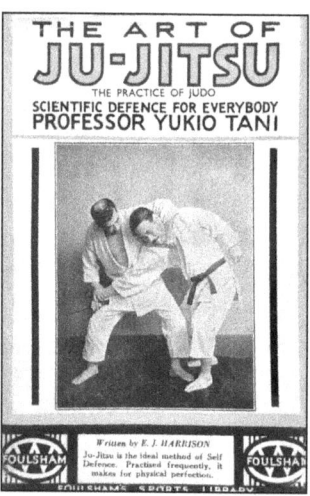

Figure 18. *The Game of Ju-jitsu* by Taro Miyake and Yukio Tani was published in 1906. (The figure shows the cover of a modern reprint).
Figure 19. *The Art of Ju-Jitsu* by E.J. Harrison was published in 1938 under the auspices of Yukio Tani.

Yukio Tani married Mary Alice Faeron, and in 1920 the couple had a daughter, Moya. Moya (who became Moya Ward on marriage) went on to both practice and teach judo, specifically at the Anglo-Japanese Judo Club in Strathmore Gardens, London, in the mid 1930s (Ito, 2001:195; Watson, 2017:4). This club was founded in 1901 by Tani's jujutsu collaborator Sadakazu Uyenishi (b. 1880–d. not known), who also had toured the music hall circuit as a prize-fighter for a time, before returning to Japan.

Tani suffered a severe and crippling paralytic stroke in 1937 which left him unable to physically perform judo. Up to that event he had still been training vigorously (Noble, 2000). Nevertheless, Tani continued to teach from the sidelines at The Budokwai and attend the Society's annual enbu.

In 1938, the British journalist, author and judoka Ernest John (E.J.) Harrison Kodokan 4th dan (1873–1961) published the book *The Art of Ju-jitsu* which he had produced with the support of Tani (Harrison, 1938; Figure 19).

Yukio Tani died on 24 January 1950, aged 69.

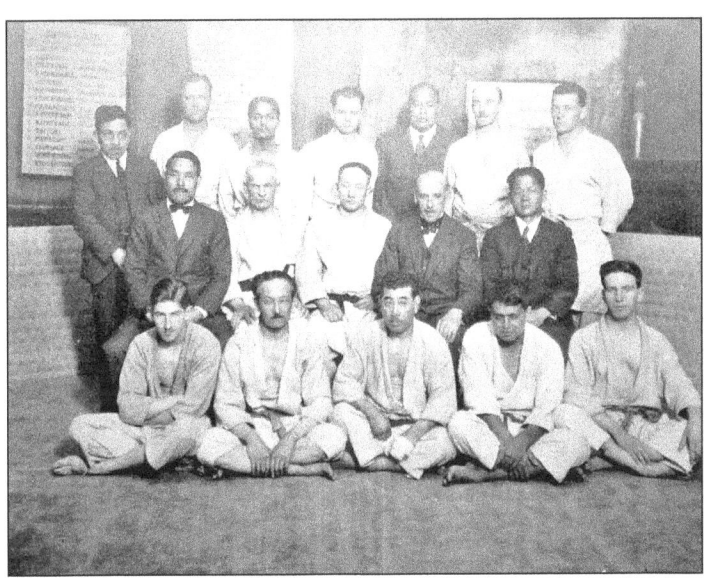

Figure 20. A group photograph containing Koizumi, Harrison and Tani taken at the original Budokwai. Gunji Koizumi is seated on the far left in the middle row and next to him is E.J. Harrison. Sitting cross-legged in the middle of the front row is Yukio Tani. Courtesy of Roger Payne.

Edward (Ted) Mossom

Edward (Ted) Mossom (Figure 21) started practicing judo at The Budokwai in 1932. He was a sales engineer by profession, and enjoyed reading and philosophy (Edwards and Menzies, 1955; Budokwai Members and Historical site, n.d.). According to R. Bowen (2011b; 151–152) Mossom was about 1.68m tall (5' 6"), weighed less than 58 kg (9 stone) and was lame in one leg because of poliomyelitis (polio). Nevertheless, he developed into a superb judoka, who was also adept at wrestling and boxing (Ibid.).

By some accounts Mossom was also a serious pub (public house) brawler and apparently, Koizumi at one point had him banned from The Budokwai, but not for brawling. During WWII, because he could not be on the front line, Mossom taught unarmed combat to troops.

One of the authors (Finch) recalls Mossom telling him a story, in a pub, of when he (Mossom) was working in an office at an electricity company, and a man entered and tried to steal cash from the till in the front office. Mossom saw what was happening and, despite his condition, chased the robber, catching and throwing him to the ground, and holding him till the police arrived.

Mossom was promoted to 1st dan in 1937, to 2nd dan in 1940 and to 3rd dan in 1943. He represented The Budokwai in international matches from about1938 onwards, and GB in international contests from around 1947 to 1949 (Ibid.). The zenith of Mossom's contest career was his 2-0 defeat of the legendary French judoka Jean de Herdt (Figure 22) in a GB versus France international team contest held in London on 2 December 1947. The format of the match was a "best of three" contest, and one of the authors (Bowen) recalls 1964 Tokyo Olympian Tony Sweeney BJA 9th dan, telling him that Mossom twice threw de Herdt with an ashi/o-guruma (leg-wheel/major-wheel) style technique.

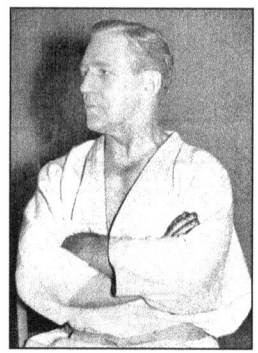 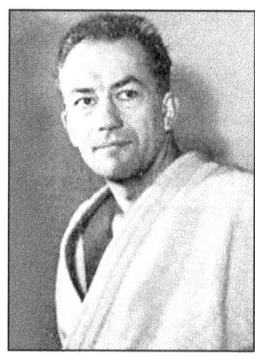

Figure 21. Ted Mossom. Figure 22. Jean de Herdt (1923–2013).

Figure 23 shows the team from The Budokwai after international matches against France and The Netherlands during the 32nd Budokwai Display on 21 March 1949. Mossom is on the far left holding a trophy. Note that one of the members of the Dutch team at that event was Jaap (Jacobus) Nauwelaerts de Agé (1917–2016) who was a co-founder of the Judo Bond Netherlands (JBN) in 1939, and later prominent, alongside Koizumi, in the activities that lead to the formation of the EJU (1948) and the IJF (1951).

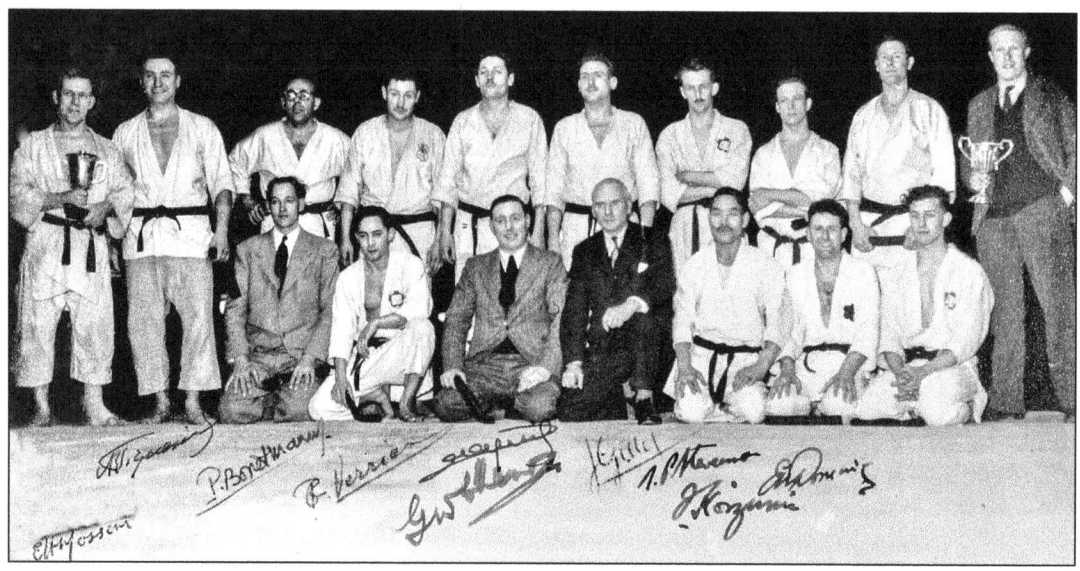

Figure 23.
The Budokwai team at the 32nd Budokwai Display on 21 March 1949.
Ted Mossom is on the far left of the photograph, holding a trophy.

Budokwai 32nd Annual Display
Seymour Hall
Monday 21st March 1949

FRENCH TEAM.		WIN	VERSUS	WIN	BRITISH TEAM
Capt. Bonnet-Maury	3 dan		-	OO	Capt. T. Mossom 3 dan (2x ogurumas)
(A) Piquemal	3 dan	O	-		N. Hyde 3 dan
(B) Verrier	2 dan		-	O	P. Sekine 3 dan (osoto).
Coquil	2 dan	X	-	X	G. Chew 2 dan (draw)
Gillet	1 dan		-	OO	I. Stevenson 2 dan (2x hanes).

(A) Former Champ. of France.
(B) Reigning " " "

HOLLAND			VERSUS	WIN	BRITAIN
J. Snijder	1 dan		-	O	C. Palmer 1 dan (seoiotoshi)
I. Nauwelaerts de Age (Kataguruma)	1 dan	O	-	O	G. Dominy 1 dan (Tai-o)

Inter-club Final.

	Budokwai			versus		Warwick J.C.
(Hold + Harai)	J. Gregory	1 Kyu	OO	-		A. Hayes 1 Kyu (x)
(Harai + Shime)	S. Wright	1 Kyu	OO	-	O	W. Heath 2 Kyu (uragoshi)
(Kosoto + Hane)	P. Foster	1 Kyu	OO			S. Hilton 2 Kyu

(x) later to be "Judo Al Hayes" - saw him get his black belt later that year at the Budokwai - R Bowen

Back Row Mossom, Piquemal, Bonnet-Maury, Verrier, Coquil, Gillet, Stevenson, Nauwelaerts, ?Snijder, Gregory.
Kneeling: H. Hyde P. Sekine G. Chew

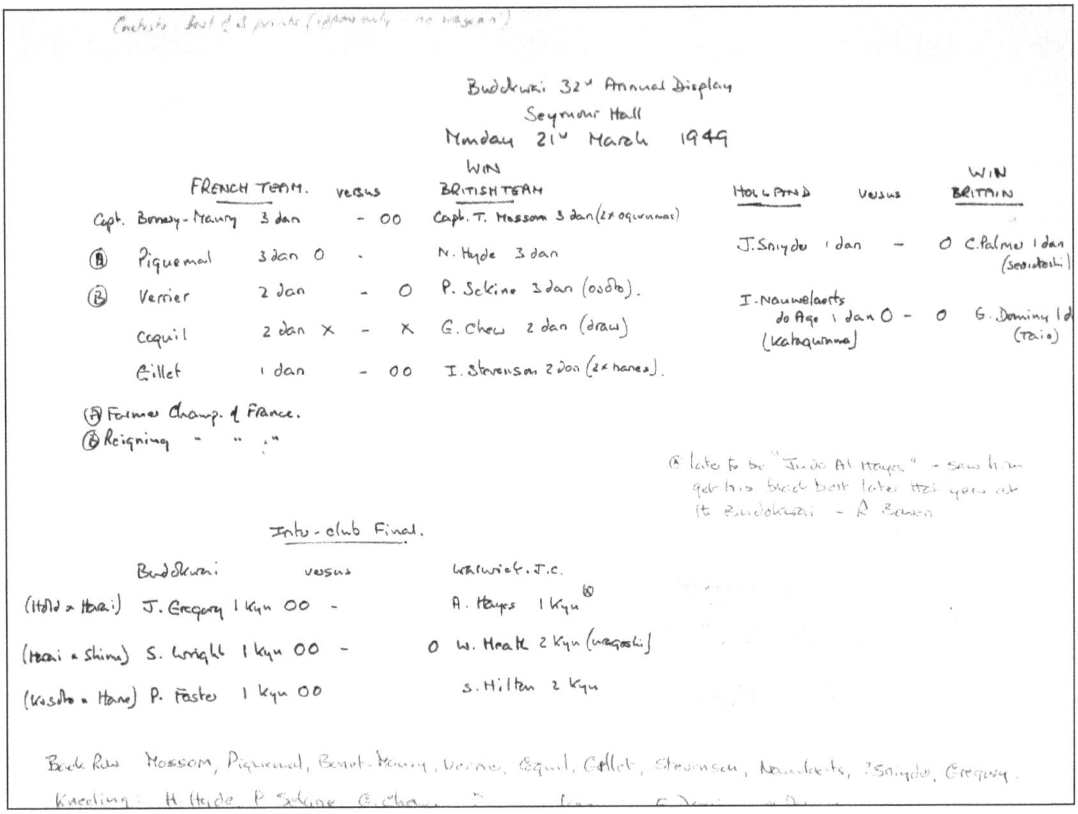

Figure 23-B.
Notes on the reverse side of the photographs of The Budokwai team at the 32nd Budokwai Display on 21 March 1949.

Mossom along with Stan Bissel featured as a demonstrator in the British edition of T. Shozo Kuwashima and Ashbel R. Welch's book *Judo: Forty-One Lessons in the Modern Science of Jiu-Jitsu* (Kuwashima and Welch, 1951; Figure 24). This book came in both an original version, entitled *Judo: Thirty Lessons in the Modern Science of Jiu-Jitsu*, and a later enlarged edition with even more judo self-defense-oriented content. Both versions have larger, clear black and white photographs and well-written text.

The late senior British judoka, Robert (Bob) Thomas, IJF 8th dan, Kodokan 6th dan (1938–2017), recalled taking instruction in *tai-otoshi* (body drop throw) from Mossom at the LJS in 1962. Thomas remembered Mossom as "a fine judoka" (Robert Thomas, personal communication, 1 April 2006). Mossom was also the instructor to the GEC (General Electric Company) and the LEB (London Electricity Board judo clubs.

One of the authors (Finch) recalls the last time he saw Mossom would have been in the late 1960s. At that time Mossom was retiring from the LJS and moving to Essex.

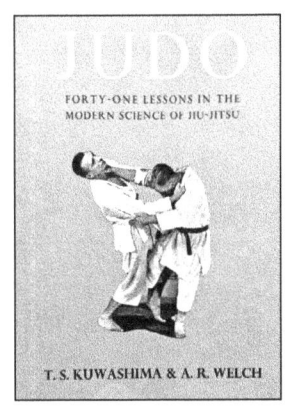

Figure 24.
Judo: Forty-One Lessons in the Modern Science of Jiu-Jitsu (British Edition) with Ted Mossom.

George Kerr

George Kerr (Figure 25 and 27) was born in 1937 and started judo in Edinburgh, UK aged eight. He achieved his 1st dan aged 15, and in 1957 received a scholarship to train in Japan where he spent the next four years. Over that period he learnt Japanese, and absorbed judo's moral code which continues to influence him to this day.

As a competitive judoka, his successes include individual European Championships silver medals in 1962 (Essen), 1963 (Geneva) and 1967 (Rome) as well as being British Open Champion in 1966 and 1968. After retiring from competition at the age of 31, Kerr developed himself as an international referee—officiating at two Olympic Games (1972 and 1976), and at three World Championships between 1969 and 1975. He retired from refereeing in 1976, and subsequently became National Coach to the Austrian judo team, where he guided Peter Seisenbacher to two Olympic gold medals in 1984 and 1988.

Kerr has also been involved actively with the BJA, British Olympic Association (BOA), EJU and IJF. He first became a BJA Director in 1981, and later Chairman from 1991 to 1997. In 2001 he became BJA President, a position he still holds. In the 1990s he was a EJU Sports Director and Vice President, and on the Sports Commission of the IJF.

Kerr was promoted to 10th dan by the IJF for services to judo in 2010, and received an Honorary Doctorate from Heriot-Watt University, Edinburgh in the same year. He was made a Commander of the Most Excellent Order of the British Empire (CBE) in 2011, and that year also received the Japanese Order of the Rising Sun, Gold Rays with Rosette, after being named in Emperor Akihito's November 2010 honors list.

In 2013, Kerr was inducted to the IJF Hall of Fame and presented with an IJF Lifetime Achievement Award. He has written a few books on judo, and his autobiography *My Journey to the 10th Dan*, co-written with Edward (Eddie) Ferrie, was published in 2017 (Kerr and Ferrie, 2017).

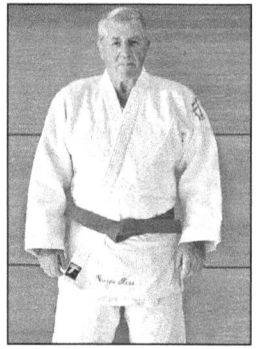 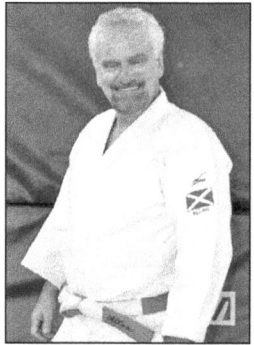

Figure 25. George Kerr (born 1937). Courtesy of Richard Goulding.
Figure 26. Maurice Allan (born 1945).

Maurice Allan

Maurice Allan (Figures 26 and 27) was born in Edinburgh, UK in 1945 and is a multiple GB and Scottish National Champion in judo. A protégé of George Kerr (Figure 27), Allan managed the Edinburgh Club and taught judo at Edinburgh University.

In addition to his prowess as a judoka, Allan is well known as a wrestler and grappler of international stature—being World Sambo Wrestling Champion in 1975, and representing GB in freestyle wrestling at the 1976 Olympic Games in Montreal. For his contributions to the grappling arts as both a competitor and a teacher, Allan was made a Member of the Most Excellent Order of the British Empire (MBE) in 1975.

Since 1976, Allan has lived in Virginia in the US, where he runs his own judo school and is responsible for defense training for all trainee law enforcement officers at the Fairfax County Criminal Justice Academy. He presently holds an 8th dan in judo awarded by both the USJA and USA Judo.

Rodger Bornowski

Rodger Bornowski (Figure 28), presently BJA 3rd dan, achieved his 1st dan in 1977 and was an active competitor for almost 20 years, winning multiple medals over that period. Bornowski has extensive knowledge of kata, which he has demonstrated on many occasions with George Kerr.

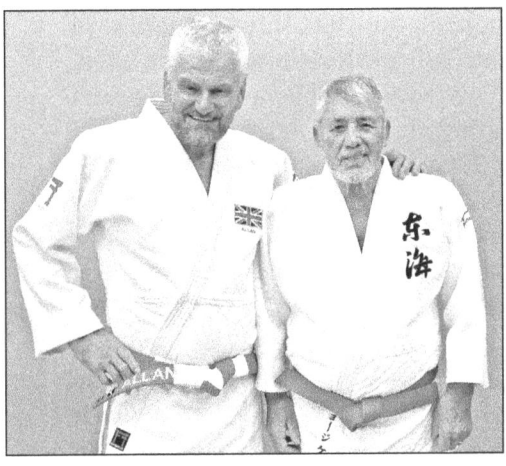

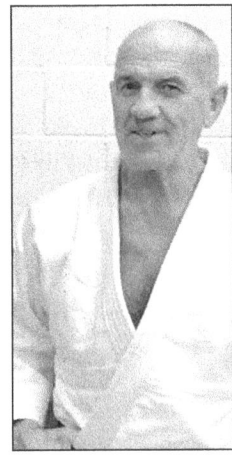

Figure 27. Maurice Allan and George Kerr. Courtesy of Eddie Ferrie.

Figure 28. Rodger Bornowski (born 1958).

BUDOKWAI KIME-NO-KATA

Creation of Budokwai Kime-no-kata

The name most often linked to Budokwai Kime-no-kata is Gunji Koizumi. He is generally considered to have been developed, refined and concluded the exercise in and around the 1930/40s, working either alone ...

> ... the Self Defence Kata—Kime no Kata—which differs from that normally shown elsewhere as Koizumi had devised it so that it could be visually pleasing, and that which is shown is known as the Budokwai Kime no Kata.
> – Budokwai, n.d.

or, as suggested by the eminent judoka and judo historian Richard (Dicky) Bowen (1926–2005), jointly with Yukio Tani.

> The Budokwai uses two kime no kata; one being the Kodokan kata, which is in many senses archaic but nonetheless is an extremely valuable training method, and one anybody professing to be a judo teacher should be able to perform and teach, along with nage no kata and katame no kata; the other is the Budokwai kime no kata, which was devised by Tani and Koizumi, and for many years the kata favoured for display work.
> – R. Bowen, 2011:333

No direct evidence is provided to underpin either of the above statements, so it will now be considered if the claims that it is the creation of Koizumi, possibly working with Tani, are correct.

Authorship of Budokwai Kime-no-kata
Attribution of the authorship of Budokwai Kime-no-kata to Gunji Koizumi is based on critically evaluating the following components:

- Koizumi is known to have been an innovator regarding judo kata. Documentation exists of his personal involvement in (i) modifying official Kodokan katas, and (ii) developing original, not officially recognized, judo katas;
- Koizumi was one of the judoka participating in the 1932 international judo gathering involving Oxford University Judo Club and a visiting German team. Recall that, to the best of the authors' knowledge, Budokwai Kime-no-kata was possibly first introduced to the general judo public at this event.
- Koizumi participates in the earliest known recorded demonstration of Budokwai Kime-no-kata, which features on The 'Budokwai' Film, produced in 1948 to mark the Society's thirtieth anniversary.
- Koizumi wrote the most detailed known technical resource on Budokwai Kime-no-kata—a multi-part instructional article published in *The Budokwai Bulletin* over 1948 and 1949;
- Koizumi is known to have had a background in koryu. Specifically, he is known to have studied Tenjin Shin'yo-ryu jujutsu—a style of jujutsu which has influenced and inspired some of the specific self-defense skills shown throughout Budokwai Kime-no-kata.

Koizumi's Kata Activities
Koizumi is known to have been a modernizer regarding judo kata. Records exist of him amending, and showing, standard Kodokan kata, and also showing original, and hence unofficial, exercises.

Concerning him modifying official Kodokan katas, T. Leggett recalled an incident during Kano Shihan's 1933 visit to The Budokwai, when Koizumi and Tani did an altered Ju-no-kata (forms of gentleness and flexibility):

> Dr. Kano watched two English Budokwai members performing Nage-no-kata, and then Mr. Gunji Koizumi and Mr. Yukio Tani performing Ju-no-kata. Koizumi had introduced some of his own ideas into the kata, and I heard that Dr. Kano remarked: 'that is a modification of Ju-no-kata'. – Leggett, 2000

Regarding Koizumi's association with innovative, unsanctioned katas, R. Bowen describes the 12 July 1927 opening of the new lower dojo at The Budokwai in front of the Japanese ambassador, Baron Matsui:

> ... various kata were performed, these included shinri no kata demonstrated by Koizumi and Tani. Lacking the Japanese characters used no meaning can be placed on the name. Shinri could mean "psychological" or "spiritual," but there are other possible meanings. The spelling is correct as it is mentioned several times in the late twenties, including in a printed programme. It was probably a kata devised by Koizumi and Tani. – R. Bowen, 2011b:8

Another occasion where Koizumi and Tani did Shinri-no-kata was the 29 November 1932 Oxford University enbu. The event program describes Shinri-no-kata as containing "locks, holds, methods of strangling, etc." (Oxford University Judo Club, 1932; De Crée, 2015). Recall from earlier that it was also at this enbu that Koizumi and Tani did their "Kime-no-kata" featuring knife, pistol and stick attacks—possibly the first public showing of Budokwai Kime-no-kata.

In November 1932 Koizumi and Tani would have been 47 and c. 51 years old, respectively. This would have been some 14 years after Tani was appointed The Budokwai's first professional jujutsu/judo teacher, and five years before his debilitating stroke. If Budokwai Kime-no-kata was by then complete and finalized, the timeline implies that Koizumi and Tani could have collaborated on its development for a maximum period of about 15 years. This would have required them to have started their joint working at the ages of 28 and 32 years old, respectively. If they continued to refine the exercise beyond the enbu, then the absolute maximum period for its joint development would be about 19 years.

However, finalizing Budokwai Kime-no-kata during this period would have required the pair to be working on the exercise at a period when Koizumi was growing his lacquerware business and philanthropic interests (and had recently become a father), and when Tani was a busy professional jujutsu teacher. It is probably unlikely that either man would have focused that much on developing a new kata during this time, however the possibility cannot be totally dismissed.

Introduction and Prominent Demonstrations of Budokwai Kime-no-kata

It is known that Gunji Koizumi participated in early demonstrations of Budokwai Kime-no-kata. As already described, Koizumi, along with Tani, did a "Kime-no-kata" featuring defenses against knife, pistol and stick attacks, at an international judo meet in Oxford in 1932. Recall also that Koizumi, along with Ted Mossom, did Budokwai Kime-no-kata in the earliest known (1948) recording of the exercise as part of The 'Budokwai' Film.

Koizumi's Kime-no-kata Article

The 1932 enbu took place 16 years before Koizumi wrote the first, and only known, technical article on Budokwai Kime-no-kata—"Kime No Kata; Decisive Combat Forms", which was serialized in three consecutive issues (October 1948 to April 1949) of the *The Budokwai Bulletin*. Koizumi's article contained an explanation of the complete Budokwai Kime-no-kata—including rudimentary line drawings of various techniques, as well as advice on their execution. However, neither in his article, nor elsewhere, does Koizumi make any explicit claim for personal authorship of the exercise. Additionally, to the best of the authors' knowledge, nowhere is it mentioned precisely when, or exactly under what circumstances, Budokwai Kime-no-kata was created. Equally, nowhere is it stated what the technical sources of inspiration for the exercise were.

Sources of Inspiration for Budokwai Kime-no-kata

Although Koizumi does not identify any external sources as inspiration for Budokwai Kime-no-kata, this does not mean that such sources do not exist. Since Koizumi had direct koryu experience—mostly in Tenjin Shin'yo-ryu jujutsu, it is useful to explore whether any links to this *ryu* (school) are evident in the exercise.

To achieve this objective, the authors posed the question to Paul Masters *shike* (teacher of the line)—the first ever Westerner to hold the highest technical credential of *menkyo kaiden* (license of full transmission and mastership) in Tenjin Shin'yo-ryu. The engagement and interaction with P. Masters was kindly facilitated by his son, Lee Masters

Shihan, who himself achieved menkyo kaiden in the ryu in 2017.

Having viewed the recording of Koizumi and Mossom doing Budokwai Kime-no-kata (Budokwai, 1948; Take Five Productions, n.d.; Whittlesea, 2013a), Paul Masters (personal communication, 23 May 2017) opined that the exercise does indeed clearly contain techniques identical to, or very like, those found in the 124 Teai Kata of Infinite Change of Tenjin Shin'yo-ryu. Most of these techniques are also found in judo, which is logical, and not surprising, as Jigoro Kano Shihan himself had studied Tenjin Shin'yo-ryu, and was greatly inspired by it when he created Kodokan Judo.

With respect to the spirit shown by Koizumi and Mossom, P. Masters (Ibid.) explained that in any Kime-no-kata, the function of uke is to be *teki* (the enemy), and that this is how uke's role is always seen within Tenjin Shin'yo-ryu. This is to ensure that the intent, serious nature, and intensity of the attack is always reflected, and that uke and tori have the correct mindset whilst performing the techniques.

P. Masters added that one expression in Tenjin Shin'yo-ryu is "*hito nage, hito shime, hito ate, hissatsu jujutsu*" (one throw, one strangle, one strike certain death jujutsu) and that this reflects the seriousness of the koryu jujutsu which was not a sport but a way of survival, as taught by, and to, the samurai. Recall that Koizumi had received jujutsu training from a former samurai, and had brought this mindset to his judo teaching.

Conclusion

Having considered and evaluated the arguments, there is little doubt that Koizumi created Budokwai Kime-no-kata. He was an outstanding individual who possessed both the technical knowledge and skills, and the charisma and leadership characteristics vital for such an endeavor. This conclusion is reinforced by the fact that no other credible, or senior, judo teacher has ever challenged the crediting of authorship of Budokwai Kime-no-kata to Koizumi.

Note also that while the involvement of Yukio Tani in the exercise's creation cannot be totally dismissed, it can readily be speculated that his role is unlikely to be as significant as that of Koizumi.

TECHNICAL CONTENTS
OF BUDOKWAI KIME-NO-KATA

Etiquette in Budokwai Kime-no-kata

The only mention of reiho in Koizumi's original 1948 article on Budokwai Kime-no-kata is:

> The partners ... take position about 15 feet [c. 4.5m] apart. After exchanging bows ... [they] advance forward in a normal walking manner ...
> – Koizumi, 1948:38

The 1948 film of Koizumi and Mossom doing Budokwai Kime-no-kata (Budokwai, 1948) shows the exercise to be very lacking in ceremony, and overall the reiho is very informal when compared with the present day (highly prescriptive) reiho standards for all the official Kodokan kata. Koizumi and Mossom begin the exercise with a *ritsurei* (standing bow), but conclude it with a *zarei* (seated bow)—see Figure 29. The authors can only speculate why this is the case, but would note that such an approach is simple and natural, as both judoka are on the ground after the *sutemi-waza* (sacrifice throw) defense of the final sequence. Additionally, as De Crée (2015: 148) notes, "... kata were never intended to become over-standardized as they often appear today", and the type of bowing chosen was simply "... proper for the occasion" (Ibid.).

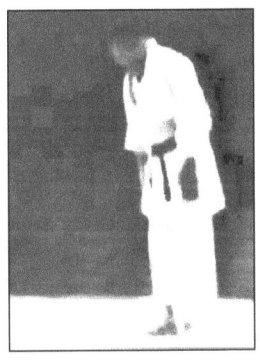 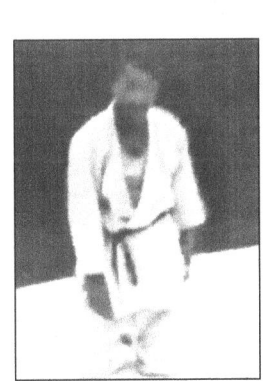 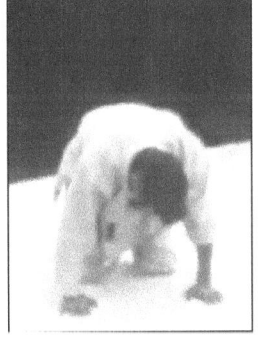 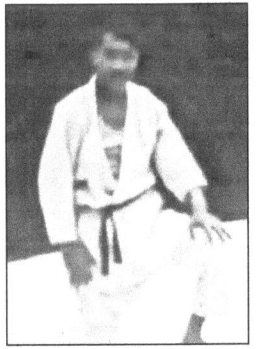

Figure 29. Opening *ritsu-rei* (standing bow) and closing *za-rei* (kneeling bow) from the 1948 demonstration of Budokwai Kime-no-kata as shown by Gunji Koizumi. Photographs are snapshots from The 'Budokwai' Film.

Structure, Names and Technical Contents of Budokwai Kime-no-kata

A schematic overview of the structure and contents of Budokwai Kime-no-kata is presented in Table 1, and simple representative illustrations of the exercise's techniques in Table 2. Instructions on how to perform the mechanical movements of Budokwai Kime-no-kata's attack and defense sequences are specified in Table 3. The source for all the information found in these tables is Koizumi's original article (Koizumi, 1948–49).

Tables 1, 2 and 3 also suggest Japanese names for the attacks in Budokwai Kime-no-kata. These names, due to the authors, follow the established and highly efficient naming convention described by John Cornish.

The Japanese names used for the techniques in the kata only describe parts of the attack. To use a comprehensive description of all the attack and the defence would make the name too long-winded and, for the non-Japanese, difficult to remember whereas these short names should prove no difficulty at all. The English... is not meant to be a transcription of the Japanese names, like them it is meant only as a memory aid.

— Cornish, 1984:3

Table 1. Structural and Functional Overview of Budokwai Kime-no-kata After Koizumi (1948–49).
Budokwai Kime-no-kata (Budokwai Forms of Decisive Techniques)

English language description	*Proposed Japanese name*	*Nature of attack*
1. Hold from behind over both arms	daki-kakae	unarmed – hold
2. Pistol in right hand	shomen-zuke	armed – pistol
3. Downward attack with knife held over the head	kiri-oroshi	armed – knife
4. Upward stab with knife	age-tsuki	armed – knife
5. Both hands hold	ryote-dori	unarmed – hold
6. Belt pull and chin push	ago-oshi	unarmed – hold / blow
7. Blow to side of chin	ago-tsuki	unarmed– blow
8. Uppercut	tsuki-age	unarmed– blow
9. Downward blow with stick	furi-oroshi	armed – stick
10. Side blow with stick	furi-mawashi	armed – stick
11. Two hand attack on throat	mae-jime	unarmed – hold
12. Dash to the side	yoko-tosshin	unarmed – rush
13. Dash to the front	shomen-tosshin	unarmed – rush

Table 2. The Budokwai Kime-no-kata. After Koizumi (1948–49)

1. Hold from behind over both arms (*daki-kakae*).

2. Pistol in right hand (*shomen-zuke*).

3. Downward attack with knife held over the head (*kiri-oroshi*).

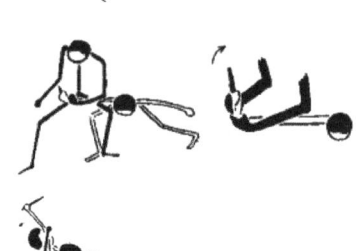

4. Upward stab with knife (*age-tsuki*).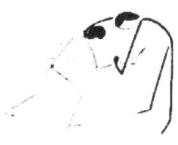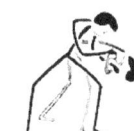

5. Both hands hold (*ayote-dori*).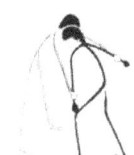

6. Belt pull and chin push (*ago-oshi*).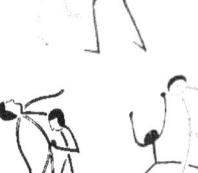

7. Blow to side of chin (*ago-tsuki*).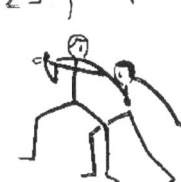

8. Uppercut (*tsuki-age*).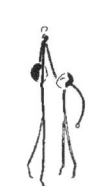

9. Downward blow with stick (*furi-oroshi*).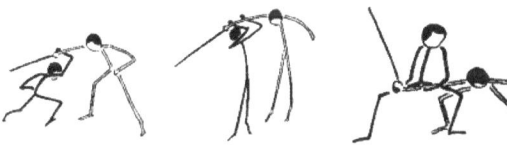

10. Side blow with stick (*furi-mawashi*).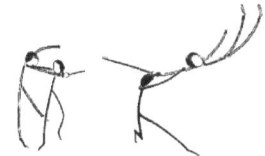

11. Two hand attack on throat (*mae-jime*).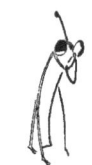

12. Dash to the side (*yoko-tosshin*).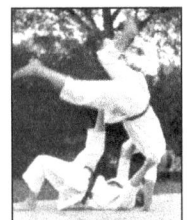

13. Dash to the front (*homen-tosshin*).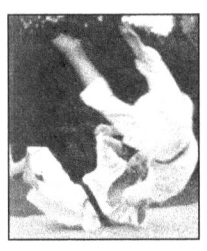

Table 3. Budokwai Kime-no-kata [Budokwai Forms of Decisive Techniques] Techniques 1 to 3. After Gunji Koizumi (1948-49)

1	Daki-kakae	Hold from behind over both arms	• Walking normally, tori and uke advance towards each other; • As they pass one another, uke attacks tori suddenly from behind, and attempts to hold him bodily over the arms; • Before the hold is tightened tori strikes uke's solar-plexus with his left elbow, and sharply turns his own body to the left; • Tori then slips his left leg behind uke's rear, and throws him with *sukui-nage* (scooping throw).
2	Shomen-zuke	Pistol in right hand	• Tori and uke swap roles; • As the new tori rises to his feet, the new uke covers him with a pistol held in his right hand; • Tori raises his hands over his head, and at a critical time drops his left hand, and with his thumb turned towards his own body grips the wrist of uke's armed hand from the top. Simultaneously tori pivots on his left toes; • Tori turns to the right, describes a semi-circle with his right foot, and brings his body in contact with uke's right side; • As he does so, tori passes his left arm over uke's right arm and applies an armlock; • Tori then applies a *tekubi-gatame* (wrist lock) and disarms uke by taking the pistol with his right hand.
3	Kiri-oroshi	Downward attack with knife held over the head	• Tori and uke swap roles; • Having released the wristlock the new uke moves away from the new tori and draws the knife that was hidden inside his jacket; • With the knife raised over his head, uke then moves towards tori; • As uke prepares to strike, tori rushes forwards—advancing on his left foot to the right of uke's right foot. tori's left arm is bent over his head and his body curved forwards, so that his left forearm meets the underside of uke's right arm at a point slightly above the elbow; • Tori then curves his body further forward by moving his hips back, and presses uke's arm towards his right ear; • Simultaneously, tori grips the back of uke's jacket with his right hand, draws uke's body forwards, and breaks his balance; • Tori then passes his right hand under uke's right upper arm, and by gripping the wrist applies a while locking uke's right elbow joint with *ude-garami* (entangled armlock); • Tori now releases his left arm and applies a *tekubi-gatame* (wrist lock); • Tori disarms uke by taking the knife with his left hand

4	Age-tsuki	Upward stab with knife	- Tori and uke swap roles;
- The new uke slowly and cautiously releases the new tori and takes a step or two backwards. As he does so he transfers the knife to his right hand and points it forward;
- Then drawing the knife back, uke prepares to stab tori upwards;
- As uke thrusts up, tori brings his left wrist sharply down onto uke's right forearm to block the upwards movement;
- Tori then moves his hips backwards and bends his body forwards to get further away from the point of the knife. Simultaneously, he applies his right hand to the back of uke's head and pulls uke forwards to unbalance him;
- Tori then pushes uke's right arm backwards with the back of his left hand, advances his left foot, and pivoting on it, turns his body to the right, describing a semi-circle with his right foot;
- As tori does so he bends uke's right arm back by passing his own left hand under uke's forearm and to the back of uke's right upper arm.
- Tori then applies *ude-garami* [entangled armlock] by bending his own left wrist, and disarms uke with a *tekubi-gatame* [wrist lock] by taking the knife with his right hand.
5	Ryote-dori	Both hands hold	- Tori and uke swap roles, and the new uke throws away the knife;
- As the new tori straightens himself up from the previous technique, uke seizes both of his (tori's) wrists with both of his hands simultaneously, and tries to hold them at the side of uke's body;
- Tori opens his arms sideways and draws back his left foot, pulling uke forwards and weakening his balance;
- Next, tori instantly turns his wrists inwards and upwards, moving his left foot forwards to break free from uke's grip;
- Continuing the upwards movement, tori places his free hands to the right of uke's left shoulder, and to the left of his right arm, and throws uke with *osoto-gari* [major outer reaping throw].
6	Ago-oshi	Belt pull and chin push	- Tori and uke swap roles;
- The new uke watches as the new tori raises himself from the ground;
- Uke then suddenly grasps the front of tori's belt with his left hand and pulls forwards. Simultaneously, Uke pushes tori's chin upwards, thereby bending his body and breaking his balance;
- Tori grips uke's right wrist with his left hand, palm turned upwards, and pushes uke's arm upwards, slightly drawing him forwards thereby removing uke's hand from his chin;
- At the same time, tori turns his body to the left and places his right hand on uke's right shoulder;
- Continuing to turn, tori bends his body forwards, raises his arms over his head and balances on his left leg, thereby weakening uke's balance to his rear right corner;
- Tori then throws uke with an *ashi-waza* [leg technique] by sweeping uke's right leg with his own right leg.

7	Ago-tsuki	Blow to side of chin	• Tori and uke swap roles; • As the new uke slowly rises from the ground he attempts to strike the left side of the new tori's jaw with his right fist; • Tori moves his head back, lets uke's fist pass by him and bends up his right arm to block and trap uke's right wrist with his own wrist. (The contact should be made at the inside of the wrists.) • Simultaneously, tori brings down his left arm over uke's upper arm, pressing uke's elbow against his chest and forming a powerful armlock; • Tori expands his chest to apply the lock.
8	Tsuki-age	Uppercut	• Tori and uke swap roles; • Having released the armlock, the new uke attacks the new tori with an uppercut using his right fist; • Tori evades the strike by bending back his head, and grips Uke's fist (or wrist) with both his hands and lifts it over his head, straightening the arms; • Retaining the contact and drawing uke with him, tori turns his body to his left and drops onto his left knee; • Uke is then thrown with an *uki-otoshi* (floating drop) style technique.
9	Furi-oroshi	Downward blow with stick	• Tori and uke swap roles; • As the new uke rises from the ground (following his application of a throw in the previous defense) he picks up a stick; • Holding the stick in his right hand, and with his arm slightly to the rear, uke contrives for an appropriate opportunity to attack. At the right moment, uke swings downwards aiming at Tori's head; • Tori dives forwards, taking a step with his right foot, and parries the blow with his right forearm, which is raised over his head. Tori's right forearm should now be directly under uke's right wrist, with the right arm bent, so that tori's forearm is horizontal over his head, meeting Uke's arm near the wrist; • Quickly and continuously, tori draws up his left foot to the front of his right, while simultaneously placing his left wrist beneath uke's arm just above the elbow. Gripping uke's right wrist with his right hand, tori pushes uke's elbow upwards to practically lock uke's arm; Pivoting on his left toes, tori turns his body to the right—describing a semi-circle with his right foot. As he does so, tori lowers his arms and locks uke's right arm between his left wrist and his own left thigh. In locking uke's arm, tori should use his *te-gatana* (hand blade) vertically against the arm; • Maintaining the armlock, tori passes his left hand over uke's elbow and holds his forearm with it to be able to control uke's arm with only his left hand; • Tori then disarms uke with a *tekubi-gatame* (wrist lock) by taking the stick with his right hand.

10	Furi-mawashi	Side blow with stick	• Tori and uke swap roles; • The new uke, having retained the stick in his right hand, carefully draws it back, and at the right opportunity, strikes sideways, aiming for the new tori's head; • Tori parries the blow with his left hand and grips uke's right wrist from the inside. Turning his body to his left, he draws uke forwards; • Continuing this turning movement tori places his right hand on uke's shoulder and dropping to the rear on his left knee throws uke with an *uki-otoshi* (floating drop) style technique.
11	Mae-jime	Two hand attack on throat	• Tori and uke swap roles; • As the new tori rises from the floor the new uke hurls himself at him— grasping at tori's throat with both hands; • Tori yields to uke's force, bends his body back and breaks uke's balance; • As he bends, tori grips uke's right sleeve with his left hand, and raises his right arm; • Tori controls uke by pressing his right arm against uke's left arm from the outside; • Pivoting on his right toes, tori turns his body to the left—describing a semi-circle with his left foot, and throws uke with *o-goshi* (major hip throw).
12	Yoko-tosshin	Dash to the side	• Tori and uke swap roles; • The new uke charges at the new tori, with his right arm outstretched; • Tori sacrifices his position by dropping down onto his side, and throws uke with *yoko-otoshi* (side drop).
13	Shomen-tosshin	Dash to the front	• Remaining in role, uke rushes at tori as soon as he picks himself up; • Tori sacrifices his position by dropping down onto his back, and throws uke with *tomoe-nage* (circle throw).

Role of Tori and Uke

Table 3 shows that throughout Budokwai Kime-no-kata, tori and uke reverse roles following every attack and defense sequence. This is apart from the final two sequences, where the roles are not swapped, and the judoka that commenced the exercise as tori, completes the twelfth and thirteenth techniques as uke. This distinctive alternating of tori and uke is usually highlighted in the limited literature that features Budokwai Kime-no-kata:

> Budokwai Kimenokata: The kata of decisive ends.
> The role of the attacker and attacked alternate.
> – Budokwai, 1968

Not of course that there is no logical reason for alternating tori and uke throughout the exercise, and indeed Koizumi suggests the approach was only introduced to make demonstrations more interesting.

> ... Generally, the parts of attacker and defender are played by the same persons throughout the whole series, but in order to make the demonstration more interesting, we arranged to act the parts alternately. – Koizumi, 1948-49:38

Technical Contents of Budokwai Kime-no-kata

Inspection of Tables 1, 2 and 3 shows that Budokwai Kime-no-kata consists of thirteen distinct attack and defense sequences—specifically, eight unarmed, and five armed attacks (by uke), which each time are overcome by a defensive technique (from tori). The unarmed attacks are four holds, two blows, and two rush attacks, whereas the armed attacks are one pistol (*kenju*), two knife (*tanto*), and two stick (*jo*) attacks. Note that in the exercise shown in the film with Koizumi and Mossom (Budokwai, 1948), the stick attacks are actually performed with a short stick (*tanbo*).

The Tables also reveal that Budokwai Kime-no-kata has few, if any, similarities with the official Kime-no-kata, and that the exercise has no obvious logical structure with respect to the ordering of the attack and defense techniques.

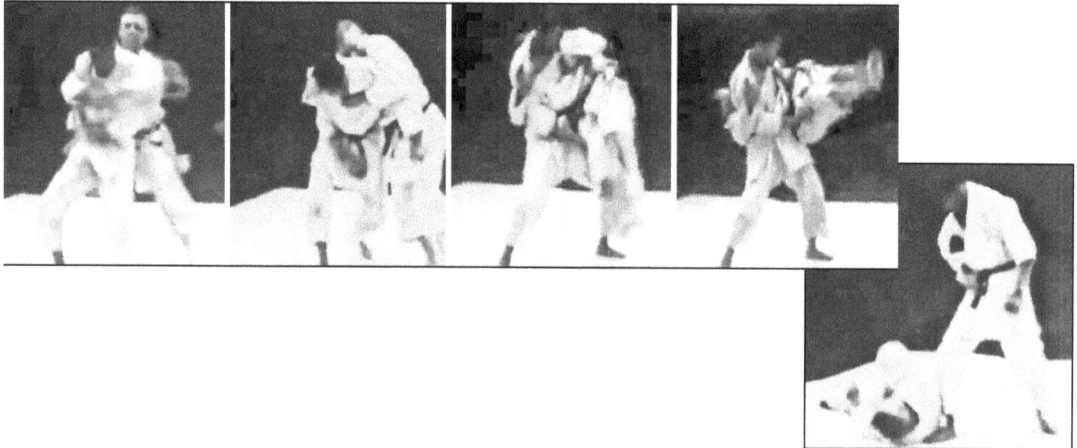

Figure 30. *Daki-kakae* (hold from behind over both arms)—the first technique in Budokwai Kime-no-kata. The attack/defense sequence commences with *uke* (the one attacking) seizing tori from behind with both arms, and concludes with tori throwing uke with *sukui-nage* (scooping throw). Gunji Koizumi is tori and Ted Mossom is uke.

The lack of logical structure to the exercise is indicated through the unarmed holding attacks being the first (Figure 30), fifth, sixth (Figure 31) and eleventh (Figure 32) attacks, and the unarmed rush attacks as the twelfth (Figure 33) and thirteenth attacks. The photographs of the attack and defense sequences shown in Figures 30 to 33, are snapshots from The 'Budokwai' Film (Budokwai, 1948).

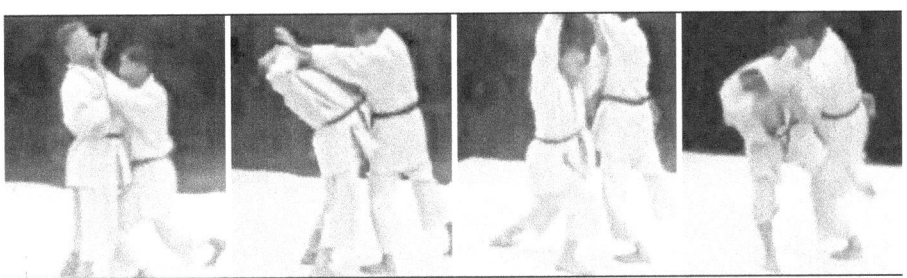

Figure 31. *Ago-oshi* (belt pull and chin push)—the sixth technique in Budokwai Kime-no-kata. The attack/defense sequence commences with uke holding tori's belt from the front and pushing up on his chin, and concludes with tori throwing uke with *osoto-gari* (major outer reaping throw). Ted Mossom is tori and Gunji Koizumi is uke.

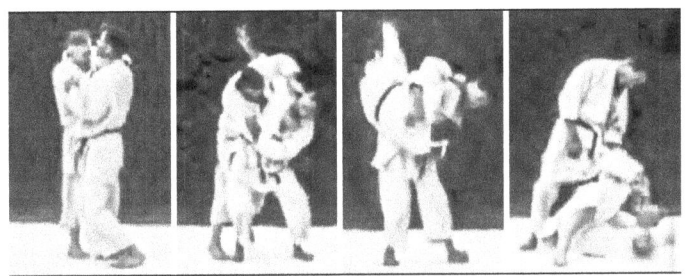

Figure 32. *Mae-jime* (choke with both hands)—the eleventh technique in Budokwai Kime-no-kata. The attack/defense sequence commences with uke attacking tori's throat with both hands from the front. Gunji Koizumi is tori and Ted Mossom is uke.

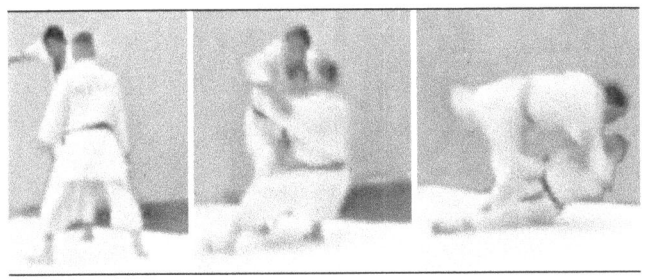
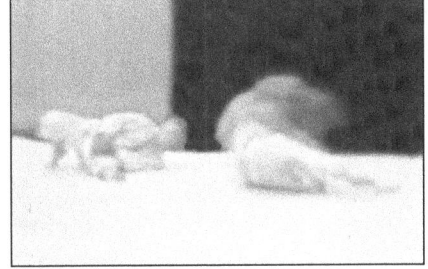

Figure 33. *Yoko-tosshin* (dash to the side)—the twelfth technique in Budokwai Kime-no-kata. The attack/defense sequence commences with uke rushing to tori's side with his right arm extended. Ted Mossom is tori and Gunji Koizumi is uke.

In a similar manner, the absence of a logical structure for the armed attacks is indicated by the pistol attack being the second technique (Figure 34), the knife attacks being the third (Figure 35) and fourth techniques, and the stick attacks being the ninth (Figure 36) and tenth attacks.

The photographs of the attack and defense sequences shown in Figures 34 to 36, are again snapshots from The 'Budokwai' Film (Ibid.).

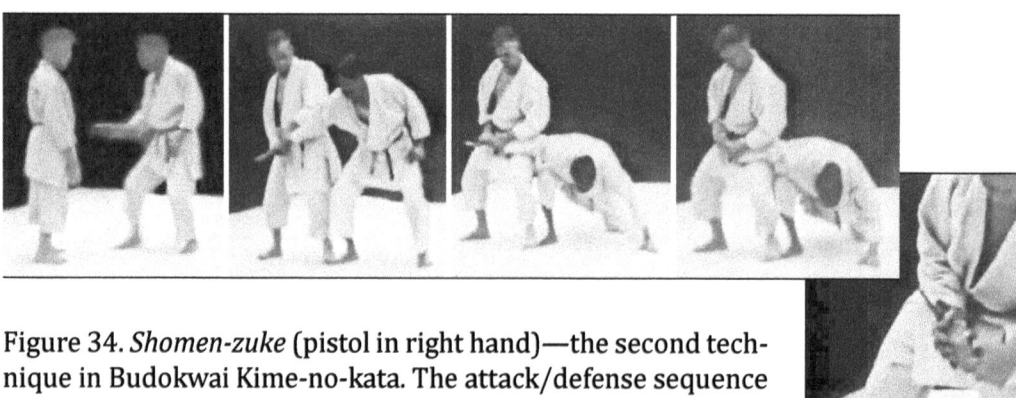

Figure 34. *Shomen-zuke* (pistol in right hand)—the second technique in Budokwai Kime-no-kata. The attack/defense sequence commences with uke covering tori with a pistol to the front, and concludes with tori disarming uke with a wrist lock. Ted Mossom is tori and Gunji Koizumi is uke.

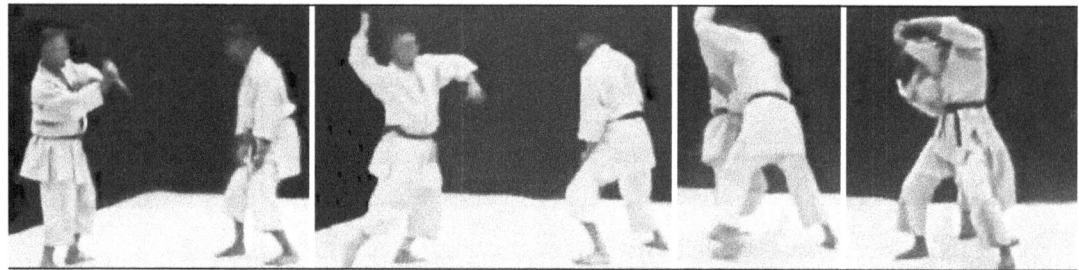

Figure 35. *Kiri-oroshi* (downward attack with knife held over the head)—the third technique in Budokwai Kime-no-kata. Gunji Koizumi is tori and Ted Mossom is uke.

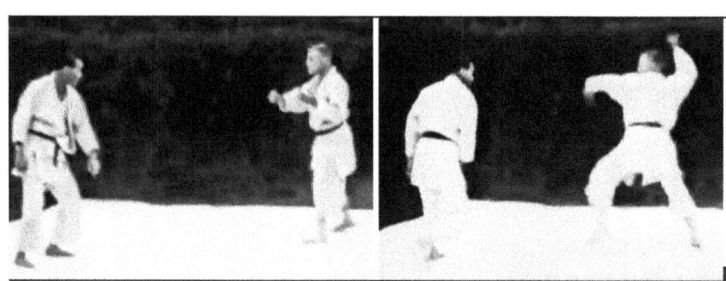

Figure 36. *Furi-oroshi* (downward blow with stick)—the ninth technique in Budokwai Kime-no-kata. Gunji Koizumi is tori and Ted Mossom is uke.

Foundations of Budokwai Kime-no-kata

It is clear that the composition and organization of Budokwai Kime-no-kata are uninfluenced by those of the official Kodokan Kime-no-kata. As has been already described in detail, there is no formal organization to the exercise, with the armed and unarmed techniques not having any logical sequence to them. On this point concerning the structure and the ordering of the techniques in a kata, Iain Abernethy explains that:

> Kata are not random collections of technique. There is a structure to them which imparts the methods in a logical and ordered way ...
> – Abernethy (personal communication, 6 September 2017)

This concern about the lack of structure in Budokwai Kime-no-kata is compounded by the interchanging of tori and uke throughout the exercise, which to the best of the authors' knowledge is not found elsewhere in any judo kata.

Moreover, Koizumi indicates that the selection rationale underpinning the included techniques was that they were "common forms of attack", with "effective and simple methods of defence" chosen "for the purpose of demonstration." This is as opposed to the attacks representing a suitably complete set of generic situations for teaching self-defense concepts and principles as part of a structured pedagogical framework in the manner of the official Kodokan kata, or even a practical means of self-defense.

> For the purpose of demonstration, the Budokwai has selected the most common forms of attack and most effective and simple methods of defence.
> – Koizumi, 1948–49:38

Given the preceding material the authors can state with a high degree of certainty that Budokwai Kime-no-kata was created primarily to be an entertaining display for showcasing, to an audience, the self-defense application of judo, and not a self-defense-oriented training system. However, this in no way diminishes its historical significance.

THE MOST RECENT BUDOKWAI KIME-NO-KATA

As part of the 27 November 1988 enbu, held at the Albert Hall, to mark the seventieth anniversary of The Budokwai's founding, a Budokwai Kime-no-kata was done by George Kerr and Rodger Bornowski (Fighting Films, 1988). As already mentioned, this exercise differed quite significantly from Koizumi's original creation (Koizumi, 1948–49) as described in *The Budokwai Bulletin*, and accordingly from the one done by Koizumi and Mossom (Budokwai, 1948). Much to their regret, the authors were unable to source the origin of these differences.

Etiquette

In the exercise shown in the 1988 film featuring Kerr and Bornowski, the etiquette is like that found in Nage-no-kata (forms of throwing), with formal *zarei* (Figure 37). Both judoka make seated bows then, after rising together, simultaneously take one (large) step forward to "open" the kata. The kata is closed by reversing this procedure.

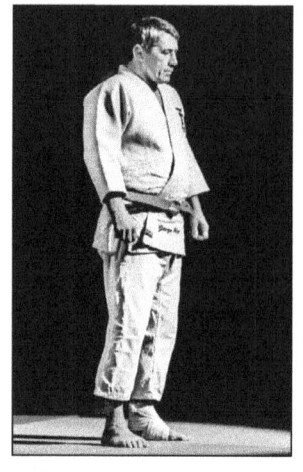
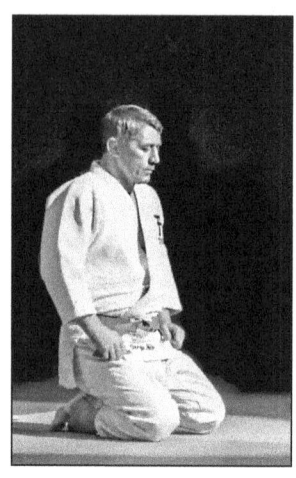

Figure 37.
Formal bowing at the start and finish of the 1988 demonstration of Budokwai Kime-no–kata, as shown here by George Kerr.

It is not known why Kerr and Bornowski elected to introduce this additional formality into the reiho in their Budokwai Kime-no-kata. The authors can speculate that perhaps it was to reflect the serious character and historical significance of the (seventieth anniversary) Albert Hall enbu.

Structure and Technical Contents of the Most Recent Budokwai Kime-no-kata

A structural and functional overview of the exercise done by Kerr and Bornowski is provided in Table 4. The Japanese names in this table were kindly suggested by Osamu Mouri Kodokan 7th dan, and based on his viewing of the Fighting Films recording (Osamu Mouri, personal communication, 11 September 2016).

Table 4:
Structural and Functional Overview of the Most Recent Budokwai Kime-no-kata. After Kerr and Bornowski (Fighting Films, 1988).

English language description	Proposed Japanese name	Nature of attack
1) Hold from behind over both arms	daki-kakae	unarmed – hold
2) Pistol in right hand	shomen-zuke	armed – pistol
3) Downward attack with knife held over the head	kiri-oroshi	armed – knife
4) Both hands hold	ryote-dori	unarmed – hold
5) Belt pull and chin push	ago-oshi	unarmed – hold / blow
6) Hold from behind	ushiro-dori	unarmed – hold
7) Blow on chin	ago-tsuki	unarmed – blow
8) Hit the face from sideways	naname-uchi	unarmed – blow
9) Downward blow with stick	furi-oroshi	armed – stick
10) Hold from behind and lift-up	daki-age	unarmed – hold
11) Dash to the front and lift-up	kakae-age	unarmed – hold
12) Side blow with stick	furi-mawashi	armed – stick
13) Two hand attack on throat	mae-jime	unarmed – hold
14) (Dash to the front and…) Push both shoulders	ryote-tsuki	unarmed – rush / push
15) (Dash to the side and…) Push left shoulder	katate-tsuki	unarmed – rush / push

Inspection of Table 4 shows that the Kerr and Bornowski demonstrated version of Budokwai Kime-no-kata contains 15 attack and defense sequences, compared with only thirteen in the Koizumi original. Specifically, the Kerr and Bornowski variant contains eleven unarmed and four armed attacks, with the unarmed attacks being seven holds, two blows, and two rush attacks, and the armed attacks being one pistol, one knife and two stick attacks.

Table 5. Comparative Overview of Various Budokwai Kime-no-kata.

Koizumi (1948-49)	Koizumi and Mossom (1948)	Kerr and Bornowski, 1988
1. Hold from behind over both arms	1. Hold from behind over both arms	1. Hold from behind over both arms
2. Pistol in right hand	2. Pistol in right hand	2. Pistol in right hand
3. Downward attack with knife held over the head	3. Downward attack with knife held over the head	3. Downward attack with knife held over the head
4. Upward stab with knife	4. Upward stab with knife	<Attack does not feature>
5. Grip on the wrists	<Attack inexplicably omitted>	4. Hold the wrists with both hands
6. Belt pull and chin push	5. Belt pull and chin push	5. Belt pull and chin push
<Attack does not feature>	<Attack does not feature>	6. Hold from behind
7. Blow to side of chin (from side-rear)	6. Blow to side of chin (from side-rear)	<Attack does not feature>
8. Uppercut	7. Uppercut	7. Uppercut
<Attack does not feature>	<Attack does not feature>	8. Blow to side of head (from front)
9. Downward blow with stick	8. Downward blow with stick	9. Downward blow with stick
10. Side blow with stick	9. Side blow with stick	<Attack features later>
<Attack does not feature>	<Attack does not feature>	10. Hold from behind and lift up
<Attack does not feature>	<Attack does not feature>	11. Dash to the front and lift
<Attack already featured>	<Attack already featured>	12. Side blow with stick
11. Two hand attack on throat	10. Two hand attack on throat	13. Two hand attack on throat
12. Dash to the side	11. Dash to the side	14. (Dash to the front and...) Push shoulders
13. Dash to the front	12. Dash to the front	15. (Dash to the side and...) Push left shoulder

For completeness, Table 5 presents a comparative overview of three Budokwai Kime-no-kata—that is those due to Koizumi (1948-49), Koizumi and Mossom (1948), and Kerr and Bornowski (1988).

Inspection of Table 5 shows that seven of uke's attacks are common across the three Budokwai Kime-no-kata. If the precise details of the rush attacks (the last two attacks in every variant) are ignored, then arguably nine attacks are common. The technical content of selected elements of Kerr and Bornowski's Budokwai Kime-no-kata are now described. The narrative will focus on where tori executes different defensive responses to identical attacks, and on where the attack and defense sequences are unique to Kerr and Bornowski's demonstration.

The images of the attack and defense sequences supporting this narrative, Figures 38 to 45, are a hybrid of photographs taken on the evening by one of the authors, professional photographer David Finch, and snapshots from the video production—The Albert Hall Show 1988 (Fighting Films, 1988). In these images, George Kerr is the judoka wearing the *kohaku-obi* (red and white belt), and Rodger Bornowski is the one wearing the *kuro-obi* (black belt).

Consider first, the second technique in the exercise, that is the pistol attack *shomen-zuke* (pistol in right hand). In the versions (Kozumi, 1948–49; Budokwai, 1948) uke is disarmed with a simple arm and wrist lock, whereas in the 1988 Kerr and Bornowski variant, Figure 38, tori takes hold of uke's right hand holding the gun, twists and lifts uke's right arm, and then throws him directly forwards by locking the arm and taking a wide stride to the front, in a manner somewhat similar to the concluding defensive action in *ago-tsuki* (uppercut) from Kodokan Goshin-jutsu. As tori steps forwards he takes the gun from uke's right hand, with his own right hand, and then discards it.

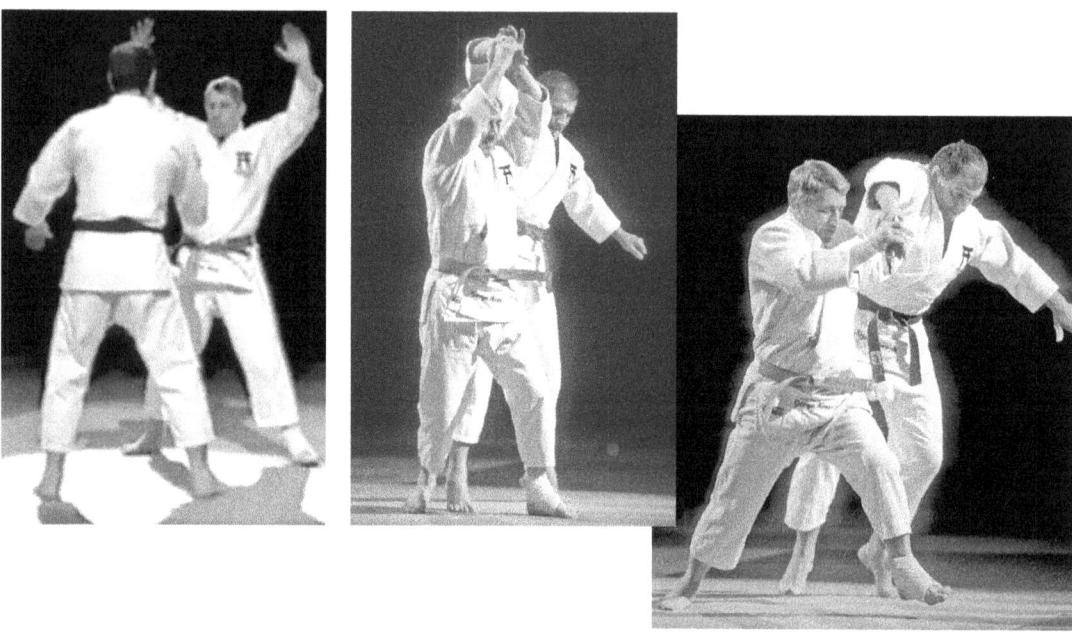

Figure 38. *Shomen-zuke* (pistol in right hand). The attack/defense sequence commences with uke covering tori with a pistol to the front, and concludes with tori throwing uke to the front. George Kerr is tori and Rodger Bornowski is uke.

For the next attack, *kiri-oroshi*, where uke attacks downwards with the knife held over his head, the way tori defends and disarms uke is common to all variants. However, in the Kerr and Bornowski variant (Figure 39), once having disarmed uke, tori pushes him down to the ground and kicks the knife away.

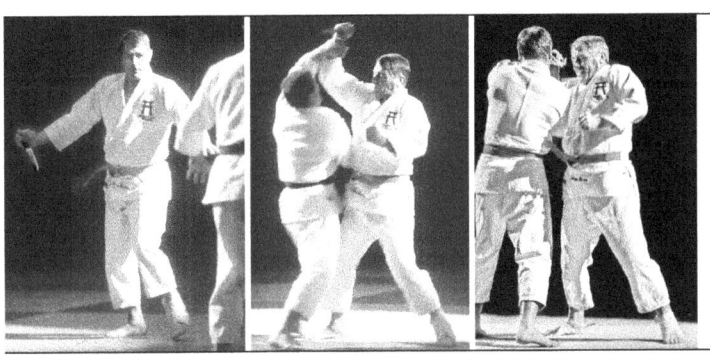

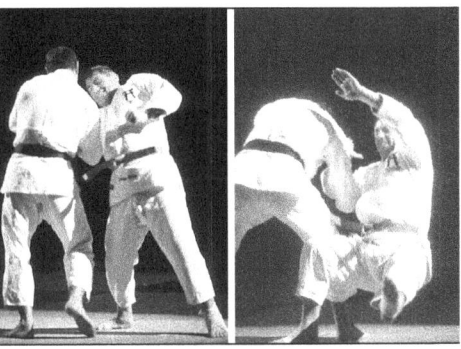

Figure 39. *Kiri-oroshi* (downward attack with knife held over the head). Rodger Bornowski is tori and George Kerr is uke.

For *ago-oshi*, uke takes hold of and pulls the front of tori's belt and then pushes up on tori's chin. In the early versions, tori escapes uke's grasp and throws him to the rear with *osoto-gari* (major outer reaping throw). However, in the Kerr and Bornowski variant (Figure 40), once having escaped uke's grip, tori turns in and throws uke with a classic *morote-seoi-nage* (two-handed back-carry throw).

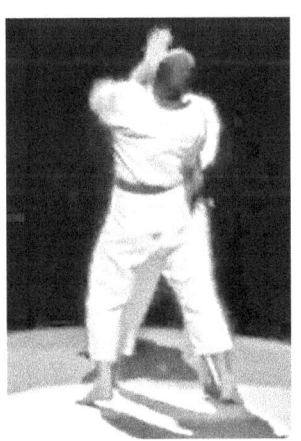
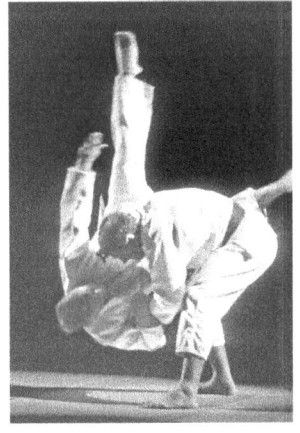

Figure 40. *Ago-oshi* (belt pull and chin push). The attack/defense sequence commences with uke holding tori's belt from the front and pushing up on his chin, and concludes with tori throwing uke with *morote-seoi-nage* (two-handed back-carry throw). Rodger Bornowski is tori and George Kerr is uke.

The first attack original to Kerr and Bornowski's Budokwai Kime-no-kata demonstration is *ushiro-dori* (hold from behind). This is the sixth technique in their exercise. Here, uke attacks tori by holding him high over the arms from behind. Tori escapes by creating space, and then responds decisively by throwing uke with *ippon-seoi-nage* (one-armed back-carry throw), dropping down onto one knee as he does so (Figure 41).

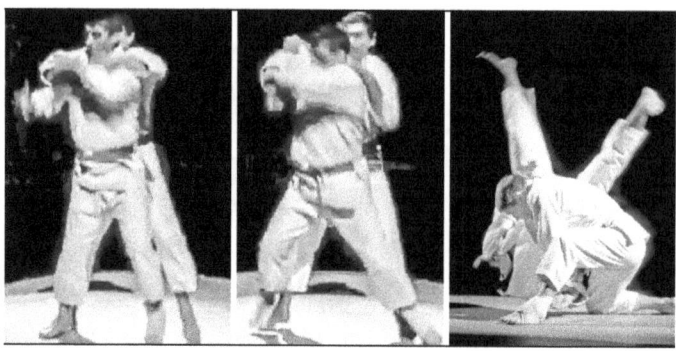

Figure 41. *Ushiro-dori* (hold from behind). The attack/defense sequence commences with *uke* (the one attacking) holding tori high over the arms from behind, and concludes with tori throwing uke with *ippon-seoi-nage* (one-armed back-carry throw]. George Kerr is tori and Rodger Bornowski is uke.

A further attack original to Kerr and Bornowski's Budokwai Kime-no-kata demonstration is *naname-uchi* (hit the face from sideways]. This is the eighth technique in their exercise. Here, tori evades uke's blow and then responds with a decisive armlock as shown in Figure 42.

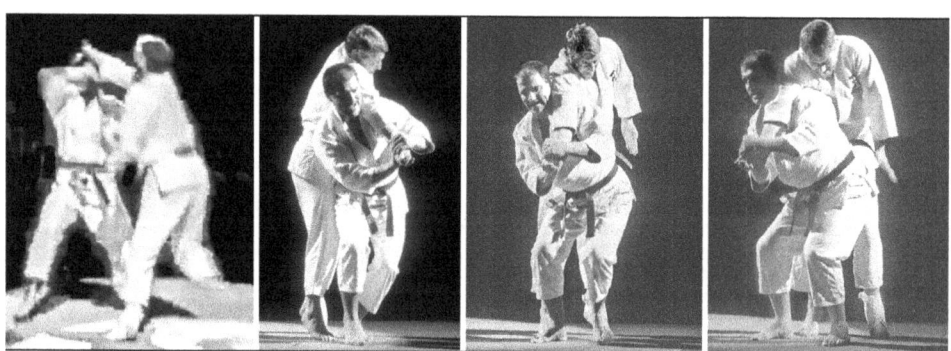

Figure 42. *Naname-uchi* (hit the face from sideways].
Rodger Bornowski is tori and George Kerr is uke.

The tenth technique in Kerr and Bornowski's Budokwai Kime-no-kata is *daki-age* (hold from behind and lift-up). Again, this attack and defense sequence (Figure 43) is not found in Koizumi's variants. Tori attacks uke from behind by holding him around the waist, and lift him up high. Tori struggles, and as he is placed back down, he grabs uke's right heel with both hands (one from the inside, one from the outside) and sweeps him down backwards in a split second with *kibisu-gaeshi* (heel trip). With uke on his back on the floor, tori executes a decisive technique by stamping on his chest with his left leg.

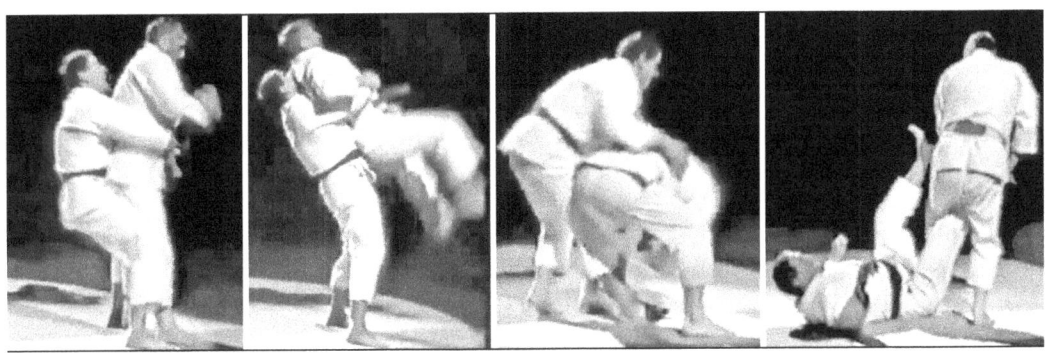

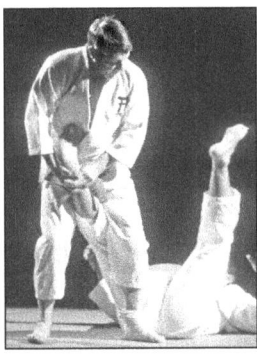

Figure 43. *Daki-age* (hold from behind and lift-up).
George Kerr is tori and Rodger Bornowski is uke.

In the mae-jime attack sequence, tori attacks uke by placing both his hands on either side of uke's neck and attempts to apply the strangle by twisting his wrists. Tori yields to uke's attack by bending slightly backwards, weakening uke's balance as he does so. In the original versions (Kozumi, 1948–49; Budokwai, 1948), tori turns in and throws uke with an *ogoshi* (major hip throw), whereas in the Kerr and Bornowski variant, once having escaped uke's grip and having turned in, tori throws uke with a *sode tsurikomi-goshi* (sleeve lifting and pulling hip throw) style technique (Figure 44).

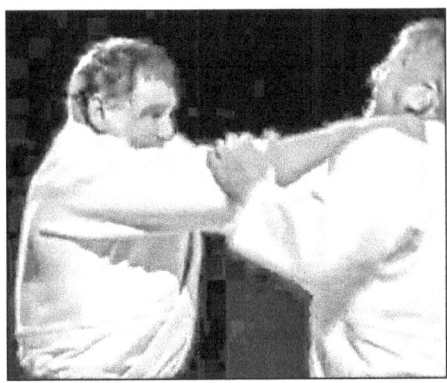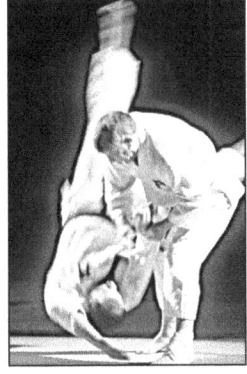

Figure 44. *Mae-jime* (two hand attack on throat). The attack/defense sequence commences with uke attacking tori's throat with both hands from the front, and concludes with tori throwing uke with a *sode tsurikomi-goshi* (sleeve lifting and pulling hip throw) style technique. George Kerr is tori and Rodger Bornowski is uke.

The final attack in Kerr and Bornowski's Budokwai Kime-no-kata demonstration is *katate-tsuki* (dash to the side and push left shoulder). In this sequence, uke rushes towards tori and attempts to push his left shoulder. Tori responds by dropping to the mat and executing a large abandonment throw—*yoko-otoshi* (side drop) (Figure 45). In the Koizumi originals, uke rushes head on towards tori, and is thrown directly over his head with *tomoe-nage* (circle throw).

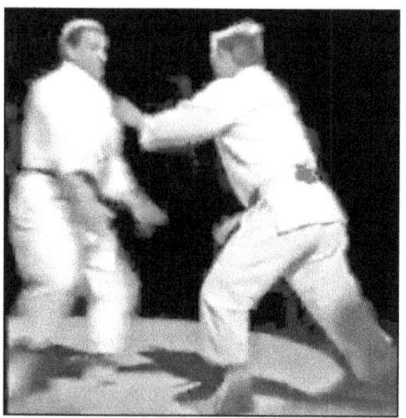 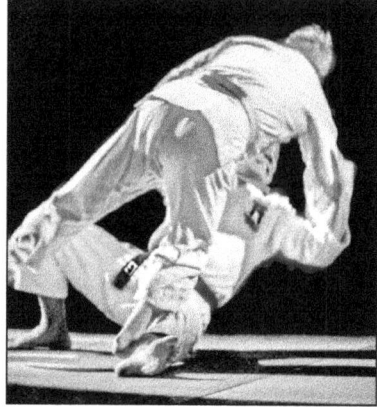

Figure 45. *Katate-tsuki* (dash to the side and push left shoulder). The attack/defense sequence commences with uke rushing towards tori and attempting to push his left shoulder, and concludes with tori throwing uke with *yoko-otoshi* (side drop). Rodger Bornowski is tori and George Kerr is uke.

CREDIBILITY OF BUDOKWAI KIME-NO-KATA FOR SELF-DEFENSE

While Budokwai Kime-no-kata is certainly spectacular, and likely to appeal to an audience, it must be examined how well (if at all) it prepares judoka for a serious combative (real) fight. As already suggested, close inspection of the films featuring Gunji Koizumi and Ted Mossom, and George Kerr and Rodger Bornowski, leads one to conclude, in both instances, that the judoka involved are simply doing Budokwai Kime-no-kata as a display, rather than as a practical training exercise for real self-defense.

Specifically, the suitability of the last two techniques of either demonstrated variant of Budokwai Kime-no-kata for real self-defense is questionable as they are *sutemi-waza* (sacrifice techniques). With such techniques, tori gives up his own position by dropping himself to the ground, either on his back or his side, to execute the throw.

Sutemi-waza can be very well applied to an attacker with strong forwards momentum, such as when he comes running towards the defender. However, deliberately going from standing to ground in a real self-defense situation is usually ill-advised, as it can place the defender in a seriously disadvantaged situation. First, giving up a standing position removes the opportunity for the defender to flee the attack by simply running away. Next, by going to the ground the defender is left with the possibility that he is confronted with attacks in this position—either from the original attacker, or his associates. Anything less than flawless execution of the sutemi-waza could well result with the attacker being on top of the defender. Finally, the ground is not a tatami, and attempting sutemi-waza in a street environment could mean dropping on to debris, stones, broken glass, etc.

POPULARITY OF BUDOKWAI KIME-NO-KATA AND AVAILABILITY OF TEACHERS FOR LEARNING THE EXERCISE

Popularity

The authors could not find any evidence in the literature of Budokwai Kime-no-kata ever being a popular or well-known exercise outside of The Budokwai itself. Even there, its popularity was restricted to a very small group of judoka. Moreover, the popularity of kata practice at The Budokwai, and elsewhere across the UK, was waning significantly towards the end of Koizumi's life, as judo was increasingly being transformed into a sport. Koizumi was known to dislike this transformation, as in his view "judo was an education" (Callan, 2011), and it is known that in January 1965, just a few months before his death, Koizumi was working on an article entitled "Judo and the Basic Human Education" (Ibid.).

Instruction in Budokwai Kime-no-kata

The authors know of no living judoka other than George Kerr, Maurice Allan and Rodger Bornowski to have performed Budokwai Kime-no-kata and publically demonstrated it to a high level. However, it is understood that none of these judoka presently have the exercise in their teaching portfolio.

As already explained, the two known film recordings of Budokwai Kime-no-kata are freely viewable on the YouTube video-sharing website, and this web-based material can readily help with learning the exercise's mechanics. The archive film footage featuring Budokwai Kime-no-kata's creator, Gunji Koizumi, is very helpful and inspiring, particularly when studied in conjunction with Koizumi's article on the exercise.

Concluding Remarks

Research into Budokwai Kime-no-kata is not a simple task. This is due to a scarceness of sources, and the exercise not featuring in any currently available judo text or film. Additionally, Budokwai Kime-no-kata is not presently taught at The Budokwai, or elsewhere—nor has it been performed in public since 1988. Notwithstanding, the authors of this paper strongly encourage the learning and practice of Budokwai Kime-no-kata as a means of preserving an important element of The Budokwai's history—specifically an original creation of its highly influential founder, Gunji Koizumi. Finally, it is the authors' hope that perhaps this chapter will serve as a worthy sequel to Koizumi's original 1948–49 work, and become the most critical resource for serious learning or research regarding Budokwai Kime-no-kata.

ACKNOWLEDGEMENTS

The authors are indebted to Dr. Michael Callan, Principal Lecturer at the Department of Psychology and Sports Sciences, University of Hertfordshire, Hatfield, UK for generously making available, from his own library, a copy of Gunji Koizumi's original three-part article on Budokwai Kime-no-kata.

Artist, author and judoka, Ian Whittlesea provided Figure 1. He also provided high quality digital media renditions of the two films containing Budokwai Kime-no-kata demonstrations. Figure 2 was supplied by judoka and Budokwai old-boy Robert John Mewett, whereas Figure 17 is used with the permission of Tony Wolf of the Bartitsu Society. Figure 20 is from the personal collection of judoka and budoka, Roger Payne, whereas Figure 25 was kindly made available by professional photographer Richard Goulding. Author, professional photographer and judoka, Eddie Ferrie provided Figure 27.

Paul Masters, and his son Lee, both holders of the menkyo kaiden license in Tenjin Shin'yo-ryu jujutsu provided expert insight into whether their koryu could have been a source of inspiration for Budokwai Kime-no-kata's attacks and defenses, whereas Osamu Mouri Kodokan 7th dan helpfully proposed Japanese names for the techniques in Kerr and Bornowski's kata. Finally, the authors would like to thank Shinro Fujita and Rie Kurashina of the International Department of the Kodokan Judo Institute for providing helpful information at all times. Kodokan-certified kata expert, Martin Savage, proofread this manuscript. Any and all errors are our own.

Note: Japanese names in this chapter are presented given name first and family name second—instead of traditional Japanese usage that places the family name first.

NOTES

1. The Kodokan (in full, the Kodokan Judo Institute) is the headquarters of the worldwide judo community. Literally, *ko* means "to lecture" or "to spread information," *do* means "the way," and *kan* is "a public building or hall," together translating roughly as "a place for the study or promotion of the way." The original Kodokan was founded in 1882 at the Eishoji Temple in the Higashi Ueno area of Taito-ku, Tokyo. Today, the Kodokan Judo Institute is in a modern eight-story building in Bunkyo-ku, Tokyo.
2. Since in judo the term *shihan* is used exclusively for Kano, it could be translated as "master."
3. The use of *Budokwai*, as opposed to *Budokai*, arises from the conversion of Japanese to the Roman alphabet using an earlier system of transliteration than the one commonly used today. To this day, the continued use of Budokwai remains the Society's preference.
4. In this context, a certain decisive finality is implied, and with the techniques of the official Kime-no-kata, one could maim, or kill, an attacker (Jones et al., 2016).
5. Kyuzo Mifune (1883–1965) Kodokan 10th dan has been categorized one of the finest ever exponents of judo, after Kano Shihan himself. He possessed sublime technical skills, and is regarded as one of the greatest judoka in history.
6. *Torite* is a type of self-defense containing technique for restraining, or escaping from, an attacker.
7. For clarity, *reigi* is the concept of etiquette and *reiho* is its physical manifestation.
8. DNBK = Dai Nippon Butokukai = Greater Japan Martial Virtue Society—a private organization established in April 1895 as part of the events marking the 1100th year of the Japanese imperial line. Its purpose was to preserve and promote Japanese martial arts,

foster martial virtue, and contribute to rousing national morale (Kawamura and Daigo, 2000: 68).

9. FFJDA = Fédération Française de Judo (jujutsu, kendo, aikido) et Disciplines Associées = French Federation of Judo (jujutsu, kendo, aikido) and Associated Disciplines—the NGB for judo in France.
10. Kawaishi was posthumously promoted to 10th dan by the FFJDA (De Crée, 2015).
11. Waseda University is a private university mainly located in Shinjuku, Tokyo.
12. This of course cannot be stated with certainty, though the authors were unable to trace any other source back further.
13. This was through the establishment of Kodokan Goshin-jutsu (Kodokan self-defense) (Tomiki, 1958)—see later.
14. This is as opposed to just an opportunistic and random demonstration of self-defense techniques.
15. *The Budokwai Bulletin* was published from 1945 to 1967—a time when judo had yet to have the overwhelming emphasis on sports-competition, and winning medals, so prevalent today. Its contents included articles on how to develop technical capabilities, news from Japan and the Kodokan, self-defense techniques, and tournament results.
16. A stickman is a human figure drawn in thin strokes.
17. The Hurlingham Club is an exclusive sports and social club located in Fulham, London, UK.
18. BJA = British Judo Association (BJA)—the National Governing Body (NGB) for judo in the UK.
19. Take Five Productions wrongly give the year of the film's creation as 1949, as opposed to 1948.
20. The Royal Albert Hall is a concert hall in South Kensington, London. It has a capacity of up to 5,272 seats.
21. Kodokan Goshin-jutsu should not be called Kodokan-Goshin-jutsu-no-kata (forms of Kodokan self-defense), though this inaccurate name quite often features in some of the less informed material on the exercise.
22. Tomiki's name is very closely associated with Kodokan Goshin-jutsu due to his strong technical contribution to its development and his authorship of the first textbook on the exercise—*Kodokan Goshin-jutsu* (Tomiki, 1958).
23. This style of aikido is referred to by several names including Tomiki Aikido, Shodokan (the place for illuminating the Way) Aikido, and Sport Aikido.
24. Note that the while the booklet lists 1988 light-heavyweight (-95kg) Olympic Bronze Medalist Dennis Stewart as representing Great Britain in the -95kg class versus the then West Germany, it was 1984 Olympian, Nicholas (Nick) Kokataylo, that fought in that category on the evening. This was a late change made after the booklet was printed.
25. Founded by Simon Hicks, and based in Bristol, Fighting Films originally transformed the way in which judo was filmed and represented. Today, it is a world's leading producer and supplier of judo DVDs, books and equipment.
26. Note, henceforth, that when discussing either of the film recordings of Budokwai Kime-no-kata that exist, only the original format will be referenced, and not the YouTube sources due to Whittlesea.
27. As the younger son, these options would have been starting his own farm, or, as per Japanese custom, being adopted into a family without a male heir.
28. Tenjin Shin'yo-ryu is one of the last schools of classical jujutsu to be formulated. It featured many choking and joint-lock techniques, many of which form the basis of several techniques in Kodokan judo.

29 Mikinosuke Kawaishi, in France, is often credited with introducing the colored belt system for early grades. However, this is incorrect as Kawaishi did not go to France until the mid 1930s.

30 Koizumi had planned to start the BJA and EJU in 1938 but had to delay for ten years because of WWII.

31 There is no date for Koizumi's promotion to 5th dan, as he was "jump promoted" to 6th dan directly from 4th dan, skipping 5th dan as a special case (Rie Kurashina, personal communication, 26 September 2016).

32 Note that Grant (1965) indicated that Koizumi had been promoted to Kodokan 8th dan before he died, whereas Fromm and Soames (1982:10) stated that his promotion was posthumous. The authors have confirmed with the Kodokan that Koizumi's promotion to 8th dan was ante-mortem (i.e. during his lifetime), and was made on 17 November 1962 (Rie Kurashina, personal communication, 12 September 2016).

33 The other two jujutsuka were Yukio Tani's brother, Kaneo Tani, and Seizo Yamamoto. These two men soon returned to Japan—apparently unhappy with jujutsu being promoted for entertainment purposes.

34 Edward Barton-Wright was the founder of Bartitsu—an eponymous and eclectic martial art system developed at the turn of the twentieth century, and immortalized (as "Baritsu") in Sir Arthur Conan Doyle's Sherlock Holmes stories.

35 E.J. Harrison was the second foreign-born person to achieve a dan grade in Kodokan Judo (13 August 1911), and was one of the earliest martial arts authors in English language. His books are still in demand to this day.

36 Someone who partakes in rough or noisy fights or quarrels in a place, especially in GB or Ireland, where alcoholic drinks can be bought and drunk on the premises.

37 In those pre-credit card days, it was routine for businesses to have relatively large amounts of cash on the premises.

38 Jean de Herdt (1923–2013) FFJDA 6th dan, was an original pupil of Mikinosuke Kawaishi, and the first Frenchman to receive the ranks of 1st, 2nd and 3rd dan. He was a double European Champion (1951), in both the 3rd dan and Open categories, and twice won a European title again (1952 and 1955) in the 4th dan category. de Herdt is also known for his 1951, 22-minute contest with Toshiro Daigo (then Kodokan 6th dan, now 10th dan) that ended in a draw.

39 R. Bowen (2011b:394) notes that Mossom sat on the first EJU Council for a few months in 1951.

40 At that time, the General Electric Company was a major player in the electrical industry. Between the wars, it had expanded to become a global corporation and national institution.

41 The London Electricity Board was the public-sector utility company responsible for electricity generation and electrical infrastructure maintenance in London prior to 1990.

42 USJA = United States Judo Association is an association for judo in the US. USA Judo is the NGB for judo in the US.

43 The authors presently know of no source that enables the exercise's creation date to be more precisely estimated.

44 Richard (Dicky) Bowen, Kodokan 4th dan, was born in Belgravia, London in 1926. In January 1949, he started judo and joined The Budokwai, where he trained under Gunji Koizumi, Percy Sekine, T. Leggett and Teizo Kawamura. In 1956, he was selected to represent GB at the first World Judo Championships, held in Tokyo, and subsequently spent three years training at the Kodokan. On his return to the UK his close association

with The Budokwai, both as a judoka and as a committee member and Vice-President, continued. He also became actively involved with the BJA.

45 As the official Kodokan kata for such techniques is Katame-no-kata (forms of grappling/holding), it can only be concluded that Shinri-no-kata is a personally created, unofficial kata.

46 Paul Masters (born 1953) received his menkyo kaiden license in 2010 directly from the late Toshihiro Kubota (1937–2013), the *shihanke* (family of head teachers) of the Torajiro Yagi lineage of Tenjin Shin'yo-ryu. Kubota Sensei was also the holder of a Kodokan 7th dan in judo.

47 Lee Masters (born 1972) received his menkyo kaiden license from his father in 2017.

48 The 124 Teai kata are the recorded techniques of Tenjin Shin'yo-ryu. The total of 124 is obtained by summing the number of *idori* (kneeling) and *tachiai* (standing) katas of the various levels of the ryu. This figure does not include the extra teaching of the *kuden gohon* (five oral transmissions) which are only taught person-to-person and usually to the next inheritor of the ryugi (Lee Masters, personal communication, 2 June 2017).

49 The "infinite change" is by *okuden* (secret, or deeper teaching) of the *ryugi* (martial tradition and techniques of a school).

50 During controlled practice, *uke* is the one who makes the initial attack, receives the decisive technique and is defeated.

51 Similarly, during controlled practice, *tori* is the one who is attacked and then applies the decisive, defensive technique.

52 Self-defense was one of the most popular and efficient methods of practicing judo around the time that Budokwai Kime-no-kata was created, with many books being published on this aspect. It was only later that self-defense came to be neglected by most judoka—especially after judo's 1964 introduction into the Olympic Games.

53 Koizumi himself only provided English language names for the attacks in the exercise.

54 John P. Cornish (born 1929) is a senior British judoka (presently BJA 7th dan) and aikidoka (presently 8th dan). He commenced his study of judo in 1952 at The Budokwai under T. Leggett.

55 One of the holds also incorporates a push on tori's chin.

56 Iain Abernethy holds the rank of 6th dan both with the British Combat Association (a dedicated group for close-quarter combat, self-protection and practical martial arts), and with the British Karate Association.

57 Note though that there is no standing bow to *shomen* (the front).

58 *Age-tsuki* (upwards stab with dagger) is omitted from the exercise done by Kerr and Bornowski.

BIBLIOGRAPHY

Bowen, R. (n.d.). R. Bowen's Archive. Personal Research Catalogue.

Bowen, R. (2011a). *100 years of judo in Great Britain – Reclaiming of its true spirit: Volume 1*. Brighton: IndePenPres Publishing Limited.

Bowen, R. (2011b). *100 years of judo in Great Britain – Reclaiming of its true spirit: Volume 2*. Brighton: IndePenPres Publishing Limited.

Bowen, R. (2002). Koizumi Gunji, 1885-1965: Judo master. In: Cortazzi, H. editor. *Britain and Japan: Biographical portraits, Volume 4*. Abingdon: Routlage, 312–322.

Brousse, M. (2015). *Judo for the world*. France: International Judo Federation.

Budokwai. (n.d.). Order form for the Take Five VHS Reissue of The 'Budokwai' Film. London: The Budokwai.

Budokwai. (1948). The 'Budokwai' Film. (16mm). London: The Budokwai.
Budokwai. (1962). Mr. N. Nishimura, 6th dan. *Judo – Budokwai Quarterly Bulletin*, 68, 25.
Budokwai. (1965). Tributes to Gunji Koizumi – 8th dan. *Judo – Budokwai Quarterly Bulletin*, 82, 1-17.
Budokwai. (2018). *100 Years of The Budokwai and British judo*. London: The Budokwai.
Budokwai Members and Historical Site. (n.d.). Past personalities. Available online from URL: http://www.budokwai.net/past_personalities.htm. (Accessed: January 2017).
Callan, M. (2011). Gunji Koizumi, the Father of British Judo. Paper presented at the 7th International Science of Judo Symposium. Paris, France.
Callan, M. (2017). 'History of the Budokwai, London: The Adoption of Kodokan Judo in the early years.' Proceedings of the Fourth European Science of Judo Research Symposium and the Third Scientific and Professional Conference on Judo: "Applicable Research in Judo", Porec, Croatia, 12 June 2017.
Cornish, J. (1984). *Go-shin-jutsu – Judo self defence kata*. United Kingdom: FJR Publishing for the British Judo Association.
De Cree, C. and Jones, L. (2009). Kodokan Judo's elusive tenth kata: The Go-no-kata – "Forms of proper use of force" Parts 1-3, *Archives of Budo, 5*, 55–73; 75–82 and 83–95.
De Cree, C. and Jones, L.C. (2011). Kodokan Judo's inauspicious ninth kata: The Joshi go-shiho – "Self-defense methods for women" Parts 1-3. *Archives of Budo, 7*(3), 105–123; 125–137; 139–158.
De Cree, C. (2015). Kodokan judo's three orphaned forms of counter techniques – Part 1: The Gonosen-no-kata – Forms of post-attack initiative counter throws; part 2: The Nage-waza ura-no-kata – Forms of reversing throwing techniques; Part 3: The Katame-waza ura-no-kata – Forms of reversing controlling techniques. *Archives of Budo*, 11, 93–123; 125–154; 155–171.
Edwards, G.A. and Menzies, A.R. editors. (1955). Judo personalities – Edward Mossom. *Judo. III*(7), April 1959, 22–23.
Fighting Films. (1988). The Albert Hall Show – The Budokwai International Judo and Karate Tournament. [VHS]. Bristol: Fighting Films.
Fromm, A. and Soames, N. (1982). *Judo – The gentle way*. London: Routledge and Kegan Paul.
Grant, C. (1965). Gunji Koizumi – A judo landmark. *Black Belt. 3*(11): 10-14.
Harrison, E.J. (1932). *Art of ju-jitsu*. London: W. Foulsham.
Ito, K. (1970). *Judo no nage-to katame-no-ura-waza* (Judo's counter throw and control techniques). Tokyo: Seibunkan Shoten. (In Japanese).
Ito, K. (2001). *The Japanese community in pre-war Britain: From integration to disintegration*. Abingdon: Routledge.
Jones, L.C., Savage, M.P. and Gatling, W.L. (2016). Kodokan judo's self-defense system – Kodokan Goshin-jutsu. *Journal of Asian Martial Arts, 25*(1), 1–46.
Kawamura, T. and Daigo, T., editors. (2000). *Kodokan new Japanese-English dictionary of judo*. Tokyo: Kodokan Institute.
Kawaishi, M. (1956). Gailhat, J., editor. *Les katas complets de judo*. Paris: Impr. de J. Cario. (In French).
Kawaishi, M. (1957). Harrison, E.J. translator. *The complete 7 katas of judo*. London: W. Foulsham and Co. Ltd.
Kerr, G. and Ferrie, E. (2017). *My journey to the 10th dan*. Edinburgh: Crawford Print and Design Limited.
Kodokan. (2015). Kime-no-kata. Tokyo: Kodokan kata textbook. Available online from URL: http://kodokanjudoinstitute.org/en/docs/kime_no_kata.pdf (Accessed: March 2017).

Koizumi, G. (1925). *Lacquer work – Full description of the process and the preparations how to identify the age and the quality of lacquer.* London: Sir Issac Pitman and Sons.

Koizumi, G. (1948-49). Kime-no-kata (Parts 1-3). *Judo – Budokwai Quarterly Bulletin,* IV(III), October 1948, 38–39; IV(IV), December 1948, 37–39; V(I), April 1949, 37–40.

Koizumi, G. (1955). A visit to my homeland after 50 years. *Judo – Budokwai Quarterly Bulletin,* X(4), January 1955, 28–30.

Koizumi, G. (1958). *Judo: The basic technical principles and exercises – Supplemented with contest rules and grading syllabus.* London: W. Foulsham and Co.

Koizumi, G. (1960). *My study of judo: The principle and the technical fundamentals.* London: W. Foulsham and Co.

Kuwashima, T. and Welch, A. (1949). *Judo: Forty-one lessons in the modern science of jiu-jitsu.* London: Putnam.

Leggett, T.P. (2000). Memories of Jigoro Kano's visit to the London Budokwai in August 1933. (Reprint). *Journal of Combative Sport.* Available online from URL: http://ejmas.com/jcs/jcsart_leggett1_0300.htm (Accessed: March 2017).

Lindsay, T. and Kano, J. (1889). Jiujutsu: The old samurai art of fighting without weapons. *Transactions of the Asiatic Society of Japan,* XVI(II). Yokohama. 1915 reprint. 202–217.

Menzies, A.R. (1964). Budokwai Show. *Judo,* IX(3), December 1964, 29–36.

Mifune, K. (1955). Mifune soen Goshin-jutsu (Mifune's personal self-defense). On: (2005). Shingi Mifune Judan (Kanzenhan): Judo no shinzui (The divine Mifune 10th dan (Complete Edition): The essence of judo). [DVD] Nihon Eiga Shinsha. Tokyo: Quest Co., Ltd. DVD SPD-3514, ca.: 06'21" (In Japanese).

Mifune, K. (1956). *Canon of judo – Principle and technique.* Tokyo: Seibundo-Shinkosha Publishing Co.

Miyake, T. and Tani, Y. (1906). *The game of ju-jitsu.* London. Hazel, Watson and Viney, Ltd.

Nakao, S. (1996). *Random House – Japanese-English, English-Japanese dictionary.* New York: Random House Inc.

Noble, G. (1999). An introduction to E. W. Barton-Wright (1860–1951). *Journal of Asian Martial Arts,* 8(2), 50-61.

Noble, G. (2000). The odyssey of Yukio Tani. Available online from URL: http://ejmas.com/jalt/jaltart_Noble_1000.htm. (Accessed: April 2017).

Otaki, T. and Draeger, D. (1983). *Judo formal techniques.* Tokyo: Charles E. Tuttle Company Incorporated.

Oxford University Judo Club. (1932). Program. Unpublished program brochure of an international judo gathering between the Oxford University Judo Club and Germany, 29th November 1932. Oxford: Oxford University Judo Club.

Pho, D.M. (writing as Ay-Leen The Peacemaker). (2011). #85 Yukio Tani and Sadakazu Uyenishi: Bringing jujitsu to the west. Available online from URL: https://beyondvictoriana.com/2011/07/31/85-yukio-tani-and-sadakazu-uyenishi-bringing-jujitsu-to-the-west/. (Accessed: April 2017).

Stevens, J. (2013). *The way of judo – A portrait of Jigoro Kano and his students.* Boston: Shambhala Publications Inc.

Tomiki, K. (1958). *Kodokan Goshin-jutsu.* Tokyo: Kodokan / Baseball Magazine. (In Japanese).

Watson, B.N. (2017). The Budokwai centennial. *Kano Society – The Bulletin.* 29, 1–6.

Whittlesea, I. (2013a). The Budokwai Film 1949. Available at: https://www.youtube.com/watch?v=vwjQqjHedwI&t=127s. (Accessed 19 May 2017).

Whittlesea, I. (2013b). The Budokwai Albert Hall 1988. Available at: https://www.youtube.com/watch?v=ytBc3vtO35E&t=1403s. (Accessed 19 May 2017).

chapter 28

"Treasure Chivalry, Despise Cowardice, and Esteem Straight-Living": Culture and the Origins of The Budokwai
by Michael Callan, Ph.D.

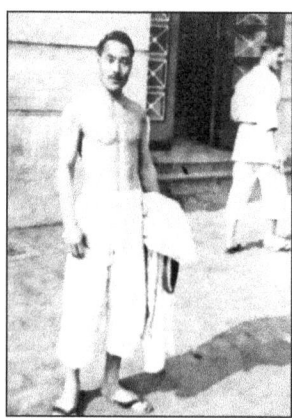 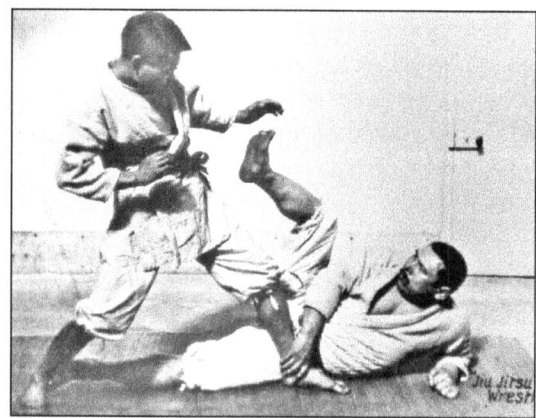

Figure 1 (left): Gunji Koizumi at the Frankfurt Summer School, 1937.
Figure 2 (right: Gunji Koizumi and Akitaro Ohno pose for publicity photographs prior to the Anglo-Japanese Exhibition, 1910.

Introduction

26 January 2018 was precisely one hundred years since the founding of The Budokwai, in London, which promotes itself as "Europe's oldest and most prestigious judo and martial arts club" (Budokwai, 2017).

The Budokwai, was founded in London by Gunji Koizumi (Figure 1 and 2) as a martial arts and cultural club for Japanese, and westerners with an interest in Japanese culture. He said "I opened a dojo for the practice of the Japanese martial arts, including kenjutsu and jujutsu, and named it The Budokwai—The Way of Knighthood Society" (Koizumi, 1965).

History of The Budokwai

Opening on a Saturday, in two empty shops at 15 Lower Grosvenor Place, London SW1 close to Buckingham Palace (Budokwai, 1931), Gunji Koizumi had leased the former dressmaker's premises from the landlords' agents on 19 December 1917 (Koizumi, 1965). The fledgling society was promoted through the Japanese newspaper, *Nichi-Ei Shinshi* (Koizumi, 1965).

An advertisement in *Health and Strength* magazine states "Budokwai (Knighthood Club) for Ju-jitsu" (Budokwai, 1918). Initially the principles of the society did not mention judo (flexible way) but included; "Be earnest in pursuance of Budo, but never boast." Many authors have drawn parallels between concepts of budo (martial way) and the chivalry of European knights in the Middle Ages (Leggett, 1998; Nitobe, 1900; Yamamoto, 1979). The third point of the "Principles of The Budokwai" stated: "Treasure chivalry, despise cowardice and esteem straight-living" (Steers, 1919) – see Figure 3.

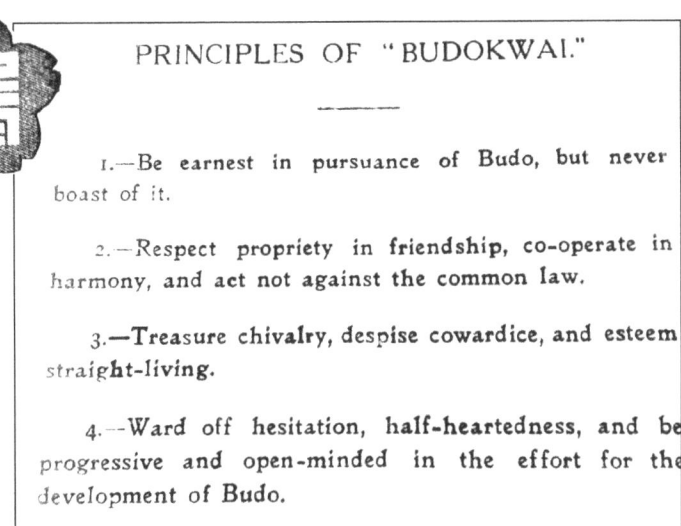

Figure 3: Principles of The Budokwai, 1918.

London was subject to night-time bombing raids during the First World War. Just two days after opening, the dojo diary [practice hall diary] notes that in the middle of the practice they could hear the air raid and the booming of guns (Koizumi, 1918). 1918 also marked a turning point for the efforts of the women's suffrage movement, when the Representation of the People Act gave the right to vote to women over the age of thirty, if they were property owners (Crawford, 2006).

The first Budokwai member was Masami Ouchiyama. The society gained fourteen members in the first five days. By the end of February, the numbers had swelled to thirty-six, all Japanese. Yukio Tani was member number seventeen. The membership fee was set at £3, worth £119 in 2018 (Budokwai, 1929; Koizumi, 1918). Initially the dojo diary was written in Japanese. The first British member was Mr. O. D. Smith, number thirty-seven who joined in February 1918. The first lady member was Miss Katharine White-Cooper, who had enrolled in a beginners' course of twelve lessons aimed at British people on 3 October 1918 (Koizumi, 1918). The activities offered embraced traditional Japanese culture. These included *kendo* (way of the sword) and *kenbu* (sword dancing).

Keen to expand the membership, the first annual Budokwai Display was held at the Lower Grosvenor Place premises, on 11 May 1918 from 3:00–7:00 pm. Koizumi had invited Sir Robert Stephenson Smyth Baden-Powell (later The Lord Baden-Powell), author of the book *Scouting for Boys* which extolled the virtues of jujutsu (Baden-Powell of Gilwell, 1908). The event attracted about 100 visitors, including the Spanish Ambassador and Consul General Yamazaki. This was also the first mention of the word "judo" in the dojo diary. The displays included demonstrations of jujutsu (flexible art), kendo, kenbu, contests between Red and White in jujutsu and offerings of sushi and monaka (Budokwai, 1931).

Earlier in 1906 Koizumi was an instructor at the Kara Ashikaga School of Jiu-jitsu (Figure 4) in Liverpool, England. There he met Sadakazu Uyenishi (Raku) and Akitaro Ohno (Daibutsu) Figure 2, who were performing in the music halls (Bowen, 2011). Then Koizumi taught at the "Piccadilly School of Ju-jutsu" in Golden Square, London in 1906, alongside Sadakazu Uyenishi, Akitaro Ohno, Mitsuyo Maeda and Yukio Tani. He had been introduced to the manager of the Piccadilly School of Ju-jutsu, Mr. William Garrud, by Uyenishi. After around three years in the United States, Koizumi return to the UK in 1910, just before the Anglo-Japanese Exhibition in White City, which he took part in with Daibutsu (Bowen, 2011).

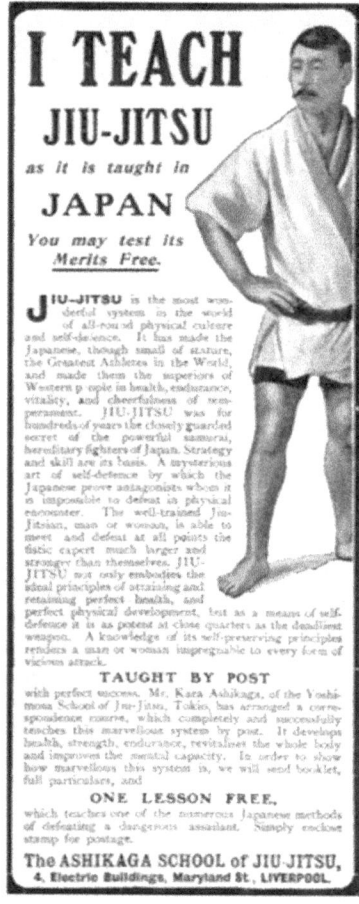

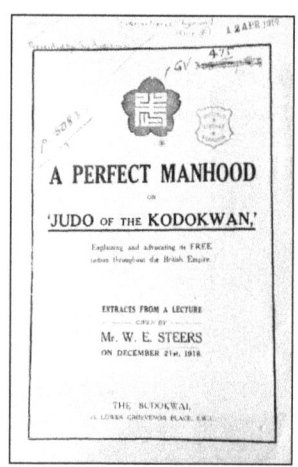

Figure 4: Advertisement for the Kara Ashikaga School of Jiu-jitsu, 1906.

Figure 5: Front cover of *A Perfect Manhood or Judo of the Kodokwan*, lecture by W. E. Steers, 21 December 1918.

Figure 6: E. J. Harrison, Gunji Koizumi and Yukio Tani with the Hyde brothers, possibly at the Japan Society, 1925 or 1926.

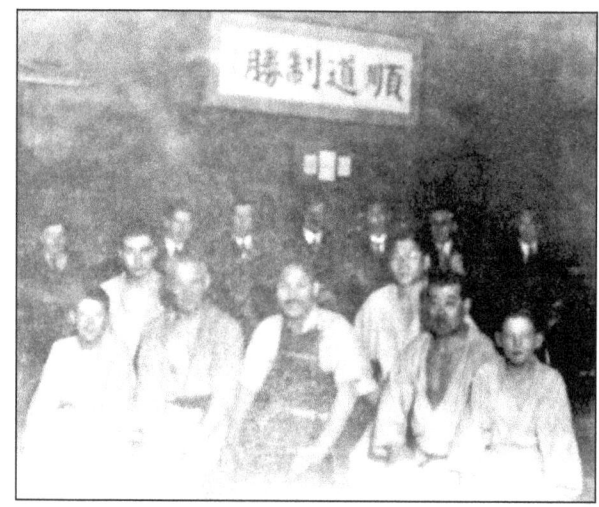

The Role of William Steers

William E. Steers had met Koizumi at the Piccadilly School of Ju-jutsu in Golden Square. He had been in Japan in 1903, and later was awarded shodan by the Kodokan at the age of fifty-five. He joined The Budokwai in November 1918, and by the end of the year had taken on the role as Honorary Secretary. Steers gave a lecture on 21 December 1918, entitled "A perfect manhood and judo of the Kodokan" (Steers, 1919)—see Figure 5. Previously the first lecture meeting on 3 November 1918, was on the topic of "Bushido and Religion."

Ernest Harrison (Figure 6), member 64, joined in May 1919. He had also studied Tenshin Shinyo-ryu in 1897 at the Ryoshinsai Hagiwara dojo in Yokohama, before he moved to Tokyo and gained a shodan at the Kodokan (E. J. Harrison, 1914).

The second annual Budokwai Display (Figures 7 and 8) on 31 May 1919, included an address entitled "Bushido" by Gonnosuke Komai. There were demonstrations of kendo, *kusarigama* (chain and sickle), *nito* (pair of swords) and *nabebuta* (saucepan lids) by Masatada Sonobe, jujutsu by Koizumi, and *naginata* (fencing with the halberd) by Yoshiko Hino (Koizumi, 1965).

JAPANESE THRILLS.

A "BUDOKWAI" AT THE ÆOLIAN HALL.

There were exciting episodes at the Æolian Hall on Saturday night, when the Japanese "Budokwai" gave its second annual display.

There was one thrilling encounter between Mme. Yoshiko Hino, a little Japanese woman who is a renowned exponent of the Japanese halberd, and Mr. Masteda Sonobe, who wielded a two-handed Japanese sword. Their weapons whirled about, and the audience broke into applause as the lady was seen cutting off her opponent's head. The halberd, it should be added, was of wood. The head did not come quite off, and the fight continued.

Towards the end of the fight the swordsman sent the halberd flying out of the little woman's hand, but she caught him by the wrist, gave it a little twist, and left him prone on the floor. He got up and pursued the combat, and once again the halberd was knocked out of the lady's hand, but this time she whipped out a little sword, struck her opponent in the ribs, and made an end of him.

There were various other kinds of Japanese fighting, and two-handed swordsmen slashed at each other until the whole audience rocked with laughter. Their swords were wooden, or neither of them would have lived to tell the tale. There was also "Judo" wrestling, and after many dashing combats a Mr. Saboe Achida gave a sword dance, accompanied by a recitation!

The principal events are illustrated on Page Eight.

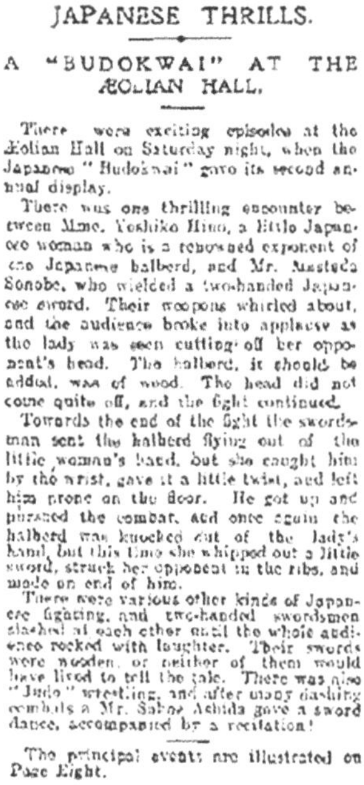

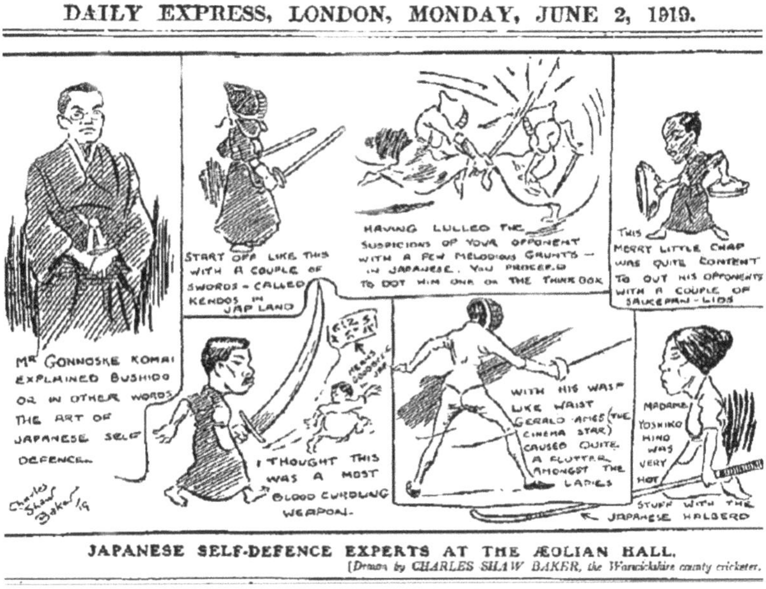

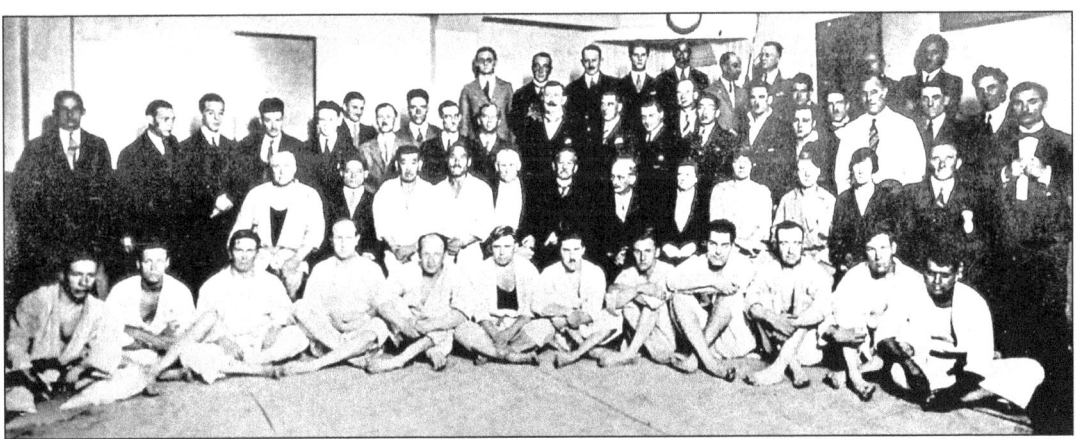

Figure 7: "Japanese Thrills" article about the Second Budokwai Display, in the Daily Express 2nd June 1919.

Figure 8: "Japanese self-defence experts at the Aeolian Hall' illustration of the Second Budokwai Display, in the *Daily Express* 2 June 1919.

Figure 9: Upper dojo at The Budokwai, 15 Lower Grosvenor Place, London SW1 where Jigoro Kano, seated in the middle, was bid farewell in July 1928. Immediately to his right is E. J. Harrison, then Gunji Koizumi and Yukio Tani.

Both Steers and Harrison were strong advocates for Kodokan judo. In May 1919 Harrison wrote a piece for *Health and Strength* magazine, entitled "The Art of Judo" (E. Harrison, 1919). Thanks to arrangements managed by Steers, on 15 July 1920 the founder of Kodokan judo, Jigoro Kano, accompanied by fourth dan instructor Hikochi Aida visited the UK and The Budokwai en-route to the Antwerp Olympic Games. A *yudanshakai* (dan grade holder association) was held at The Budokwai, in December 1920 when Kano awarded second dan to both Koizumi and Tani. After this The Budokwai adopted Kodokan judo (Bowen, 2011), and Kano went on to make more visits to the club in the years that followed (Figures 9).

▼▲▼

ACKNOWLEDGEMENTS

Figures 1 to 9 reproduced by kind permission of the Richard Bowen Collection at the University of Bath Library. Figure 10, by permission of David Finch.

NOTES

[1] This chapter formed the basis of a conference presentation given on 8 Sept. 2017, at the 2nd International Budo Conference, and the Japanese Academy of Budo, 50th Anniversary Conference held at Kansai University, Osaka.

[2] Japanese names in this chapter are presented given name first and family name second—instead of traditional Japanese usage that places the family name first.

BIBLIOGRAPHY

Baden-Powell of Gilwell, R.S.S.B.-P.B. (1908). *Scouting for boys. A handbook for instruction in good citizenship ... Illustrated.* London: Horace Cox.

Bowen, R. (2011). *100 years of judo in Great Britain.* Brighton: IndePenPress.

Budokwai. (1918). Advertisement for Budokwai (Knighthood Club). *Health and Strength.*

Budokwai. (1929). 8pp typescript transcript entitled 'Appendix' listing members of the Budokwai, 1918–1929. Bowen Collection, (B64). University of Bath.

Budokwai. (1931). Hardback volume containing minutes of meetings of the Budokwai General Committee, January 1918-December 1931. Loose material intercalated. Bowen Collection, (B8). University of Bath.

Budokwai. (2017). Europe's oldest and most prestigious martial arts club. Retrieved from http://budokwai.co.uk/

Crawford, E. (2006). *The women's suffrage movement in Britain and Ireland.* London: Routledge.

Harrison, E. (1919). The art of judo; Japanese physical culture explained. *Health and Strength.*

Harrison, E. J. (1914). *The fighting spirit of Japan.* London: T. Fisher Unwin.

Koizumi, G. (1918). 10pp typescript entitled 'Dojo Diary', 26 January–10 November 1918. Bowen Collection, (C13). University of Bath.

Koizumi, G. (1965). 21pp manuscript with amendments entitled 'Introduction' giving biographical details of Koizumi's early life, nd. Bowen Collection, (B238). University of Bath.

Leggett, T. (1998). *The spirit of budo: Old traditions for present-day life.* London: Kegan Paul.

Nitobe, I. (1900). *Bushido: The soul of Japan. An exposition of Japanese thought.* Philadelphia: Leeds and Biddle Co.

Steers, W. E. (1919). A perfect manhood or, Judo of the Kodokwan ... : extracts from a lecture given by Mr. W.E. Steers on Dec. 21st, 1918. University of Birmingham. London: The Budokwai.

Yamamoto, T. (1979). *Hagakure: The book of the samurai* (1st ed.). Tokyo: Kodansha International.

chapter 29

One Hundred Years of The Budokwai
by John B. Goodbody, M.A.

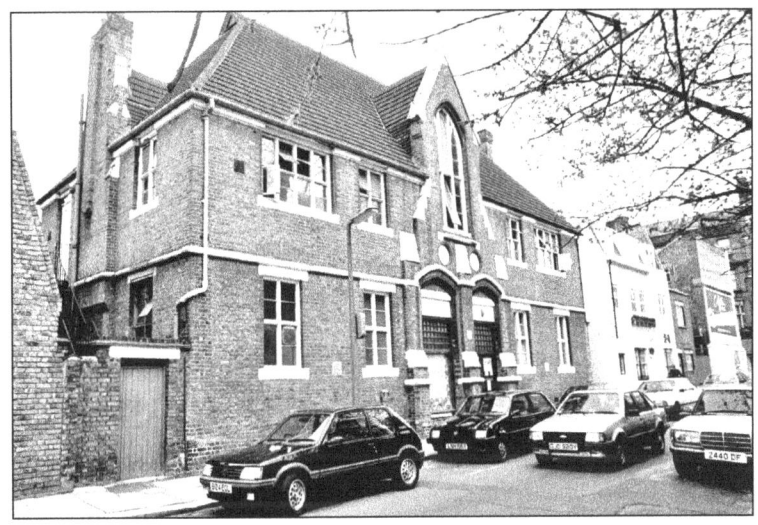

London, England, 8 May 1986: The Budokwai at GK House looking down
Gilston Road towards the main Fulham Road, Kensington, London.
Photo © by David Finch. All rights reserved.

Origins of The Budokwai

The Budokwai in London celebrates its centenary in 2018, the first judo club to be founded not only in Britain but also in Europe. The club has remained a center of excellence in the Japanese martial arts ever since.

It was part of the first-ever international event in Europe when its members fought against German clubs in 1929, while its founder, Gunji Koizumi (1895-1965), was a driving force in establishing the European Judo Union (EJU), initially before the Second World War and then, more lastingly, in 1948, as well as the setting up of the International Judo Federation (IJF) in 1951.

Koizumi, a Japanese immigrant, founded The Budokwai to teach judo and kenjutsu [sword fighting] wishing to help his adopted country. He wrote: "I hoped that rendering my service in promoting such training would be a means of pacifying my conscience, which was pricked by the fact that we Japanese, especially students, had been recipients of the kindness and generosity bestowed by the people of this country, without making any tangible return."

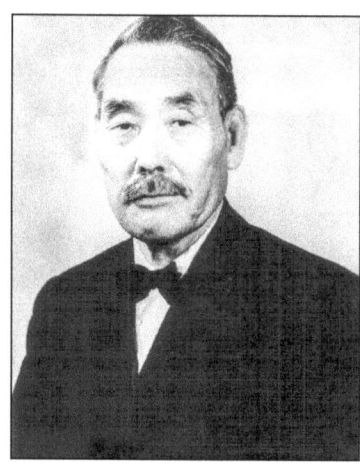 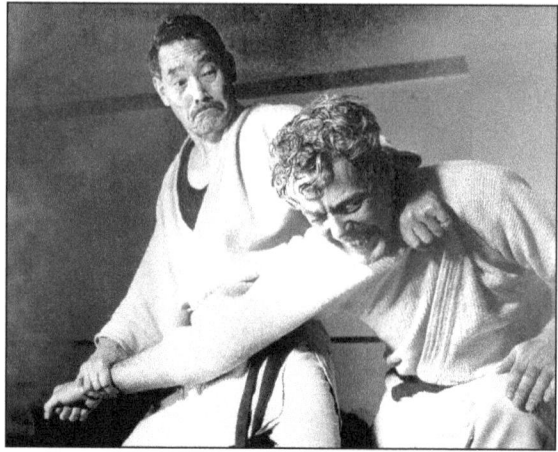

Left: Gunji Koizumi poses for the camera in 1960 during his 75th year. From "The Bowen Collection." Right: Gunji Koizumi realistically strangles Trevor Leggett for the camera and a national newspaper article in 1960. From "The Bowen Collection."

As Michel Brousse wrote in the book, *Judo for the World*:

> British judo holds a special place in the history of world judo, both unique and typical of the emergence of judo in Europe. The specificity of the history of early British judo is due to the country, to the context and to the pioneering vision, the unflagging energy of the key figure: Gunji Koizumi.

The club was established on the ground floor and basement of what had been a German dressmaker in premises backing onto a wall surrounding Buckingham Palace, the London residence of the kings and queens of the United Kingdom. It officially opened on 26 January 1918 with 12 members, and with Yukio Tani (1881–1950), as its first professional instructor.

The Name

Koizumi adopted the name "The Budokwai" for the club, or strictly speaking "society", in the following manner: "*bu*" means martial, "*do*", meaning way and "*kwai*" meaning society.[1] He always emphasised the character-training of judo, saying that pupils came into the sport wanting to throw but the first thing they were taught was how to fall. In other words, one cannot lead a successful life until one has met failure and recovered.

There were three main principles in judo for Koizumi, namely:
1) In pursuance of judo: be earnest, sincere and open-minded for mutual assistance.
2) Treasure chivalry, despise cowardice, and esteem straight-living.
3) Never boast of, or misuse, one's skill in judo or other arts.

Early Days and Japanese Teachers

An early tradition was the club's annual show, the first of which was held at The Budokwai on 11 May 1918. These continued, often annually, until 1968 when, with the growth of international and national competitions, the rehearsing for the regular shows distracted members from preparing for these events.

In 1926, Jigoro Kano (1860-1938), the founder of judo, visited The Budokwai and gave his approval to Koizumi's work, so beginning the long association of the club with the Kodokan. In 1929, The Budokwai was invited to Germany by the Frankfurt club. Marcus Kaye, a member of the team, said that uppermost in his mind was how the Budokwai methods would manage against the "husky Teutons." In fact, The Budokwai won both matches against Frankfurt and also against Wiesbaden.

During the 1930s, Mikinosuke Kawaishi (1899-1969), who was to have such a significant influence on the development of judo in France, came to Britain for four years, spending two of them practising at The Budokwai. When he returned to France, he linked up with Moshe Feldenkrais (1904-1984), who had been teaching jujutsu for many years, and between them, the pair devised a judo syllabus. They also followed The Budokwai's innovation of having kyu grades with different coloured belts, white, yellow, orange, green, blue, brown before the black belt dan grades.

One of the leading figures at The Budokwai in the 1930s was Trevor Pryce (TP) Leggett (1914-2000), Figure 4, who in 1938 went to Japan and was, for some time, employed by the British Embassy in Tokyo. Continuing his judo studies at Kodokan, his promotion history with this Institute was 3rd and then 4th dan (1940), 4th dan (1948) and 6th dan (1955)—at the time the highest graded non-Japanese judoka in the world. Leggett later became Head of the Japanese Service of the BBC. At the time of his death in 2000, he had reached the grade of seventh dan, having been promoted to this rank by the BJA in 1955.

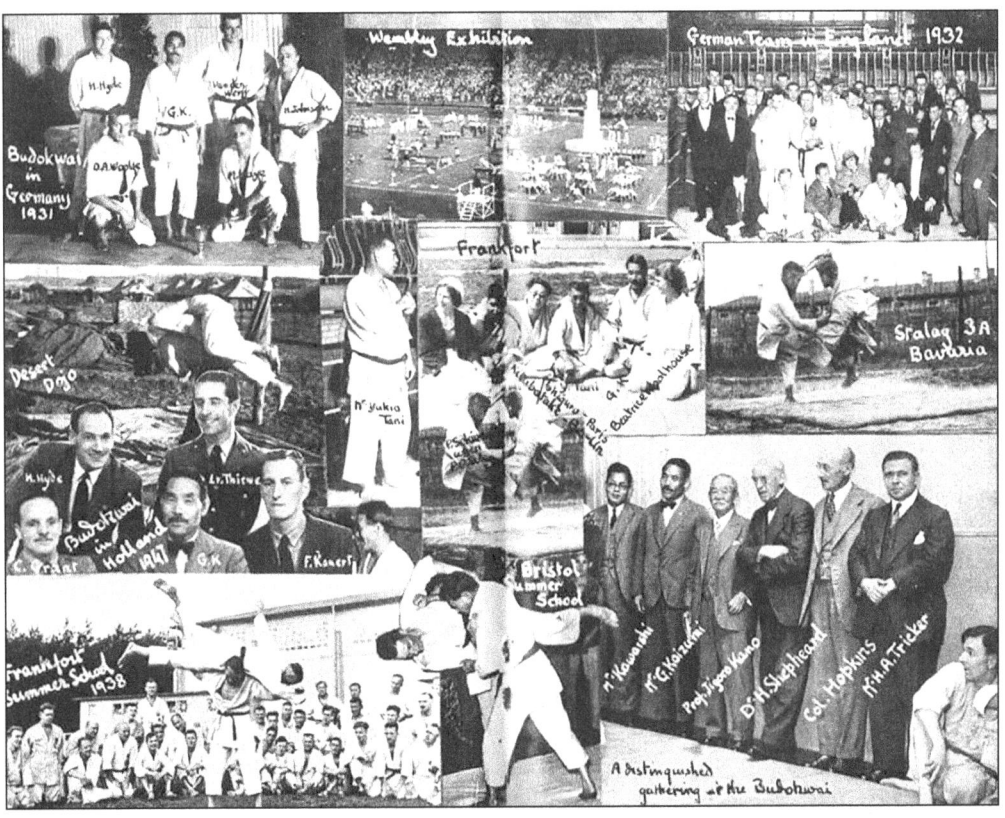

Figure 4: Collage of pictures to celebrate the thirtieth anniversary of the *Budokwai Quarterly Bulletin* in 1975. Included at the far right are Jigoro Kano, Gunji Koizumi, Mikinosuke Kawaishi, E.J. Harrison and others at The Budokwai in the 1930s. From "The Bowen Collection."

The club moved to its current premises in Kensington, one of the most fashionable areas of London in 1954. It has benefitted enormously from the instruction given by visiting Japanese, most recently by Yasuhiro Yamashita, Kenzo Nakamura, Hidetoshi Nakanishi, Hirotaka Okada, Maki Tsukada and Kosei Inoue.

The British Team and the Olympic Games

One of the leading figures of The Budokwai in the 1950s and 1960s was Charles Palmer (1930–2001), Figure 6, the first non-Japanese to be President of the International Judo Federation, or IJF Captain of the British team, when it won the European team title, he was a referee at the 1964 Tokyo Olympics, when judo first appeared on the Games programme as the selected sport by the Japanese hosts. As Brousse has pointed out this was 24 years after judo had been originally included in the Olympic programme for 1940—Games that were cancelled because of the War. Three Budokwai members were part of the first British Olympic team—Brian Jacks (born 1946), Syd Hoare (1939–2017) and Tony Sweeney (born 1938).

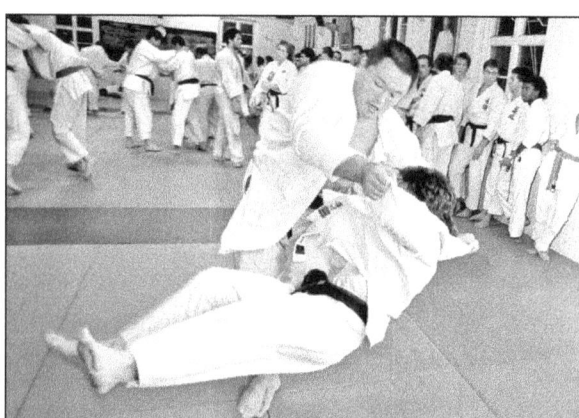 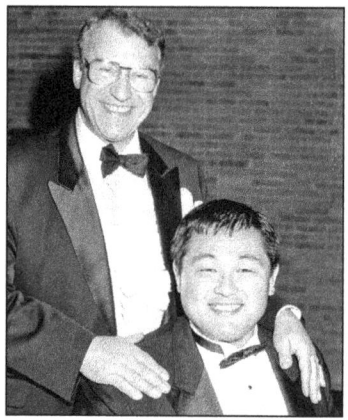

Left: World and Olympic champion Yasuhiro Yamashita throwing at The Budokwai in 1986. Right: Former IJF President, Charles Palmer and Yasuhiro Yamashita, 1984 Olympic Open Champion at the 1986 Sports Writers Dinner where both were guests of honour.

Although judo was dropped from the Olympics in 1968, Palmer campaigned ceaselessly and successfully to get it readmitted by the International Olympic Committee, or IOC, for 1972 and it has remained on the programme ever since. Palmer had also supported having females fighting at the Olympics, supporting the holding of the first Women's World Championships in New York in 1980 and before his death was delighted to see women's judo become a medal sport at the 1992 Barcelona Olympics.

In 1972, Britain had won three medals at the Olympics, two of them by Budokwai members, middleweight Brian Jacks (born 1946) and also Angelo Parisi (born 1953). Parisi, who was born in Italy, came to Britain as a young boy, and after winning European junior titles took the senior European light-heavyweight gold medal in 1972 and, aged 19, an Olympic bronze medal in the Open class in 1972.

He then married a French girl and switched nationalities, representing France from 1977 onwards, becoming Olympic heavyweight champion in 1980 and a silver medallist in the Open class in 1984, when he was the flag-bearer for the French team at the Opening Ceremony in the Los Angeles Coliseum. Parisi was renowned for his superb throwing techniques, especially *seoi-otoshi* [(shoulder drop throw), a technique that he used to win the final in Moscow at the Olympics, hurling the Bulgarian Dimitar Zaprianov to the mat for ippon.

Other Olympic medallists who were members of The Budokwai were Keith Remfry (1976), Arthur Mapp (1980), Neil Adams (1980 and 1984) and Ray Stevens (1992). Adams was, like Parisi, another marvellous technician, especially with *tai-otoshi* (body drop throw) and also used *juji-gatame* (cross armlock) in *ne-waza* (ground techniques) an armlock with which he forced the Japanese, Jiro Kase, to submit in the light-middleweight final at the 1981 World Championships in Maastricht. Stevens, the last British male to win an Olympic medal is now an instructor at the club.

Recently, British judo has had a centralised training base for the National Squad in Walsall, near Birmingham. So, The Budokwai has become no longer the place where many of the British team train every week. However, it is open seven days a week for both junior and adult judo. Its current premises have a main *dojo* (training hall) with two contest mats, a small dojo, a gym, changing rooms, a club room and offices.

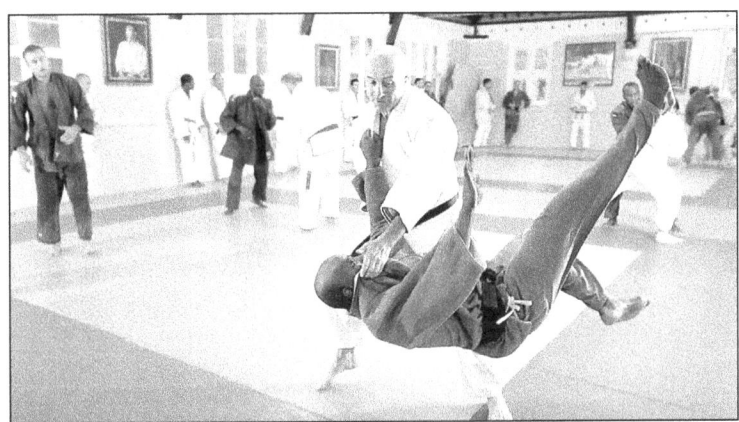

Top: General and Advanced class at The Budokwai's main dojo.

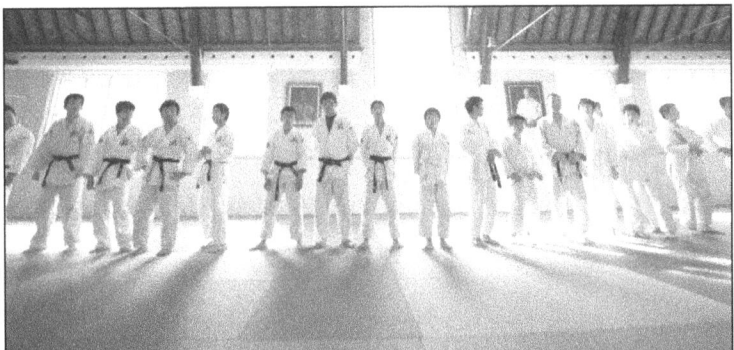

Middle: The visiting Nada High School judo team at The Budokwai's main dojo in 2012. Photos by David Finch.

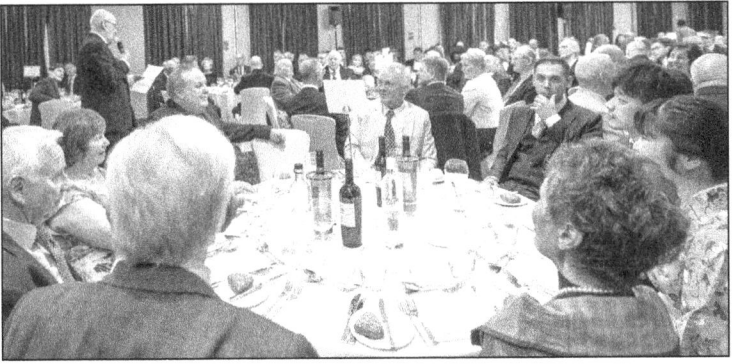

Bottom: 1964 Olympian, 9th dan and President of The Budokwai, Tony Sweeney, addresses the 23 tables and 240 guests during the 2018 Budokwai Centenary Celebratory Dinner at the Rembrandt Hotel held on 3 February 2018 in Kensington, London, United Kingdom.

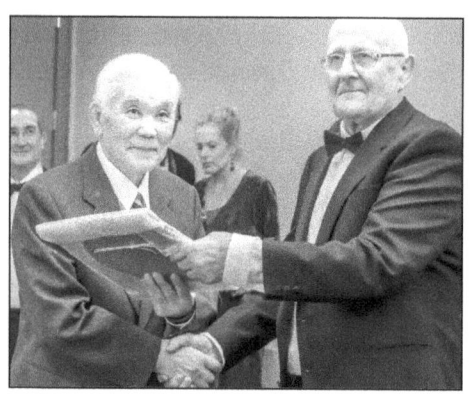 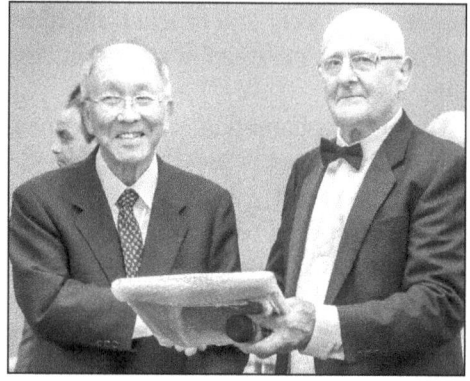

At the Budokwai Centenary Celebratory Dinner, President Sweeney presents an Honorary Membership to legendary Budokwai coach, Kisaburu Watanabe (left) and to Meiji Watanabe (right) of Japan. Photos by David Finch.

The Centenary

The Budokwai celebrated its centenary by hosting a gala dinner for 240 people at the Rembrandt Hotel in Kensington, London on 3 February 2018. The guests at the sell-out event included leading figures in British and international judo, as well as representatives from the Japanese Embassy in London. Several former British judo team managers attended the dinner, along with a host of Olympians and ex-international judo players, many of whom had undertaken significant international travel to be present. Guests were particularly thrilled to see that Kisaburo Watanabe (born 1936), and Chief Instructor at The Budokwai from 1961 to 1966, had flown in with his family, from Japan, to join the celebrations.

A very special guest at the evening was Gunji Koizumi's daughter, Hana (born 1920), who is now in her late 90s and still very lucid and sprightly. Hana, who went on to marry Percy Sekine (1920–2010), is a tangible link with the founding of British judo. All present were in agreement that the evening was an outstanding success, and a very fitting event to say, "Happy Birthday to The Budokwai and to European judo."

NOTE

[1] The use of Budokwai, as opposed to Budokai, arises from the conversion of Japanese to the Roman alphabet using an earlier system of transliteration than the one commonly used today.

BIBLIOGRAPHY

Brousse, M. (2015). *Judo for the world*. France: International Judo Federation.
Budokwai. (2018). *100 Years of The Budokwai and British judo*.

Sources of Original Publication

Articles in this anthology were originally published in Via Media Publishing's *Journal of Asian Martial Arts,* and from two books titled *Asian Marital Arts: Constructive Thoughts and Practical Applications* (2013) and *Jujutsu & Judo in the West* (2018). Listed according to original date of publication:

Smith, R,W. (1996)	Vol. 5 No. 3, pp. **60–65**
Long, J. (1997)	Vol. 6 No. 4, pp. **62–75**
Svinth, J. (1998)	Vol. 7 No. 1, pp. **28–47**
Svinth, J. (1999)	Vol. 8 No. 1, pp. **30–43**
Bowen, R. (1999)	Vol. 8 No. 3, pp. **42–53**
Finch, D. (2001)	Vol. 10 No. 3, pp. **92–99**
Behrendt. J. (2001)	Vol. 10 No. 4, pp. **88–91**
Finch, D. (2003)	Vol. 12 No. 1, pp. **40–47**
Wingard, G. (2003)	Vol. 12 No. 2, pp. **16–25**
Webb, J. (2003)	Vol. 12 No. 2, pp. **64–73**
Finch, D. (2003)	Vol. 12 No. 4, pp. **82–87**
Gutiérrez, C., and Espartero, J. (2004)	Vol. 13 No. 2, pp. **8–31**
Finch, D. (2004)	Vol. 13 No. 3, pp. **82–85**
Finch, D. (2004)	Vol. 13 No. 4, pp. **56–59**
Jones, L. (2005)	Vol. 14 No. 3, pp. **72–85**
Finch, D. (2006)	Vol. 15 No. 2, pp. **60–69**
Ebell, S.B. (2008)	Vol. 17 No. 1, pp. **28–37**
Gatling, W.L. (2008)	Vol. 17 No. 1, pp. **68–77**
Wingard, G. (2009)	Vol. 18 No. 1, pp. **8–21**
Hlinak, M. (2009)	Vol. 18 No. 2, pp. **8–19**
Jones, L., and Hanon, M. (2010)	Vol. 19 No. 4, pp. **8–37**
Yiannakis, L. (2011)	Vol. 20 No. 3, pp. **92–107**
Jones, L. (2012)	*Asian Martial Arts*, pp. **86–89**
Yiannakis, L. (2014)	Vol. 23, pp. **1–13**
Jones, L., Savage, M., & Gatling, W.L. (2014)	Vol. 25, pp. **1–46**
Callan, M. (2018)	*Jujutsu & Judo in the West*, pp. **109–114**
Watson, B. (2018)	*Jujutsu & Judo in the West*, pp. **115–126**
Jones, L., Bowen, H.J. and Finch, D. (2018)	*Jujutsu & Judo in the West*, pp. **135–193**
Goodbody, J. (2018)	*Jujutsu & Judo in the West*, pp. **127–123**

INDEX

A

advanced foot sweep (de ashi barai), 226
aiki-jujutsu, 239, 244, 264, 275 note 15, 276 note 34
aikido, 12, 238-239, 242-244, 255, 257, 262, 268, 276 note 34, 277 notes 41 and 46, 299, 337 notes 9 and 23, 339 note 54
Aizawa, Yasushi, 173
All-Japan Judo Federation, 156-157
almost ippon (wazari), 72, 150
Araki, Muninsai, 243
Araki-ryu, 243
archery techniques (kyu-jutsu), 170, 221, 243
arm crush (ude gatame), 284
arm crushing armpit armlock (ude-hishigi-waki-gatame), 252, 256
arm crushing hand armlock (ude-hishigi-te-gatame), 263, 272
arm crushing stomach armlock (ude-hishigi-hara-gatame), 240
armed attacks (buki-no-bu), 239, 249-250, 253, 257-260, 268, 299, 324, 326, 329
armlock (kote hineri), 121-123, 133, 240, 252, 263, 272, 308, 332, 351
arresting art (taiho-jutsu), 264
attacked from a distance (hanareta-baai), 249-250, 253, 260
Awazu, Shozo, 3

B

back-carry throw (seoi-nage), 194-195, 226, 331-332
balance breaking (kuzushi), 194, 212, 214, 228-229, 243, 252-253, 256, 258, 268, 271, 277 note 54, 283
bare-knuckle boxing, 167, 172
basic technique (kihon), 13, 157
being gentle and pure (seiboku), 199-200
Blackwell, Edward, 168-169
Blonk, Mas, 267
body control (tai-sabaki), 4, 131, 194, 222, 232, 239, 252-254, 256, 258, 271, 275 note 17
break-falling (ukemi), 147, 229
Bregman, Jim, 87, 92
British Judo Association (BJA), 49, 52-53, 57, 128, 132, 200, 238, 262, 275 notes 12 and 13, 277 note 46, 298-305, 310, 312-313, 337 note 18, 338 notes 30 and 44, 339 note 54, 347 note 18, 349
broken top four-corner hold (kuzure kami shiho-gatame), 284
Budokwai (London), 49-52, 55, 58, 77-78, 191, 262, 265, 275 note 12, 277 note 60, 285, 287-292, 297-302, 304-311, 313-315, 327, 335, 336 note 3, 338 note 44, 342-352
Budokwai Judo/Quarterly Bulletin, 4 note 1, 54, 290, 292, 297-298, 300, 314-315, 327, 337 note 15, 349
Budokwai Kime-no-kata, 294-302, 313-319, 324-335, 337 note 26, 339 note 52
Burns, Martin "Farmer", 169
Butokukai, 17, 31 note 1, 239, 276 note 27, 296, 336 note 8

C

Camp Harmony (Puyallup, WA), 29, 89
catch-as-catch-can, 6-7, 14, 106, 114-116, 169-170, 179-180
Chicago Yudanshakai (black belt association), 90
Chicago's Jiu-Jitsu Institute, 43
choking techniques (shime-waza), 4, 10, 15, 117, 243, 252, 259, 262, 337 note 28
circle throw (tomoe-nage), 2, 4, 96, 202, 334
Colgan, Jim, 91
commitment (genshitsu), 199
comprehensive martial arts (sogo bujutsu), 243
contest (shiai), 1, 4 note 1, 129, 139, 150-151, 157, 191, 201, 239, 295
continuousness (renzoku), 213-214, 224, 228
controlling techniques (katame waza), 239, 251-253, 256, 258, 266
Cornish, John, 206 note 4, 248-249, 252, 256-258, 260-262, 268-269, 277 note 46, 278 note 67, 317-318, 339 note 54
Cornish-style wrestling, 179
counterattacking techniques (kaeshi-waza), 4, 239, 295-296
criteria of Western sports advocates, 81-83, 84 note 4, 153, 171-173
Cuevas, Jorge, 265
Cumberland-style wrestling, 179

D

Dabauza, Pedro Rodríguez, 264-265
Daigo, Toshiro, 4, 4 note 5, 95-97, 150, 160, 162, 164, 192-193, 198-200, 202, 206 note 5, 235-238, 248, 264, 274 note 4, 278 note 70, 338 note 38
de Bijl, Richard, 267
Devonshire-style wrestling, 179
distance control (maai), 213, 252-253, 256, 277 note 51
double foot sweep (okuri ashi barai), 226
downswing (furi-oroshi), 250, 318-319, 326, 328
downward slask/cut (kiri-oroshi), 154, 277 note 55

E

eight directions unbalancing (happo-no-kuzu-shi), 253
English small-sword, 166, 168
etiquette (reiho), 248, 259, 277 note 47, 296-297, 302, 317, 328, 336 note 7
European Judo Union (EJU), 49-59, 163, 200, 288, 305, 347

F

Fife Dojo, 35-45, 45 note 2, 47 note 12, 89
floating drop (uki-otoshi), 194-195, 215, 231-232
following or countering (gonosen), 230, 247, 296
forms of decision (Kime Shiki), 193, 197, 236, 247
forms of gentleness (Ju Shiki), 193, 197, 236
free practice (randori), 3, 129, 138-139, 149, 157, 163, 191-195, 205, 207 note 7, 224, 235, 237-239, 247, 253, 256, 282, 294-295
Fujoshi Goshin-jutsu no Kata, 246-247, 276 note 40
Fukuda, Hashinosuke, 147
Fukuda, Keiko, 91

G

Geesink, Anton, 54, 90, 96, 98, 289
generating momentum (hazumi), 212-213
Giunta, Jeff, 161-163
Go-no-kata, 132, 193, 196, 238, 247, 251
Gokyu-no-waza, 149
Goshin-jutsu, 131, 133, 195, 234-235, 237-239, 241-273, 275 note 22, 277 notes 44 and 59, 278 notes 67 and 73,
Goshin Waza, 229, 237-238, 247
Gotch, Frank, 180
Goto, Ichizo, 1
gouging, 169-170, 174
grade advancement (batsugun), 128-129, 151
grappling techniques (ne-waza), 2, 23, 31 note 1, 147, 351,
grasping hands (torite), 241, 276 note 28, 296, 336 note 6
Greater Japan Martial Virtue Society (Butoku-kai), 17, 31 note 1, 239, 267 note27, 336 note 8

H

Habersetzer, Roland, 255, 266, 277 notes 56 and 57
Hackenschmidt, Georg, 177, 180
halberd techniques (naginata-jutsu), 243, 345
Hamana, Tomoo, 270

hand techniques (te-waza), 194, 283
Harris, George, 87, 92
Heike-ryu Jujutsu, 87-94
Hirohito, Michinomiya (Emperor), 1, 17
Hoare, Syd, 191, 238, 275 note 12, 350
holding techniques (osae-waza), 4 note 3, 284
horse-riding techniques (ba-jutsu), 221, 243

I

Iikubo, Tsunetoshi, 147
Iizuka, Kunisaburo, 21
immovable mind (fudoshin), 197
initiative strategies (sen), 213-214, 230, 296
inner thigh throw (uchi-mata), 4, 61-62, 66, 73, 75, 89, 142, 145, 230, 284
International Judo Federation (IJF), 49, 55-57, 64-66, 96, 128, 141, 145, 151, 153, 192, 200-201, 207 notes 13 and 15, 269-270, 278 notes 65 and 68, 305, 310, 312, 347, 350
International Olympic Committee (IOC), 27, 152-154, 285, 288-289, 350
International Sports Federation, 152-153
Isogai, Hajime, 1-3
Ito, Tokugoro, 183-185
Itsutsu-no-kata, 131, 194, 197, 207 note 10, 251, 265
Iwakiri, Ryoichi, 35-45, 46 note 10, 89

J

Japanese immigrant (issei), 21, 28, 36, 38, 41, 178, 182, 184, 186, 347
Japanese Ministry of Education, 182
jigotai (a defensive posture), 223
Jiu-Jitsu Institute of America, 45
Job, Michael, 162
joint-locking technique (kansetsu-waza), 4 note 3, 251-252, 284
Jomantas, Nicole, 202-203
Joshi Goshin Ho,
Ju-no-kata (flexible form),

K

Kaeshi-no-kata, 132
kake (finishing a throw), 205, 212, 228, 283
Kano, Jigoro, 3, 7, 18, 25, 27, 39, 42, 44, 49, 58-59, 82, 89, 91, 98, 127-128, 139, 146-147, 156-157, 160, 172-173, 181, 184, 190-191, 193-194, 197, 199, 201, 204-205, 205 note 1, 207 notes 6 and 16, 219, 234, 236, 238, 255, 259-260, 263, 275 note 14, 276 note 25, 277 note 45, 285-286, 294, 316, 345-346, 349
Kano, Risei, 3, 56-57, 244-245
Kano Society, 268
Kano, Yukimitsu, 157, 207 note 16

Katame-no-kata (grappling form), 130, 138, 158-159, 194-195, 231, 238, 251, 262, 266, 271, 274 note 5, 282-284, 313, 339 note 45
Kato Hiroshi, 22-24, 26-27
Kaufman, Bill, 90-91
Kawabe, Kazuhiko, 263
Kawaishi, Mikonosuke, 3
Kime-no-kata (decision form), 131, 154, 158, 160, 195, 197, 205, 238-241, 244-246, 248, 251-253, 259, 262, 264, 272, 275 notes 21 and 22, 276 notes 25 and 27, 277 note 58, 295, 297, 299, 313, 324, 327, 336 note 4
Kimura, Mitsuo "Mits", 42, 90
Kito Kata, 197
Kito-ryu Jujutsu, 132, 147, 149, 158, 191, 197, 199, 241
knee strike (hiza-ate), 256
kneeling (idori), 131-132, 239-240, 277 note 49, 295, 339 note 48
Kodokan, 1, 3, 17, 20-22, 29-30, 31 note 1, 55, 98, 127, 149, 154, 156-157, 163, 179, 181, 190-191, 193-194, 206 note 1, 215, 234-235, 238, 240-241, 244, 246, 274 note 1, 285, 287
Kodokan All-Japan Kata Competition, 163
Kodokan Goshin-jutsu, 131, 133, 195, 205, 234-273, 275 note 22, 277 notes 44 and 59, 278 notes 67 and 73, 299, 330, 337 notes 13, 21 and 22
Koiwai, Eichi (Ei'ichi), 19, 24, 26, 30
Koshiki-no-kata, 132, 194, 197, 205, 207 note 10, 237-238, 251, 265
Kotani, Sumiyuki, 69, 234, 241-242, 247, 260-261, 287
Koyasu, Masao, 241, 259
Kudo, Kazuzo, 241-242
Kuhara, Yoshiyuki, 247
Kumagai, Yasuyuki, 24, 27, 29, 37, 42-43, 89
Kumitsukareta-baai, 249
Kuniyuki, Kaname "Ken", 19-21, 23-26, 29-30, 41
Kurihara, Tamio, 1-3, 234, 241-242
Kurosaka Dojo, 17-20
Kurosaka, Hiroshi, 17, 19

L
large outer reap (osoto-gari), 2, 4, 97, 214, 217-218, 221, 225-227, 231, 325, 331
large wheel throw (oguruma), 213, 217, 226
leading (sen sen no sen), 230
lectures (kogi), 38, 77, 84 note 1, 191, 235, 294
leg techniques (ashi waza), 284
leg wheel (ashi guruma), 3, 216-217
Leggett, Trevor, 29, 52-54, 58, 78, 132, 191, 232, 262, 288-291, 298, 302, 314, 338 note 44, 339 note 54, 348-349

lift-pull hip throw (tsurikomi-goshi), 2, 283, 333
lifting-drawing foot sweep (harai tsurikomi ashi), 226

M
major hip throw (ogoshi), 142-143, 216, 226, 333
major outer drop twist (osoto-otoshi), 250
major outer wheel throw (osoto-guruma), 217-218
manly arts, 80, 166-172, 174, 177
Maruyama, Paul, 87
Masamoto, Iso, 147
maximum efficiency (seiryoku zen'yo), 132, 148, 236, 245
Mifune, Kyuzo, 1-33, 70, 90, 200, 207 note 12, 234, 239, 241, 244, 296, 335 note 5
Mifune Soen Goshin-jutsu, 239, 241, 296
Minidoka Relocation Center, 29-30, 34 note 84, 43
minor outer hooking throw (ko soto gake), 215, 226
Mochizuki, Minoru, 239, 275 note 14
modern martial ways (shin budo), 149, 173
modern sport, 7, 78-79, 81-83, 167, 170-174, 175 note 6, 187, 201, 271
Murata, Naoki, 163, 191, 204-205
Musashi, Miyamoto, 221, 232
muscular Christians, 79, 167, 171

N
Nadi, Aldo, 170
Nagao, Hic, 90-91
Nagaoka, Hideichi, 234, 240-241, 276 notes 26 and 27, 287-288
Nagaoka, Hidekazu, 17, 276 note 26
Nagaoka, Shuichi, 1, 276 note 26
Nage-no-kata (throwing forms), 130, 138, 158, 162-163, 194-195, 202, 215, 231, 237-238, 251, 271, 274 note 5, 282-284, 314, 327
Nakano, Shozo, 234, 241-242
Nakat Packing Corporation, 24
naked choke (hadaka-jime), 242, 284
Nanka Kodokan Judo Yudanshakai, 30
Nippon Kan Theater, 19-23, 26-27
nisei, 17, 20-22, 24, 26, 28, 30, 32 notes 34 and 47, 41, 43, 46 note 6
Nitta, Susumu, 21-25, 28, 30
no-mindness (mushin), 198, 252, 277 note 52
Nogaki, Paul, 199

O
Oba, Hideo, 255, 260
Ochiai, Toshiyasu, 247

Okamura, Henry, 90-91
Oltremari, Alessio, 192, 200-201
Olympic judo, 66, 154,
Omori, Chigusa, 164
Onozawa, Koshi, 162, 265, 268
opportunity (debana), 194, 224-225, 229, 232, 252-254, 271, 334
optimization (sei-ryoku), 199
Osako, John, 88, 90-91
Osawa, Yoshimi, 260-261
Oshu-no-bu, 259
Otaki, Tadao, 234, 241-242, 261, 299

P
Pan-Am Judo Union, 163
partnered practice (sotai renshu), 196
Parulski, George, 262
Pelletier, Guy, 198, 262
pistol at the back (haimen-zuke), 250, 254-256, 258-260, 263
pistol attacks, 241, 324
Pojello, Karl, 90
practice drills (uchi-komi), 129, 149, 228-229, 256

R
race factor, 183
Randori-no-kata, 194, 198, 248, 274 note 5, 276 note 30, 282-283
rear sacrifice techniques (ma-sutemi-waza), 202
rear throw (ura nage), 284
remaining mind (zanshin), 194, 252
renraku waza (combinations), 228
Rentai-no-kata (forms of physical education), 196, 274 note 5
repetitive throwing practice (nagekomi), 229
rhythm (hyoshi), 221-232, 277 note 51
Ri-no-kata (forms of theory), 197-199, 274 note 5
Rommelmann, Heiko, 161-163
Roosevelt, Theodore, 8-10, 14-15, 169, 175 note 3, 184, 186, 285
rough and tumble, 168-169
Russo, Miguel, 162
Russo-Japanese War, 178

S
Sakata, Chuji, 18, 23-24, 26-27, 32 note 34
Samura, Kaichiro, 1, 3, 241, 244
Sato, Masaru, 248, 251
Seattle Dojo, 17-21, 23-24, 26-30, 31 note 14, 37, 40
Sei-ryoku-zen'yo Kokumin-Taiiku, 193, 196, 207 note 9, 236
Sei'ichi Shirai, 241
Seinan Judo Dojo, 25
Sengoku, Tsueno, 251, 263-265
sense of positioning (tsukuri), 194, 205, 211-212, 214, 222, 226, 228, 231, 253, 283
Shin-Kime-no-kata, 245, 247-248
Shinken Shobu, 195, 257, 275 note 16
Shinken Shobu-no-kata (combat forms), 131, 154
Shinmeisho-no-waza (newly accepted techniques), 237
Shobu-no-kata (kata of self-defense), 131-132, 154, 195, 198, 274 note 5
short staff techniques (jo-jutsu), 243-244
shoulder wheel (kata-guruma), 124-126, 194-195, 283
shu-ha-ri (educational process), 198-199, 270, 278 notes 69 and 70
side hook (yoko-gake), 284
side sacrifice throw (yoko-sutemi), 2-4, 258, 284
side separation throw (yoko wakare), 226
side thrust (yoko-tsuki), 240
side wheel throw (yoko guruma), 226, 213-214, 226
single-wing choke (kataha-jime), 240
slanting strike (naname-uchi), 250, 328, 332
social class, 100, 172
solo practice (tandoku renshu), 196
Sone, Taizo, 226
Sosuishi-ryu, 238
Sosuishitsu-ryu, 243
spear techniques (so-jutsu), 243
staff techniques (bo-jutsu), 243, 276 note 25
standing techniques (tachiai), 239-240, 252, 277 note 55, 70, 295, 339 note 48
stereotypes, 15, 119, 178, 186
stick, 131, 168-170, 295, 297, 299, 315, 318-319, 324, 326, 328-329
striking techniques (atemi waza), 11, 13, 147, 229-230
Sugiyama, Shoji, 162
supine sacrifice techniques (ma-sutemi-waza), 202, 284
Suzuki, Kiyoji, 259
Suzuki, Kiyoshi, 241
sweeping loin throw (harai goshi), 226
swimming techniques (sui-jutsu), 243
sword techniques (ken-jutsu), 243
sword unsheathing (nuki-gake), 240, 47 note 12

T
Tabata, Shotaro, 1-3
Tacoma-Fife Dojo, 44-45

Taira Clan, 87-88
Taira, Shu, 266-267
Takahashi, Toshimitsu, 163
Takeda, Jiro, 239
Takenaka-ha, 197
Takenouchi, Hisamori, 243
Takeuchi Santo-ryu, 241
Tamura, Hikaru, 37, 40, 42-43, 45
Tamura, Hiroshi, 38, 40, 42-43, 45
Tamura, Masato, 22, 24-25, 27-28, 32 note 44, 35-45
Tamura, Vince, 44-45, 86-94
Tanto-no-baai (knife attacks), 250, 260, 271-272, 326
Tenshin Shinyo-ryu, 91, 158, 345
Tentoku Kan, 17-30, 31 note 12, 33 note 55, 40-41
throwing techniques (nage-waza), 147, 149, 253, 256
Tokyo Metropolitan Police, 163, 182, 264, 272
Tomiki, Kenji, 234, 238-239, 241-245, 251, 253-255, 258-260, 262, 268, 270, 272, 274, 276 note 35, 277 notes 44 and 46, 299, 337 notes 22 and 23
Treaty of Amity and Commerce, 181-182
traditional 18 martial arts (bugei juhappan), 243
traditional school (koryu), 234, 239, 241, 243, 264, 274 note 3, 276 notes 27 and 32, 294, 296, 307, 314-316, 336
Tsue-no-baai (staff attacks), 250, 258, 260
tsukkake, 252, 271, 277 note 55
Tsukuri, 194, 205, 211-212, 222, 228, 283
two-hands hold (ryote dori), 133, 215

U
Uemachi Dojo, 25
Ueshiba, Morihei, 238-239, 243-244, 275 note 14, 276 notes 34 and 35, 299
unarmed attacks (toshi-no-bu), 99, 241, 158, 249-250, 263, 268, 299, 324, 329
underlying principles (riai), 237, 256, 258, 275 note 7
undivided attention (senshin), 199
uppercut (ago tsuki),

V
van Dijk, Ferry, 267

W
Waseda University, 243, 245, 254, 259, 274, 276 note 31, 286, 296, 337 note 11
water wheel (mizu guruma), 133, 136-137
Waza no Ri, 205
Westmorland-style wrestling, 179

White River Dojo, 20-21, 27
World Masters Judo Association (WMJA), 200, 265, 278 note 65
World War II, 43, 89, 165-166
wrestling, 5-7, 9, 12-15, 17, 23, 26, 40-41, 46 note 6, 59, 65, 80-81, 83, 99-119, 129, 154, 167-172, 175 note 5, 177-180, 182-184, 187, 309, 312
wrist reversal (kote-gaeshi), 254-255, 260, 263, 270
wrist techniques (tekubi-waza), 242

Y
Yagyu, Munenori, 224
Yagyu Shinkage-ryu, 224
Yamashita, Yoshitsugu, 2-3, 8-9, 44, 240, 275 note 24, 285-286
Yamazaki, Masayoshi, 270
Yoda, Fumikazu, 163
Yokoyama, Estuko, 164
Yoshida, Jim, 23-24, 26-30, 32 note 40, 33 note 55, 65
Yoshimatsu, Yoshihiko, 4, 4 note 4
Yoshin-ryu, 191

Other Titles by Via Media Publishing

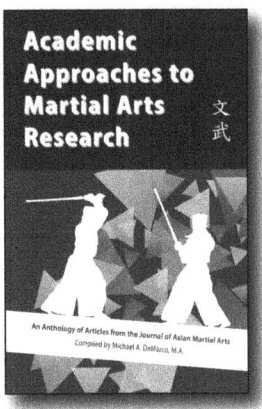
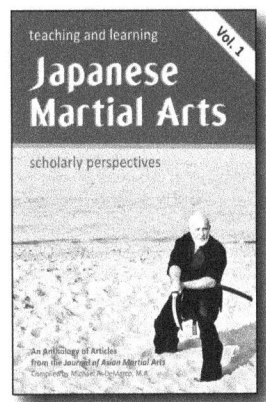
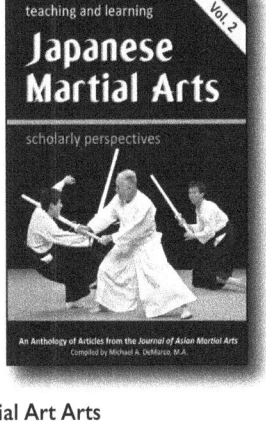

Academic Approaches
to Martial Art Research

Teaching and Learning Japanese Martial Art Arts
Volume I and Volume II

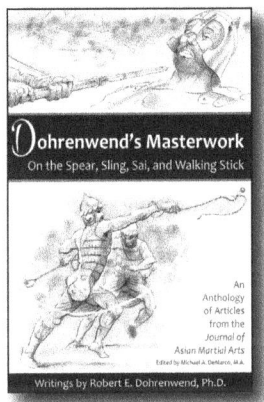
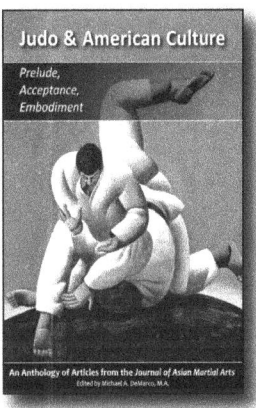

Conditioning for
Martial Art Practice

Dohrenwend's Masterwork
spear, sling, sai, walking stick

Judo and
American Culture

Fiction

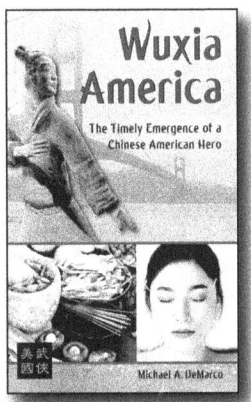
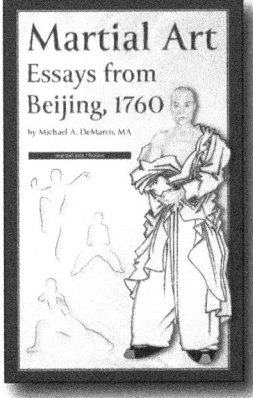
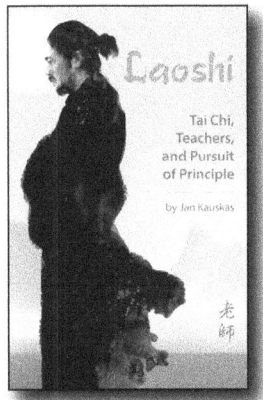

Wuxia America - Emergence
of a Chinese American Hero

Martial Art Essays
from Beijing, 1760

Laoshi: Tai Chi, Teachers,
and Pursuit of Principle

www.viamediapublishing.com

www.ingramcontent.com/pod-product-compliance
Lightning Source LLC
Chambersburg PA
CBHW061351010526
44107CB00011B/904